NurseThink® for Students

NCLEX-RN®
Conceptual Review Guide

Clinical-Based for Next Gen Learning

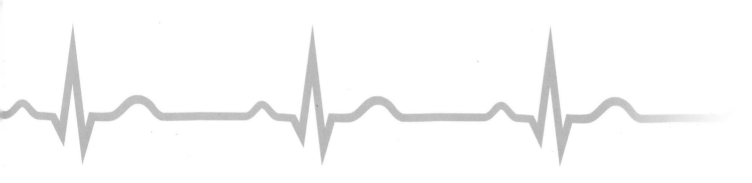

Tim J. Bristol
PhD, RN, CNE, ANEF, FAAN

Judith W. Herrman
PhD, RN, ANEF, FAAN

Winsome Stephenson
PhD, RN, CNE

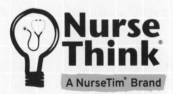

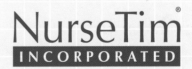

Follow Us On Social Media 🅕 🅞 @NurseThink / NurseThink.com / Help@NurseThink.com

Executive Editor: Tim Bristol
General Manager: Mitch Fisk
Project Coordinator: Rebecca Synoground
Design Account Director: Cory Dammann
Design, Layout, & Production: Shayla Johnson
Marketing Manager: Kelly Christian
Video Production Assistant: Hans Bristol
Photography: © Shutterstock

Published by NurseTim, Inc., P.O. Box 86, Waconia, MN 55387

Additional copies of this publication are available at www.NurseThink.com.

ISBN: 978-0-9987347-4-3

ebook ISBN: 978-0-9987347-5-0

Printed in the United States of America

First Edition

Brief Contents

General Table of Contents ii

NurseThink® Focused Specialties Table of Contents v

NurseThink® Focused NCLEX-RN® Client Needs Table of Contents................. vi

About the Authors..viii

Acknowledgements ix

Letter from the Authors x

Reviewers and Contributors.. xi

CH 1: Save Time Studying..1

CH 2: What is NCLEX-RN® all about? 5

CH 3: What can I expect?...13

CH 4: How can I prepare?..19

CH 5: Sexuality...25

CH 6: Circulation 61

CH 7: Protection 93

CH 8: Homeostasis 137

CH 9: Respiration 167

CH 10: Regulation 199

CH 11: Nutrition 235

CH 12: Hormonal...293

CH 13: Movement 339

CH 14: Comfort...391

CH 15: Adaptation 421

CH 16: Emotion...447

CH 17: Cognition 475

CH 18: Health Promotion 495

CH 19: Role of the Nurse in Quality and Safety...................................521

CH 20: Where do I go from here?...539

Table of Contents

SECTION 1

Introduction

CH 1: Save Time Studying 1
NurseThink® *THIN Thinking, 2*
Prioritization Power, 3
Alternate Item Formats, 4
NurseThink® for Clinical Judgment, 4

CH 2: What is NCLEX-RN® all about? 5
National Council of State Boards of Nursing, 5
Cognitive Level of Exam Questions, 5
NCLEX-RN® Client Needs, 7
Integrated concepts, 10
Focus: Priority setting, safety, and clinical judgment, 12

CH 3: What can I expect? 13
The Exam, 13
Application, 14
Before and the day of the exam, 15
Staying calm in the cubicle, 16
Calming yourself in the cubicle!, 17
Scoring the exam and passing standards, 17
Getting my results, 18

CH 4: How can I prepare? 19
Know what you don't know with the 20/50 Rule!, 19
Test-taking Strategies, 20
Terms to know, 22
Healthy lifestyle for healthy testing, 22

SECTION 2

Priority Exemplars

CH 5: Sexuality 25
Go To Clinical Case 1, 26
Hypertensive disorders of
    pregnancy, 28
Go To Clinical Case 2, 30
Newborn care, 32
Contraception, 34
Erectile dysfunction (ED), 35
Pregnancy, 36
Abortion/miscarriage, 38
Preterm labor, 39
Stages of labor, 40
Dystocia, 43
Placental abruption, 44
Placenta previa, 45
Postpartum hemorrhage, 46
Breastfeeding, 47
STI: Chlamydia, 48
STI: Human papillomavirus (HPV),
    49
STI: Syphilis, 50
NurseThink® Quiz Questions, 51
NurseThink® Quiz Answers, 54

CH 6: Circulation 61
Go To Clinical Case 1, 62
Shock, 64
 Go To Clinical Case 2, 66
Heart failure, 68
Cardiomyopathy, 70
Coronary artery disease (CAD), 71
Myocardial infarction (MI)/acute
    coronary syndrome, 72
Peripheral artery disease (PAD), 73
Buerger's Disease and Raynaud's
    Phenomenon, 74
Hypertension, 75
Stroke-cerebrovascular accident
    (CVA), 76
Valvular heart disease, 78
Venous thromboembolism (VTE), 79
Pulmonary embolism (PE), 80
Disseminated intravascular
    coagulation (DIC), 81
NurseThink® Quiz Questions, 82
NurseThink® Quiz Answers, 85

CH 7: Protection 93
Go To Clinical Case 1, 94
Meningitis, 96
Go To Clinical Case 2, 100
Pancreatitis, 102
Appendicitis/peritonitis, 104
Cellulitis/wound infection/
    septicemia, 106
Gout, 108
Systemic lupus erythematosus, 110
Rheumatoid arthritis, 112
HIV/AIDS, 114
Hypersensitivity reactions, 116
Influenza, 118
Polycystic kidney, 119
Urinary tract infection, 120
Pyelonephritis, 122
Methicillin-resistant Staphylococcus
    Aureus/vancomycin resistant
    Enterococcus, 124
NurseThink® Quiz Questions, 126
NurseThink® Quiz Answers, 129

CH 8: Homeostasis 137

Go To Clinical Case 1, 138
Overhydration/fluid overload, 140
Go To Clinical Case 2, 142
Dehydration/fluid deficit, 144
Hyper/hypocalcemia, 146
Hyper/hypokalemia, 147
Hyper/hypomagnesemia, 149
Hyper/hyponatremia, 150
Hyper/hypophosphatemia, 151
Metabolic acidosis, 152
Metabolic alkalosis, 153
Respiratory acidosis, 154
Respiratory alkalosis, 155
NurseThink® Quiz Questions, 156
NurseThink® Quiz Answers, 159

CH 9: Respiration 167

Go To Clinical Case 1, 168
Chronic obstructive pulmonary
    disease (COPD), 170
Go To Clinical Case 2, 172
Cystic fibrosis (CF), 174
Chest trauma/pneumothorax, 176
Asthma, 177
Acute respiratory distress syndrome
    (ARDS), 178
Tuberculosis, 179
Pneumonia, 180
Bronchiolitis/lower airway infections,
    181
Upper airway infections, 182
Croup syndromes/epiglottitis, 183
Pulmonary hypertension, 184
Iron-deficiency anemia, 185
Sickle cell anemia (SSA), 186
NurseThink® Quiz Questions, 188
NurseThink® Quiz Answers, 191

CH 10: Regulation 199

Go To Clinical Case 1, 200
Hydrocephalus, 202
Go To Clinical Case 2, 204
Blood-borne cancers, 206
Skin cancers, 208
Lymph cancers, 210
Other cancers, 211
Acute traumatic brain injury, 214
Polycythemia, 216

Thrombocytopenia, 218
Hyperthermia, 219
Hypothermia, 220
NurseThink® Quiz Questions, 222
NurseThink® Quiz Answers, 226

CH 11: Nutrition 235

Go To Clinical Case 1, 236
Inflammatory bowel disease: Crohn's
    disease/ulcerative colitis, 238
Go To Clinical Case 2, 242
Cleft lip and palate, 244
Gastroesophageal reflux, 246
Gastritis, 248
Peptic ulcer disease, 250
Celiac disease, 253
Gallbladder conditions, 254
Constipation, 256
Intestinal obstruction, 258
Diverticular disease, 260
Colorectal cancer, 262
Cirrhosis, 264
Hepatitis, 266
Pyloric stenosis, 269
Obesity, 270
Benign prostatic hypertrophy/
    prostate cancer, 272
Chronic kidney disease/end-stage
    renal disease, 275
Acute kidney disease/injury, 280
NurseThink® Quiz Questions, 282
NurseThink® Quiz Answers, 285

CH 12: Hormonal 293

Go To Clinical Case 1, 294
Diabetic ketoacidosis, 296
Go To Clinical Case 2, 298
Diabetes mellitus – type 2, 300
Diabetes mellitus – type 1, 302
Gestational diabetes, 304
Hyperglycemic hyperosmolar
    syndrome, 306
Hyperparathyroidism, 308
Hypoparathyroidism, 310
Hyperthyroidism, 312
Hypothyroidism, 314
Cushing's syndrome, 316
Addison's disease, 318
Syndrome of inappropriate
    antidiuretic hormone (SIADH), 320

Diabetes insipidus, 322
Wilms tumor, 324
Metabolic syndrome, 326
NurseThink® Quiz Questions, 327
NurseThink® Quiz Answers, 331

CH 13: Movement 339

Go To Clinical Case 1, 340
Cerebral palsy, 342
Go To Clinical Case 2, 344
Seizures, 346
Osteoporosis, 348
Osteoarthritis, 349
Fractures, 350
Peripheral neuropathy, 352
Trigeminal neuralgia, 354
Carpal tunnel, 356
Amputation, 357
Amyotrophic lateral sclerosis, 358
Guillain-Barré syndrome, 359
Multiple sclerosis, 360
Myasthenia gravis, 362
Parkinson's disease, 364
Cataracts, 366
Glaucoma, 367
Conjunctivitis, 368
Macular degeneration, 369
Hearing impairment, 370
Scoliosis, 371
Labyrinthitis/Meniere's disease, 372
Otitis media/externa, 374
Spina bifida, 376
Spinal cord injury, 378
NurseThink® Quiz Questions, 380
NurseThink® Quiz Answers, 383

CH 14: Comfort 391

Go To Clinical Case 1, 392
Pressure ulcers, 394
Go To Clinical Case 2, 396
Burns, 398
Acute pain, 400
Chronic pain, 402
Contact dermatitis/ impetigo, 404
Fatigue, 405
Sleep disorders, 407
NurseThink® Quiz Questions, 409
NurseThink® Quiz Answers, 413

Table of Contents

SECTION 2
Priority Exemplars

CH 15: Adaptation 421
Go To Clinical Case 1, 422
Eating disorders, 424
Go To Clinical Case 2, 426
Post-traumatic stress disorder (PTSD), 428
Trauma: Abuse, rape, and sexual assault, 430
Crisis intervention, 432
Substance abuse, 434
Obsessive-compulsive disorder (OCD), 436
NurseThink® Quiz Questions, 437
NurseThink® Quiz Answers, 440

CH 16: Emotion 447
Go To Clinical Case 1, 448
Anxiety disorders, 450
Go To Clinical Case 2, 452
Schizophrenia, 454
Depression, 456
Postpartum depression (PPD), 458
Bipolar disorders, 460
Death and dying, 462
Bereavement, 463
NurseThink® Quiz Questions, 464
NurseThink® Quiz Answers, 467

CH 17: Cognition 475
Go To Clinical Case 1, 476
Delirium, 478
Go To Clinical Case 2, 480
Dementia/Alzheimer's disease, 482
Autism spectrum disorders (ASD), 484
Attention-deficit/hyperactivity disorder (ADHD), 485
NurseThink® Quiz Questions, 486
NurseThink® Quiz Answers, 489

SECTION 3
Closing

CH 18: Health Promotion 495
Infants, 496
Toddlers, 498
Preschoolers, 500
School-age children, 502
Adolescents, 504
Adults, 506
Older adults, 508
NurseThink® Quiz Questions, 510
NurseThink® Quiz Answers, 513

CH 19: Role of the Nurse in Quality and Safety 521
Patient-centered care, 522
Teamwork and collaboration, 522
Evidence-based practices, 524
Quality Improvement, 524
Safety, 525
Informatics, 525
NurseThink® Quiz Questions, 527
NurseThink® Quiz Answers, 531

CH 20: Where do I go from here? 539
Next steps: Set your study goals— Plan your study time and stick with it, 539
Your healthy NCLEX® lifestyle, 540
Be Successful!, 542

NURSETHINK® FOCUSED

Specialties

Children's Health

Acute pain, 400
Adolescents, 504
Asthma, 177
Attention-deficit/hyperactivity disorder (ADHD), 485
Autism, 484
Breastfeeding, 32
Bronchiolitis/lower airway infections, 181
Cerebral palsy, 342
Chronic pain, 402
Cleft lip and palate, 244
Croup syndromes/epiglottitis, 183
Cystic fibrosis, 174
Dehydration/fluid deficit, 144
Diabetes mellitus – type 1, 302
Eating disorders, 424
Gastroesophageal reflux, 246
Heart failure, 68
HIV/AIDS, 114
Hydrocephalus, 202
Infants, 496
Iron-deficiency anemia, 185
Meningitis, 96
Newborn care, 32
Otitis media/externa, 374
Overhydration/fluid overload, 140
Preschoolers, 500
Pyloric stenosis, 269
Scoliosis, 371
Seizures, 346
Sickle cell anemia, 186
Spina bifida, 376
Toddlers, 498
Upper airway infections, 182
Valvular heart disease, 78
Wilms tumor, 324

Mental Health

Anxiety disorders, 450
Attention-deficit/hyperactivity disorder (ADHD), 485
Autism, 484
Bereavement, 463
Bipolar disorders, 460
Crisis intervention, 432
Death and dying, 462
Delirium, 478
Dementia/Alzheimer's disease, 482
Depression, 456
Eating disorders, 424
Obsessive-compulsive disorder, 436
Post-traumatic stress disorder, 428
Schizophrenia, 454
Substance abuse, 434
Trauma: Abuse, rape, and sexual assault, 430

Women's Health

Abortion/miscarriage, 38
Acute pain, 400
Adults, 506
Breastfeeding, 47
Chronic pain, 402
Constipation, 256
Contraception, 34
Disseminated intravascular coagulation, 81
Dystocia, 43
Eating disorders, 424
Fatigue, 405
Gestational diabetes, 304
Hypertensive disorders of pregnancy, 28
Iron-deficiency anemia, 185
Newborn care, 32
Obesity, 270
Older adults, 508
Osteoporosis, 348
Placental abruption, 44
Placenta previa, 45
Postpartum hemorrhage, 46
Pregnancy, 36
Preterm labor, 39
Shock, 64
Stages of labor, 40
STIs, 48–50
Trauma: Abuse, rape, and sexual assault, 430
Urinary tract infection, 120

Table of Contents

NURSETHINK® FOCUSED

NCLEX-RN® Client Needs

Priority Exemplars that emphasize different parts of the NCLEX-RN®.

Management of Care

Acute respiratory distress syndrome (ARDS), 178
Blood-borne cancers, 206
Burns, 398
Cardiomyopathy, 70
Cerebral palsy, 342
Chest trauma/pneumothorax, 176
Chronic kidney disease/end-stage renal disease, 275
Cleft lip and palate, 244
Cystic fibrosis, 174
Diabetes mellitus – type 1, 302
Diabetes mellitus – type 2, 300
Fractures, 350
Hypersensitivity reactions, 116
Hyperthermia, 219
Hypothermia, 220
Lymph cancers, 210
Multiple sclerosis, 360
Myocardial infarction (MI)/acute coronary syndrome, 72
Other cancers, 212
Pneumonia, 180
Postpartum hemorrhage, 46
Pyloric stenosis, 269

Safety and Infection Control

Appendicitis/peritonitis, 104
Cellulitis/wound infection/septicemia, 106
Cerebral palsy, 342
Cleft lip and palate, 244
Croup syndromes/epiglottitis, 183
Dystocia, 43
Gastroesophageal reflux, 246
HIV/AIDS, 114
Hydrocephalus, 202
Hypersensitivity reactions, 116
Influenza, 118
Meningitis, 96
Peripheral artery disease, 73
Pneumonia, 180
Postpartum hemorrhage, 46
Pressure ulcers, 394
Pyelonephritis, 122
Seizures, 346
Spina bifida, 376
Spinal cord injury, 378
STIs, 48–50
Stroke, 76
Thrombocytopenia, 218
Tuberculosis, 179
Urinary tract infection, 120

Health Promotion and Maintenance

Breastfeeding, 47
Celiac disease, 253
Cellulitis/wound infection/septicemia, 106
Constipation, 256
Contraception, 34
Fatigue, 405
Gestational diabetes, 304
Growth and development-ages and stages, 496–508
Hearing impairment, 370
Hypertension, 75
Iron-deficiency anemia, 185
Newborn care, 32

Obesity, 270
Osteoarthritis, 349
Osteoporosis, 348
Postpartum depression, 458
Pregnancy, 36
Sleep disorders, 407
Stages of labor, 40
STIs, 48–50
Upper airway infections, 182
Urinary tract infection, 120

Basic Care and Comfort

Amyotrophic lateral sclerosis, 358
Cataracts, 366
Celiac disease, 253
Chronic obstructive pulmonary disease, 170
Constipation, 256
Dehydration/fluid deficit, 144
Fractures, 350
Gastroesophageal reflux, 246
HIV/AIDS, 114
Hyperthermia, 219
Hypothermia, 220
Newborn care, 32
Osteoarthritis, 349
Overhydration/fluid overload, 140
Parkinson's disease, 364
Pressure ulcers, 394
Rheumatoid arthritis, 112
Sleep disorders, 407
Spina bifida, 376
Spinal cord injury, 378
Stroke, 76
Urinary tract infection, 120

Pharmacological and Parenteral

Acute pain, 400
Asthma, 177
Burns, 398
Chronic pain, 402
Contraception, 34
Diabetes mellitus – type 1, 302
Diabetes mellitus – type 2, 300
Diabetic ketoacidosis, 296
Erectile dysfunction, 35
Gastroesophageal reflux, 246
Gout, 108
Heart failure, 68
Hypersensitivity reactions, 116
Hypertension, 75
Hypothyroid, 314
Iron-deficiency anemia, 185
Methicillin-resistant Staphylococcus Aureus/vancomycin resistant Enterococcus, 124
Myasthenia gravis, 362
Parkinson's disease, 364
Peptic ulcer, 250
Postpartum hemorrhage, 46
Shock, 64
STIs, 48–50
Tuberculosis, 179

Reduction of Risk Potential

Acute kidney disease, 280
Amputation, 357
Appendicitis/peritonitis, 104
Blood-borne cancers, 206
Burns, 398
Cirrhosis, 264
Cystic fibrosis, 174
Diabetic ketoacidosis, 296
Disseminated intravascular coagulation, 81
HIV/AIDS, 114
Hydrocephalus, 202
Inflammatory bowel disease: Crohn's disease/ulcerative colitis, 238
Lymph cancers, 210
Meningitis/encephalitis, 96
Multiple sclerosis, 360
Other cancers, 211
Placental abruption, 44
Placenta previa, 45
Preterm labor, 39
Seizures, 346
Sickle cell anemia, 186
Spinal cord injury, 378
Thrombocytopenia, 218
Valvular heart disease, 78
Venous thromboembolism, 79
Wilms tumor, 324

Physiological Adaptation

Acute respiratory distress syndrome, 178
Acute traumatic brain injury, 214
Burns, 398
Cardiomyopathy, 70
Cirrhosis, 264
Diabetes insipidus, 322
Diverticular disease, 260
Gallbladder conditions, 254
Gout, 108
Guillain-Barré syndrome, 359
Hydrocephalus, 202
Hyperglycemic hyperosmolar syndrome, 306
Metabolic acidosis/alkalosis and Respiratory acidosis/alkalosis, 152–155
Myasthenia gravis, 362
Myocardial infarction/acute coronary syndrome, 72
Pancreatitis, 102
Pneumonia, 180
Polycystic kidney, 119
Postpartum hemorrhage, 46
Pulmonary embolism, 80
Pulmonary hypertension, 184
Rheumatoid arthritis, 112
Scoliosis, 371
Syndrome of inappropriate antidiuretic hormone, 320
Systemic lupus erythematosus, 110

About the Authors

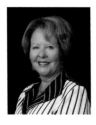

Dr. Judith W. Herrman is a nurse, educator, and researcher with a passion for learning and teaching. Judy's experiences in and love for nursing education provide context for work in creative teaching strategies, curriculum development, evaluation and test development, building positive workplaces, preparing for NCLEX®, and applying the principles of brain science to clinical decision-making. Judy's research interests include healthy decision-making across the lifespan, enhancing sexual health and promoting access to sexual education and healthcare, and advocacy for marginalized populations, especially children with health issues, young parents, and vulnerable youth. Judy has published widely and is excited that the team's hard work on these resources may help students join the great profession of nursing!

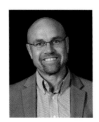

Dr. Tim Bristol is a nurse educator from Minneapolis, Minnesota. He has taught students at all levels to include LPN, ADN, BSN, MSN, and PhD. Through NCLEX® reviews and coaching, NurseTim® brings clinical judgment to life for students and faculty at all levels. He works with programs and organizations internationally on everything from student remediation and retention to exams and curricular success. He helps ensure that clinical is the focus of everything that happens in nursing education. He also enjoys working internationally and leads many service learning trips each year with his wife and four children. Over the past 12 years his family has led over 600 travelers abroad. These trips focus on nursing and community empowerment in developing countries.

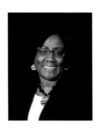

Dr. Winsome Stephenson is a Nurse Educator whose expertise includes test item writing, NCLEX® student success, use of transformative learning strategies in the classroom and faculty development. She has taught students at both undergraduate and graduate levels and trained faculty on all levels. Dr. Stephenson is passionate about nursing education and ensuring that the next generation of nurses are fully trained to use clinical judgment in the provision of quality patient care. She believes in giving back to the community and has coordinated a health ministry to serve the health needs of congregants in her church. She has served as a community member on the IRB of two local hospitals and in her free time, she enjoys travelling and spending time with her family.

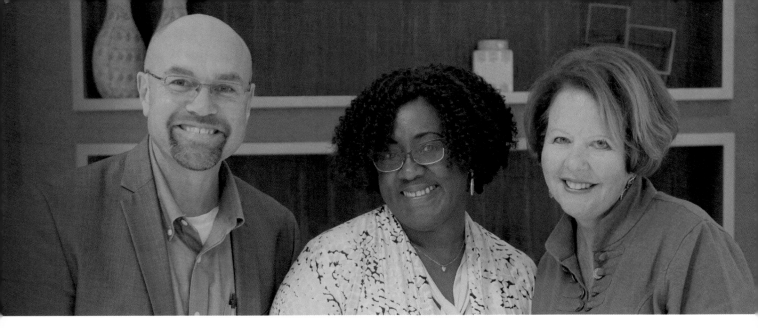

Acknowledgements

I would like to thank the entire Nurse Tim, Inc. team, especially Tim and Winsome, for their tireless work and sincere desire to assist nursing students become nurses! I wish to thank Dan, my husband, for his unwavering support, love, and encouragement. I would also like to acknowledge the energy, enthusiasm, and inspiration that comes from our three sons, their three wives, and our six fantastic grandchildren! They bring joy to our lives and provide hope for the future!

- Dr. Judith W. Herrman

My family sacrificed so much for me to be able to be a part of this book. So I must first and foremost say thank you to my best friend Christina and my four amazing children. Then I have to acknowledge our team to include Judy, Winsome, Rebecca, Kristofer, Kelly, Cory, Shayla, Mitch, Sharon and the army of contributors, item writers, and reviewers. We wanted this book to change the way students study and that could only happen with the best team in the world. I have the pleasure of being on that team.

- Dr. Tim Bristol

I would like to express sincere gratitude to Tim and Judy for the opportunity to co-author this book. My thanks also to those who provided support and constructive feedback. I would be remiss not to extend my profound thanks to the contributors and reviewers who took the time to review the chapters. Finally, thank you to all the many students and faculty who will purchase, and be benefited by this book.

-Dr. Winsome Stephenson

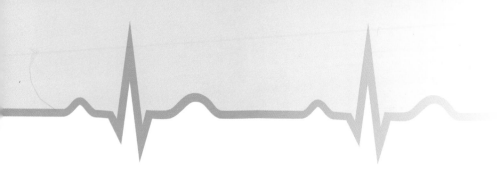

Letter From the Authors

Wherever you are in your nursing career...early in nursing school...about to graduate... already done with school, you have one more hurdle! Passing NCLEX® is your next challenge. We wrote this book to help you be successful on NCLEX® and with YOUR learning needs in mind! We hope the Go To Clinical cases, the Priority Exemplars, the NurseThink® quizzes, and the other features help on your NCLEX® journey! We wish you well and we are anxious to join you in the profession of nursing. Being a nurse is indeed a privilege. We love nursing and we hope you do too!

- Dr. Judith W. Herrman

Nursing school is one of the most transformative experiences one can ever pursue. What you have to remember as you reach for the milestones of graduation and licensure is that it is all about the patient. This one fact can propel you into that dream career you have been pursing for so long. Ohhh yeah, it can also help you graduate and pass the NCLEX-RN®. Whether you are approaching a patient in the hospital, or a question on the exam, make the patient the center of your focus as they are the center of NurseThink®.

- Dr. Tim Bristol

You should be very proud of yourself for making the decision to embark upon a profession that is highly respected and where you will have significant impact on the lives of patients every day. Regardless of the area of nursing that you chose upon graduation, you will effect change, provide quality and enrich lives. This book is aimed at helping you prepare for and achieve success on the NCLEX®. The Priority Exemplars, Go To Clinical Cases and NurseThink® Quizzes are geared towards helping you realize that goal but more importantly, they will assist you to use clinical judgement as you care for patients. Remember, nursing will not be what you do, but truly who you are so live it well!

- Dr. Winsome Stephenson

Reviewers and Contributors

Reviewers

Anne Brett, PhD, RN
Consultation Manager
NurseTim, Inc.
University of Phoenix, College of
Doctoral Studies
Faculty
Germantown, WI

Kris Douglass, DNP, RN-BC
Associate Professor
Brady School of Nursing
Shorter University
Rome, GA

Lawrence Fisher, MSN, RN
Instructor
Stark State College
North Canton, OH

Jennifer S. Graber, EdD, PMHNP-BC
Assistant Professor
University of Delaware
Newark, DE

Mark C. Hand, PhD, RN, CNE
Department Chair BSN Nursing
East Carolina University
Greenville, NC

Barbara Horning, ASN, RN
Registered Nurse
Good Samaritan Society
Waconia, MN

Paige J. Lodien
Nursing Student
Crown College
St. Bonifacius, MN

Shanna Miko, MSN, RN-BC, CPN, CCRN
Registered Nurse
Children's Minnesota Minnetonka
Surgery and Specialty Center
Minnetonka, MN

Kathy Mixson, JD, MS, RN
Recurrent Faculty
Texas Tech Health Science Center
School of Nursing
Melissa, TX

Christy L. Skelly, DNP, APRN
Assistant Professor of Nursing
Florida Southern College
Lakeland, FL

Kathy Van Eerden, PhD, RN, CNE
Associate Dean
Ruth S. Coleman College of Nursing and
Health Sciences
Cardinal Stritch University
Milwaukee, WI

Contributors

Wenona B. Bell, MSN, RN
Assistant Professor
Franciscan Missionaries of Our Lady
University
Baton Rouge, LA

Anne Brett, PhD, RN
Consultation Manager
NurseTim, Inc.
University of Phoenix, College of
Doctoral Studies
Faculty
Germantown, WI

Kristofer Bristol, BSN, RN
Registered Nurse
University of Minnesota Medical Center
Minneapolis, MN

Elise Dando, MSN, RN
Registered Nurse
Phoenix, AZ

Emily R. Day, MPH, BSN, RN, PHN
Assistant Professor of Nursing
Bethel University
St. Paul, MN

Carla A. Harmon, PhD, MSN, RN
Associate Professor
Franciscan Missionaries of Our Lady
Undergraduate Nursing Program
Baton Rouge, LA

Christy L. Skelly, DNP, APRN
Assistant Professor of Nursing
Florida Southern College
Lakeland, FL

**Kim Leighton, PhD, RN, CHSE, CHSOS,
ANEF, FAAN**
National Curriculum and Instruction
Developer
Chamberlain University College of Nursing
Downers Grove, IL

Michelle D. Myles, DNP, RN, CNE
National Academic Success Specialist
Chamberlain University College of Nursing

Belinda B. Munson, MSN, RN
Assistant Professor
Franciscan Missionaries of Our Lady
University
Baton Rouge, LA

Nicole C. Orent, MSN, RN, CNE
Nursing Faculty
Scottsdale Community College
Scottsdale, AZ

**Karin J. Sherrill, RN, MSN, CNE, CHSE,
ANEF, FAADN**
Faculty Educator and Consultant
MaricopaNursing at GateWay
Community College
Phoenix, AZ

Introduction

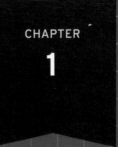

Save Time Studying

Focus on Clinical

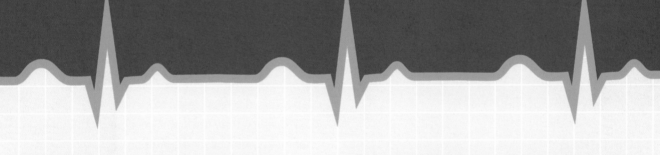

You knew about this exam before you started nursing school—in fact, you may have picked your school based partly on its NCLEX® pass rate. But, now that the exam is near, you realize how little you know about the exam, what it means, and how to be successful. This book is designed to help you. By knowing more about the exam—what it looks like, what it measures, and how it is scored—you can be more prepared and be successful on the exam.

You've been successful in nursing school and you have used your thinking skills to help you achieve that success! You learned early on that multiple-choice questions in nursing often have four right answers— and you needed to choose the highest priority or the best answer! That was your clinical judgment skills at work! While you were in nursing school you learned NurseThink® and how to process information to perform well on tests AND in the clinical area.

Some of you completed a nursing program based on concepts (perfusion, oxygenation, comfort, homeostasis, etc.). Others learned based on units or medical models. Nonetheless, you learned about concepts in caring for clients clinically. The NCLEX-RN® is all about clinical judgment and that is why NurseThink® is clinically-based.

Experienced nurses, when walking into a client's room, may be aware of the client's medical diagnosis. However, the nurse provide high-level care based on priority needs of the client. For example, the nurse considers: How is the client oxygenating? What about the client's perfusion? How about the client's pain level? What do the client's vital signs and laboratory data tell us about the client's homeostasis? **Remember, the NCLEX-RN® does not test what you know, it tests how you think.**

As you answer questions, consider the concepts in the item—how would a nurse provide care for the client in the question? This book provides **Priority Exemplars** to assist you in building your clinical judgment skills. Simultaneously, this book offers several tools and resources to help you succeed on NCLEX-RN®.

NurseThink® *THIN Thinking*

THIN Thinking is a unique clinical judgment strategy from NurseThink®. *THIN Thinking* allows for processing of the information essential to providing high-level and complex client care. This method promotes higher-order mental processing, rather than memorization. On the exam, students often select an answer based on recognition of material rather than analyzing an item for priority client needs. *THIN Thinking* encourages the student to read the question and focus on the client.

The student will apply the **"THIN"** mnemonic to guide the decision towards the highest priority answer. This strategy is especially valuable when confused by a question or stuck between two answers. To implement *THIN Thinking*, consider this process:

T: TOP THREE

What are the three priority needs, concepts, questions, components, or elements noted in this question? Ask yourself: What is this question addressing? What are the top three needs?" This is where to apply **Prioritization Power**! Consider these prioritization options.

> **Maslow's Hierarchy of Needs:** This is a theory that places basic physiological needs as a higher priority than psychological needs. A greater challenge occurs when comparing the priority of safety to physiological needs. For example, if a client is not breathing, that is the priority. But, if the client is not breathing from a car accident and the car is on fire, moving the client to a safe environment should occur before addressing the fact that they are not breathing (making safety a higher priority).

> **ABC's:** This is everyone's favorite. Is there a time when circulation is a higher priority than airway or breathing? Yes, consider a client with diabetic ketoacidosis with a respiratory rate of 28 breaths per minute. Although alarming, this is a good thing as it indicates that they are attempting to compensate for the metabolic acidosis from the ketosis state. In this case, airway and breathing are not a problem, move on the circulation.

> **Actual versus Potential:** In most cases an actual problem will take precedence over a potential problem, unless the actual problem offers low risk, while the potential problem offers a high-risk for safety or injury. For example, an alert client may have an actual problem of vomiting, but the client that is nauseated, in c-spine precautions is a higher priority, since if they begin vomiting there are concerns of airway safety and spinal injuries.

Acute versus Chronic: Acute will be the higher priority. An example would be the client suffering from chronic obstructive pulmonary disease being managed with medication and oxygen. This client is considered chronic until there is evidence of respiratory distress (respiratory rate, ABGs, pulse ox, etc.) at which time the client becomes acute (shows change in their baseline condition).

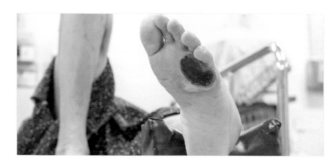

Image 1-1: When is a foot wound acute and when is it chronic?

> **Least Invasive First:** It is important for the nurse to consider less invasive options before increasing the client risk of injury with an invasive option. For example, standing a male client at the bedside every two hours to use a urinal is a better option than applying protective briefs. Applying protective briefs is a better option than applying a condom catheter. Applying a condom catheter is a better option than placing a Foley catheter.

> **Safe Practice:** Safety concerns may include evaluation of the risk for falls, prevention of injury when performing a skill, reduction of risk for hospital-acquired infections (HAI), and more.

H: HELP QUICK

What can the nurse do quickly to relieve the problem? What strategies can the nurse use quickly while waiting for another intervention or healthcare professional? What interventions may be implemented quickly? Will it help to elevate the head of the bed? What if oxygen is applied? Will the dizziness be improved if the client sits down? How can the nurse act now to help the client?

I: IDENTIFY RISK TO SAFETY

What are the top safety concerns of the client? The National Council Licensure Examination (NCLEX®) is an exam about safety – many questions are going to address client safety or discuss a threat to client safety. Because of this, it is important to consider the highest concerns for safety experienced by the client. Safety concerns may include evaluation of the risk for falls, prevention of injury, reduction of risk for hospital-acquired infections (HAI), and more.

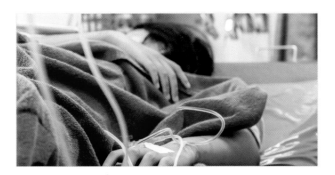

Image 1-2: Any patient receiving intravenous therapy is at risk for multiple safety concerns. Can you list three safety concerns?

N: NURSING PROCESS

Many questions represent a step of the nursing process. Although it is possible for a test question to refer to any step of the nursing process the NCLEX® exam is focused on nursing action related to assessment and intervention. Reflect on "what action should the nurse take next?" knowing that an action can be an assessment or intervention. When determining a priority action, ask yourself, "Have I fully assessed what I need to in order to safely perform this intervention?" For example, a client with surgical pain of 8 out of 10 needs pain medication (intervention). A higher priority would be to assess the vital signs to confirm that the medication can be safely delivered without injury to the client.

Prioritization Power

Let's discuss more about **Prioritization Power**. When you looked up your medications for clinical, you tried to learn all twenty side effects or all six indications for a medication. Now that you are preparing for NCLEX-RN®, you want to use **Prioritization Power**. That means you will need to analyze the options and identify the TOP THREE side effects and indications for each medication. In each chapter of this book, you will read the Go To Clinical case and practice **Prioritization Power** with multiple medications.

For each clinical case you will read the details of care for a specific client. Then, you will be asked to identify the TOP THREE: Priority Assessments, Priority Labs/Diagnostics, Priority Potential and Actual Complications, Priority Interventions, Priority Medications, Priority Nursing Implications, and Priority Education/Discharge issues. In the following pages, you will find the answers to the TOP THREE **represented by NurseThink®** in the related **Priority Exemplars**. As you progress through the book you will identify concepts, consider key components of nursing care, and develop your clinical judgment skills. This guide will lead you through 20 chapters, over 160 **Priority Exemplar**s requiring nursing care, and more than 1000 exam questions. You will be able to check your answers and review extensive rationale for correct/incorrect answers and NurseThink® *THIN Thinking.*

> NurseThink® is a tool to develop habits of clinical judgment through prioritization and conceptual processing to meet client needs.
>
> Clinical judgment is the observed outcome of critical thinking and decision making (NCSBN, 2018).

To help you develop your clinical judgment skills, each question is categorized to competencies listed by the Quality and Safety Education for Nurses (QSEN) institute at QSEN.org. These competencies include Patient-Centered Care, Teamwork and Collaboration, Evidence-based Practice, Quality Improvement, Safety, and Informatics. The NCLEX-RN® Patient Needs for each question are also identified. They include Management of Care, Safety and Infection Control, Health Promotion and Maintenance, Psychosocial Integrity, Basic Care & Comfort, Pharmacological and Parenteral Therapies, Reduction of Risk Potential, and Physiological Adaptation. More discussion of these components of the NCLEX-RN® test plan categories is in Chapter 2 and online at www.NCLEX.org.

Alternate Item Formats

To ensure you have the most up-to-date information on the mechanics of the NCLEX-RN®, be sure to visit www.NCLEX.org. In addition to the customary multiple-choice format (e.g. four options with one correct answer), the National Council of State Boards of Nursing (NCSBN) implements other question types using what they call alternate item formats. These questions assess critical thinking and clinical judgment in different ways. They take a little more time and sometimes cause stress for students. Therefore, we will explain them briefly. In addition, you can go on the NCLEX-RN® website to learn more about the different formats (more about that in Chapter 2). Alternate format questions include:

> **Chart exhibit questions:** Computer tabs allow you to view client records, including healthcare provider prescriptions, client flow sheets, diagnostic results, progress notes, and other documents. You will then answer an item about this information.

> **Select all that apply:** These questions, sometimes referred to as multiple response, include a stem and usually more than four options. You will need to pick one or more options as the correct answer.

The best strategy is to treat each option as a true/false question. There is no partial credit for these items. These questions are reported to appear frequently on NCLEX-RN®.

> **Ordered Response / Drag and Drop:** Perhaps the hardest of all question formats—these questions ask you to read an item and put the answer options in order of rank or occurrence. You need to have a good understanding of the steps needed and the correct order! Again, there is no partial credit.

> **Fill-in-the-blank:** These options are primarily reserved for math calculations (drug dosages, intravenous drip rates, conversions). You will be provided the unit of measurement and rounding instructions to type the answer into the provided field.

> **Hot spot:** These questions ask you to use the cursor to identify one or more places on the screen that answers the question. These can be locations on the body, elements of the environment, components of a medical record, or any other graphic depiction of the question that you are asked to interpret and identify a key spot or location on the picture.

> **Varied multiple choice:** Audio or graphic files may provide information about which candidates must make decisions in related test items.

NurseThink® for Clinical Judgment

We know that NCLEX-RN® tests how you think, not what you know! Therefore, one of the things we know about clinical practice in nursing, and the NCLEX-RN® exam, is that they require us to Think! Think hard from a clinical perspective! The **Priority Exemplars**, **Go To Clinical** cases, and **NurseThink® Quizzes** will contribute to your NCLEX-RN® preparation! In addition, **Next Gen Clinical Judgment** boxes, and **Clinical Hints** will continue to grow your decision-making skills. Remember, that focusing on the **Top-Three** helps you save time studying. We hope you find this book valuable on your road to NCLEX-RN® success!

CHAPTER 2

What is NCLEX-RN® all about?

National Council of State Boards of Nursing

To start out, NCLEX® stands for the National Council Licensure Examination. This exam is written, regulated, and evaluated by the National Council of the State Boards of Nursing (NCSBN). In fact, one of your greatest tools is the NCSBN website (www.nclex.org). You want to be familiar with their website since this organization is responsible for WRITING THE EXAM! There are many resources on this site, including details about the exam, the process of applying, specific policies, and frequently asked questions (FAQs). These FAQs are especially informative! In addition, the website includes important information about exam security and what you will be asked to do and provide as part of your exam experience. For example, there is a strict "No phones" policy such that it is best if you leave it in your car! If not, it will be put in a sealed bag and locked in a locker but you are to have no contact with your phone during the exam. There are also practice tests, alternative item tests, and details about computer adapted testing (CAT). CAT is unique in that it is able to estimate the clinical decision-making and clinical judgment skills of a candidate in as few as 75 questions—candidates will answer between 75 and 265 questions. We'll talk more about that in Chapter 3! Let's discuss the questions first before we address the exam.

Cognitive Level of Exam Questions

There was a time when test-taking "tricks" were shared when teaching about the preparation for standardized exams. These "tricks" were thought to give students the advantage when they confronted information they did not know or with which they were not comfortable.

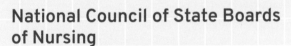

Current testing practices warrant that you must **know** the material and be able to **think critically** about that material in order to pass the exam. Although "tricks" don't work, we will share some strategies in Chapter 4 to help you along!

Before we launch into the exam and the details of how you can be successful, we want to share with you a little more about the NurseThink® approach to critical thinking and answering higher level questions. What are higher level questions? You may have heard through nursing school that, early in your program, you are learning content. You are memorizing, remembering, and comprehending content about the human body, alterations in body systems, and the fundamentals of nursing science. Knowledge level questions ask about these facts and concepts. Building on that, a comprehension level question has you use information you learned to demonstrate how something works or how it is used. For example, a Knowledge/Comprehension level question could be:

Q: **An 80-year-old client enters the emergency room with shortness of breath and fatigue. The nurse plans care based on which client factor?**
1. The client is Asian American and is underweight for height
2. The client prefers to sleep flat in his bed
3. 💡 The client with a history of three myocardial infarctions
4. The client expresses a fear of dying

These knowledge and comprehension questions are important. You needed to learn this information so that, as you progress in your education and in your nursing career, you are able to critically think about that information to make important clinical decisions—both in professional practice and on NCLEX-RN®. So, there was a place for knowledge and comprehension level questions early in your education. In fact, there are some knowledge and comprehension questions in this text.

As you progressed through nursing school the focus changed from learning information to using the nursing process to address and treat conditions, essentially asking the question "What would the nurse do about it?" These questions identified nursing actions, whether assessments, interventions, or evaluations, that were indicated by information given in the test item. These questions are known as application and analysis questions and *these* are the items you will see on NCLEX-RN®. NCSBN tells us that questions will only be at this level, so we want to make sure you are comfortable with these questions and the thinking involved in answering higher level questions.

First, let's talk about application questions. These questions are more than just about a client or clients—they ask what a nurse would do based on the information or case portrayed in the question:

Q: **A client enters the emergency department with shortness of breath, pedal edema, and reports sleeping in a recliner chair for the past two nights. Which would the nurse do first?**
1. Obtain a blood sample for BNP
2. 💡 Elevate the head of the stretcher
3. Prepare for a 12 lead EKG
4. Auscultate heart sounds

This question gives you information and you need to establish the highest priority—first thing to do—again, what a nurse would do in this situation. If you remember, back in Chapter 1, we presented the *THIN Thinking* model. This question is a great example of *THIN Thinking*—**Help Quick** is the first thing to do for this client.

Next Gen Clinical Judgment

According the National Council of State Boards of Nursing (NCSBN) clinical judgment is the **doing** part of critical thinking and decision making. As you answer test items, be sure to try and envision what the nurse would be doing. They want to know what you are going to do as a nurse.

The highest level projected on NCLEX-RN® is the Analysis level. These items require reviewing a set of data, analyzing that data, and coming to a conclusion about a nursing action. They tend to include more data than application questions and require high level thinking. These analysis questions may ask you to set priorities between several clients or several competing priorities within one client. Here is an analysis question:

Q: A client enters the emergency department with shortness of breath, pedal edema, and a productive cough. In triage the client is assessed and blood for laboratory studies are drawn. The client's BNP levels are elevated, there are crackles throughout the lung fields, and the client's arterial blood gases include a PaO2 of 60 mmHg. Which would the nurse anticipate administering first to this client?

1. A normal saline fluid bolus
2. Morphine intravenously
3. 💡 A stat dose of furosemide
4. A digitalizing dose of digoxin

You can see these higher level questions cause you to use **NurseThink**®! Many experts believe that it is not as important for you, as a student, to differentiate between application and analysis questions. Instead, you need to be able to recognize higher level questions from lower level items. The alternative format items you read about in Chapter 1 may be higher or lower level questions. Although alternative items are often thought of as more difficult, and certainly are more time-consuming than standard items, they are not always at the higher cognitive level. It is important to know about alternative items, to be able to differentiate between knowledge/comprehension and application/analysis ones, and be able to answer these higher level items before you sit down to take the exam.

NCLEX-RN® Client Needs

The NCLEX-RN® exam is computer adapted such that each candidate gets a unique exam experience based on their ability. Items are chosen for the candidate based on level of difficulty of the previous question and the blueprint (see Table 2-1).

Safe and effective care environment	
Management of care	17-23%
Safety and infection control	9-15%
Health promotion and maintenance	6-12%
Psychosocial integrity	6-12%
Physiological integrity	
Basic care and comfort	6-12%
Pharmacological/Parenteral Therapies	12-18%
Reduction of risk potential	9-15%
Physiological adaptation	11-17%

Table 2-1: See www.NCLEX.org for more information.

What this means is that every student will answer questions along this blueprint, but each student will receive unique questions. Questions are assigned a level of difficulty. If a student answers a question correctly, the next question is either the same level of difficulty or a little harder. If the student answers it incorrectly, the subsequent question is the same level of difficulty or a little easier.

The blueprint is an excellent example of evidence-based practice! The NCSBN conducts a practice or job analysis and this information, in addition to other analyses, is used to develop the blueprint. For the practice analysis, surveys are sent to newly working registered nurses with a list of tasks. These new practitioners are asked to consider- "What do you do all day?" They rank this list of activities and these rankings inform the components of the blueprint. The exam is reviewed every three years and items undergo rigorous review to ensure accuracy, validity, lack of bias, and readability. In addition, each candidate takes 15 pretest items and the performance on these items by the large pool of candidates inform further revision and validity of the questions. These questions don't count but nor do you know which ones they are in your exam—so do your best on every item! We do know that these pretest questions ensure that each question that counts on the exam is truly valid and that pilot questions are posed to every candidate in the first 75 questions. We usually say, use strategies and knowledge to the best of your ability to answer every question. Even though you don't know which questions "don't count," you may feel some solace in knowing that a truly obscure or difficult question may be a pretest question!

Sometimes the categories of the NCLEX-RN® blueprint may seem hard to understand—they may not mesh with how you learned or studied in nursing school. Let's take a question through the process to show you how the Client Needs work. We'll describe a case and consider the types of questions that could be under each domain.

Case

We are caring for a client who enters the Emergency Department with abdominal pain. The woman states she is about 8 months pregnant. She presents with dizziness, "spots in front of her eyes," and epigastric pain. If we look at the Client Needs, we can come up with questions that might be seen in each category.

Safe and effective care environment:

> **Management of care:** We are working with an Unlicensed Assistive Personnel (UAP)—a question could refer to delegation of vital signs. We would know to carefully ask about and interpret blood pressure in this delegation because it is such a critical assessment in the care of this client.

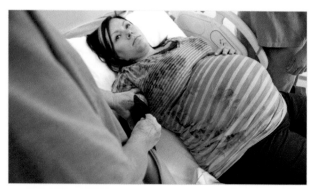

Image 2-1: If you were caring for this woman, would you delegate blood pressure to an UAP?

> **Safety and infection control-**We know that the client's symptoms may indicate pregnancy-induced hypertension/preeclampsia. We may have a question on seizure precautions and keeping the client and fetus safe.

Health promotion and maintenance:

We discover that this is our client's first baby and she did not receive prenatal care. We may have a question on the third trimester of pregnancy or on preparing the woman for labor and delivery.

Psychosocial integrity:

It is easy to develop a question related to the stress this client may be feeling and appropriate nursing interventions to enhance coping.

Physiological integrity:

> **Basic care and comfort:** How about the comfort needs of this client? We will need to create a quiet and restful environment to keep her calm, position the client on her side to enhance fetal circulation, and maintain NPO restrictions as part of comfort and safety care.

> **Pharmacological/Parenteral Therapies:** A test question could be developed based on our anticipation to administer magnesium sulfate or intravenous fluids.

> **Reduction of risk potential:** We could write a test question that discusses our need to avoid the complications of a potential seizure or the impact of the hypertension on the fetus. This may include laboratory data that we need to interpret within the context of the test question.

> **Physiological adaptation:** Finally, questions may be asked about the protein in the client's urine, the physiology of the client's condition, and how these contribute to the clinical picture.

You can see how this blueprint or test plan covers the spectrum of professional nursing care and may apply to any specialty or setting. Clients in NCLEX-RN® questions are from across the well-illness continuum, across the lifespan, and in a variety of clinical settings, including homes, community agencies, hospitals, schools, workplaces, long-term care facilities, and anywhere nurses provide care!

Examples of Topics in each Client Need

Students are encouraged to go to the NCSBN website to review topics under each category and the complete test plan, but they are briefly discussed here for your review.

Safe and effective care environment:

This larger category speaks to the role of professional nurses in leadership, priority setting, and keeping clients safe.

> **Management of care:** This section highlights the aspects of client care related to leadership, conflict management, priority setting, delegation, and working with the healthcare team. Candidates are asked to establish priorities within a single client and also to juggle competing priorities between several clients. Consider the laws, policies, and research that govern nursing's scope of practice as questions ask about delegation.

> **Safety and infection control:** As indicated in this title, this section discusses injury and infection prevention and the nurse's role in keeping clients safe. One great way to study for this section is to take note of the precautions in the clinical area— these are essentially agency care plans to keep clients safe. Neutropenic, fall, aspiration, suicide, seizure, flight risk, bleeding, and other precautions keep clients safe. These agency precautions are like safety "care plans" and reinforce what we know about client-centered care.

Health promotion and maintenance:

This is the wellness aspect of the exam and includes such content as normal labor and delivery, developmental milestones including changes of aging, physical assessment, risk behaviors, screening, and keeping clients healthy across the lifespan. One key component here is vocabulary. Consider the meanings of the words: lie, station, orientation, and position in establishing the placement of a fetus in a woman's abdomen—these words have unique meanings in this specialty. Similarly, there are other areas of the test plan that require you to be able to know and use specific terms. This area of the exam questions may ask about wellness concepts as they may occur concurrently with acute or chronic illness and as they impact individuals, families, and populations.

Psychosocial integrity:

Although a lower percentage of the exam than other areas, the skills tested in this area are critical components of professional nursing! Therapeutic communication, substance use and abuse, defense mechanisms, dealing with crisis and stress, persistent/chronic mental illness, grief and bereavement, and psychotropic medications are included in this section. Establishing therapeutic relationships and communication questions may be asked in this domain where answers appear in quotation marks and reflect client or nursing statements. Communication questions may be difficult because the response choices may not reflect your usual communication style. Remember that the goal of therapeutic communication is to open up the reciprocal communication pathway and encourage the client to respond. Even if you personally would not say something, you want to follow the accepted styles that reinforce therapeutic communication. Options that foster communication include open-ended questions, and those that reflect empathy, respect, genuine caring, and therapeutic boundaries. Closed-ended questions, that can be answered with a yes or no, do not promote rich discussion.

Physiological integrity:

This section, about one-half of the exam, focuses on physiological components of care.

> **Basic care and comfort:** We frequently discuss that, although the quality of today's healthcare is augmented by technology and advances in science, one cannot forget the importance of the basics. Skills you learned in fundamentals, like activities of daily living, hygiene, assistive devices, sleep, body mechanics and moving clients, comfort measures, and nutrition are also critical components and basics of client care. Basic nutrition and therapeutic/condition-specific dietary recommendations are part of this category. This section also includes alternative/complementary therapies and the professional nurse's role in ensuring client safety with these treatments.

> **Pharmacological/Parenteral Therapies:** This section, about one-fifth of the exam, is often the most dreaded of all sections! It includes questions about specific medications and classes of drugs, routes of administration, calculations of doses, and priority nursing implications of medications. Medication therapeutic actions and side effects, contraindications, potential interactions, client teaching, and details about administering the medication may be the subjects of these items. In addition, questions pertaining to parenteral therapies are asked in this section, including fluid choices, blood product and fluid administration, intravenous therapy, total parenteral nutrition, and associated nursing care.

> **Reduction of risk potential:** This section, although perhaps the most abstract of all the blueprint, speaks to the essential role of nursing in monitoring for and preventing complications. Untoward effects from infection, surgery, injury, illness, interventions, immobility, and other conditions may be prevented or reduced in severity if detected and intervened upon early. Here, questions discuss diagnostic procedures, unexpected effects of care, and therapeutic procedures, including psychomotor skills and policies. One recent change made in this section is the reduced emphasis on the intraoperative phase for nurse generalists although questions may still be asked about the preoperative and postoperative periods.

> **Physiological adaptation:** This section mirrors what you learned in pathophysiology and about disease processes. Expected signs and symptoms, and therapeutic measures, related to conditions are addressed, along with unexpected responses to treatments, illness management, hemodynamics, and fluid and electrolytes.

Integrated concepts

NCLEX-RN® items are also written by attending to what the NCSBN calls the **Integrated Concepts**. These concepts are woven throughout your exam and reflect the beliefs and philosophy of the exam. These provide the foundation for the exam such that each item has some elements addressed as these integrated concepts. The integrated concepts are:

> **The Nursing Process** is the assessment, analysis, planning, implementation and evaluation of nursing care. Remember that nursing diagnosis is limited on NCLEX-RN® and that the exam is focused on "What would a nurse do?" so the emphasis is on ACTION—assessment and intervention.

> **Caring** is the interaction of the nurse and client in an attitude of mutual respect and trust. It may seem like common sense but choose answers that demonstrate this level of caring!

> **Communication and Documentation** includes both the verbal and non-verbal messages between clients, client's significant others, and members of the healthcare team as well as written/electronic health records.

> **Teaching and Learning** is the facilitation of knowledge, skills, and attitudes designed to assist to promote changes in behaviors. The role of the nurse as teacher is critical part of professional nursing practice and is reflected in the NCLEX-RN®. Questions on the exam may refer to situations in which nurses may be teachers and learners. We have seen many questions in the literature, and on faculty tests, about teaching. These questions may have two purposes—to test the candidate's knowledge of the content to be taught and to assess the candidate's ability to adapt material to level of understanding of the client. It is critical to read the stems of the questions several times, as in all item stems you experience, because the stem itself indicates the type of answer for which you are looking. For example, if a stem states "Which option indicates a need for more teaching?" you are looking for a wrong or incorrect statement or answer. If the stem states: "Which indicates a good understanding of teaching?" you are looking for a correct or valid statement or answer. These questions reinforce the need for careful reading in the NCLEX-RN® exam and the role of the nurse as teacher and learner.

> **Culture and Spirituality** is the interaction of nursing with clients (individuals, families/significant others, groups, and populations) which recognizes and considers client-reported, self-identified unique and individual preferences in client care, within parameters of standards of care and legal implications. The Integrated Concept of Culture and Spirituality was added in 2016. Prior to this, these questions were under Psychosocial Integrity. The NCSBN realized that, in many cases, culture and spirituality may infuse any question and that this elevation to an Integrated Concept reinforced the importance of considering aspects of culture and spirituality in every area of nursing and client care. Cultural awareness, cultural influences on health, spiritual influences on health,

and spiritual factors impacting care all infuse the NCLEX-RN® exam. How language and religious and spiritual client needs are met are integral nursing considerations in holistic client care. Culture and spirituality may influence rituals, customs, holidays, dietary practices, manner of dress, relationships with authority, social interactions, gender roles, communication, and decision-making. Critical to this is the need to focus on the client as an individual and respect the client's choices and needs.

Next Gen Clinical Judgment

You are a nurse in the Emergency Department. You are triaging a 19-year-old African American male client brought in by his partner. The client discussed with his partner that he wanted to kill himself by taking a bottle of prescription antidepressant medications. The partner was able to "talk him out of it." The client had disclosed to his parents the night before that he was a homosexual. His parents, especially his father, became angry and "kicked him out of the house." The family is dedicated to their religion and believe homosexuality is a sin. They also stated that they don't ever want to see the client again.

1. How might the client's culture and spirituality impact the client's health and healthcare?

Next Gen Clinical Judgment

You are a nurse on an inpatient pediatric unit. You are caring for an 8-year-old child with a history of asthma who is being admitted in respiratory distress. The client's grandmother was watching the child and brought the child to the hospital. The client's mother and father burst into the room saying "Stop the breathing treatment, Stop everything. We don't believe in this. Our religion does not allow all this. We want to take our son home. We will heal him our way!"

1. How might the client's culture and spirituality impact the client's health and healthcare?

2. How is the client's care influenced by his age?

Focus: Priority setting, safety, and clinical judgment

To summarize, the NCLEX-RN® exam is individually developed for each person to ensure that successful individuals provide safe and competent entry-level nursing care. By using higher level thinking questions, along the guidelines of the exam blueprint, the candidate's clinical decision-making and priority setting skills are measured. We'll end this chapter with a graphic that might help you as you set priorities. See the higher priority assessments and interventions on the left and the lower priority assessments and interventions on the right. This is a great schematic to help you consider priorities on the NCLEX-RN® exam!

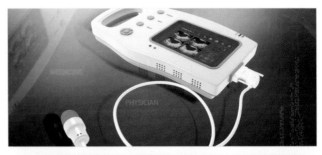

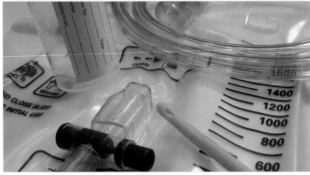

Image 2-2: When setting priorities for assessing a patient with urinary retention, should the nurse use a bladder scanner or insert a urinary catheter?

Next Gen Clinical Judgment: How do you set PRIORITIES?

Higher Priorities:

Priority Assessments or Cues

> ABCs
> Acute - Unstable
> Early Findings
> Old and young

Lower Priorities:

Priority Assessments or Cues

> Chronic - Stable
> Late Findings

Priority Interventions or Actions

> Least invasive
> Fast action
> Client-centered
> Basic Maslow needs
> Assessment > Intervention
> Safety

Priority Interventions or Actions

> More invasive
> Slow action
> Nurse focused
> Teaching
> Emotional needs

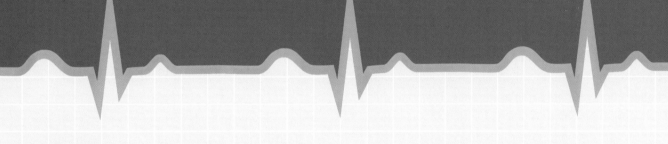

CHAPTER
3

What can I expect?

The Exam

The NCLEX-RN® exam experience is different for each candidate. Let's talk a little about the exam itself. The exam for each student is unique but based on standardized content and is directed toward assessing clinical decision-making skills. You will answer between 75 and 265 questions and will have up to 6 hours to complete the exam. This time period includes time for the tutorial and optional breaks. Breaks are offered to each candidate at the two-hour and three and one-half hour point, but it is up to you if you want to take a break or keep on testing! Although this is plenty of time for most people you may want to keep your review of each question to less than three minutes. Studies tell us that if you think about a question for more than three minutes you risk the potential to "overthink" a question. Make sure you consider the options and answer confidently—moving on to the next question!

As discussed earlier, in Computer Adapted Testing (CAT), the exam is constructed for each candidate based on items' levels of difficulty and to represent the appropriate percentages of the test plan. If the candidate gets a question correct, the next question is the same or a higher level of difficulty. If the question is answered incorrectly, the next item is the same or an easier difficulty level. Once you have answered the item and press "enter," that item disappears and will not be seen again. You must answer every question, there is no ability to skip or leave a question blank, and there is no penalty for guessing. This means of administration is good news for most people, especially for individuals who often change their answers. Research tells us that we often change correct to incorrect options; a good rule to follow is to change you answer with confidence, not with doubt. In other words, if you have a brainstorm that another answer is correct—then change the answer with confidence. On the other hand, if you doubt your thoughts or judgment—leave it! Your first inclination or hunch is often correct. Remember, your educated guess is often correct and, for traditional multiple choice items, you have a 25% chance of getting the question right! The process of elimination is your ally as you take the test, that will enable you to increase this percentage even higher! Some candidates use the dry erase board to write down the numbers signifying the answer options (Details about the dry erase board later). These test-takers cross out options as they proceed to think through an item, ultimately yielding a visible reminder of their answer option.

You do not need to have special computer skills for this exam and you will be taken through a tutorial at the beginning of the exam. You can also go to the NCSBN (www.nclex.org) website to watch the tutorial video. You will be able to use the drop-down calculator on the computer and the computer has the customary mouse, keyboard, and monitor. There is also a clock/timer on the computer which may be turned on or off based upon your personal preference. The computer will show the number of each question. If you require specific accommodations related to your health, testing skills, or specific abilities/disabilities, you should check the NCSBN website (www.nclex.org) and you are encouraged to contact the testing center well in advance to ensure the best testing situation for you and to allow the center to meet your needs.

You are encouraged to do your best the FIRST TIME you take the exam. We have heard of people taking the exam the first time, without studying, as a way to "try it out" and see how the exam looks and feels. Candidates may do this with the intent of then studying and passing the second time. Not only is this a waste of money, and prolongs the time before you can practice a nurse (and maybe, pay back your school loans!), but there is research that indicates that the passing rate on those taking the second exam is ONE HALF the rate for the first exam. In other words, if 85-89% of NCLEX-RN® candidates pass the first time, studies demonstrate that around 45% pass the

second time! It is important that you focus on passing the FIRST TIME you take NCLEX-RN®. Not only is that critical for you and your career, but schools, as you may remember, are evaluated based on their first-time pass rates, among other criteria! On the other hand, if you are not successful the first time, despite your hardest efforts, we hope this text can continue to build your clinical judgment, competence, knowledge, and skills such that you are successful in subsequent testing experiences!

Application

You are in your last semester of school and are getting ready to graduate and take the NCLEX-RN® exam. The best source of information about your applying for the exam is the NCSBN website (www.nclex.org) and the state/location board of nursing where you plan on living. We will generally summarize the general principles, although the application process varies slightly.

> The NCSBN website (www.nclex.org) offers the NCLEX-RN® Exam Candidate Bulletin. Make sure you download that first to make sure you get off to the right start!

> You will need to apply for a nursing license with the state in which you are living or plan to be living. If the state you live in or plan to live in is part of the multistate compact, you will be able to work in other compact states, but you must have the license in your state of residence. If you plan to work in a state that is not part of this compact, you will need to get a license for that state. International candidates should check the NCSBN website and their local nursing boards to ensure compliance with procedures. Although it seems very confusing, check your state board of nursing's website and you will be on your way. Many schools provide this information to students prior to graduation. You will need to pay a fee and complete an application. Each application process is unique and some states/locations require passport-size pictures. Be very careful completing this application and follow the directions completely. You may experience significant delays if the application needs to be returned to you to correct errors.

> You will also need to apply to Pearson Vue or the exam setting (for locations not using Pearson Vue) to take the exam. There is also a fee for this application.

> Once you have graduated, your school provides the information to the state board of nursing indicating that you have graduated and meet the requirements for taking the exam.

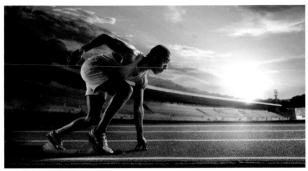

Image 3-1: Graduation is just part of the picture. How will you continue your clinical judgment training until the day of NCLEX®?

> Once "all the planets align" (your school, the state/location board of nursing, and Pearson Vue) you will be sent an authorization to test (ATT). You can call the Pearson Vue or other exam setting (for locations not using Pearson Vue) and enter your ATT. Many sites also provide a mechanism to make an appointment online. You cannot make an appointment without an ATT.

Things you want to consider when making an appointment:

> > Think about the time of day when you are at your best! Make a morning appointment if you are an early riser… an afternoon appointment if that is when you perform at your peak! You will be asked to make an appointment at least six hours prior to the site's closing time because that is the maximum time allowed for the exam.

> > Consider life events and other scheduling variables—big events, time commitments, your work schedule, and your prospective employment's requests for your start date.

> Pay attention to the policies related to changing your appointment or if you miss the appointment. If you do not call to cancel your appointment, and don't show up, you will lose your application fees and will need to pay and schedule again.

> Research studies indicate that candidates who take the exam within 45-90 days after graduation experience the highest success rates. The information is more "fresh in your mind," you are still in the studying/test-taking groove, and there is less of a chance for life and other distractions to divert you from your NCLEX-RN® goals.

Before and the day of the exam

Chapter 4 and Chapter 20 will address how to set study goals, prepare yourself, and get you closer to NCLEX-RN® success. The day before the exam, you may want to do a "trial drive" to make sure you know where you are going and are comfortable with the location, the traffic patterns, and parking options. The night before the exam you want to put your books away and consider means to pamper yourself, clear your mind of distractions, and feel the best about yourself! Many go to a movie, get a massage, spend time with friends or family, read a book, or hunker down in front of the television for some intense relaxation. Make sure you get enough rest—go to bed early and set your alarm, or maybe a few alarms, to ensure that you wake up on time.

The morning of the exam, no matter what time you are scheduled to take the exam, eat a nutritious, light meal. Do not overdo caffeinated or other beverages and make sure you are comfortable but not hungry. There are a few differing thoughts on dressing for the exam. Some recommend the "dress for success" option where you wear professional clothes to gain confidence and positive self-thoughts. Others dictate that comfort is the key such that one small step above pajamas is the best idea! You decide—but make sure you dress in layers to adapt to the climate of the testing center.

Arrive at the testing center thirty minutes early to provide a buffer if you encounter traffic congestion or problems with parking. Bring your ATT and government-issued identification (ID) with you. Make sure this ID matches the name on your application exactly and, if it doesn't match, call the testing center **before you arrive to test** to allay any test day worries! Leave your phone, watch, books, and any other materials out in your car. Anything you bring with you into the testing center will be placed in a locker and you will not be able to access these during testing time. You will not be able to bring any food or water into the setting; if you have medical requirements for a snack or beverage you are encouraged to contact the testing center and you may need to apply for special accommodations. Water is available and may be accessed during breaks. Most centers have you wear a lanyard indicating that you are a testing candidate to curb any access to the lockers during testing and to curtail any conversations. Because centers have very small waiting rooms, and friends or family are not able to wait for you, candidates are encouraged to drive themselves or to be dropped off at the center.

At the testing center you will undergo significant security procedures to confirm your identity and preclude any test compromise. You will be finger-printed and have palm vein scanning, in addition to being videotaped, photographed, and audio-recorded during the examination. You will receive a dry erase board and marker; should you run out of room on the board you must turn in that board and get a new one rather than erasing your board. You will be placed in a cubicle with a computer with adequate lighting. Because multiple examinees are in the same room, some candidates find the ambient noise disruptive. You may ask for ear plugs from the exam proctor. Anytime you wish to contact the proctor, you are encouraged to raise your hand rather than getting out of your seat. Once you have completed the exam, your will receive a message that "Exam ENDED." There is a brief survey after the exam is completed.

Although the test pool available to NCSBN is large, there are a finite number of questions that make up the NCLEX-RN® examinations for a vast number of candidates. For this reason, and to preserve the examination pool for future candidates, each examinee will sign a confidentiality statement. In this document you promise not to discuss specific topics or items on the exam or to provide any information to others that would compromise the integrity of the exam. It is human nature to talk about the experience. It is an important, as you begin your professional career, that you adhere to the principles and policies of this confidentiality agreement. In kind, it is critical that you refrain from asking these details of other candidates and ensure that this exam remains a sound mechanism to determine and validate entry-level nursing practice.

Staying calm in the cubicle

We will talk again, in Chapters 4 and 20, about dealing with the stress of life and NCLEX-RN® in the weeks and months prior to the exam. Here we are briefly going to address "calming yourself in the cubicle."

For example, you have just answered #39—it was a really hard question and you start to feel yourself panic. You know your personal, early signs of stress and anxiety. Do you feel a fluttering in your stomach? Perspiration EVERYWHERE? A headache coming on? Are your hands shaking? Do you feel nauseous? Do you feel like you can't think?

These feelings have happened to all of us and we know NCLEX-RN® is stress producing. But this is your chance to demonstrate how much you have learned, how much you know, and how you can use clinical judgment! Rather than letting stress cloud your thoughts and get the best of you, take control in the cubicle and keep on testing.

Instead of seeing stress as a liability in exam taking, think of stress as your friend. That may sound crazy to you, so let us explain. Without any stress, it would be hard for you to take the exam seriously and be primed to do your best! Instead, you may daydream during the exam or be distracted by other competing priorities. Here is where stress helps you out. A moderate level of stress ensures that you are focused and able to fully attend to the task at hand—taking the exam. You filter out distracting thoughts and focus on each question with enthusiasm and peak performance in test-taking. This stress keeps your brain oxygenated and helps you not worry about hunger, fatigue, or other concerns. On the other hand, stress may exceed this moderate level and start to interfere with your ability to think and make connections. Higher levels of stress impair your reasoning and distract you from a complete level of focus. Your physical and emotional symptoms detract from your abilities to rationally think through questions, retrieve memories, and make cogent decisions. Rather than allowing these symptoms to persist, you have to handle them---calm them (and yourself) in the cubicle!

Only you know the EARLY signs of stress you are most likely to manifest and when stress levels start to exceed moderate levels. Take a moment now to write down your symptoms. What do you feel when you first feel stress set in? How do these feelings progress? What goes on in your mind as these symptoms and feelings become apparent during testing? Now that you have that information in mind, consider what you can and should do to address rising stress levels and ensure that you are functioning at your peak level. You may already have a successful means to deal with stress during testing. You were successful in nursing school, so keep it up! If you are not sure you have a favorite method, you aren't confident your method will work with this level of high stakes testing, or you want to try something new, see this list to continue to foster stress reducing techniques. Practice a few before the exam, pick a favorite one, and master the technique prior to the exam. When you FIRST feel stress rising during NCLEX-RN® with the early signs identified previously, call your new stress management strategies into play and then, when you are calm, continue with your testing!

Calming yourself in the cubicle!

> Conjure up and use affirmations, or positive thoughts and messages, and rehearse them prior to the exam. Say to yourself—I am smart! I am qualified! I am competent! I am confident! I am ready! Some

candidates "picture themselves a nurse," wherein they envision the stethoscope around their neck or their name badge with a big RN!

> Use muscle relaxation to calm your nerves. For some this is as simple as a neck roll. For others they conduct an ascending, progressive total body muscle contraction and relaxation. Beginning with the toes and ending at the neck, individuals using this strategy contract and relax every muscle in the body as a means to provide respite from the exam and refocus energy to thinking and decision-making.

> For many individuals, prayer or calming chants (silently, of course) may allow for brief interruptions from testing and allow you to reset your testing mindset.

> Research tells us that deep breaths enable us to lower our heart rate, focus our mind, and calm negative messages. Consider embracing yoga principles or other breathing techniques that allow for optimal focus and control.

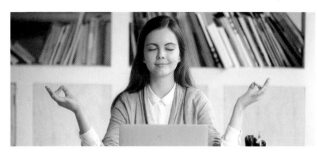

Image 3-2: When studying for NCLEX®, practice OFTEN relaxation techniques that you can use during the actual exam.

Scoring the exam and passing standards

We believe that gone are the days that you can pass NCLEX-RN® without studying! It is a difficult exam and is more difficult than it used to be. In fact, the NCLEX-RN® exam has been progressively getting more difficult. We don't say this to scare you—but to mobilize you into action to create your own study plan for NCLEX-RN®! One great resource to use to better understand the scoring of the exam is located on the NCSBN website. (https://www.ncsbn.org/356.htm). This brief video explains how items are selected and how performance is scored by comparing exam candidates with individuals working out in a gym—we encourage you to watch it a few times!

When you sit down to NCLEX-RN® you will take between 75 and 265 questions. As discussed, you will be exposed to questions at various levels of difficulty and your computer adapted test will assess your level of clinical decision making based on your answers to the test questions. Once you "prove" to the computer that you are above the passing standard and have completed at least 75 questions, the test will end. In converse, if a candidate is consistently well below the passing standard the exam will turn off. Many believe that it is a good sign if you are experiencing difficult items—the computer is pushing you to your limit!

The NCSBN describes three scenarios to describe how candidates may pass or fail the exam:

> The 95% confidence interval rule: In this scenario, the computer will end the examination after 75 questions if the candidate is, with 95% confidence, clearly above or below passing standard.

> The maximum length rule: This rule presides when the candidate reaches item 265. If the candidate is above the passing standard at this point, the candidate passes. If the candidate is below the passing standard at this point, the candidate fails.

> The run out of time rule (ROOT): This principle governs the status of the candidate if the candidate uses up the entire 6 hours allowed for the exam. If the candidate completes fewer than 75 items or is below the passing standard for the last 60 items, the candidate will fail. If the candidate was above the passing standard for the last 60 items, the candidate will pass.

Getting my results

Although you will be most eager to get your results after the exam, the testing center will not have any knowledge of your score. Rumors exist about—If you get only 75 questions, you definitely passed—If you get all 265 questions you definitely failed—If you get 265 questions but you knew you passed at question 100, you were a test subject. None of these statements

are true and NCSBN has repeatedly refuted the urban legend that some people are randomly selected to take all 265 questions! Make sure you routinely consult the NCSBN website with questions and be discriminating about believing erroneous rumors about the exam. Instead, here is what we know about getting your results:

> The exam is graded twice before releasing your findings.

> The results are sent to the state or other location board of nursing and mailed to the candidate within one month of the examination.

> Some states have access to unofficial, quick results services which make results available to candidates within 2 days for an additional fee.

> Some states or locations have a verification of licensure pathway, where candidates, employers, and schools can determine if a registered nurse license has been issued under a specific participant's name—this would indicate that the candidate passed.

Candidates who pass the exam will receive a document with the pass determination and indicate the number of items completed. Those examinees who did not pass will receive a candidate report indicating that they failed and documenting personal strengths and weaknesses. The NCSBN website notes that areas of strength or weakness are not provided to individuals passing the exam to avoid employers, schools of higher learning, or individuals using this information to compare successful NCLEX-RN® candidates or provide a means to discriminate between successful candidates. Candidates that are not successful on NCLEX-RN® are guaranteed, depending upon the state or location, to obtain a retake appointment within 45 to 90 days of receiving a new ATT.

Now that we have a firm foundation of knowledge about the exam, let's proceed to Chapter 4 and discuss how you can prepare for NCLEX-RN®: Study what you don't know and the 20/50 rule, test-taking strategies, terms to know, and an introduction to principles of a healthy lifestyle to ensure your success!

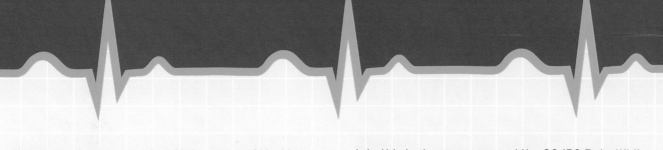

How can I prepare?

Know what you don't know with the 20/50 Rule!

It is important to think about your preparation for NCLEX-RN® as a marathon, not a sprint. Every experience you had in nursing school, in simulation and clinical, and all your preparation add to your clinical judgment and your abilities on the exam. A colleague of ours was once known to say: "We tend to study what we like and are good at knowing and doing." The converse is also true. We tend to avoid those things we find difficult or less than interesting. Our recommendation is that you identify your weaknesses through test-taking and study those topics with which you struggle or on which you perform poorly.

To do this, now is the time to discover what your areas of weakness are and to address them. As you launch into this text, we recommend the 20/50 Rule. While in nursing school, each day you need to take a 20-item quiz and review the questions you get wrong. In addition, once a week take a 50-item test and pursue those topics that you were less sure of or did not answer correctly. When you are in your study phase consider increasing this to 50 items each day with 100 item weekly tests. In Chapter 20, we will discuss more about NCLEX-RN® preparation but this text will continue to help you-so read further! Whether you are still in nursing school, or are in your intense study phase, another strategy is to use E3—what we call Expand Every Event. This strategy helps you engage in material—as you sit in class write down three words that help you understand every question, client, or case you discuss. Reflect on these terms later and try to determine if you have questions about the topic.

E3 helps you perform "mental aerobics" or engage in material three times. Brain research tells us that we need to interact with material three times for us to make a memory about, or essentially learn, content. Reading and preparing before class provides you one opportunity. Hearing information in class provides another opportunity. Engaging in material using a creative teaching strategy, like E3, will further assist you to make memories and learn material. During your study phase, make conscious efforts to actively engage in learning material—write it down, say it out loud, or compose exam questions about the material. This is so much better than memorization—it is about learning material and thinking about it to make sound clinical decisions. In Chapter 20, we are going to talk more about using the "mental aerobics" principles to learn and succeed for NCLEX-RN®.

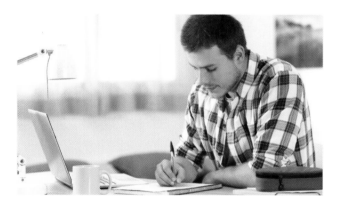

Image 4-1: When taking a practice exam, be sure to create a quiet and calm environment to replicate the actual exam.

Test-taking Strategies

As we discussed, there are no "tricks" to taking NCLEX-RN®--but there are some strategies you can use to identify correct answers.

> We believe your greatest asset for the exam is **careful** and **calm** reading! We often misread questions and the human brain has the capacity to misinterpret questions to get them to be what we want them to be! We have all looked at exams after we completed them and said, "Why did I answer that?" It is often because we misread the question or the answer options. Read questions for critical words and concepts. Words and phrases like

changes in level of consciousness, restlessness, lethargy, increased work of breathing, a threatened airway, or significant deviations in vital signs may influence how you answer a question! These keywords or concepts may describe a change in client status, so important to recognize on NCLEX-RN®. It is critical to carefully read questions!

> Often students do well to visualize the client—and use your intelligent intuition! We often second-guess ourselves and, luckily, on NCLEX-RN® you will not be able to change answers. But often you question your initial, intuitive response. Remember, a good rule of thumb is to "Change your answer with confidence, not with doubt." In this way, you change the answer if you have an ah-hah and come to the right answer, but leave an answer, with your initial response, if you doubt whether the previous or changed answers are correct.

> Think about how those keywords in a question might influence your answer. As we said, words like restlessness, dyspnea, changes in levels of consciousness, floppy, or lethargy may assist you in visualizing the client in the question and indicate a client change in status that might appear in the correct answer.

> Remember the client is always a higher priority than the equipment—when a question tells you that a client's monitor is alarming, it is always critical to assess and attend to the client first then deal with the alarm.

> Sometimes it is hard to understand a question the way it is written—try to rephrase the question in your own words and then try to answer it. In contrast, do not misinterpret the question. It is important to read and verify the meaning of a question when trying to answer. The human brain is amazing in its ability to rewrite a question to the way you "want" the item to look or the way you have seen the concept posed in the past. Make sure you accurately read the question several times. Picture in your mind what the answer might be. Then look at the options and see if it is there. Make sure you don't "read into" a question.

- If the question asks for the "First Nursing Action" it is often a nursing assessment. We know that assessment is the first step of the nursing process and more information is often needed before one can intervene. When you look at a question, do you need more information? Did a registered nurse conduct the assessment or is one still needed? Could additional assessments lead to a more appropriate intervention?

- When questions ask for the "Essential Nursing Action," think safety. We will repeat the **safety message** several times in this text—NCLEX-RN® is an exam of safety! Keeping clients, other healthcare professionals, and ourselves safe is critical on the exam.

- You will be given a piece of paper and pencil or a dry erase board and marker. Use this help you use your test-taking strategies—whether it is the process of elimination, completing calculations, making notes to yourself or writing down formulas or memorized information for later use.

- Be careful about passing client responsibilities quickly on to other healthcare professionals. It is very rare that a nurse stands at a client's side and does nothing, only to call the healthcare provider. Nor do nurses initiate a social work consult without communicating with the client. We will assess, intervene, reassure, and communicate with clients and then make the emergency call or referral. NCLEX-RN® is a test of nursing practice and, as such, will ask what the nurse would do!

- Questions about delegation may be difficult. As a testing strategy, one thing to remember is that you delegate away the simplest task. A registered nurse should retain duties that reflect the scope of practice and require nursing judgment, including assessments, teaching, and evaluation—these cannot be delegated away!

- If numbers are included in a question, take them seriously—interpret them and choose the correct nursing action. Are the numbers telling you the client is stable or unstable? Are the vital signs normal? How do they relate to the client's age?

This may be critical information! A client's age may influence an answer based on developmental level, susceptibility to medication or illness, vulnerability, or treatment. For example, urinary tract infections and dehydration are far more grave if they occur in infants or older adults.

- Consider the time frame in every question! Is the client young or old? Did the surgery happen one hour ago or last year? What is the time frame since surgery, injury, admission, diagnosis, or other event? All of these variables may critically inform the decision-making in a test item!

- The NCLEX-RN® exam takes place in "NCLEX® WORLD." In this world, you have enough time, supplies, money, and help to accomplish tasks according to the highest of standards and in exact adherence to policies. That is not to say that, in real nursing practice, these standards are not important—but they are adapted to the capacities and capabilities of the real world. So, do not answer questions on the exam after considering the limitations what you may have seen in practice or heard stories of in class or clinical. Instead, keep to the high level of care you learned about and consider what is SAFEST for the client!

- Questions will not include proper names and will only include the level of detail needed to answer the question. If the question cites an age, ethnicity, race, or gender, that information is important to answer the question.

- Questions are all "stand-alone." Except for those questions that are part of the Next Gen of NCLEX-RN®, which we will explain at the end of this book, all questions are unrelated so, do not be tempted to answer a question based on a previous question's answer. All questions are chosen randomly and are based on your personal performance.

- Questions on medications may be perceived as difficult. One strategy to consider is that side effects of medications are often accentuated expected therapeutic effects. For example, if a medication is prescribed to bring blood pressure down for clients with hypertension, then side effects include hypotension and orthostatic hypotension.

- Make sure you focus on normal values **and** critical values of laboratory studies. Although it is tempting to memorize lab studies norms, remember to focus on when lab values may yield critical signs and symptoms. For example, although a value of 126 mg/dL for blood glucose is not within the normal range, it is not a critical value that warrants emergency care. Consider when lab abnormalities may cause critical changes in status or require nursing care. They are more important to address than lab values that are marginally abnormal.

- Professional nurses are devoted to supporting clients with the utmost respect and encouraging as must self-care as possible. Although it may seem like common sense, pick an answer that supports respect and self-care for the clients. In this sense, the least invasive measures are often correct. There are times we implement a "least invasive" intervention while preparing for subsequent actions. Remember the *THIN Thinking* Help Quick option. In addition, nurses provide client-centered/family-centered care, this is important to remember as you answer questions!

Terms to know

There are certain words that are used on NCLEX-RN® to communicate to those taking the exam. They include:

- UAP: Unlicensed assistive personnel, or UAPs, is the term for any healthcare provider who does not have a license, including nurse's aides, assistants, or other titles.

- HCP: Healthcare Providers include all professionals with prescriptive privileges, including physicians, nurse anesthetists, physician assistants, nurse practitioners, and nurse midwives.

- Prescriptions is the term used for any "orders" coming from those professionals noted above. In addition to medications, prescriptions may be for diagnostic and lab studies, activity restrictions, diets, procedures, and treatments.

- Rather than saying "complains of" the exam will use another term, thought to be with less judgmental than this phrase such as "presents with" or "states has these symptoms."

- The word "client" will refer to the subject of the question and may refer to the individual, family, group, or population.

- Medications will only be listed by their generic names, not their trade names. No proprietary names will be used.

- There is limited discussion of nursing diagnosis—but concepts and themes important to nursing are included.

Healthy lifestyle for healthy testing

Although it is hard to focus on yourself or your own health while going through nursing school and preparing for the exam, we just want to briefly mention how important it is to stay healthy and engage in healthy habits. A healthy body and healthy mind will best be able to think and make connections during the exam. Researchers identified the components of success, calling it "NCLEX-RN® Boot Camp". In this model, candidates focus on personal health (physical, emotional, and spiritual), practice questions, and treat exam preparation like a job—full time and full effort! So, what can you do to prepare?"

- Questions, questions, and more questions! Research tells us that you need to complete 2000-3000 questions to be prepared for the NCLEX-RN® exam. There was a time when 5000 questions were recommended, but the evidence now points to the more conservative number. Hooray for science!

- Consider your time and balance your time with work, questions, rest, exercise, and play

- Research tells us the you need to take the exam within 45-90 days from graduation and you need to devote designated time to study for the exam—we'll talk more about this in Chapter 20.

The research also affirms that having a healthy lifestyle and health-promoting habits contribute to NCLEX-RN® Success. Here are some hints to get you started and to launch into the content sections of this book:

> Remember—you have been successful! You succeeded in nursing school—you have made it this far and you are eligible to take the exam—you are getting **ready**!

> Consider a standard place for studying—set yourself up—with or without music, with or without beverages and snacks, with or without interruptions of your phone and people in your world. Have this book available with plenty of sharpened pencils, your nursing textbooks, and a computer to search for information.

> Try to consider your diet and sleep habits. Studies tell us that a high protein, moderate carbohydrate diet fosters thinking and clear decision-making. A balanced diet with adequate fiber and water is optimal. Research indicates that the memories we make and the concepts we learn during the day are processed and organized during our sleep cycles. Adequate sleep is required to lay down memories for retrieval later. Consider your sleep and diet habits as you establish a study plan.

> Make sure you take time to play and have fun—spend time with your family and with yourself in activities that are fun and allow you to relax—and recharge—to go back to studying! Make smart decisions about alcohol, caffeine, and nicotine during this time—you want your mind to be sharp and at its best!

> Remember your affirmations!

> > You are smart!
> > You are ready!
> > You will be a Registered Nurse!

> Let's dive into the content sections of the book. Each chapter discusses a set of concepts or a system. **Within each chapter there are:**

> > The **Go To Clinical Cases**—read these and use **Prioritization Power** to complete the **Top Three** Priority Assessments, Priority Labs/Diagnostics, Priority Potential and Actual Complications, Priority Interventions, Priority Medications, Priority Nursing Implications, and Priority Education/Discharge issues.

> You can check your answers by looking at the related **Priority Exemplars**—the **Top Three** will designated by a 💡.

> Review the other **Priority Exemplars**. Consider the material you know and don't know. Try to come up with potential exam questions related to that material. Use **Priority Exemplars** as references as you work through the chapters.

> In addition, Next Gen Clinical Judgment Boxes and **Clinical Hints** will continue to enhance your decision-making skills.

> At the end of most chapters are **NurseThink®️ Quizzes**. Take the Quizzes, check your answers, and, for the ones that are incorrect, take a minute to assess what you don't know. This is where you can go back to the **Priority Exemplars** or your other resources to continue to grow your mastered content.

> Use the online quizzing and testing resources to continue to hone your skills, identify what you don't know, and direct your studies and ongoing NCLEX®️ preparation!

So, let's get started!

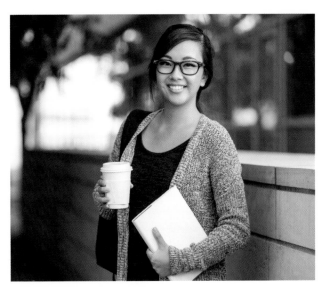

Image 4-2: How will you think positively and build your confidence?

Priority Exemplars

Sexuality

Reproduction / Sexuality

This chapter addresses pregnancy, labor, and delivery along with conditions that impair or interfere with sexuality and reproduction. Sexuality is a basic human trait and need. Reproduction is a routine process in which nurses support pregnancy, labor, and delivery.

Nurses play a significant role in teaching and supporting clients during the reproductive cycle and in conditions that interfere or impair reproduction or sexual functioning.

Study Hint: Remember, the birth process often needs little intervention. But nurses need to know their role when working with clients who need assistance!

Study Hint: (GTPAL)

> Gravida: # of pregnancies
> Term pregnancy: 37 weeks or greater
> Preterm pregnancy: 20 weeks to 36 6/7 weeks
> Abortion/miscarriage: Stillborn
> Living: Living at time of birth

Priority Exemplars:

> Hypertensive disorders of pregnancy
> Newborn care
> Contraception
> Erectile dysfunction
> Pregnancy
> Abortion/miscarriage
> Preterm labor
> Stages of labor
> Dystocia
> Placental abruption
> Placenta previa
> Postpartum hemorrhage
> Breastfeeding
> STI: Chlamydia
> STI: Human papillomavirus
> STI: Syphilis

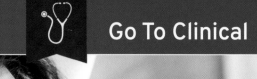

Go To Clinical

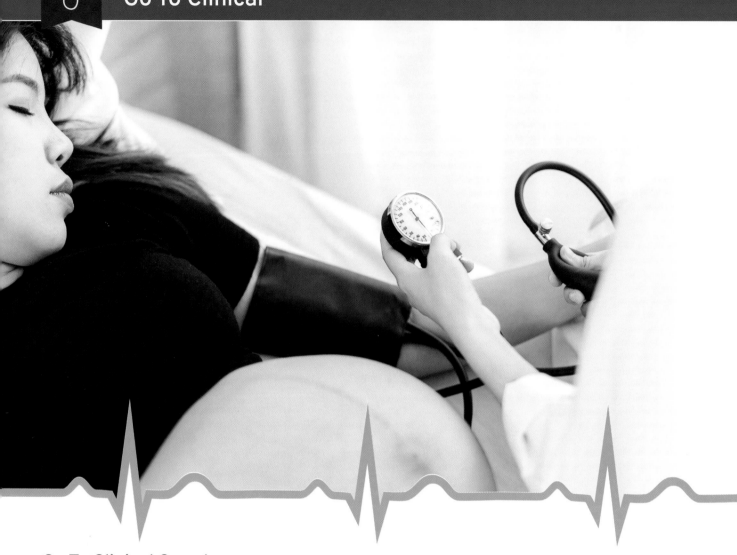

Go To Clinical Case 1

You are a registered nurse working in the emergency department. A client bursts into the triage area. The woman is noticeably pregnant and being supported by a man and the taxi driver that drove them to the agency. The woman reports that she is dizzy, seeing double, and has severe upper abdominal pain. You attempt to escort her to a wheelchair and the woman begins to have a seizure. She is incontinent of urine and is having rhythmic, tonic-clonic movements in her upper and lower extremities. The client is safely lowered to the floor and the seizure lasts 20 seconds.

The client is moved to a stretcher after the seizure and the client's vital signs are 99°F–120-22-166/122. Baseline blood pressure is not available. The client is sleepy but alert. The client is asking what happened and about her baby. The client is put on a fetal

monitor and the fetus's heart rate is strong at 130-140 bpm with good variation. She is not contracting at this time. Vaginal examination reveals that she is one fingertip dilated without effacement. The client states she is 8 months pregnant. She did not receive prenatal care because she newly immigrated to this country and does not have health insurance. She states her eyes and hands have been swollen and that she has been feeling very tired lately. The client is admitted to the high-risk pregnancy unit. Her partner is at her side.

NurseThink® Time

Using the NurseThink® system, complete the priorities. Check your answers designated by 💡 in the Hypertensive disorders of pregnancy Priority Exemplar.

NurseThink® Time

✎ Priority Assessments or Cues

1.

2.

3.

⚗ Priority Laboratory Tests/Diagnostics

1.

2.

3.

⚠ Priority Interventions or Actions

1.

2.

3.

⚑ Priority Potential & Actual Complications

1.

2.

3.

℧ Priority Nursing Implications

1.

2.

3.

◖ Priority Medications

1.

2.

3.

▣ Priority Education/Discharge Issues

1.

2.

3.

Hypertensive disorders of pregnancy

📋 Pathophysiology/Description

> Hypertension occurs in 5-10% of all pregnancies
  • Gestational hypertension is defined as increased blood pressure without proteinuria after 20 weeks gestation; BP >140/90 mmHg , 2 readings 4 hours apart, generally resolves within 12 weeks postpartum
  • Preeclampsia (pregnancy-induced hypertension—PIH) is hypertension after 20 weeks gestation, may or may not include proteinuria. Clients may have no previous history of hypertension and may occur postpartum. May include thrombocytopenia, liver dysfunction, renal insufficiency, pulmonary edema, and cerebral or visual changes
  • Eclampsia is seizures and/or coma not due to other causes
  • Chronic hypertension is when hypertension exists before pregnancy
  • Superimposed preeclampsia is chronic hypertension with preeclampsia

> Pathophysiology includes changes in placental perfusion, vasospasm, decreased liver and kidney perfusion, cerebral edema, central nervous system irritability

> Major cause of morbidity and mortality by uteroplacental insufficiency and preterm birth

> Risk factors include primipara, < 19 or > 40 years, preeclampsia in previous pregnancy, African American descent, multifetal gestation, maternal infection, preexisting chronic hypertension, renal disorders, diabetes mellitus, obesity, connective tissue disorders/systemic lupus erythematosus, chronic hypertension increases risk of eclampsia, pregnancy onset of snoring

> May be associated with HELLP defined as hemolysis, elevated liver enzymes, low platelets (may occur without blood pressure changes); diagnosed third trimester; often misdiagnosed; high rate of maternal death and poor perinatal outcomes

✏️ Priority Assessments or Cues

💡 Assess blood pressure, compare to baseline values. BP 30 mmHg over systolic or diastolic baseline are diagnostic for preeclampsia

💡 Ask about symptoms: Headache, epigastric pain, visual changes (scotoma, photophobia, double vision), dizziness

🧪 Priority Laboratory Tests/Diagnostics

💡 24-hour urine collection for protein most accurate assessment. Value > 300 mg in 24 hours contributes to diagnosis

💡 Urine dipstick of +1 also noted (may be less reliable)

💡 Platelets < 100,000/mm³

💡 Liver enzymes may be twice normal value

> Serum creatinine > 1.1 mg/dL or doubling of the normal serum creatine, prolonged creatinine clearance

⚠️ Priority Interventions or Actions

> Prevention for high-risk clients includes low dose aspirin therapy
> All clients: Monitor blood pressure and for seizures
> Maintain a restful and calming environment
> Preeclampsia
  • Monitor fetal and maternal health status—fetal monitoring
  • Assess for growth restriction
  • <37 weeks and a BP <160/110—mother and fetus are monitored and mother kept on bed rest
  • > 37 weeks—vaginal induction/cervical ripening
> Chronic hypertension/gestational hypertension
  • Administer medications to decrease blood pressure (Methyldopa—safest with breastfeeding)
> Eclampsia
  • Observe for warning symptoms-headache, blurred vision, epigastric/right upper quadrant pain, changes in level of consciousness
  💡 Seizures or convulsions
    💡 Stay with client/call for help
    💡 Assess fetal heart tones/heart rate patterns as able
    - Raise and pad side rails
    - Maintain a patent airway-turn and position, prevent aspiration
    - Assess pulse oximetry, oxygen by mask as able/needed
  💡 Assess blood pressure
    - Monitor and document seizure (tonic/clonic) and other signs
    - Obtain IV access with a large bore needle
    - Administer magnesium sulfate
    - Prepare for delivery as indicated
  • After seizure
    - Assess for hypotension, halted respirations, twitching, amnesia, post-ictal sleep, and potential for falls after sleep
    - Assess for stability
    - Assess fetal heart tones/uterine activity/cervical status
    - Prepare for delivery as indicated

Clinical Hint

Seizure precautions: Nurses often need to implement precautions to keep clients safe during a seizure. Precautions include: Raising side rails, padding side rails, having oxygen and suction at the bedside, ensure loose clothing, seizure record at the bedside.

⚑ Priority Potential & Actual Complications

- 💡 Severe hypertension
- 💡 Eclampsia
- ❯ Pulmonary edema
- 💡 Fetal demise/decline
- ❯ Placental abruption
- ❯ Disseminated intravascular coagulation (DIC)
- ❯ Stroke

℧ Priority Nursing Implications

- ❯ Assist the client in dealing with the stress of pregnancy and high-risk status, may feel guilt over lifestyle issues, negative outcomes, or fear related to outcomes
- 💡 Create a non-stimulating/low-stress environment—lower lights, maintain quiet, keep away from high activity on the unit or at home
- 💡 Assess for risk of seizures. Maintain seizure precautions including suction and oxygen at bedside, padded side rails, call button available
- 💡 Have emergency medication and emergency birth pack available

⬤ Priority Medications

- 💡 betamethasone
  - Steroid to mature fetal lungs in the event of an emergency or early delivery
  - Given IM every 24 hours times two
  - Works 24 hours after first dose for 7 days
- 💡 nifedipine
  - Calcium channel blocker/antihypertensive
  - To decrease blood pressure
  - Avoid with magnesium sulfate
  - May cause a headache, flushing of skin, may slow or interfere with labor
  - Must be delivered slowly
- ❯ methyldopa
  - Antihypertensive
  - To decrease blood pressure
  - Watch for CNS sedation
  - May cause drug-induced fever
  - Monitor fetal heart rate
- 💡 magnesium sulfate
  - Magnesium supplement/prevent seizures
  - IV piggyback via IV pump

- IM avoided due to pain or give with anesthetic
- Assess serum magnesium levels (toxic level will be greater than 4 mEq/L)
- Assess for magnesium toxicity/serum hypermagnesemia. Signs include absence of patellar deep tendon reflexes, decreased level of consciousness, low urine output, bradypnea, and cardiac dysrhythmias
- Antidote for hypermagnesemia is calcium gluconate
- May be given for 24-48 hours postpartum

👤 Priority Education/Discharge Issues

- ❯ Home management for hypertension (BP > 150/100) as long as no protein in urine, normal platelets, normal liver enzymes
  - 💡 Teach about BP and urine monitoring
  - 💡 When to call MD, symptoms to report, and routine appointments
  - 💡 Tracking of fetal activity by assessing daily fetal movement count-kick counts
  - Maintain partial bed rest, means to avoid venous thrombosis, and types of gentle exercise
  - Diversional activities, maintaining calm, and stress management
  - Encourage side-lying position
  - Diet should be regular with increased water and fiber, decreased caffeine, decreased sodium, and no tobacco or alcohol
- ❯ Provide education about blood pressure management and lifestyle patterns that may contribute to preeclampsia, chronic/gestational/superimposed hypertension, and eclampsia

Go To Clinical Answers

Text designated by 💡 are the top answers for the Go To Clinical related to Hypertensive disorders of pregnancy.

Next Gen Clinical Judgment

When studying hypertensive disorders, it often helps for you to pause and create a set of vitals that would be consistent for a given scenario. Try to create a set of vitals for a client struggling with pregnancy-induced hypertension (PIH). Then watch the Concepts at Work: Sexuality video in the online resources. How did you do?
📀 Nursethink.com/NCLEX-RN-book/

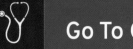
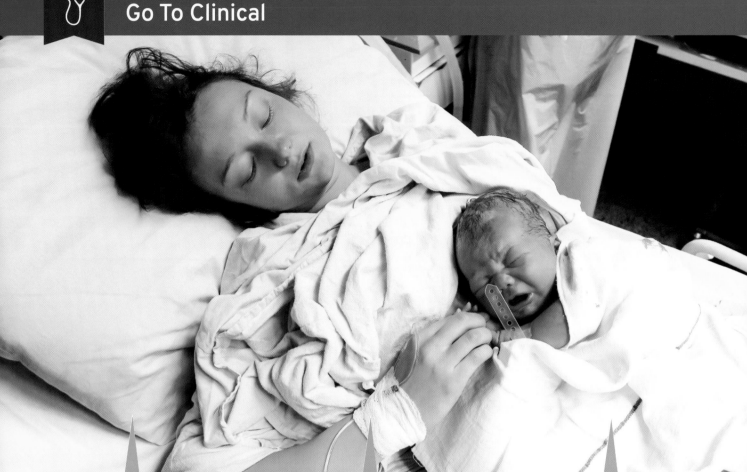

Go To Clinical Case 2

A 38-year-old woman enters triage indicating that she is 39 weeks pregnant and has been in labor for several hours. This is her fourth child and, when examined, she is 8 cm dilated and 100% effaced.

While completing the admission interview, the mother exclaims that "I have to push, the baby is coming." When she is transferred to a stretcher the baby is crowning and the baby is delivered rapidly.

Some meconium is noted in the amniotic fluid. The baby is placed on the woman's abdomen and the woman/infant are rushed to the labor/delivery/postpartum room.

The nurse anticipates the newborn's needs based on this precipitous delivery. The baby boy is 7 lb. 12 oz. and is 21 inches long. The child's APGAR is 7 at one minute, 9 at five minutes (acrocyanosis persists). The client's vital signs are 95.2°F—152-48-82/40. The infant's respirations are rapid and shallow, with some crackles and excessive mucus noted. The infant is noted to have tremoring of hands, arms, and legs. The mother plans to breastfeed and is Rh negative. Her husband, who is the father of all her children, is Rh positive. The nurse plans the care of the newborn.

NurseThink® Time

Using the NurseThink® system, complete the priorities. Check your answers designated by 💡 in the Newborn care Priority Exemplar.

✏ Priority Assessments or Cues

1.

2.

3.

⚗ Priority Laboratory Tests/Diagnostics

1.

2.

3.

⚠ Priority Interventions or Actions

1.

2.

3.

⚑ Priority Potential & Actual Complications

1.

2.

3.

⚕ Priority Nursing Implications

1.

2.

3.

⬤ Priority Medications

1.

2.

3.

👤 Priority Education/Discharge Issues

1.

2.

3.

Newborn care

Pathophysiology/Description

> Newborn/neonatal period is initial birth to one month of age
> Care of the newborn includes assessments and assisting with adaptation to extrauterine environment

Priority Assessments or Cues

- Assess for spontaneous respirations and describe cry (lusty, high-pitched, weak)
- Assess APGAR score is a 10 point scale, each of 5 criteria given a 0, 1, or 2—at 1 and 5 minutes (10 minutes if score indicates)
  - Heart rate
  - Respiratory rate and effort
  - Muscle tone
  - Reflex irritability
  - Skin color
- Assess general appearance including respiratory effort and for signs of distress, overt anomalies or trauma, level of alertness
> Assess vital signs(axillary temperature), body weight, length, and head circumference
> Initiate or observe Ballard scale for gestational assessment based on neuromuscular maturity (posture, range of motion, recoil, limberness) and physical maturity (breast, genitalia, palmar wrinkling, lanugo, ear mobility, eye opening)
> Assess periods of reactivity at birth to 30 minutes and 2 to 8 hours after birth (between a period of decreased responsiveness/sleep)
> Initial physical assessment
  - Assess head—sutures, fontanels, molding, masses (caput succedaneum, cephalohematoma), subgaleal hemorrhage
  - Eyes—symmetry, pupils, tracking
  - Ears—symmetry, height compared to eyes
  - Mouth—intactness of soft and hard palates, tongue (connection), ability to suck/gag/swallow
  - Neck—range of motion, midline, torticollis (contraction of one side)
  - Chest—respiratory effort, adaptation to extrauterine environment, patency of nares (newborns breathe mostly through the nose), coughing and sneezing to clear airway, symmetry of thorax/barrel chest, nipples, clavicles for fractures; infant heart sounds
  - Skin—vernix caseosa (cheese-like substance), lanugo (downy hair), milia (small pustules), peeling skin, skin turgor, color (central cyanosis, acrocyanosis, plethoric [deep red color]), lesions, bruising, petechiae, birthmarks Mongolian spots, nevus vasculosus [strawberry mark], nevus flammeus [port-wine stain], telangiectatic nevi [stork bites], forceps or vacuum marks, Harlequin's sign (transient unilateral erythema of newborn, usually benign)

> Assess for jaundice/bilirubin (normal < 5.2 mg/dL)
  - Physiological in 60% of newborns
  - Pathological appears within the first 24 hours and requires treatment, if untreated-leads to kernicterus/ acute encephalopathy
  - Breastfeeding 2-5 days, related to low milk supply, encourage frequent feeding
  - Breastmilk 5-10 days
  - Measured by transcutaneous bilirubinometers/serum levels
  - Treatment with phototherapy beds or lights (values at which treatment is initiated vary)
> Abdomen—assess umbilical cord (3 vessels—2 arteries, one vein), bleeding, cord site for infection, umbilical hernia, symmetry, bowel sounds, distention
> Genital/Anus—assess patency of anus, labia (pseudomenstruation, smegma), penis/scrotum: placement of meatus (hypospadius, epispadius), for hernia, descent of testes, for void of urine in first 24 hours (uric acid crystals may produce a rust colored urine), for meconium (black/ green jelly-like pasty stool)
> Spine—assess tone (hypotonicity/hypertonicity), hair tufts or dimples, neonates should have some head control, movement of all extremities
> Hips—for developmental dysplasia of the hip (no clicks when abducting hips)
> Assess for hypoglycemia—jitteriness, tremors—treat/ prevent with early feeding
> Reflexes
  - Sucking/rooting
  - Swallowing
  - Tonic neck/fencing
  - Palmar/plantar grasp
  - Moro
  - Startle
  - Pull-to-sit response
  - Babinski
  - Stepping/walking
  - Crawling

Priority Laboratory Tests/Diagnostics

> Audiometry screening
> CBC-hemoglobin/hematocrit
- Serum glucose level
> Serum bilirubin/correlate with transcutaneous bilirubinometer
- Arterial blood gases (if warranted)
> Universal newborn screening
  - Varies based on region and state law
  - Many include screening for sickle cell anemia, phenylketonuria, galactosemia, severe combined immunodeficiency—heel sticks
  - Critical congenital heart disease screen-via pulse oximetry
- Culture if infections are suspected

⚠ Priority Interventions or Actions

- 💡 Results of APGAR if 8-10 (no intervention, supportive care), 4-7 (stimulate the infant, backrub, provide oxygen), 0-3 (full resuscitation)

- 💡 Suction mouth and then nares with bulb syringe

- 💡 Dry, stimulate, and wrap infant, place cap on head (need to maintain/support thermoregulation—avoid cold stress due to lack of brown fat—infants generate heat via non-shivering thermogenesis)

- ❯ Avoid hyperthermia because of neonates' immature sweat gland function

- ❯ Initiate skin-to-skin contact or breastfeeding as soon as feasible, if not feasible, place infant in a radiant warmer

- ❯ Encourage parental bonding

- ❯ Follow agency policy for identification-wrist/ankle bands, foot and hand printing, matching ID bands

⚑ Priority Potential & Actual Complications

- ❯ Respiratory distress syndrome
- 💡 Meconium aspiration syndrome
- ❯ Bronchopulmonary dysplasia
- ❯ Intraventricular hemorrhage
- ❯ Retinopathy of prematurity
- ❯ Necrotizing enterocolitis
- ❯ Hyperbilirubinemia
- ❯ Erythroblastosis fetalis
- ❯ Fetal alcohol spectrum disorders
- ❯ Addiction/neonatal abstinence syndrome
- ❯ Vertical transmission of HIV
- 💡 Hypoglycemia
- 💡 Transient tachypnea of the newborn

℧ Priority Nursing Implications

- 💡 In cases of infant or maternal change in condition, nurses provide support to partners, support persons, and mothers

- 💡 Ensure infant safety and identify, protection from abduction

- ❯ Gestational age including assess preterm (before 37 weeks), small for gestational age, large for gestational age

- 💡 Support early attachment, skin-to-skin (use overbed warmer as needed) contact, and feeding (breast or bottle)

- ❯ Support parents' choice related to circumcision

🩸 Priority Medications

- 💡 phytonadione
  - Vitamin K injection IM vastus lateralis injected in the delivery room
  - Sterile gut of the newborn-bacteria does not produce coagulants

- 💡 hepatitis B vaccine
  - Given IM prior to newborn discharge
  - If mother is Hep B antigen positive, administer hepatitis B immune globulin within 12 hours of birth along with immunization. Provide injections in separate thighs
  - Document on immunization record, obtain parental consent

- 💡 erythromycin
  - Eye prophylaxis
  - Prevent ophthalmia neonatorum-gonorrhea/chlamydia (not as effective treating chlamydia—treated with oral erythromycin)
  - Allow bonding before ointments
  - Required by law

👤 Priority Education/Discharge Issues

- 💡 Teach parents about cord care-check agency protocol for cleaning, antibiotics for infection

- ❯ Teach parents how to manage circumcision or care of uncircumcised penis

- 💡 Teach parents about preferred method of feeding either formula or breastfeeding

- ❯ Teach parents infant care including bathing, dressing, nail care, diaper changes, consoling infant, bonding, infant stimulation

- ❯ Discuss maternal and infant return to healthcare providers

- ❯ Teach about infant behaviors including consolability, cuddliness, irritability, crying, use of non-nutritive sucking (pacifiers), and cues

- 💡 Teach infant safety including car seats, safe sleep ("back-to-sleep," in own bed, without stuffed animals or pads, "tummy time" to prevent plagiocephaly (abnormal head shape), holding and carrying, cardiopulmonary resuscitation and management of airway obstruction

- ❯ Teach parents to bathe infant in warm water (test with elbow), dress infant appropriate for weather, and to avoid actions that cause hyper/hypothermia.

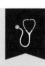

Go To Clinical Answers

Text designated by 💡 are the top answers for the Go To Clinical related to Newborn care.

Contraception

Pathophysiology/Description

> Many contraceptive methods are available to clients who choose to prevent or delay childbearing. Cultural, religious, and personal preferences will influence method choice

> Methods are largely described as barrier methods (may be used by women and men) and hormonal methods (largely used by women)

> Contraceptive methods vary in effectiveness, cost, reversibility, effort needed, and use of hormones

> Contraceptive methods require varying levels of capacity for adherence to a schedule, association with sexual activity, participation of sexual partners, ability for discretion, and comfort with body

> Male and female condoms, along with the use of barrier dental dams, are able to prevent exposure to sexually transmitted infections

> Cost may be a factor for some clients

> Hormonal contraceptives may be indicated to treat menstrual irregularities

Priority Assessments or Cues

> Assess blood pressure (hormonal methods are contraindicated/used cautiously with hypertension). Assess blood pressure frequently while on hormonal birth control

> Assess client's weight (some methods contraindicated with obesity)

> Assess desire to prevent pregnancy, level of motivation, and knowledge level

> Assess health status and presence of pre-existing conditions, including thromboembolic disease, history of estrogen feeding cancers, hypertension, cardiac disease, and pregnancy, that contraindicate some hormonal contraceptives

> Assess woman's lifestyle, habits, and risk behaviors, including tobacco smoking and multiple sexual partners

> Assess client's current medications (antibiotics may decrease the effectiveness of oral contraceptives, hormonal methods may interact with anticoagulants)

Priority Laboratory Tests/Diagnostics

> Screen for sexually transmitted infections based on age, symptoms, risk factors, and sexual history

Priority Interventions or Actions

> Many healthcare providers now prescribe oral and injectable contraception without a vaginal examination, but clients are encouraged to have routine screenings, including clinical breast examinations, based on age, health history, and risk factors

> Nursing interventions with contraception focus on teaching about self-administration, side effects, adverse reactions, and when to consult healthcare providers

Priority Potential & Actual Complications

> Clients with a latex allergy may react to latex condoms

> Complications differ based on method (intrauterine devices complications may include ectopic pregnancy, uterine perforation) and implanted contraceptive rods may migrate

> Complications differ based on client health history (oral contraceptives may increase blood glucose levels in clients with type 1 diabetes)

> Non-barrier methods increase the risk for sexually transmitted infections

Priority Nursing Implications

> Nurses need to ensure that contraceptive methods match the client's needs and that the client is able to safely adhere to the method or medication regimen

> Assist client to develop methods for reminders (phone alarm for daily pills, calendar for injection every 3 months, etc.)

> Need to ensure client's knowledge of, comfort level with, and ability to access a birth control method

> Ensure that the method's effectiveness coincides with client's desire to prevent pregnancy and sexually transmitted infections

> Encourage clients using hormonal methods to wear condoms with all sexual activity

> Assess each client for potential birth control sabotage, reproductive coercion, or intimate partner violence

Priority Education/Discharge Issues

> Ensure that clients are aware that they need to use back up contraception during initial period of starting contraception

> Teach clients what to do if a pill or injection is missed (depends upon method) and to use backup method of contraception until birth control levels are re-established

> Teach client to conduct self-breast exams monthly

> Make sure clients are aware of need to have blood pressure assessed and for follow-up

> Instruct client on method-specific recommendations related to cessation of method if they desire to become pregnant (for example, the client is recommended to be off of oral contraceptives for one to two months prior to attempting to become pregnant)

Next Gen Clinical Judgment

Helping clients may be about helping them find resources. Find an app on your phone that you would recommend to a client needing resources related to contraception.

Erectile dysfunction (ED)

Pathophysiology/Description

> Inability to attain and/or sustain an erection to engage in satisfying sexual activity

> More than 10 million men affected, 50% of men 40-70 years have some level of ED

> Lack of blood flow (vascular impairment) associated with ED

> May be from primary or secondary causations including recreational drug use, alcohol use, smoking, illnesses, or medications (antihypertensives, antilipemics, sedatives, others)

> Causes may also include vascular (hypertension, peripheral vascular disease), endocrine (diabetes, obesity, reduced testosterone level), genitourinary (prostatitis, renal failure, history of a radical prostatectomy), neurological (Parkinson's, stroke, trauma/spinal cord injury, tumors), psychological (depression, stress, fear/anxiety)

> May occur at any age, more prevalent as men age

Priority Assessments or Cues

> Ask client about ability to attain and sustain an erection

> Ask about frequency and onset and may be episodic, may be gradual onset (illness/medications), or may occur suddenly (fear, anxiety, or emotionally related)

> Ask about emotional impact of ED on intimate relationships

> Conduct a thorough medical, sexual, and psychosocial assessment; screening may include erectile function, orgasmic function, sexual desire, intercourse satisfaction, and overall satisfaction with sexual experiences

> Assess genitalia for lesions, masses, changes in structure

Priority Laboratory Tests/Diagnostics

> Medical history profile to include serum glucose, lipid profile, complete blood count

> Hormone levels (testosterone, prolactin, luteinizing hormone, thyroid hormone)

> Prostate specific antigen levels

> Non-invasive testing include nocturnal penile tumescence/ rigidity testing, penile blood flow/angiography, and ultrasound

Priority Interventions or Actions

> Address causative factors that are modifiable-change medications, manage illnesses, counseling
> Medications are the most common treatment
> Vacuum constriction device (VCD)
> Penile implants
> Intraurethral medication pellets
> Intracavernosal self-injection
> Sexual counseling

Priority Potential & Actual Complications

> Sexual dysfunction

> Impaired relationships

> Mental health issues-stress, depression

> Use of erectogenics with nitrates may cause hemodynamically significant hypotension/bradycardia, cardiopulmonary arrest

Priority Nursing Implications

> Ensure that clients have realistic expectations of treatment—if sensation or function were absent, ejaculation or tactile sensation may not be resumed

> Ensure client safety related to hypotension/dizziness with first doses of medication

> Ask all clients with chest pain about use of erectogenic medications

Priority Medications

> sildenafil/ tadalafil/ vardenafil

- Relaxes smooth muscle and increases blood flow/ erectogenic
- Take 30-60 minutes before anticipate intercourse
- Do not take more than once per day
- Potentiates hypotension with nitrates—should not be used with nitroglycerin
- Side effects include headache, flushing, GI upset, and nasal congestion
- Tadalafil may be safer with clients with cardiac history
- All erectogenic drugs may cause priapism (sustained erection for 4 hours or more) and require medical attention
- Alcohol should be avoided—increases hypotension

Priority Education/Discharge Issues

> Safe administration and use of erectogenic medications
> Refer clients for assistance with sexual communication with partners and counseling for clients and partners

Clinical Hint

Reinforce safety precautions—Do not take erectogenic drugs more than once per day, stay with prescribed dose, and do not take with nitrates.

Pregnancy

Pathophysiology/Description

> Described as gestation (approximately 280 days) from fertilization to implantation to birth

> Nagele's rule—subtract 3 months and add seven days to the first day of the last menstrual period—add one year-yields date of delivery

Priority Assessments or Cues

> Pregnancy outcomes terminology
  - Gravidity—number of pregnancies (nulligravida-no pregnancies, multigravida-two or more pregnancies)
  - Parity—numbers of births (nullipara, primipara, multipara)
  - GTPAL—gravidity, term births, preterm births, abortions/miscarriages, living children

> Signs of pregnancy
  - Presumptive—amenorrhea, nausea/vomiting, breast changes, urinary frequency, quickening, fatigue, change in color of vaginal mucosa
  - Probable—uterine enlargement, Hegar's sign (softening of uterine segment), Goodell's sign (softening of cervix), Chadwick's sign (violet discoloration of the cervix), Ballottement (rebounding of uterus when fetus is unengaged), Braxton Hicks contractions, positive hCG
  - Positive—fetal heart tones, fetal movements, ultrasound confirmation

> Fundal height
  - From 18-30 weeks, fundal height = gestational age

> Maternal physical changes
  - Increase in circulating blood volume, physiological anemia of pregnancy, retention of sodium/water
  - Nausea and vomiting, constipation
  - Urinary frequency
  - Skin changes—linea nigra (dark line down abdomen), melasma (mask of pregnancy), striae gravidarum (stretch marks), vascular spider nevi, palmar erythema pruritis gravidarum
  - Increased lordosis, relaxed muscle tone, posture changes, carpal tunnel syndrome, tingling of hands and feet, diastasis recti abdominis (separation of abdominal muscles), syncope
  - Emotional changes—ambivalence, acceptance, emotional lability, body image changes, preparing emotionally for motherhood

> Assess the mother's history
  - Chronic or acute illness/disease and current health status (hypertension, diabetes, cardiac disease, asthma, rubella, other infections: STIs and HIV)
  - Assess family history
  - Assess reproductive history

- Assess history of or risk for intimate partner violence
- Assess for substance use or abuse/cigarette smoking
- Assess risk associated with age (< 18 years, > 35 years)
- Ask about genetic issues
- Assess nutritional history
- Assess use of medications, herbal therapies, and complementary/alternative therapies

Priority Laboratory Tests/Diagnostics

> Pregnancy test for human chorionic gonadotropin (hCG)-appears 8-10 days after conception-via blood, urine, or home urine testing (variations in accuracy of home tests)

> Blood type and Rh factor

> Rubella titer

> Hemoglobin/hematocrit/complete blood count

> Pap smear

> Cultures for STIs (gonorrhea, syphilis, HPV, Chlamydia, trichomoniasis, herpes simplex, HIV)

> Sickle cell screening as indicated

> Tuberculosis screening

> Hepatitis B titer

> Urinalysis and urine culture

> Ultrasounds—gestational age, fetal outlines, amniotic fluid volume, multiple fetuses (abdominal or transvaginal)

> Biophysical profile—assess fetal breathing movements, fetal movements, fetal tone, amniotic fluid volume, and fetal heart patterns

> Doppler blood flow analysis—blood flow in fetus, umbilical cord, and placenta

> Percutaneous umbilical blood sampling—needle aspiration of blood guided by ultrasound

> Alpha-fetoprotein screening—assesses for spina bifida and Down syndrome

> Lecithin-sphingomyelin (L/S ratio)—maturity of fetus

> DNA testing—assess for genetic abnormalities

> Chorionic villi sampling—assess for genetic abnormalities via villi in chorion

> Amniocentesis—aspiration of fluid between 15 and 20 weeks

> Kick counts—fetal movement counting and recording

> Fern test—microscopic slide test to ascertain if vaginal leakage is amniotic fluid

> Nitrazine test—assess pH of vaginal secretions—amniotic fluid is 7.0-7.5; vaginal secretions are 4.5-5.5

> Fetal-Fibronectin-cervical swab, assesses risk for preterm labor

> Non-stress test—for fetal well-being, assesses changes in heart rate as related to fetal movement

> Contraction stress test—for fetal well-being, assesses changes in heart rate as related contractions or simulated contractions

> Group B streptococcus—vaginal and rectal cultures at 35-37 weeks gestation

⚠ Priority Interventions or Actions

> Establish healthcare provider visit schedule—every 4 weeks until 32 weeks, every 2 weeks until 36 weeks, every week until delivery

> Nausea and vomiting—most in first trimester, elevated hCG levels, eat dry crackers, small/frequent meals, drinking liquids apart from meals, if unmanageable-hyperemesis gravidarum-treated with IV fluids or total parenteral nutrition (antiemetics with caution)

> Supine hypotension—side sleeping and caution during examination, change positions slowly, ensure safety

> Breast discomfort—wear a supportive bra, wash nipples carefully

> Fatigue/backache—rest periods, regular exercise, yoga, optimal hydration and nutrition

> Heartburn—tailor sitting, upright after meals, small/frequent meals

> Ankle edema—elevate legs, supportive hose, ankle exercises, sleep on side

> Varicose veins—supportive hose, elevate legs, move/exercise often

> Headaches—drink water, change positions slowly, snacks, cool cloth

> Hemorrhoids/constipation—sitz baths, high fiber foods/water, exercise

> Leg cramps—increase calcium intake, regular exercise, dorsiflex foot

> Shortness of breath—rest, sleep with HOB elevated, pace activities

> Pica—eating non-food substances, may result in anemia, nutrition counseling

> Anemia—ensure prenatal vitamins and, if prescribed, iron supplementation, take with vitamin C, nutrition counseling

⚑ Priority Potential & Actual Complications

> Hypertensive disorders/gestational hypertension
> Abortion/miscarriage/fetal demise
> Gestational diabetes and DIC
> Infection-TORCH-assess and manage
  • Toxoplasmosis
  • Other infections: HIV, HBV, STIs, Group B strep, pyelonephritis, UTI, tuberculosis
  • Rubella
  • Cytomegalovirus
  • Herpes simplex
> Ectopic pregnancy is implantation outside of uterus
> Hydatidiform mole is peripheral cells of fertilized ovum proliferate, may be benign or malignant-must be vacuum extracted, pregnancy not recommended for one year
> Incompetent cervix is treated with cervical cerclage

⚕ Priority Nursing Implications

> Nurses provide a key role in educating, counseling, and offering support to women during pregnancy

> Nurses may provide sexuality counseling. Pregnancy does not limit intercourse but may require position or activity changes, pregnant women may have decreased desire or body image changes that warrant teaching and discussion

> Pregnancy can offer challenges for women who are obese with complications in pregnancy, delivery, post-delivery

> Assess and intervene related to the emotional tasks of pregnancy including transitioning to motherhood/parenthood/fatherhood, changes in family dynamics, and dealing with body image changes

> Attend to needs of non-pregnant partners/co-mothers

> Assess and intervene with extended family adaptation including siblings, grandparents, etc.

> Counsel mothers that the expected weight gain in pregnancy is 25-35 pounds, increase to 300 kcal/day during pregnancy (may be based on pre-pregnancy BMI)

💧 Priority Medications

> Prenatal vitamins
  • High iron may cause constipation
  • High in folic acid (preconceptual and prenatal recommended to prevent neural tube defects)
  • Taken throughout pregnancy and breastfeeding

👤 Priority Education/Discharge Issues

> Provide education about the importance of nutrition and hydration during pregnancy—instruct to avoid high mercury fish (swordfish, tuna), raw or undercooked fish and meat (sushi), cold cuts, soft cheeses, raw eggs, uncooked batter (avoid salmonella, listeria)

> Provide instruction on expected physical and emotional changes of pregnancy, anticipatory guidance for pregnancy, labor, and delivery

> Teach about the prevention of urinary tract infections including fluid intake, frequent emptying of bladder, cranberry juice or capsules, Kegel exercises, hygiene

> Ensure attention to dental health including cleaning, examinations, and treatment, gingival health

> Explore birth plan and potential alternatives with client and family including care givers (physician, midwife, doula) and setting (hospital, birth center, home)

> Encourage exercise as tolerated. Mothers may continue exercises that they were accustomed to until later in pregnancy, not time to start a new exercise regimen; stop exercise if feel shortness of breath, dizzy, numbness, contractions, or vaginal bleeding

> Counsel client on avoidance of alcohol, unprescribed medications, cigarettes, and caffeine

Abortion/miscarriage

📋 Pathophysiology/Description

> Spontaneous loss of products of conception prior to period of viability, defined as before 20 weeks gestation (also called miscarriage)

> About 10-15% of pregnancies end in miscarriage, 80% before 12 weeks

> Spontaneous abortions in the first 12 weeks are thought to be related to chromosomal abnormalities, endocrine/thyroid deficiencies, varicella exposure/contraction, genetic factors, type 1 diabetes, systemic conditions (lupus)

> Spontaneous abortions 12-20 weeks (second trimester loss) are more common in mothers <18 or >40 years or with poor outcomes from previous pregnancies, or related to diet, obesity, alcohol/caffeine consumption

> Differentiated as:

- Induced—therapeutic or elective ending of pregnancy

- Spontaneous—occurring by natural causes

- Threatened—spotting or cramping without cervical changes

- Inevitable—spotting or cramping and cervix begins to dilate and efface

- Incomplete—loss of some products of conception, some (usually the placenta) is retained

- Complete—loss of all products of conception

- Missed—products of conception retained in the uterus after fetal demise

- Recurrent/habitual—3 or more pregnancy losses at < 20 weeks gestation in successive pregnancies

- Septic—spontaneous abortion with infected products of conception

✏️ Priority Assessments or Cues

> Assess vital signs—focusing on heart rate and blood pressure/related to blood loss

> Assess for bleeding—history, amount, pad count, clots, tissue

> Assess pain—cramping, lower abdominal pain

> Assess woman's emotional state, support systems, coping abilities, screen for depression

🧪 Priority Laboratory Tests/Diagnostics

> Pregnancy test—hCG—human chorionic gonadotropin to confirm pregnancy/maintained pregnancy along with progesterone levels

> Complete blood count-assess hemoglobin and hematocrit following blood loss and to assess for infection

> Ultrasound (abdominal or transvaginal) of uterus to detect contents

> Genetic evaluation of clients with recurrent miscarriages

⚠️ Priority Interventions or Actions

> Maintain bedrest

> Monitor for bleeding including patterns, amount, pad count, clot count, weigh pads as per agency policy

> Monitor cramps

> Assess for hemorrhage

> If inpatient, save tissue and clots for healthcare provider observation and to allow mother the option of viewing remains

> Ensure IV access, administer prescribed fluids and blood products

> Prepare for dilation and curettage/suction curettage if suspected to be an incomplete abortion

> Administer Rho (D) immune globulin if client is Rh negative

> Prophylactic cerclage of the cervix may be done if cause is cervical insufficiency

🚩 Priority Potential & Actual Complications

> Incomplete abortions without procedure include infection, sepsis

> Emotional and relational implications include depression and anxiety

🩺 Priority Nursing Implications

> Clients often report that at less than six weeks pregnancy, the miscarriage may feel like a period. From 6-12 weeks clients report some discomfort along with more substantial blood loss. Greater than 12 weeks, clients usually report severe pain/cramping along with substantial blood loss

> Assess for risk factors and assist with potential identification of future prevention efforts

> Provide emotional support and assist with potential guilt, depression, and anger felt by the client

💧 Priority Medications

> misoprostol
- To medically ensure complete miscarriage if incomplete
- Side effects include nausea, vomiting, diarrhea

> oxytocin
- Administered post-curettage to prevent hemorrhage

👤 Priority Education/Discharge Issues

> Encourage rest after miscarriage

> Avoid tampons, sexual intercourse, or douching for two weeks

> Ensure follow-up with healthcare provider for birth control, timing of subsequent pregnancies, and importance of prenatal care

> Refer for potential underlying health issues

> Ensure emotional needs of client and family are addressed to support groups and/or counseling

Preterm labor

Pathophysiology/Description

> Labor that occurs after the 20th week but before the 37th week

> Risk factors include history of ongoing or chronic medical conditions, substance use, lack of prenatal care, infection, social and environmental factors, previous preterm labor or other obstetrical complications, multiparity and overdistention of the uterus, anemia, age younger than 18 or over 40 years

Priority Assessments or Cues

> Assess risk factors for preterm labor

> Assess gestational age of infant

> Assess uterine contractions (painful or painless)

> Assess for abdominal cramping, low back pain, pelvic pain or heavy feeling, discharge (color, consistency, odor, presence of blood)

> Assess for intactness of membranes

> Assess for presence of fetal fibronectin in vaginal canal

> Assess shape and dilation of cervix

Priority Laboratory Tests/Diagnostics

> Urine culture and sensitivity

> Monitor blood glucose levels

> Monitor complete blood count including WBC

> Ultrasound for fetal position and cervical shape

> Fetal fibronectin (via vaginal swab) associated with placental inflammation/collect specimen before lubricant

Priority Interventions or Actions

> Focus on ceasing contractions

> Treat infections with antibiotics

> Hydrate via oral and intravenous routes

> Maintain bed rest in lateral position

> Provide for continuous fetal monitoring

> Provide steroids to mature fetal lungs

> Provide antibiotics if septic abortion

Priority Potential & Actual Complications

> Issues associated with infant prematurity

> Precipitous delivery

> Postpartum hemorrhage

> Fetal demise

Priority Nursing Implications

> Support the mother during the stress associated with preterm labor

> Carefully assess fetal monitoring and infant responses to or impact of preterm labor

Priority Medications

> magnesium sulfate
  - Relaxes smooth muscles and halts preterm labor, prevents preterm birth
  - Assess for respiratory depression and depressed deep tendon reflexes
  - Monitor magnesium levels
  - Should be administered via infusion pump
  - Have calcium gluconate available-antidote
  - Monitor urine output throughout infusion

> nifedipine
  - Relaxes smooth muscles, including the uterus
  - Watch for maternal hypotension, dizziness, headache, facial flushing, fatigue, nausea, nervousness, tachycardia
  - Do not use with magnesium sulfate

> betamethasone
  - Increases production of surfactant to accelerate fetal lung maturity
  - Watch for hyperglycemia and maternal immunosuppression
  - Administer deep intramuscular injection

> 17 alpha hydroxyprogesterone caproate
  - Intramuscular injections to prevent preterm labor

> terbutaline
  - SQ injection
  - Relaxes smooth muscle
  - Duration of not more than 24 hours
  - Contraindicated with cardiac disease, hypertension, hyperthyroid, or hemorrhage

> Antibiotics may be indicated with septic abortions

Priority Education/Discharge Issues

> Provide support and information about course of labor and birth

> Provide support for infants who are in a NICU due to prematurity

> Encourage maternal and family bonding, breastfeeding, and infant care to support a thriving newborn

> If labor is stopped, provide client with guidelines on bedrest, pelvic rest (no sexual intercourse/vaginal exams/douching), tocolytics, hydration, emptying bladder frequently, and parameters for calling/returning to healthcare provider

> Notify healthcare provider of heavy, bright red vaginal bleeding, elevated temperature, or foul-smelling vaginal drainage

Stages of labor

Pathophysiology/Description

> Process of moving fetus, placenta, and membranes out of the uterus and through the birth canal

> Onset of labor
  - Increased estrogen and decreasing progesterone, increased uterine pressure and distention
  - Mechanisms not completely understood
  - Beginning of contractions, effacement/dilation, and descent

> Mechanisms of labor
  - Powers-contractions, pushing, or bearing down
  - Passage
  - Passenger
    - Attitude-flexion, extension
    - Lie-longitudinal or transverse
    - Presentation-cephalic/vertex, breech, shoulder, brow
    - Position-presenting part as compared to maternal pelvis
    - Station-0 at ischial spine (engagement), negative (above), positive (below)
  - Position-mother's position/activity
  - Psychological-fear, anxiety, etc.

Priority Assessments or Cues

> Assessments preceding labor
  - Ask about lightening (dropping of infant into the true pelvis) client will feel less pressure on rib cage, and more pressure on bladder
  - May experience low backache or Braxton Hicks contractions
  - Increase in vaginal mucus ("bloody show")
  - Weight loss
  - Increase of energy ("nesting")
  - Rupture of membranes (TACO-Time, amount,color, odor)
  - Diarrhea
  - Differentiate true and false/prodromal labor

> Assessments of first stage of labor
  - Onset of labor to full dilation and effacement
  - Longest stage—usually occurs before mother seeks healthcare
  - Latent phase (0-3 cm cervical dilation)
  - Active phase (4-7 cm cervical dilation)
    - Usually indicates entry to the clinical agency
    - Seek out client history-prenatal data, screening assessment, vital signs, general review of systems, abdominal palpation, vaginal examination, support systems/birth coaches, preparedness for labor
  - Transition phase (may not be identified with epidural anesthesia)-(8-10 cm cervical dilation) dilation & descent
  - Pain during contractions/relief between/low back pain with posterior position

> Assessments of second stage
  - Full dilation to birth
  - Latent-passive fetal descent and rotation to anterior position
    - Processes include: Engagement, descent, flexion, internal rotation, extension, restitution, external rotation, and expulsion
  - Active-pushing and bearing down; strong urge to push and provide pressure on stretch receptors in the pelvic floor
    - Assist mother into position/assess position of comfort
    - Observe for crowning
    - Assist with delivery and assess status of mother and fetus/infant
  - Most intense pain level-abdominal and pelvic
  - Observe for shaking extremities, vomiting, restlessness, increase in bloody show

> Assessments of third stage
  - After birth of the fetus to the delivery of the placenta
  - Placenta separates and is delivered 3-4 contractions after birth of infant
  - Pain in perineal area and uterus

> Assessments of fourth stage
  - After delivery of placenta to 2 hours after birth
  - Provide skin-to-skin time with infant (Kangaroo care) bonding/breastfeeding
  - Physical recovery from delivery
  - Provide supplies for episiotomy/repairs as needed
  - Provide newborn care and assessment
  - Assess for bleeding/hemorrhage and risk factors for postpartum bleeding
  - Assess lochia (red, pink-brown, yellow-white)/involution of the uterus

> Assessments throughout the labor process
  - Fetal adaptation
    - Fetal heart rate
    - Fetal circulation (pressure on umbilical cord, impact of contractions)
    - Fetal respiration (preparing for and adapting to extrauterine environment)
  - Maternal adaptation
    - Circulatory (increases in cardiac output, supine hypotension, flushing, hemorrhoid protrusion, hot or cold feet)
    - Respiratory (tachypnea, increased oxygen consumption, potential for hyperventilation)
    - Renal (difficulty voiding, proteinuria)
    - Tearing around the vaginal opening
    - Muscle cramping
    - Diarrhea
    - Nausea/vomiting
    - Low blood glucose levels
  - Assess maternal comfort and the many factors that impact pain perception-anxiety, culture, previous experiences, and support

- › Fetal monitoring
  - For low-risk women
  - Every 15-30 minutes in first stage of labor
  - Every 5-15 minutes in second stage of labor
  - Continuous monitoring encouraged for high-risk deliveries
  - Electronic fetal monitoring may be external or internal/fetal scalp monitoring
  - Baseline heart rate/responses to labor-tachycardia/bradycardia
  - Variability—absent, minimal, moderate, or marked (absent or minimal may indicate fetal distress, anomalies, or sleep state-[limited to 30 minutes at a time])
  - Accelerations—periodic or episodic, indicate fetal well-being
  - Decelerations
    - Early—in response to uterine contractions
    - Late—does not begin until after contraction started, does not return to baseline until after contraction, may indicate uteroplacental insufficiency-ominous sign with absent/minimal variability. May occur with tachysystole caused by oxytocin
    - Variable—any time in contraction cycle—cord compression; sometimes benign; repetitive may indicate fetal hypoxia
    - Prolonged—fetal hypoxia
- › Observe amniotic fluid after rupture of membranes
- › Observe vaginal fluids for abnormal bleeding or meconium (could indicate fetal distress)

Priority Laboratory Tests/Diagnostics

- › Ultrasound to assess fetal head size to determine feasibility of vaginal delivery
- › X-ray of maternal pelvis
- › Urinalysis to assess hydration, infection
- › Complete blood count/Rh testing
- › Rapid screen HIV test (unless mother opts-out)
- › Group B streptococcus rapid test (if status not known)

Priority Interventions or Actions

- › Provide non-pharmacologic pain management
  - Cutaneous stimulation—counterpressure, massage, heat or cold, water therapy, acupressure, acupuncture, intradermal water block
  - Sensory stimulation—music, imagery, aromatherapy, breathing techniques
  - Cognitive strategies—childbirth education, hypnosis, biofeedback
- › Provide pharmacologic pain management
  - Sedatives
    - Diazepam—relieve anxiety (may hamper thermoregulation in infant)
  - Metoclopramide—relieve nausea and potentiate analgesics

- Analgesia
  - Opioid agonists/agonist-antagonists
  - Patient-controlled analgesia (PCA)
  - May have intense impacts on neonate-respirations, FHR, contractions
  - Administered after labor is well established
  - Should not be administered if delivery expected in 1-4 hours
- Anesthesia
  - Nerve blocks-epidural, spinal, pudendal
  - Nitrous oxide/general anesthesia
- C-sections
  - Spinal/epidural blocks
  - General anesthesia
- › Provide supplemental oxygen as indicated
- › Provide intravenous fluids as prescribed/observe for overhydration
- › Provide antibiotics if client is positive for group B streptococcus
- › Encourage voiding every two hours
- › Care with nonreassuring heart patterns
  - Identify cause
  - Discontinue oxytocin
  - Change mother's position
  - Increase/apply oxygen
  - Provide IV fluids
  - Ensure continuous fetal monitoring
  - Prepare for C-section as indicated
  - Document events with strips

Priority Potential & Actual Complications

- › Respiratory depression of mother and fetus secondary to opioids
- › Postpartum hemorrhage
- › Infection
- › Non-progression of labor
- › Precipitous delivery
- › Fetal hypoxia/asphyxia

Priority Nursing Implications

- › Maintain safety precautions with any medication and during active labor
- › Support, within agency protocol, women's activity, showering, use of birthing ball, walking, and use of non-pharmacological pain relief
- › Maintain mother's hygiene
- › Watch for contraction patterns—too rapid contractions, or those without rests in between, may be less effective in dilating cervix
- › Although controversial, sources indicate allowing laboring mothers to choose oral food and fluid intake to ensure adequate energy for labor

Priority Medications

> Meperidine
> - Less respiratory depression than morphine
> - Rapid onset when administered IV
> - Causes neonatal depression-must be given prior to 1-4 hours from delivery
> - May be used after C-section
> - Have naloxone available

> Fentanyl
> - Fewer neonatal and maternal side effects and less respiratory depression
> - Short half-life, quick action and more frequent dosing

> Nalbuphine
> - Opioid agonist-antagonist
> - Less respiratory side effects for mother and fetus, causes sedation
> - Not with those addicted to opioids—stimulates withdrawal in mother and fetus
> - High ceiling medication (higher doses do not increase effect)

> Naloxone
> - Opioid antagonist
> - Administer if birth proceeds rapidly to address impact of narcotics
> - Pain will return with reversal of opioid
> - May delay breastfeeding

> Oxytocin
> - Encourage contraction/tone of uterus
> - 10-40 units/1000 lactated ringers or normal saline solution

Priority Education/Discharge Issues

> Assess parents and teach about baby care including feeding, bathing, diaper care, care of umbilicus, circumcision (if done), assessing for jaundice, and follow-up to pediatrician

> Postpartum use of copper intrauterine devices, progestin implants, and progestin-only birth control pills are optimal for first contraception when breastfeeding. Many sources recommend avoiding estrogen methods for 3-6 weeks postpartum in nursing mothers to ensure breast milk supply

> Provide mother with instructions on self-care including avoiding constipation, hygiene, sitz baths, resuming sexual activity, contraception, follow-up, nutrition, pain relief, and hydration

> Assess and refer for postpartum "blues"

> Assist with transition to parenting for co-mother, father/co-parent, grandparents, and siblings

Next Gen Clinical Judgment

Supine hypotension occurs when a pregnant woman lies on her back, causing pallor, dizziness, breathlessness, nausea, faintness, sweating, cool, clammy skin, and tachycardia. It is caused by uterine pressure on vena cava and aorta. The nurse quickly turns the client on her left side.

1. What would the client's vital signs be during the episode?

2. What would the client's vital signs be if the issue was resolved after turning the client?

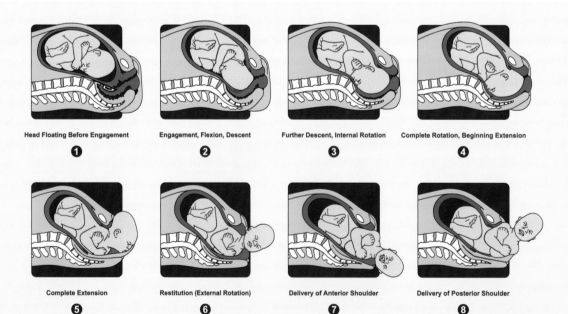

1 Head Floating Before Engagement

2 Engagement, Flexion, Descent

3 Further Descent, Internal Rotation

4 Complete Rotation, Beginning Extension

5 Complete Extension

6 Restitution (External Rotation)

7 Delivery of Anterior Shoulder

8 Delivery of Posterior Shoulder

Image 5-1: When studying the stages of labor, make sure you fully understand all terms involved. What terms in this image are unfamiliar to you?

Dystocia

Pathophysiology/Description

> Dysfunctional, long, difficult, or abnormal labor

> Lack of progress of dilation, descent, and/or expulsion

- 8-11% of labors, it is most common indication for C-section

> Related to alterations in function or parts of the birth process

1. Powers-ineffective contractions, pushing, or bearing down
   - Maternal fatigue or dehydration
   - Epidural or early analgesia
   - Overstimulation of uterus, uterine dysfunction, hypotonic (short, irregular, weak) or hypertonic (painful, frequent, and uncoordinated) uterine contractions

2. Passage-pelvis/soft tissue obstruction
   - Cephalopelvic disproportion
   - Fetopelvic dystocia

3. Passenger
   - Size, presentation
   - Multiparity

4. Position
   - Maternal body position during labor
   - Restriction of normal activity

5. Psychological
   - Negative past experiences and fear inhibit progress in labor
   - Childbirth preparation and support may allow childbirth to progress more quickly

> Risk factors include obesity, short stature, previous dystocia, malpresentation, malposition, advanced maternal age, infertility

Priority Assessments or Cues

> Assess vital signs for maternal tachycardia, monitor maternal temperature

> Assess fetal heart tones for fetal tachycardia and response to contractions and progress of labor

> Assess cervical effacement and dilation

> Assess contraction patterns

> Determine Bishop score which is maternal readiness for labor/induction, (dilation of cervix, effacement of cervix, consistency of cervix, position of cervix, and station of presenting part—each of 5 parameters are scored 0-3, 6 or more is readiness for labor induction)

> Assess fetal position and presentation—palpate using Leopold's maneuvers

> Assess intactness of amniotic membranes

> Assess for risk for dystocia throughout labor

> Assess maternal pain level and effectiveness of management strategies

Priority Laboratory Tests/Diagnostics

> Ultrasound

> Non-stress tests to ensure fetal well-being

Priority Interventions or Actions

> Encourage maternal rest between contractions to ensure energy to deal with labor, provide comfort measures, back rubs, position changes, and encourage ambulation and frequent voiding

> Assist mother in learning breathing and relaxation strategies

> Pain relief may allow client to deal with contractions and allow labor to progress

> Administer prophylactic antibiotics as prescribed

> Administer fluids as prescribed, assess intake and output

> Monitor color of amniotic fluid

> Assess for prolapse of cord after membranes break or are ruptured

> Internal or external version to turn a fetus in breech or shoulder presentation

> Cervical ripening
- Chemical agents
- Physical and mechanical methods-balloon catheter, hydroscopic dilators, amniotic membrane sweeping
- Other methods-intercourse, nipple stimulation, walking

> Amniotomy—rupture of membranes

> Episiotomy—incision of posterior vagina/perineum

> Forceps assisted birth or vacuum assisted birth

> Cesarean birth with spinal, epidural, or general anesthesia

Priority Potential & Actual Complications

> Maternal dehydration and infection

> Fetal hypoxia, injury, asphyxia, or demise

> Post-vaginal delivery complications: infection, hemorrhage

> C-section complications include anesthesia reactions, hemorrhage, bowel/bladder injury, aspiration pneumonia, drug reaction, air embolism, amniotic embolism, urinary tract infections, wound hematoma/infection, dehiscence, bowel dysfunction, venous thrombosis. For the neonate, tachypnea, asphyxia, injuries, prematurity

> Complications associated with procedures (forceps, etc.)

Priority Nursing Implications

> Continually monitor mother's comfort, fetal heart tones, and mother's vital signs in response to procedures

> For mothers who are Rh negative, prepare to administer Rho (D) immune globulin

Priority Education/Discharge Issues

> Assist client and family/partners to review and debrief birth process, although it may not have replicated the birth plan

> Ensure that client gets the rest needed to heal and provide mothering, feeding, and affection to infant

Placental abruption

Pathophysiology/Description

> Detachment of all or part of the placenta from the uterus after implantation
> Occurs between 20 weeks gestation and birth
> High level of morbidity and mortality
> Accounts for 1/3 of antepartum bleeding
> Risk factors include maternal hypertension (chronic or pregnancy-related), multiparity, cocaine use (vascular constriction), abdominal trauma/motor vehicle accident/domestic violence, cigarette smoking, history of abruptio or premature rupture of membranes with previous pregnancies

Priority Assessments or Cues

> Assess for risk factors
> Categorized on grade:
>   • Grade 1 (10-20% abruption)—minimal bleeding, dark red blood, without tenderness, upper uterine placement
>   • Grade 2 (20-50% abruption)—absent to moderate bleeding, dark red blood, increased uterine tone/rigidity without relaxation, pain, mild shock, potential DIC, may impact fetal heart tones
>   • Grade 3 (>50% abruption)—absent to moderate bleeding, dark red blood, sudden, significant shock, board-like abdomen, agonizing pain, impacts fetal heart tones, may lead to fetal demise
> Assess maternal vital signs and fetal heart tones
> Assess fundal height

Priority Laboratory Tests/Diagnostics

> Abdominal and transvaginal ultrasound
> Coagulation studies
> Fetal non-stress test—assess heart rate patterns in response to fetal movement, uterine contractions, or stimulation
> Biophysical profile—real-time ultrasound assessing amniotic fluid volume, fetal movements, fetal heart tones, fetal breathing movements, and fetal muscle tone
> Type and cross match as needed prior to transfusion
> Kleihauer-Betke test—to detect fetal blood in maternal circulation

Priority Interventions or Actions

> From 20-34 weeks gestation, if there are normal fetal heart tones
>   • Client is hospitalized and large-bore intravenous access and a urinary catheter placed to check urine output. Oxygen applied as needed. If there is mild bleeding bedrest is recommended. With no bleeding, bedrest with bathroom privileges is indicated

> > 34 weeks gestation
>   • Client is hospitalized and managed as above.
>   • Betamethasone is administered to mature the fetal lungs
> Large volume bleeding-above, plus:
>   • Mom and fetus may be in jeopardy
>   • Position Trendelenburg to decrease pressure on placenta or lateral if client hypovolemic
>   • Birth-vaginal preferred, C-sections are not done with coagulopathy
> All cases: External fetal monitoring, assess for bleeding, monitor coagulation studies

Priority Potential & Actual Complications

> Fetal loss/demise
> Shock
> Couvelair uterus-decreased contractility
> Disseminated intravascular coagulation (DIC)
> Transplacental hemorrhage
> Renal failure
> Rh sensitization
> Intrauterine growth retardation
> Preterm birth

Priority Nursing Implications

> Nurse provide support and care in the event of fetal demise
> Provide emotional support to deal with stress of critically ill mother and/or fetus
> Provide pain management and replacement fluids

Priority Medications

> betamethasone
>   • Enhance fetal lung maturity
>   • Steroid

Priority Education/Discharge Issues

> Educate family as status of mother and fetus changes
> Provide support of client and infant if preterm
> Support family with an ill neonate and premature infant—neonatal intensive care unit and routines

Next Gen Clinical Judgment

Compare and contrast can help you save a lot of time studying. List 2 similarities and 2 differences in placental abruption and placenta previa.

Placenta previa

Pathophysiology/Description

> Placenta is implanted lower than optimal in the uterus—completely or partially/marginally covers the cervix

> Bleeding occurs with dilatation and effacement of the cervix

> Occurs in second and third trimester

> Risk factors include history of C-section, suction curettage, and previous placenta previa; advanced maternal age, multiparity, smoking, and living in a high altitude

Priority Assessments or Cues

> Ask about risk factors

> Assess vaginal bleeding—bright red with placenta previa

> Assess pain—bleeding with placenta previa is usually painless

> Assess abdomen—soft, relaxed and non-tender, fundal height may be greater than expected, often with breech/transverse/oblique lies

> Assess fetal heart tones—usually normal unless major deterioration

> Assess urine output

Priority Laboratory Tests/Diagnostics

> Transabdominal ultrasound (check for placental placement—if low than transvaginal)

> Transvaginal ultrasound—done with select cases, avoid uterine stimulation

> Blood studies—Hemoglobin/hematocrit, platelets, coagulation studies, type and screen/crossmatch

> Kleihauer-Betke test to detect fetal blood in maternal circulation

Priority Interventions or Actions

> Closely monitor vital signs and assess for a rapid hemorrhage

> Large bore intravenous access-prepare for fluids and blood products

> Position side-lying, bed rest

> Refrain from unneeded vaginal exams

> < 34 weeks-betamethasone to mature fetal lungs

> Without bleeding and < 36 weeks without labor, implement expectant management including limited activity, pelvic rest, assess for bleeding, nonstress test, biophysical profile-twice/week—if no bleeding for 48 hours/stable-may discharge to home with restrictions

> > 36 weeks and no major bleeding—active management including birth. If previa is within 2 cm of cervix, a C-section is indicated; > 2cm away, a vaginal birth is recommended

Priority Potential & Actual Complications

> Hemorrhage (bleeding may also occur postpartum)

> Abnormal placental attachment

> Hysterectomy

> C-section (with concurrent potential side effects)

> Fetal death secondary to preterm birth

> Fetal abnormalities/intrauterine growth retardation

Priority Nursing Implications

> Emotional support for potential stress associated with high-risk pregnancy

> Assess for degree of bleeding by estimating milliliters of blood loss of spots or stains

Priority Medications

> magnesium sulfate

  • Have available for tocolysis (relax uterus)

  • To prevent preterm delivery

  • Assess serum magnesium levels (4-7 mEq/L)

  • Assess for magnesium toxicity/serum hypermagnesemia. Signs include absence of patellar deep tendon reflexes, decreased level of consciousness, low urine output, bradypnea, and cardiac dysrhythmias

  • Antidote for hypermagnesemia is calcium gluconate

> beclomethasone

  • Steroids administered to mature fetal lungs

  • Given if risk of delivery prior to 34 weeks

> ferrous sulfate

  • Increase iron stores in the event of bleeding

  • May cause constipation and gastric upset

Priority Education/Discharge Issues

> If discharged, home care includes activities restrictions and client must have access to a phone, must be within 20 minutes of the hospital, must have access to transportation, and must have friends/family to assist in care. Clients are told to proceed to the hospital in the event of any vaginal bleeding

> Ensure that mothers understand precautions of pelvic rest-no exams, no sexual intercourse, limited transvaginal ultrasounds

> Counsel client about ways to keep busy and diversional activities—activity restrictions may be very boring and raise anxiety levels

Postpartum hemorrhage

Pathophysiology/Description

> Leading cause of morbidity and mortality in US and worldwide

> Bleeding of 500 mL or more post-vaginal delivery or 1000 mL or more after a C-section

> May occur as early hemorrhage (first 24 hours) or late hemorrhage (after 24 hours to 6 weeks)

> May be caused by uterine atony, lacerations of the cervix or vagina, retained portions of the placenta, or rupture of hematomas

> Risk factors include history of previous hemorrhage after birth; placental abruption; placenta previa; distended uterus related to multiparity birth, large baby, or polyhydramnios; dystocia or prolonged labor; oxytocin induction or augmentation; administration of magnesium sulfate; operative/invasive delivery; or infections

Priority Assessments or Cues

> Assess vital signs. Attend to blood pressure and heart rate

> Assess perfusion including skin temperature, capillary refill, peripheral pulses, motor/sensory function, and pallor

> Assess bleeding including source (lacerations, hematomas, or episiotomy), pattern, amount, perineal pad count/weight, assess and count clots, duration, color (dark red-venous; bright red-arterial/lacerations), and consistency

> Assess signs of hypotension including restlessness, tachycardia, tachypnea, hypotension, cool/clammy skin, pale or grey skin color

> Assess for complaints of dizziness, weakness or dyspnea

> Evaluate contractability of uterus (hypotonic/boggy)

> Assess fundal height, firmness, and position

> Assess bladder for distension

Priority Laboratory Tests/Diagnostics

> CBC—Hemoglobin or hematocrit levels

> Ultrasound of uterus for retained placenta

> Blood type and screen

> Coagulation studies/platelet counts

Priority Interventions or Actions

> Ensure safety precautions and reinforce bedrest

> If lack of uterine tone, gently massage fundus, encourage client to empty her bladder if condition warrants. Healthcare provider may do bimanual compression, put baby to breast

> Insert a urinary catheter to assess renal perfusion and output and empty bladder

> Position client on right side with hips lifted and legs elevated (elevate legs 20-30 degrees to increase venous return)

> Administer oxygen-non-rebreather 10-12 L/min, monitor pulse ox

> Access two IV sites and provide fluids, bolus, or transfuse as prescribed (PRBCs preferred)

> Prepare for surgery as indicated-surgical or bedside repair of lacerations or evacuation of hematomas, uterine packing, suturing, surgical or manual removal of retained placenta, or insertion of tamponade balloon

> If indicated, critical care monitoring and hemodynamic monitoring

Priority Potential & Actual Complications

> Hypovolemic shock/hemorrhagic shock

> Acidosis

> Uterine inversion

> Disseminated intravascular coagulation

> May be fatal

Priority Nursing Implications

> Provide support to client and family with care of critically ill client

> Ensure maternal contact with infant as able

> Consider interventions to address interruption in infant/maternal bonding

Priority Medications

> oxytocin
  - To decrease bleeding
  - 10-40 units/1000 lactated ringers or normal saline solution
  - Increases tone of uterus to decrease bleeding

> prostaglandins
  - To decrease bleeding
  - misoprostol-per rectum, sublingual, or oral
  - 15-methyl prostaglandin F2 alpha
    - Intramuscular injection
    - Contraindicated with asthma and hypertension
  - prostaglandin E2 -oral or per rectum

> methylergonovine
  - IM uterine stimulant
  - Contraindicated with hypertension

Priority Education/Discharge Issues

> Reinforce the increased importance of rest in mother after blood loss-superimposed on care of infant/assistance with baby care

> Encourage a high iron diet to include green, leafy vegetables, meats, and supplements as prescribed

> With lacerations and while on iron prevent constipation, encourage fluids and high fiber diet

> May have difficulty with delays in breastfeeding, refer to lactation counselor

Breastfeeding

Pathophysiology/Description

> Benefits of breastfeeding including physical and psychological health advantages for mother and baby, convenience, along with economic and environmental advantages

> Preferred method of nutrition, in accordance with the wishes and abilities of the mother, for the first six months of life

Priority Assessments or Cues

> Assess mother's level of knowledge about breastfeeding

> Assess mother's comfort level with breastfeeding and support from others, including partner and family

> While observing breastfeeding, assess the ability of the infant to latch on to the nipple on both breasts, the sucking and swallowing sequence, the optimal position for the mother to hold the infant during feeding, the condition of the nipple and surrounding tissue after feeding, and the mother's expressed comfort and satisfaction with each feeding

> Assess infant weight gain

> Assess infant color for breast milk jaundice

Priority Interventions or Actions

> Mothers who choose breastfeeding should be given the opportunity to put the baby to breast as soon as stable, preferably in the delivery room

> Provide hygiene care and instruct mothers on breast hygiene

> Provide support and coaching during each of the early feeding, referrals to a lactation counselor for every breastfeeding mother are encouraged

> Encourage feeding on each side for 15-20 minutes and to begin each feeding on the side last nursed upon. Mothers often develop creative ways to remember this, including double breast pads on the last used side, hair elastics on the wrist of the side last used, etc

> Encourage use of breast pads to deal with leaking between feedings

> Provide education and support for minor and major issues with breastfeeding

> Teach mothers methods to encourage latching on: Brush lower lip with nipple, stimulate the lips to open the mouth wide, release suction by placing a clean finger into the infant's mouth or pull down on the infant's chin

> Seek out healthcare provider's views on Vitamin D supplementation for exclusively breastfed infants

> Ensure iron supplementation for exclusively breastfed infants as iron stores are depleted around 4 months

Priority Potential & Actual Complications

> Breast engorgement to treat between feedings use ice packs or chilled cabbage leaves, manually express milk. Immediately before feedings, use warm soaks or a warm shower to encourage let-down during the early days of feeding

> For cracked nipples, leave nipples open to air between feedings, rub nipples with dry washcloth to toughen nipples, ensure that the infant latches onto entire areola of breast and not just nipple, ensure that the mother rotates breast and limits time on each side, and use lanolin cream as needed

> For inverted or flattened nipples, use breast shields

Priority Nursing Implications

> Encourage breastfeeding moms to wear supportive bras (without underwires) after delivery and throughout breastfeeding, even when sleeping

> Educate moms about the potential for uterine cramping during early breastfeedings

> Encourage mothers to assess foods which the infant may not tolerate in breastmilk including strawberries, caffeine, brussels sprouts, chocolate, cauliflower, onions, garlic, etc.

> Encourage mothers to avoid over-the-counter, other medications, and alcohol unless approved by healthcare provider

Priority Education/Discharge Issues

> Discuss nutrition and hydration—breastfeeding women should increase intake of water/fluids, continue prenatal vitamins, and consume about 300-500 more calories/day

> Reinforce the value of handwashing to prevent infection transmission

> Encourage mothers to burp the infant after each breast

> Reinforce the role of the partner/co-parent/parent to change diapers, burp, console, and cuddle with infant before and after feedings

> Inform client/parents that infants who breastfeed often have loose, frequent, yellow, seedy stools

> Assist client, infant, and family to develop a feeding schedule

> Provide mother with information and teaching on breastmilk pumping and storage, many insurance companies provide breast pumps

> Teach mom about feeding readiness cues and means to deal with a fussy or sleepy baby or nursing multiple infants

> Teach mother symptoms of and means to prevent plugged milk ducts and mastitis

> Provide access to breastfeeding support groups in the community

STI: Chlamydia

📋 Pathophysiology/Description

> Bacterial infection caused by *Chlamydia trachomatis*

> Most commonly reported STI in American women, 2 ½ times the rate for men

> Difficult to diagnose, symptoms nonspecific

> Highest rates among sexually active women 15-24 years, peaks at 18-20

> Highest risk among women with multiple sexual partners, nonuse of barrier methods, lower socioeconomic status (less treatment-seeking behaviors)

> Neonatal infection occurs in 25-60% of vaginal births in infected mothers, may also occur with C-sections

✏️ Priority Assessments or Cues

> May have "silent symptoms"

> Assess for risk factors and obtain a culture from women with 2 or more risk factors; screen all women 20-25 years or women with multiple sexual partners

> Screen at first prenatal visit and repeat in late third trimester if women previously tested positive, has a new sexual partner, has multiple sexual partners, had a previous pregnancy complicated with chlamydia, or is < 25 years of age

> May be asymptomatic but ask about potential symptoms including spotting, post-coital bleeding, pelvic pain, mucoid or purulent cervical drainage, or dysuria

> Neonatal chlamydial conjunctivitis includes redness and edema of eyes, untreated may lead to chronic conjunctivitis, scarring, and micro-granulations

> Neonatal chlamydial pneumonia at 4-11 weeks of age, symptoms include progressive rhinorrhea, tachypnea, and coughing

🧪 Priority Laboratory Tests/Diagnostics

> Laboratory culture (expensive and more effort)

> DNA probe (less expensive but less sensitive)

> Enzyme immunoassay (less expensive but less sensitive)

> Nucleic acid amplification tests (expensive, sensitive) via urine samples—first void and mid-stream samples detect chlamydia

℧ Priority Nursing Implications

> Provide education to clients at risk

> Screen high-risk clients

> Provide emotional support and encourage client to make all sexual partners aware of infection

🚩 Priority Potential & Actual Complications

> Acute salpingitis

> Pelvic inflammatory disease

> Pelvic abscess

> Increased risk of ectopic pregnancy

> Increase incidence of tubal factor infertility

> Cervical ulcerations which increase susceptibility to HIV

> Neonatal chlamydia conjunctivitis (ophthalmia neonatorum) or pneumonia

> May be associated with premature labor, premature rupture of membranes, stillbirth, and pregnancy loss

> May be related to postpartum endometritis

💧 Priority Medications

> neonatal ocular prophylaxis
  - Silver nitrate solution or antibiotic ointment
  - May not prevent transmission
  - May not treat infection

> azithromycin
  - Single dose for issues with adherence
  - May be more expensive
  - May be used with pregnancy (retest in 3 weeks)
  - May be used with breastfeeding
  - Treatment may be used with clients who are HIV+

> doxycycline
  - BID for 7 days
  - Avoid during pregnancy

> erythromycin
  - Ointment for eyes
  - For prophylaxis—not always effective but is part of routine, preventive newborn care

> erythromycin
  - Oral
  - For neonatal conjunctivitis/pneumonia
  - May be associated with hypertrophic pyloric stenosis-watch for projectile vomiting, feeding intolerance

> amoxicillin
  - May be used during pregnancy
  - May be used when breastfeeding

👤 Priority Education/Discharge Issues

> Encourage use of male or female condoms with every sexual encounter even when on birth control

> Teach client and sexual partners about the potential complications associated with infection and the need for repeated screening

> Treat all sexual partners

> Teach clients the importance of rescreening during pregnancy

STI: Human papillomavirus (HPV)

Pathophysiology/Description

> Also known as *condylomata acuminata* or genital warts; common viral STI
> Estimate 50% of sexually active women will contract HPV
> Transmitted via sexual contact
> Highest rate in women 20-24 years of age
> HPV has 40 serotypes that are STIs
> May be more common in pregnant women, lesions may enlarge during pregnancy—may affect urination, defecation, mobility and fetal descent

Priority Assessments or Cues

> Ask client about itching, vaginal discharge, dyspareunia, pruritis, post-coital bleeding, or "bumps" on the labia (or urethra or scrotum in men)
> Assess for lesions around posterior part of the vaginal introitus, around the buttocks, vulva, vagina, anus, and cervix (lesions are 2-3 mm in diameter, 10-15 mm in height)—lesions occur singly or in clusters (cauliflower-like mass)
> Cervical lesions—flat topped papules 1-4 cm in diameter
> Lesions are brown to black and are painless but uncomfortable
> Lesions may resolve spontaneously without treatment but warts or cancer may develop later

Priority Laboratory Tests/Diagnostics

> Although viral screening is available, diagnosis is generally done based on history and physical examination
> Papanicolaou (Pap) test to rule out cervical cancer
> HPV-DNA in woman over 30 years
> Histologic evaluation of a biopsy of HPV
> If pregnant, cultures done weekly from 35 weeks until delivery

Priority Interventions or Actions

> No curative therapy exists
> Requires multiple treatments (see medications below)
> Cryotherapy, laser, electrocautery, cytoxic agents or surgical removal of lesions during pregnancy

Priority Potential & Actual Complications

> 2 types of HPV responsible for cervical cancers
> May impede a vaginal delivery and require a C-section
> Neonatal contraction of HPV
> Children may sustain epithelial tumors on the larynx

Priority Nursing Implications

> Because lesions may exist on the labia/vagina and anus, gloves should be changed to avoid cross-contamination
> Lesion care includes bathing with oatmeal solution, blow with cool hair dryer, keep the area clean and dry, cotton underwear/loose-fitting clothing
> Clients need to assume a healthy lifestyle, including rest, diet, and hydration to maximize immune function

Priority Medications

> imiquimod
  • Not during pregnancy
  • Immune response modifier
> trichloroacetic acid (TCA) and bichloroacetic acid (BCA)
  • Applied to warts
  • Use petroleum jelly to protect surrounding skin
  • May be painful upon application
> podofilox liquid gel
  • Apply to affected area BID x 3 days weekly x 3 to 4 weeks
  • Not for use in pregnancy/breastfeeding

Priority Education/Discharge Issues

> Teaching about transmission and the importance of prevention are critical since there is no cure
> HPV vaccines are recommended for 11 and 12-year-old girls and boys—protects against some HPV – three doses over 6 months
> Clients may be taught about barrier methods (male/female condoms) and the benefits of limiting numbers of sexual partners to prevent disease transmission
> Avoid sexual contact until lesions healed

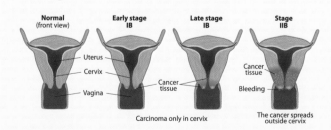 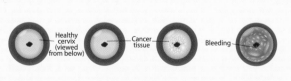

Image 5-2: As you study the stages of cervical cancer, how would you describe it to a patient with no medical or healthcare background?

STI: Syphilis

📋 Pathophysiology/Description

> Syphilis was one of the earliest STIs identified caused by *Treponema pallidum*

> Known as a chronic infectious disease

> Transmitted via physical contact with subcutaneous lesions that occur during sexual intercourse—kissing, biting, or oral-genital sex (skin, mucous membranes of mouth, anus, and genitals)

> May be transmitted in utero

> Highest risk among women 20-24 years of age

✏️ Priority Assessments or Cues

> Assess risk factors

> Assess syphilitic lesions—manifestations related to phase of syphilis infections

- Primary—most infectious
  - Lesion or chancre at point of entry of the spirochete
  - 5-90 days after infection
  - Painless papule becomes a flat, indurated ulcer
- Secondary—highly infectious
  - 6 weeks to 6 months after infection
  - Maculopapular rash localized on palms, soles, and/or skin and mucous membranes, non-pruritic rash. Mucous patches on mouth, tongue, or cervix
  - Generalized lymphadenopathy
  - Generalized symptoms of fever, headache, and malaise
  - Condylomata lata (wart-like lesions)
- Tertiary
  - Early latent phase-may be asymptomatic
  - 10-30 years after untreated primary lesion
  - Later-spirochete enters internal organs-neurological (Meningitis, paresis, ataxia, CNS deterioration), cardiovascular (aorta and aortic valve damage), musculoskeletal, and multiorgan system complications
  - Permanent organ damage

🧪 Priority Laboratory Tests/Diagnostics

> Microscopic examination of lesion tissue

> Serology during latency and late infection

> VDRL (venereal disease research laboratory test) or rapid plasma reagin

⚠️ Priority Interventions or Actions

> Penicillin

> Limit sexual contacts/treat sexual contacts

> Symptomatic care for damaged organs

🚩 Priority Potential & Actual Complications

> May be fatal

> Systemic implications

> Spontaneous abortion or premature labor if pregnant

> Crosses placenta at 18 weeks-congenital syphilis-physical anomalies, CNS damage, neonatal syphilitic lesions, hearing loss

☋ Priority Nursing Implications

> Screening indicated for all women diagnosed with another STI or HIV

> Provide emotional support for all clients, especially those who are pregnant

> Contact precautions when handling affected infants, most infectious until 24 hours after initiation of antibiotics

> Ensure treatment of all sexual contacts

💧 Priority Medications

> penicillin
- May cause GI upset in high doses
- May lead to superinfections—encourage eating yogurt or buttermilk
- High rate of hypersensitivity
- Encourage fluids to enhance excretion

👤 Priority Education/Discharge Issues

> Teach importance of treating in the early stages to avoid permanent damage to organs

> Encourage all partners to be treated

> Ensure pregnant women are tested at first prenatal visit and at 36 weeks gestation if infection is questioned

> Provide teaching about medications and prevention using barrier methods (male or female condoms)

_____

_____

_____

_____

_____

_____

1. A 39-week pregnant client has been admitted to labor and delivery with a potential placenta previa. As the nurse prepares for the examination which nursing action in the client's exam is omitted?
   1. Conducting the vaginal exam.
   2. Using Leopold's maneuvers.
   3. Placing the client on her side.
   4. Placing the client in a high Fowler's position.

2. A nurse has just administered 2 mg of butorphanol intravenously to a laboring client. Which assessment changes should the nurse recognize as the most significant?
   1. A neonatal respiratory rate of 40 breaths per minute after birth.
   2. Maternal nausea and vomiting.
   3. Maternal drowsiness.
   4. A decrease in the fetal heart rate's fluctuation from baseline.

3. During the second day postpartum, a client states that she keeps crying for no apparent reason. What is the best response by the nurse?
   1. "You are just tired from having a baby."
   2. "I am sure it will be better tomorrow."
   3. "This is called the postpartum or baby blues and it is very common."
   4. "You are showing signs of postpartum depression."

4. Magnesium sulfate is being administered intravenously to a client for pregnancy-induced hypertension. Which assessment finding should the nurse identify as a complication of this treatment?
   1. Deep tendon reflex of +2.
   2. Urine output of 70 mL/hour.
   3. Blood pressure of 148/94 mmHg.
   4. Respiratory rate of 10 bpm.

5. A 14-week pregnant primigravida client reports that she is extremely nauseous. What is the best nursing response?
   1. "You should try to avoid eating between meals."
   2. "This is reassuring that the pregnancy is developing."
   3. "You should try to eat a diet high in fat."
   4. "You should try to eat something bland every 2 -3 hours."

6. A laboring client is being prepared for an emergency cesarean section. The nurse should immediately report which client data?
   1. The client's membranes ruptured 2 hours ago.
   2. The client's platelets are 200,000/mcl.
   3. The client reported having a meal 4 hours ago.
   4. The client is RH negative.

7. Which statement made by a client with human papillomavirus (HPV) should the nurse correct?
   1. "There is a vaccination available for some strains of this virus."
   2. "There are not always symptoms associated with HPV."
   3. "I can only shed the virus when I have lesions present."
   4. "HPV can be transferred to an infant during delivery."

8. A client delivered a baby 2 months ago. The significant other calls into the office to report that his wife is angry, confused, and having conversations with herself. What is the appropriate response that the nurse should make?
   1. "Please take your wife to the emergency room for evaluation.".
   2. "Please bring your wife to the office for medication."
   3. "Your wife will require outpatient care."
   4. "Your wife will require behavioral therapy."

9. An infant is breastfeeding for the first time. Which nursing statement will reduce the client's risk for skin breakdown?
   1. "You should wear waterproof pads inside your bra."
   2. "You should insert your finger into the baby's mouth before removing the baby from your breast.".
   3. "You should breastfeed every four hours."
   4. "You should only breastfeed from one breast at each feeding and begin feeding with the opposite breast at the next feeding."

10. A nurse is preparing to administer Rho (D) immune globulin to a client who delivered a baby yesterday. The nurse recognizes that the treatment is indicated by which client data?
    1. The indirect Coombs test is negative.
    2. The mother is RH positive.
    3. The infant is RH negative.
    4. The indirect Coombs test is positive.

11. A laboring client has been prescribed Nitrous Oxide for pain management during labor. To ensure that the client will not overdose, what action will the nurse make?
    1. Instruct the client to self-administer the medication.
    2. Instruct the client to inhale every 30 minutes.
    3. Assess if the client is experiencing nausea.
    4. Ensure that the medication antidote is available.

12. When should a nurse instruct a client in the second stage of labor to start pushing?
    1. Once the infant's head is below the ischial spines.
    2. When the client feels the urge to push.
    3. When early decelerations are seen on the fetal monitor.
    4. When late decelerations are seen on the fetal monitor.

13. A pregnant client is asking a nurse about how she should wear her seatbelt while in the car. Which should be the nurse's response?
    1. "You should wear the lower lap belt across the middle of your abdomen and the upper shoulder belt above the top of your pregnant belly."
    2. "You should not wear the seatbelt because it can harm the baby if an accident occurs."
    3. "You should wear the lower lap belt below your belly and push the shoulder belt across your abdomen."
    4. "You should wear the lower belt below your belly and push the upper shoulder belt above your belly."

14. A nurse is caring for a client with Chlamydia Trachomatis. Which statement is true about this infection?
    1. It is the most commonly reported sexually transmitted infection in American women.
    2. It is more common in men than in women.
    3. The infection causes a thick white discharge.
    4. It is most common in women over 30 years of age.

15. A nurse observes a client sitting and watching a visitor hold her baby. The client states that her son "looks just like his daddy". Which bonding behavior should the nurse document?
    1. Mutuality.
    2. Claiming.
    3. En-Face position.
    4. Rhythm.

16. A nurse documents assessment changes that occur in the integumentary system with pregnancy. Select all the pregnancy related integumentary changes below: Select all that apply.
    1. Diastasis Recti.
    2. Striae Gravidarum.
    3. Linea Nigra.
    4. Lordosis.
    5. Melasma.

17. A nurse is caring for a client in the fourth stage of labor. Which nursing interventions are appropriate for a client who is experiencing postpartum hemorrhage? Select all that apply.
    1. Weigh the client's pads.
    2. Administer a uterotonic drug.
    3. Massage the client's fundus.
    4. Discontinue the client's indwelling urinary catheter.
    5. Express any clots in the uterus.

18. Which nursing interventions for a non-breastfeeding postpartum client will hinder the milk production? Select all that apply.
    1. The client is wearing a tight-fitting bra.
    2. The client is using warm compresses on her breasts.
    3. The client is wearing a loose-fitting bra.
    4. The client is using ice or cold compresses to her breasts.
    5. The client massages her breasts in the shower.

19. Which nursing interventions are appropriate for a client with syphilis? Select all that apply.
    1. Educate the client that this infection cannot be cured.
    2. Educate the client that there is a cure for syphilis at any stage.
    3. Assessment for a maculopapular rash on the palms, trunk or soles.
    4. Assess the client for adenopathy.
    5. Educate the client that this infection is caused by a fungus.

20. A client is admitted to labor and delivery and experiences a gush of fluid coming from her vagina. In which order should the nurse implement these interventions? Rank order the responses.
    1. Assess the color of the fluid.
    2. Assess the fluid with nitrazine paper.
    3. Assess the fetal heart rate.
    4. Document the assessment findings.
    5. Place the client on bedrest.

21. Using the client chart exhibit below, determine which client information is accurate.

    Today's date – 4/10
    Client – J. M.
    D.O.B – 2/28/1995
    G – 4 T-2 P-0 A-2 L-2
    Estimated date of delivery – 6/1
    Rubella titer 1:8

    1. The client may need a plan for childcare at home while she is in the hospital.
    2. The client will need a Rubella vaccination after the delivery.
    3. The client will need education on basic infant care.
    4. The client's baby is due in February.

22. A prescription for nalbuphine hydrochloride 10 mg IV every 3 hours for pain has been ordered for a laboring client. The medication is available in 20 mg/mL vials. How many mL(s) should the nurse administer each dose?

    _____

23. A prescription for methylergonovine 0.2 mg IM has been ordered for a client in stage three of labor who is hemorrhaging. Using the chart exhibit below, determine why this medication is contraindicated.

> Client – J.L.
> DOB – 4/2/1990
> Allergies – Penicillin
> G-5- T-4 P-0 A-0 L-4
> Vitals – T-98.6°F P-128 R-22 B/P-155/95
> Medications–Methyldopa 250 mg orally every 8 hours

   1. The medication is contraindicated due to the multigravidity of the client.
   2. The medication is contraindicated due to the client's drug allergy.
   3. The medication is contraindicated due to the client's blood pressure.
   4. The medication is contraindicated due to the client's heart rate.

24. A client delivers quickly, and a preheated infant warmer is not ready. The infant is placed on the cool surface. The nurse recognizes that the infant will lose heat by which mechanism?
   1. Convection.
   2. Conduction.
   3. Evaporation.
   4. Radiation.

25. A nurse is implementing a non-stress test on a 37-week pregnant client. She observes a baseline fetal heart rate of 140-145 bpm. The heart rate raises to 160 bpm for 3 different 20 second periods over 30 minutes. What is the next nursing action?
   1. Administer a vibro-acoustic stimulation to the maternal abdomen.
   2. Offer the client some juice to drink.
   3. Instruct the client that you will have to continue to monitor her.
   4. Remove the client from the fetal monitor.

26. A male client with a history of diabetes asks the nurse if his diabetes can affect his ability to get an erection. The correct nursing response is?
   1. "Yes, diabetes can increase the risk of erectile dysfunction."
   2. "No, there is no correlation between diabetes and erectile dysfunction."
   3. "Diabetes can affect erectile dysfunction if you are taking insulin."
   4. "Most causes of erectile dysfunction are not related to physical causes."

27. The fetal monitor of a laboring client shows that the fetal heart rate decreases after the peak of a contraction and does not recover until after the contraction is over. The nurse interprets this pattern as what type of fetal deceleration?
   1. Early fetal deceleration.
   2. Variable fetal deceleration.
   3. Prolonged fetal deceleration.
   4. Late fetal deceleration.

28. Which client would be appropriate to assign to a maternity nurse who has been pulled to the medical-surgical unit?
   1. A client post-appendectomy.
   2. A client after a cesarean section on a ventilator.
   3. A postoperative client with chest tubes.
   4. A client post-stroke receiving tissue plasminogen activator.

29. The nurse is counseling a client who is asking about sildenafil. The client wants to know how this works. What is the best response by the nurse?
   1. Sildenafil helps to increase the production of male hormones.
   2. The medication protects against sexually transmitted infections.
   3. This medication prevents unintended pregnancy.
   4. Sildenafil increases blood flow and sustains an erection.

30. A nurse is discussing body changes during menopause with a group of women. One woman asks why sexual intercourse is painful in menopause. Which is the best response by the nurse?
   1. "The woman's testosterone levels drop making the vaginal tissue dry and irritated."
   2. "Sexual intercourse happens less during this age which leads to painful penetration."
   3. "Many women believe intercourse is more painful but these is no physiological reason for this."
   4. "The vaginal tissue loses it elasticity and becomes dry making penetration painful.".

1. A 39-week pregnant client has been admitted to labor and delivery with a potential placenta previa. As the nurse prepares for the examination which nursing action in the client's exam is omitted?
   1. 💡 Conducting the vaginal exam.
   2. Using Leopold's maneuvers. *This is an external test and would not complicate the diagnosis.*
   3. Placing the client on her side. *Positioning would not complicate the diagnosis.*
   4. Placing the client in a high Fowler's position. *Positioning would not complicate the diagnosis.*

   Rationale: A placenta previa occurs when the placenta is covering or near the cervical opening. No internal vaginal exams should be made until further assessment is completed. Performing Leopold's maneuvers or client position will not complicate this diagnosis.

   THIN Thinking: Identify Risk to Safety – *Avoiding vaginal exams will decrease the risk for damage to the placenta and prevent it from dislodging from the uterine wall. Understanding the placenta covers the cervical opening in placenta previa helps the nurse understand the risk for bleeding if placenta becomes dislodged.* NCLEX®: Reduction of Risk QSEN: Safety

2. A nurse has just administered 2 mg of butorphanol intravenously to a laboring client. Which assessment changes should the nurse recognize as the most significant?
   1. A neonatal respiratory rate of 40 breaths per minute after birth. *This is a normal rate.*
   2. Maternal nausea and vomiting. *This is a manageable side effect.*
   3. Maternal drowsiness. *This is a manageable side effect.*
   4. 💡 A decrease in the fetal heart rate's fluctuation from baseline.

   Rationale: A decrease in fetal variability, maternal nausea and vomiting, and drowsiness may occur after the administration of a narcotic. The decrease in fetal variability is the most significant side effect. A neonatal respiratory rate of 40 is normal.

   THIN Thinking: Top Three – *Looking at ABC's, Circulation is the priority concern for the infant. Decrease in fetal heart rate fluctuation indicates poor perfusion.* NCLEX®: Safety and Infection Control QSEN: Safety

3. During the second day postpartum, a client states that she keeps crying for no apparent reason. What is the best response by the nurse?
   1. "You are just tired from having a baby." *Does not educate client on cause of crying.*
   2. "I am sure it will be better tomorrow." *False reassurance.*
   3. 💡 "This is called the postpartum or baby blues and it is very common."
   4. "You are showing signs of postpartum depression." *Depression is different than "blues" and needs to be diagnosed by a mental health specialist.*

   Rationale: The postpartum or baby blues are experienced by 50-80% of women. These women experience emotional lability and often cry very easily.

   THIN Thinking: Nursing Process – *Implementing education based on assessment data helps clients understand why they have vacillating emotions during this period. Postpartum depression is common and needs to be discussed with clients to help promote healthy interventions during postpartum depression.* NCLEX®: Psychosocial Integrity QSEN: Evidence-based Practice

4. Magnesium sulfate is being administered intravenously to a client for pregnancy-induced hypertension. Which assessment finding should the nurse identify as a complication of this treatment?
   1. Deep tendon reflex of +2. *This is an expected finding.*
   2. Urine output of 70 mL/hour. *This is normal.*
   3. Blood pressure of 148/94 mmHg. *This is elevated but would not be caused by the magnesium sulfate.*
   4. 💡 Respiratory rate of 10 bpm.

   Rationale: Magnesium Sulfate toxicity can cause a depressed respiratory rate and respiratory arrest. Respirations of 10 bpm are below the normal rate of 12 bpm.

   THIN Thinking: Identify Risk to Safety – *Respiratory rate of 10 bpm indicates inadequate oxygenation due to respiratory depression as a side effect of magnesium sulfate. Early identification of adverse side effects will improve client outcomes and decrease risk for injury.* NCLEX®: Pharmacological and Parenteral Therapies QSEN: Safety

5. A 14-week pregnant primigravida client reports that she is extremely nauseous. What is the best nursing response?
   1. "You should try to avoid eating between meals." *Frequent small meals is best.*
   2. "This is reassuring that the pregnancy is developing." *Nausea is unrelated to how the pregnancy is developing.*
   3. "You should try to eat a diet high in fat." *High-fat diet will not affect nausea.*
   4. 💡 "You should try to eat something bland every 2 -3 hours."

Rationale: Small, frequent and bland meals will reduce nausea. A diet high in fat and avoiding snacks will not affect nausea. Although nausea is a side effect of the hormone Human Chorionic Gonadotropin from the developing pregnancy, this does not address the client's need.

THIN Thinking: Help Quick – *Eating bland food in small amounts more frequently will help decrease nausea. High-fat diet or not eating will not resolve the problem and may increase the duration of nausea.* **NCLEX®:** Basic Care and Comfort **QSEN:** Evidence-based Practice

6. **A laboring client is being prepared for an emergency cesarean section. The nurse should immediately report which client data?**
   1. The client's membranes ruptured 2 hours ago. *This does not cause a complication for surgery.*
   2. The client's platelets are 200,000/mcl. *This is a normal value.*
   3. 🔘 The client reported having a meal 4 hours ago.
   4. The client is RH negative. *This does not cause a complication for surgery.*

Rationale: The client is at risk for aspiration if general anesthesia is utilized. The health care provider should be notified. The rupture of membranes, platelet level, and RH status do not need to be reported immediately.

THIN Thinking: Identify Risk to Safety – *Clients should not eat before surgery because of risk for aspiration related to general anesthesia. Identifying that the client ate 4 hours ago will allow proper interventions to be implemented.* **NCLEX®:** Reduction of Risk Potential **QSEN:** Safety

7. **Which statement made by a client with human papillomavirus (HPV) should the nurse correct?**
   1. "There is a vaccination available for some strains of this virus." *Vaccine is available.*
   2. "There are not always symptoms associated with HPV." *HPV does not always have symptoms.*
   3. 🔘 "I can only shed the virus when I have lesions present."
   4. "HPV can be transferred to an infant during delivery." *HPV can be transmitted to an infant during delivery.*

Rationale: The HPV virus can be shed even when there are not lesions present. The other options are all correct.

THIN Thinking: Nursing Process – *Education is needed that HPV can be transmitted despite the absence of lesions. Educating the client about the spread of HPV will help the client understand the need to use protection to decrease the spread of the virus.* **NCLEX®:** Health Promotion and Maintenance **QSEN:** Evidence-based Practice

8. **A client delivered a baby 2 months ago. The significant other calls into the office to report that his wife is angry, confused, and having conversations with herself. What is the appropriate response that the nurse should make?**
   1. 🔘 "Please take your wife to the emergency room for evaluation."
   2. "Please bring your wife to the office for medication." *Client requires hospitalization.*
   3. "Your wife will require outpatient care." *Client requires hospitalization.*
   4. "Your wife will require behavioral therapy." *Client requires hospitalization.*

Rationale: The symptoms are consistent with postpartum psychosis. The client is at risk to harm herself or others and needs immediate supervision and hospitalization.

THIN Thinking: Identify Risk to Safety – *Knowing the symptoms of postpartum psychosis will allow for early identification and treatment to prevent injury to self or others. Educating family members what adverse signs to be aware of is also important in implementing early interventions.* **NCLEX®:** Psychosocial Integrity **QSEN:** Safety

9. **An infant is breastfeeding for the first time. Which nursing statement will reduce the client's risk for skin breakdown?**
   1. "You should wear waterproof pads inside your bra." *Retains moisture which can cause skin breakdown.*
   2. 🔘 "You should insert your finger into the baby's mouth before removing the baby from your breast."
   3. "You should breastfeed every four hours." *Should breast feed every 2-3 hours.*
   4. "You should only breastfeed from one breast at each feeding and begin feeding with the opposite breast at the next feeding." *Both breasts should be nursed at each feeding.*

Rationale: Before removing a baby from her breast, the mother should break the seal by inserting her finger into the baby's mouth. Failure to do this technique will cause skin trauma. Waterproof pads will harbor moisture and cause skin breakdown. Breastfeeding should be done every 2 to 3 hours and each feeding should include both breasts.

THIN Thinking: Nursing Process – *Education will promote healthy habits to prevent skin break down which will decrease risk for further complications.* **NCLEX®:** Basic Care and Comfort **QSEN:** Evidence-based Practice

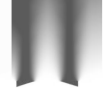

10. **A nurse is preparing to administer Rho (D) immune globulin to a client who delivered a baby yesterday. The nurse recognizes that the treatment is indicated by which client data?**
    1. 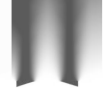 The indirect Coombs test is negative.
    2. The mother is RH positive. *Only needed if mom is Rh negative.*
    3. The infant is RH negative. *Only needed if infant is Rh positive.*
    4. The indirect Coombs test is positive. *Only needed if test is negative.*

    Rationale: Rho (D) immune globulin is indicated when the mom is RH negative, the infant is Rh positive, and the indirect Coombs test is negative.

    THIN Thinking: Nursing Process – *Collecting information from assessments and understanding Rh labs values will help the nurse identify a negative Coombs test as warranting administration of the Rho (D) immune globulin.* **NCLEX®:** Pharmacological and Parenteral Therapies **QSEN:** Evidence-based Practice

11. **A laboring client has been prescribed Nitrous Oxide for pain management during labor. To ensure that the client will not overdose, what action will the nurse make?**
    1. Instruct the client to self-administer the medication.
    2. Instruct the client to inhale every 30 minutes. *Would not provide sufficient pain management.*
    3. Assess if the client is experiencing nausea. *Not related to over dosing.*
    4. Ensure that the medication antidote is available. *No antidote.*

    Rationale: Nitrous Oxide is administered by inhaling the gas and an Oxygen mix through a mask. Self-administration makes it nearly impossible for the client to overdose.

    THIN Thinking: Identify Risk to Safety – *Through self-administration of nitrous oxide, the risk for overdose decreases significantly. Self-administration allows the client to use the nitrous during contractions or intense times of pain.* **NCLEX®:** Pharmacology **QSEN:** Safety

12. **When should a nurse instruct a client in the second stage of labor to start pushing?**
    1. Once the infant's head is below the ischial spines. *This is not an indication.*
    2. When the client feels the urge to push.
    3. When early decelerations are seen on the fetal monitor. *Decelerations do not impact timing to push.*
    4. When late decelerations are seen on the fetal monitor. *Decelerations do not impact timing to push.*

    Rationale: A client in the second stage of labor should begin pushing when she feels the Ferguson reflex or the urge to push. The infant's station or decelerations are not an indication for the client to push.

    THIN Thinking: Nursing Process – *Proper education during labor ensures the highest-quality care possible for the mother and baby.* **NCLEX®:** Health Promotion **QSEN:** Evidence-based Practice

13. **A pregnant client is asking a nurse about how she should wear her seatbelt while in the car. Which should be the nurse's response?**
    1. "You should wear the lower lap belt across the middle of your abdomen and the upper shoulder belt above the top of your pregnant belly." *This positioning could cause injury.*
    2. "You should not wear the seatbelt because it can harm the baby if an accident occurs." *Seatbelts are important for safety.*
    3. "You should wear the lower lap belt below your belly and push the shoulder belt across your abdomen." *This positioning would not provide good protection.*
    4. "You should wear the lower belt below your belly and push the upper shoulder belt above your belly."

    Rationale: During pregnancy the mother should wear her seatbelt. The lower lap belt should be placed below her abdomen and across the pelvic bones. The upper shoulder belt should be worn above the gravid uterus.

    THIN Thinking: Identify Risk to Safety – *Educating on proper belt placement will help the mother safely protect herself and the baby during car rides.* **NCLEX-RN®** Safety and Infection Control **QSEN:** Safety

14. **A nurse is caring for a client with Chlamydia Trachomatis. Which statement is true about this infection?**
    1. It is the most commonly reported sexually transmitted infection in American women.
    2. It is more common in men than in women. *More common in women.*
    3. The infection causes a thick white discharge. *Not a common symptom.*
    4. It is most common in women over 30 years of age. *Most common in women ages 15-24.*

    Rationale: Chlamydia Trachomatis is the most commonly reported sexually transmitted infection in American women. The infection is more common in sexually active women ages 15 to 24. The infection can cause a purulent discharge but is often asymptomatic.

THIN Thinking: Nursing Process – *Through knowledge and assessments the nurse will understand the prevalence of chlamydia infections in American women.* **NCLEX®:** Health Promotion and Maintenance **QSEN:** Evidence-based Practice

15. **A nurse observes a client sitting and watching a visitor hold her baby. The client states that her son "looks just like his daddy". Which bonding behavior should the nurse document?**
    1. Mutuality. *This is not the behavior demonstrated.*
    2. 💡 Claiming.
    3. En-Face position. *This is not the behavior demonstrated.*
    4. Rhythm. *This is not the behavior demonstrated.*

    Rationale: Claiming is a bonding behavior that occurs when the client claims a trait or characteristic looks like a member of the family's trait or behavior.

    THIN Thinking: Nursing Process – *Understanding of different bonding behaviors will help the nurse identify the client is experiencing claiming through the client's comment.* **NCLEX®:** Psychosocial Integrity **QSEN:** Evidence-based Practice

16. **A nurse documents assessment changes that occur in the integumentary system with pregnancy. Select all the pregnancy related integumentary changes below: Select all that apply.**
    1. Diastasis Recti. *This is a musculoskeletal change.*
    2. 💡 Striae Gravidarum.
    3. 💡 Linea Nigra.
    4. Lordosis. *This is a musculoskeletal change.*
    5. 💡 Melasma.

    Rationale: Pregnancy related integumentary changes include striae gravidarum, linea nigra, and melasma. Diastasis recti and lordosis are changes that occur within the musculoskeletal system during pregnancy.

    THIN Thinking: Nursing Process – *Understanding the physical changes during pregnancy and the outcome of those changes will help the nurse identify the integumentary changes. Melasma is because of hormone changes; striae gravidarum and linea nigra are due to the expansion of the abdomen.* **NCLEX®:** Health Promotion **QSEN:** Evidence-based Practice

17. **A nurse is caring for a client in the fourth stage of labor. Which nursing interventions are appropriate for a client who is experiencing postpartum hemorrhage? Select all that apply.**
    1. 💡 Weigh the client's pads.
    2. 💡 Administer a uterotonic drug.
    3. 💡 Massage the client's fundus.
    4. Discontinue the client's indwelling urinary catheter. *Removing the catheter would not help control the hemorrhage.*
    5. 💡 Express any clots in the uterus.

    Rationale: Nursing care for a client who is experiencing postpartum hemorrhage should include weighing the pads to obtain a more accurate blood loss level. A massaged fundus, expression of clots and the administration of a uterotonic drug will cause the uterus to contract. The bladder should be kept empty and so an indwelling urinary catheter should remain inserted to avoid the bladder placing pressure on the uterus.

    THIN Thinking: Top Three – *Decrease bleeding as soon as possible to prevent further complications. It also important to note how much blood is being lost, therefore, the client's pad needs to be weighed.* **NCLEX®:** Physiologic Adaptation **QSEN:** Safety

18. **Which nursing interventions for a non-breastfeeding postpartum client will hinder the milk production? Select all that apply.**
    1. 💡 The client is wearing a tight-fitting bra.
    2. The client is using warm compresses on her breasts. *This increases blood flow and helps with milk production.*
    3. The client is wearing a loose-fitting bra. *Tight-fitting bras or tops reduce breast swelling and milk production.*
    4. 💡 The client is using ice or cold compresses to her breasts.
    5. The client massages her breasts in the shower. *This increases blood flow and helps with milk production.*

    Rationale: A non-breastfeeding client should avoid warmth on her breasts. Cold compresses or ice, and a tight-fitting bra, will all decrease breast swelling and the promotion of further milk production.

    THIN Thinking: Nursing Process – *Educating the mother on what hinders milk production helps the client avoid bad habits and produce an adequate amount of milk for the baby. Tight fitting bras and cold compresses will decrease milk production. Loose fitting bras will not provide the support needed.* **NCLEX®:** Reduction of Risk Potential **QSEN:** Evidence-based Practice

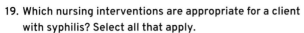

19. **Which nursing interventions are appropriate for a client with syphilis? Select all that apply.**
    1. Educate the client that this infection cannot be cured. *This disease can be cured if detected in first stage.*
    2. Educate the client that there is a cure for syphilis at any stage.
    3. Assessment for a maculopapular rash on the palms, trunk or soles.
    4. Assess the client for adenopathy. *Does not occur in first stage.*
    5. Educate the client that this infection is caused by a fungus.

    Rationale: Syphilis is caused by a bacterial spirochete. If treated in the first stage it can be cured. If allowed to progress to the secondary stage, a maculopapular rash can appear on the palms, trunk, or soles and adenopathy can occur.

    THIN Thinking: Nursing Process – *Implementing the nursing process suggests that assessments need to be done to know what interventions need to be implemented. Knowing what assessment findings to expect when a client has a diagnosis of syphilis will help the nurse focus on priorities.* **NCLEX®:** Safety and Infection Control **QSEN:** Evidence-based Practice

20. **A client is admitted to labor and delivery and experiences a gush of fluid coming from her vagina. In which order should the nurse implement these interventions? Rank order the responses.**
    1. Assess the fetal heart rate.
    2. Place the client on bedrest.
    3. Assess the color of the fluid.
    4. Assess the fluid with nitrazine paper.
    5. Document the assessment findings.

    Rationale: Because there is risk of prolapse cord with the rupture of amniotic membranes, the nurse should assess the fetal heart rate first. The color of the fluid should be assessed to determine if there is meconium staining or infection. The nitrazine paper will turn blue when placed in amniotic fluid. These assessment findings should be documented after the appropriate care is administered.

    THIN Thinking: Top Three – *Understanding the ABCs when prioritizing is critical when working with a client who is pregnant. Always assess the fetal heart rate first with any signs of bleeding. Bleeding (circulation) could be an indicator of hemorrhage or possible buildup of blood in the uterus which would put stress on the baby or pressure on the umbilical cord.* **NCLEX®:** Physiological Adaptation **QSEN:** Safety

21. **Using the client chart exhibit below, determine which client information is accurate.**

    > Today's date – 4/10
    > Client – J. M.
    > D.O.B – 2/28/1995
    > G – 4 T-2 P-0 A-2 L-2
    > Estimated date of delivery – 6/1
    > Rubella titer 1:8

    1. The client may need a plan for childcare at home while she is in the hospital.
    2. The client will need a Rubella vaccination after the delivery. *Titer is positive indicating immunity.*
    3. The client will need education on basic infant care. *Client is an experienced mother.*
    4. The client's baby is due in February. *Baby is due in June.*

    Rationale: The GTPAL indicates the prenatal history including pregnancies, term pregnancies, preterm births, abortions, and living children. This client has 2 living children. She is immune to rubella and has experience in infant care with her previous 2 deliveries. The client's due date is June 1st.

    THIN Thinking: Nursing Process – *Assessment is key to understanding that the client already has a rubella titre which renders her immune and has two living children. Therefore, educating the client that planning ahead for childcare during the hospitalization may be needed.* **NCLEX®:** Management of Care **QSEN:** Evidence-based Practice

22. **A prescription for nalbuphine hydrochloride 10 mg IV every 3 hours for pain has been ordered for a laboring client. The medication is available in 20 mg/mL vials. How many mL(s) should the nurse administer each dose?**

    Answer: 0.5 mL

    Rationale: The medication is supplied 20 mg per mL. 10 mg will be 0.5 mL.

    THIN Thinking: Identify Risk to Safety – *Careful calculation of medications reduces the risk for overdosing or not providing adequate medication to reach a therapeutic effect. Safety is always the priority with medication administration.* **NCLEX®:** Pharmacological and Parenteral Therapies **QSEN:** Safety

23. A prescription for methylergonovine 0.2 mg IM has been ordered for a client in stage three of labor who is hemorrhaging. Using the chart exhibit below, determine why this medication is contraindicated.

> Client – J.L.
> DOB – 4/2/1990
> Allergies – Penicillin
> G-5- T-4 P-0 A-0 L-4
> Vitals – T-98.6°F P-128 R-22 B/P-155/95
> Medications—Methyldopa 250 mg orally every 8 hours

1. The medication is contraindicated due to the multigravidity of the client. *Not a contraindication.*
2. The medication is contraindicated due to the client's drug allergy. *No allergy to drug noted.*
3. 💡 The medication is contraindicated due to the client's blood pressure.
4. The medication is contraindicated due to the client's heart rate. *Heart rate not a contraindication.*

Rationale: Methylergonovine is contraindicated if the client's blood pressure is 140/90 or higher.

THIN Thinking: Identify Risk to Safety – *Methylergonovine causes uterine contractions which slow or stop bleeding. It also increases blood pressure. Assessing blood pressure before administering the medication can identify risk for possible hypertensive crisis with the medication.* **NCLEX®:** Pharmacological and Parenteral Therapies **QSEN:** Safety

24. A client delivers quickly, and a preheated infant warmer is not ready. The infant is placed on the cool surface. The nurse recognizes that the infant will lose heat by which mechanism?
1. Convection. *Movement of heat through movement.*
2. 💡 Conduction.
3. Evaporation. *Change in temperature from water evaporating.*
4. Radiation. *Emission of heat from a heated body.*

Rationale: The mechanism of heat loss when the infant is placed on a cool surface is conduction.

THIN Thinking: Nursing Process – *Understanding how conduction effects the infant's temperature is crucial because of their sensitivity to temperature, especially in neonates. Placing a baby on a cool surface will cause heat loss through conduction which is dangerous for the baby.* **NCLEX®:** Physiological Adaptation **QSEN:** Evidence-based Practice

25. A nurse is implementing a non-stress test on a 37-week pregnant client. She observes a baseline fetal heart rate of 140-145 bpm. The heart rate raises to 160 bpm for 3 different 20 second periods over 30 minutes. What is the next nursing action?
1. Administer a vibro-acoustic stimulation to the maternal abdomen. *Unnecessary.*
2. Offer the client some juice to drink. *Unnecessary.*
3. Instruct the client that you will have to continue to monitor her. *Test is completed.*
4. 💡 Remove the client from the fetal monitor.

Rationale: The non-stress test is reactive because the fetal heart rate rose by at least 15 bpm and lasted for 15 seconds at least twice in a 20- minute period. The test is complete.

THIN Thinking: Nursing Process – *Analyzing the data provided from the non-stress test, the nurse identifies that the results are expected. Educating the pregnant client about the results along with removing the fetal monitor from the client are the actions the nurse should take at this time.* **NCLEX®:** Physiological Adaptation **QSEN:** Evidence-based Practice

26. A male client with a history of diabetes asks the nurse if his diabetes can affect his ability to get an erection. The correct nursing response is?
1. 💡 "Yes, diabetes can increase the risk of erectile dysfunction."
2. "No, there is no correlation between diabetes and erectile dysfunction." *False statement.*
3. "Diabetes can affect erectile dysfunction if you are taking insulin." *Doesn't matter if client is insulin dependent or not.*
4. "Most causes of erectile dysfunction are not related to physical causes." *Untrue.*

Rationale: Diabetes is an organic cause of erectile dysfunction.

THIN Thinking: Nursing Process – *Educating the client about the causes of erectile dysfunction helps the client understand that diabetes may be related to erectile dysfunction. Not all people with diabetes have erectile dysfunction but it increases the risk of the problem.* **NCLEX®:** Health Promotion and Maintenance **QSEN:** Evidence-based Practice

27. The fetal monitor of a laboring client shows that the fetal heart rate decreases after the peak of a contraction and does not recover until after the contraction is over. The nurse interprets this pattern as what type of fetal deceleration?
    1. Early fetal deceleration. *This would occur before peak of contraction.*
    2. Variable fetal deceleration. *It is consistent.*
    3. Prolonged fetal deceleration. *No prolonged affect.*
    4. 💡 Late fetal deceleration.

    Rationale: The fetal monitor pattern described is a late fetal deceleration. The deceleration began after the peak of the contraction and did not recover until the contraction was over.

    THIN Thinking: Nursing Process – *Understanding the differences between early, late, prolonged and variable decelerations helps the nurse identify any problems with the infant. Late decelerations indicate the infant may be hypoxic; therefore, quick identification of the deceleration is crucial.* NCLEX®: Reduction of Risk Potential QSEN: Evidence-based Practice

28. Which client would be appropriate to assign to a maternity nurse who has been pulled to the medical-surgical unit?
    1. 💡 A client post-appendectomy.
    2. A client after a cesarean section on a ventilator. *This nurse would not have expertise in caring for a ventilator.*
    3. A postoperative client with chest tubes. *This nurse would not have experience with chest tubes.*
    4. A client post-stroke receiving tissue plasminogen activator. *This nurse may not be familiar with how to monitor this client.*

    Rationale: Maternity nurses are capable of providing care to abdominal surgery client due to their experience with cesarean sections. A maternity nurse should not take care of client on a ventilator or have chest tubes or is receiving TPA.

    THIN Thinking: Identify Risk to Safety – *When delegating clients to nurses floated to a different unit, the best choice would be clients with similar medical conditions as they are used to on their home unit. Assigning the maternity nurse a client with ventilators, chest tubes or TPA could put the client at risk because of the lack of recent training.* NCLEX®: Management of Care QSEN: Teamwork and Collaboration

29. The nurse is counseling a client who is asking about sildenafil. The client wants to know how this works. What is the best response by the nurse?
    1. Sildenafil helps to increase the production of male hormones. *False.*
    2. The medication protects against sexually transmitted infections. *Has no effect on STIs.*
    3. This medication prevents unintended pregnancy. *Drug does not prevent pregnancy.*
    4. 💡 Sildenafil increases blood flow and sustains an erection.

    Rationale: Sildenafil increases penile engorgement to attain and maintain an erection. It increases blood supply and does not impact pregnancy, STIs, or hormone levels.

    THIN Thinking: Nursing Process – *Educating the client about the medication is important and is a primary responsibility of the nurse. Explaining the reaction of the medication in addition to the fact that it does not protect the client from STIs or prevent pregnancy helps the client identify the need for further actions if necessary.* NCLEX®: Pharmacological and Parenteral Therapies QSEN: Evidence-based Practice

30. A nurse is discussing body changes during menopause with a group of women. One woman asks why sexual intercourse is painful in menopause. Which is the best response by the nurse?
    1. "The woman's testosterone levels drop making the vaginal tissue dry and irritated." *This does not affect vaginal dryness.*
    2. "Sexual intercourse happens less during this age which leads to painful penetration." *This would not lead to thinner, dryer vaginal walls.*
    3. "Many women believe intercourse is more painful but these is no physiological reason for this." *This is a real issue, with physiological origins, for many women.*
    4. 💡 "The vaginal tissue loses it elasticity and becomes dry making penetration painful."

    Rationale: Dyspareunia may occur during hormonal changes of menopause. The vaginal walls become thinner, drier, and less lubricated.

    THIN Thinking: Top Three – *Since menopause causes thinning of the vaginal walls and dryness of membranes the clients need to be advised that precautions need to be taken to prevent damage during sexual intercourse. Education is important in this situation.* NCLEX®: Health Promotion and Maintenance QSEN: Patient-centered Care

Circulation

Perfusion / Clotting

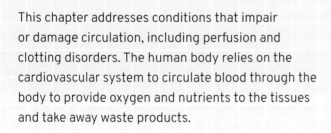

This chapter addresses conditions that impair or damage circulation, including perfusion and clotting disorders. The human body relies on the cardiovascular system to circulate blood through the body to provide oxygen and nutrients to the tissues and take away waste products.

Next Gen Clinical Judgment

Priority focused assessments are an essential part of nursing practice and clinical judgment. Recognizing cues quickly and responding accordingly are central to nursing care. Find a mirror and note three assessment findings that indicate you have effective central perfusion (e.g. brain, heart, and renal). The observe two of your limbs for effective peripheral perfusion. Now try this out with a friend. Remembering these basics of perfusion can help with many exam questions.

Nurses play a significant role in assessing for changes in circulation and perfusion, anticipating changes in clotting and circulation, and providing interventions to enhance or restore circulation.

Priority Exemplars:

> Shock
> Heart failure
> Cardiomyopathy
> Coronary artery disease
> Myocardial infarction/Acute coronary syndrome
> Peripheral artery disease
> Buerger's/Raynaud's
> Hypertension
> Stroke
> Valvular heart disease
> Venous thromboembolism
> Pulmonary embolism
> Disseminated intravascular coagulation (DIC)

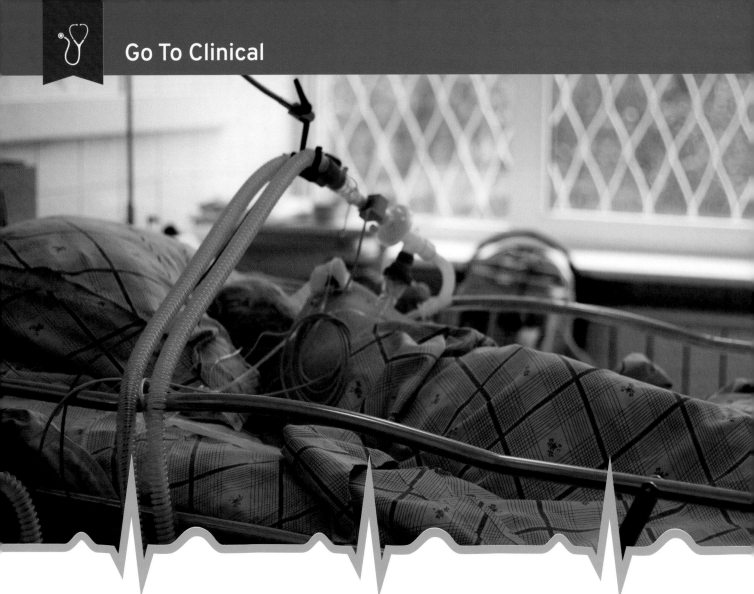

Go To Clinical Case 1

A client is admitted to the post-anesthesia care unit (PACU) following a posterior spinal fusion. The client sustained a 2300 mL estimated blood loss, with 1000 mL blood product replaced in the operating room. The client has stable vital signs and is on a mechanical ventilator when arriving. The client has a large back incision and is prescribed to remain on his back (in supine position) for eight hours post-surgery.

He has a urinary catheter in place (no urine output noted since the surgery), 2 peripheral intravenous lines, and an arterial line in place. He has clear breath sounds, good aeration to all lobes, and his pulse oximeter reads a pulse of 86 beats/minute and a saturation of 94%.

The client is pale and is nasally intubated. The client's admission BP was 118/76 mmHg. His baseline BP in the electronic health record is 130/80 mmHg.

The nurse is conducting an assessment and notes that the arterial line wave is dampened and the client's blood pressure is now 96/82.

Additional vital signs include temperature of 99.6°F and a pulse of 110 beats per minute. Ventilator set at 15 breaths/minute. The client is not breathing spontaneously.

NurseThink® Time

Using the NurseThink® system, complete the priorities. Check your answers designated by 💡 in the Shock Priority Exemplar.

✏ Priority Assessments or Cues

1.

2.

3.

⚗ Priority Laboratory Tests/Diagnostics

1.

2.

3.

⚠ Priority Interventions or Actions

1.

2.

3.

⚑ Priority Potential & Actual Complications

1.

2.

3.

℞ Priority Nursing Implications

1.

2.

3.

◌ Priority Medications

1.

2.

3.

👤 Priority Education/Discharge Issues

1.

2.

3.

Shock

Pathophysiology/Description

> Shock is decreased perfusion yielding inadequate blood flow to the tissues with decreased oxygen and nutrients, impaired cellular metabolism, and buildup of CO_2

> Stages include compensatory, progressive, and irreversible

> Cardiogenic includes reductions in cardiac output, largely related to left ventricular failure (MI), inability of the heart to fill, dysrhythmias, and structural factors

> Hypovolemic includes decrease in circulating blood flow related to loss of blood or other body fluids, fluid shifts, or internal bleeding (may be absolute or relative)

> Septic/Neurogenic/Anaphylactic are secondary to vasodilation related to infection, spinal cord injury/anesthesia, or hypersensitivity

Priority Assessments or Cues

> Identify early and manage clients at risk to prevent shock

> General shock signs/symptoms

> > Early signs include tachycardia, anxious appearance, confusion, tachypnea, restlessness, impaired end organ perfusion (prolonged capillary refill, weak peripheral pulses, changes in sensation/motor function, skin color and temperature changes), hypoactive bowel sounds

> > Later signs include tachycardia, hypotension, changes in level of consciousness, changes in urine output, narrowing pulse pressure

> - Assess mean arterial pressure (MAP). Calculated=SBP+ (2 X DBP)/3. Value of 70 ensures adequate cardiac output and peripheral vascular resistance

> Cardiogenic

> - Crackles in the lung fields, may have chest pain, nausea or vomiting

> Hypovolemic

> > Tachypnea may progress to bradypnea

> Distributive: Septic/Neurogenic/Anaphylactic

> - Septic signs include bradycardia, skin may be warm and flushed

> - Neurogenic signs include dysfunction will correlate with level of insult or injury (bladder dysfunction)

> - Anaphylactic signs include shortness of breath, stridor, wheezing, incontinence, swelling

Priority Laboratory Tests/Diagnostics

> General: Assess CBC, electrolytes, and arterial blood gases

> Hemodynamic monitoring: Arterial pressure, central venous pressure, PA pressure

> Cardiogenic

> - BNP (brain natriuretic protein levels) (< 100 pg/mL–HF unlikely; >400 pg/mL–HF likely; 100-400 pg/mL–use clinical judgment)
> - ECG (dysrhythmias)
> - CXR
> - Echocardiogram

> Hypovolemic

> > Decreased Hgb and Hct
> > Elevated urine specific gravity

> Septic

> - Elevated white blood cell count, glucose, lactate levels
> - Positive blood cultures
> - Elevated urine specific gravity
> - ABC's to rule out pulmonary embolus or disease

Priority Interventions or Actions

> General: Early identification and eliminate cause

> > Provide high flow oxygen and ventilatory support

> > IV access and fluid resuscitation with crystalloids (normal saline and, less commonly, lactated ringers) and colloids (albumin), insert nasogastric tube and urinary catheter-provide bolus of fluids along with maintenance fluids

> - Warm fluids to prevent hypothermia and dysrhythmias

> Hypovolemic

> > Replace blood volume with packed RBCs and clotting factors

> Septic

> - Antibiotics

> Control of dysrhythmias

> Increase cardiac contractility with sympathomimetics and vasodilators

> Early initiation of enteral feedings and monitor client weight

Priority Potential & Actual Complications

> Systemic inflammatory response syndrome (SIRS)

> Multiorgan system failure

> Renal failure

> Dependence on mechanical ventilation

> Neurological changes secondary to anoxia

> May be fatal (high mortality rate)

Priority Nursing Implications

- 💡 Be attuned for subtle changes in client's neurological status that may be a result of poor perfusion—early signs may be agitation and restlessness—safety measures with changes in level of consciousness

- 💡 Assess I & O and hydration status/perfusion status and assess urine output (0.5 mL/kg/hour)

- 💡 Assess bowel sounds and abdominal girth

- ❯ Assess nasogastric tube drainage and stools for occult blood—stress ulcer prophylaxis as needed

- ❯ Early nasogastric/enteral feedings are associated with improved prognosis

- ❯ Assess client's temperature and manage environmental temperature closely

- ❯ Provide basic care (bathing, oral hygiene, and turning/positioning) to avoid complications

- ❯ Assess allergen in cases of anaphylactic shock

Priority Medications

- ❯ dobutamine
  - With cardiogenic/septic shock-increases cardiac output
  - Use a central line to avoid tissue sloughing
  - Monitor vital signs-watch for hypotension
  - Assess for tachyrhythmias

- ❯ dopamine
  - Cardiogenic and septic shock
  - Use a central line to avoid tissue sloughing
  - Monitor vital signs-watch for hypotension
  - Assess for changes in peripheral circulation (vasoconstriction)

- ❯ epinephrine
  - Cardiogenic, anaphylactic, and septic shock
  - Monitor for tachycardia
  - Assess for changes in respiratory status (dyspnea, chest pain)
  - Assess renal function

- ❯ sodium nitroprusside
  - Cardiogenic shock
  - Monitor blood pressure
  - Protect from light, wrap tubing with foil
  - Administer with D_5W

- ❯ atropine
  - To treat bradycardia with septic shock

- ❯ corticosteroids
  - To reduce inflammation after acute period

Priority Education/Discharge Issues

- ❯ Depending upon etiology of shock, instruct client on: Allergies/allergy bracelet, safety and injury prevention, hydration and monitoring of fluids, rest and activity moderation with cardiac disease

- ❯ Engage multidisciplinary team to recondition the client after a critical illness

- ❯ Engage family and support systems to set goals and motivate client with long-term recovery

Go To Clinical Answers

Text designated by 💡 are the top answers for the Go To Clinical related to Shock.

Type	Result	Goals of Medical Treatment
Cardiogenic	↓ Contractility	Medications to improve left ventricular function and improve perfusion
Hypovolemic	↓ Preload	Isotonic fluids for hydration; Blood if hemorrhaging; stop bleeding
Anaphylactic	↓ Afterload from histamine release	Medications to decrease further histamine release and support constricting airway
Septic	Systemic inflammatory response leads to vasodilation	Decrease toxins, treat infection while maintaining perfusion to vital organs
Neurogenic	Disruption of autonomic pathways from spinal cord injury that leads to vasodilation	Medications to counteract the loss sympathetic tone while improving perfusion to the body

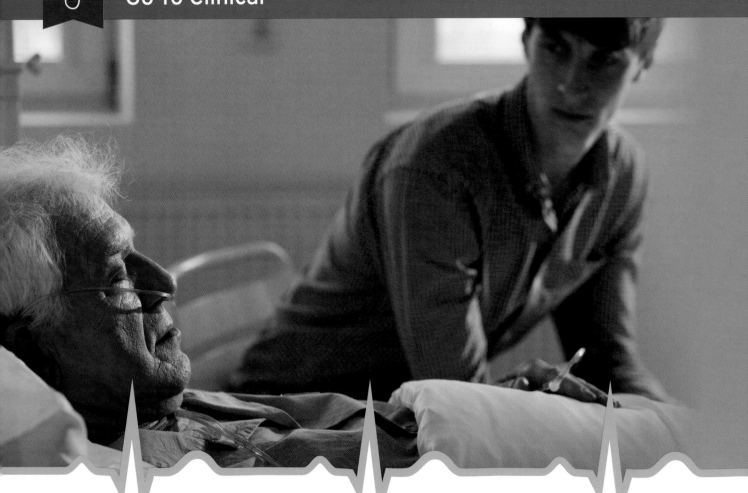

Go To Clinical Case 2

T.G. is a 93-year-old man who was diagnosed with heart failure at 85 years of age. He has a 50 year history of hypertension that has been well managed with spironolactone with hydrochlorothiazide. He has been treated with simvastatin for 30 years secondary to his high cholesterol levels. T.G. lives alone and is independent. He provides for all his own ADLs and IADLs and, although he no longer drives, he uses a subsidized transportation bus for his shopping, errands, and appointments.

For the last 10 days, T.G. has been feeling increasingly fatigued, short of breath, and displays marked edema in his ankles. He reports that he has been sleeping on 4-5 pillows at night, has little appetite, and when he coughs his "chest rattles."

T.G. has 4 children who live locally (one son with Down syndrome died at age 53), 16 grandchildren, and 4 great-grandchildren. His 2 sons are active in his care but are also busy with their careers.

Upon admission, T.G. is noted to weigh 12 pounds more than his baseline weight and is able to say 4-5 words without pausing. His color is pale and he has a stooped posture. T.G. receiving oxygen at 2 l/min. via nasal cannula.

The client's vital signs are 98.9°F—96-20-138/84. His oxygen saturation is 92%.

NurseThink® Time

Using the NurseThink® system, complete the priorities. Check your answers designated by 💡 in the Heart failure Priority Exemplar.

✏️ Priority Assessments or Cues

1.

2.

3.

🧪 **Priority Laboratory Tests/Diagnostics**

1.

2.

3.

⚠️ **Priority Interventions or Actions**

1.

2.

3.

🚩 **Priority Potential & Actual Complications**

1.

2.

3.

🩺 **Priority Nursing Implications**

1.

2.

3.

💧 **Priority Medications**

1.

2.

3.

👤 Priority Education/Discharge Issues

1.

2.

3.

Heart failure

Pathophysiology/Description

> Inadequate pumping/filling of the heart, insufficient blood to meet the oxygen needs of tissues. Impaired cardiac output from changes in preload, afterload, contractility, and heart rate

> Related to untreated hypertension/hypertension of long duration, coronary artery disease, myopathies and history of myocardial infarction, also age and health of the ventricles

> Increased incidence/increased life expectancy and improved survival rates of cardiac disease; equally in men and women, higher in African Americans

> Related to advanced age, obesity, high serum cholesterol, and tobacco use

> Described as systolic, diastolic, or mixed failure or left and right failure
> - Left-sided failure results in fluid in lung tissue/pleural circulation
> - Right-sided failure results in fluid in the periphery/systemic circulation

Priority Assessments or Cues

> Vital signs. Watch for increased respiratory rate (to increase oxygenation), increased heart rate (compensate for decreased cardiac output-blocked with clients on beta-blockers), monitor for hypotension (increased tissue perfusion or medication side effects) and hypertension (anxiety/history)

> Increased respiratory effort, cough (may be first sign), later-productive cough of blood-tinged sputum; breath sounds-decreased sounds, crackles, wheezes, rhonchi

> Edema may be dependent/peripheral, ascites, pulmonary edema/pleural effusion, pitting edema (1 kg. weight/1 liter fluid), assess perfusion in edematous extremities

> Variables from history including sleeps on several pillows or in a reclining chair (orthopnea; may experience paroxysmal nocturnal dyspnea), shortness of breath with exertion (dyspnea), levels of fatigue, history of nocturia, chest pain, or rapid fluid weight gain

> Appearance such as anxiety, paleness, cyanosis, confusion, restlessness

Priority Laboratory Tests/Diagnostics

> BNP (brain natriuretic protein levels) (< 100 pg/mL—HF unlikely; >400 pg/mL—HF likely; 100-400 pg/mL—use clinical judgment) NT-proBNP-< 300 ng/mL-HF unlikely

> Chest X-ray/arterial blood gases in acute phase

> ECG may show hypertrophy

> Cardiac ultrasound/cardiac catheterization

> Endomyocardial biopsy

> Ejection fraction studies

Priority Interventions or Actions

> Oxygen, support ventilation as needed, elevate head of bed to relieve dyspnea

> Monitor vital signs, ECG, oxygen saturation, urine output, daily or more frequent weights

> Cardiac rehabilitation, rest

> Cardiotonic/inotropic drugs

> Diuretics to reduce edema

> Fluid restrictions (based on hydration status)

> Low sodium diet

> Support and counseling for depression and anxiety

Priority Potential & Actual Complications

> Respiratory Distress secondary to pleural effusion

> Cardiac dysrhythmias

> Cardiogenic shock

> Skin breakdown with edema

> Left ventricular thrombus

> Hepatomegaly

> Renal failure

> Cardiopulmonary failure

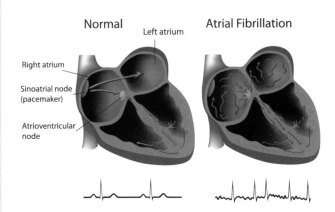

Image 6-1: Atrial fibrillation is often a part of heart failure. Describe the differences in the electrocardiogram with atrial fibrillation. List assessment findings you would expect if your client's ECG revealed atrial fibrillation.

_____

_____

_____

_____

Priority Nursing Implications

> Assess client for over- and dehydration, provide fluid restrictions if prescribed

> If on potassium-wasting diuretics, assess potassium levels, monitor serum electrolytes

> Comfort interventions and skin care with edema, elevate legs to relieve edema, use of compression stockings

> Provide information on a low-sodium, adequate potassium diet

> Provide a calm environment, reduce anxiety

> Prevention-management of hypertension and other coronary artery diseases

Priority Medications

> digoxin
  - Slow heart rate and strengthen contractility
  - Apical pulse for one minute prior to administration-hold for low heart rate (< 60 bpm for adults, <100 bpm for infants, as prescribed by healthcare provider for children)
  - Assess for signs of digoxin toxicity

> furosemide
  - Diuretic-reduce fluid volume
  - Assess output-diuresis
  - Serum potassium levels
  - Potassium chloride supplements or K+ rich foods

> milrinone
  - Phosphodiesterase inhibitor (PDE inhibitor)
  - Positive inotrope and vasodilator
  - Assess for ventricular dysrhythmias and hypotension

> lisinopril
  - Ace-inhibitor
  - Assess for cough
  - Assess for angioedema

> vasodilators
  - Nitroglycerine-decrease venous return and decrease preload and afterload, increase myocardial oxygen supply in acute heart failure
  - Watch for orthostatic hypotension

> potassium chloride
  - Potassium supplement

> In acute phases:
  - Provide morphine
  - Sedation and vasodilation

Priority Education/Discharge Issues

> Teach client to watch for FACES including fatigue, limitation of activity, cough and congestion, edema, and shortness of breath and based on client understanding, teach about disease and bodily changes

> Oxygen at home including portable devices, compressor, indications for use, assessing oxygen saturation

> Provide education about safe use of oxygen therapy

> Maintain weight within normal range for the individual and based on cultural insights

> Eat a potassium rich food each day including banana, orange juice in absence of potassium supplement

> Teach client to avoid high-sodium food sources including processed meats, canned foods, baked goods, snacks—teach about non-sodium flavor enhancers

> Rest and pace activities

> Daily weights on same scale with similar clothing/home blood pressure monitoring

> Reinforce collaborative plan to include smoking cessation, limiting alcohol, mild exercise, low sodium diet, moderate caffeine, and reduced saturated fats in foods

> Check with healthcare provider when considering over-the-counter medications and herbal preparations

> Educate on fall prevention and accessing emergency assistance

Clinical Hint

Congenital heart diseases are common causes of heart failure in infants and children related to abnormalities in structure and function (whether by shunting or obstructing blood flow or some combination of the two). Many are repaired or closed in surgery while using cardiopulmonary bypass or with cardiac catheterization.

Go To Clinical Answers

Text designated by 🔍 are the top answers for the Go To Clinical related to Heart failure.

Cardiomyopathy

Pathophysiology/Description

> Affects myocardial structure and function

> Disease of the heart muscle that makes it less able to pump blood to meet the needs of the body

> May be subacute or chronic

> May be primary or secondary (related to myocardial infarction, drug toxicity, hypertension, or infections)

> Three major types: Dilated, hypertrophic, and restrictive

> Leads to cardiomegaly, heart failure, valvular incompetence, dysrhythmias, and decreased cardiac output; leading indication for heart transplantation

Priority Assessments or Cues

> Ask client about fatigue, weakness, dyspnea, angina, palpitations, syncope, and exercise intolerance

> Assess heart sounds include S3 and S4 gallops, murmurs, dysrhythmias, exaggerated or displaced apical impulse (hypertrophic)

> Ask about history of infectious myocarditis or alcohol abuse (dilated), being an athlete (hypertrophic)

Priority Laboratory Tests/Diagnostics

> CXR may show cardiomegaly, pleural effusion

> ECG may show hypertrophy or dysrhythmias

> BNP(brain natriuretic protein levels) (< 100 pg/mL—HF unlikely; >400 pg/mL—HF likely; 100-400 pg/mL—use clinical judgment)

> Doppler echocardiography

> Endomyocardial biopsy, nuclear imaging studies (MUGA scan) to determine ejection fraction, or cardiac catheterization

Priority Interventions or Actions

> Often palliative, rather than curative treatment including management of heart failure

> Surgery with hypertrophic

> Nitrates and diuretics to reduce preload, ACE inhibitors to reduce afterload

> In late cases use of ventricular assist device or heart transplantation

> AV pacing-hypertrophic

Priority Potential & Actual Complications

> Heart failure may occur with all types of cardiomyopathy

> Varies with type including acute pulmonary edema (restrictive), emboli (dilated, restricted), sudden death (nonobstructed hypertrophic), atrial fibrillation (obstructed hypertrophic, ventricular dysrthythmias (dilated)

Priority Nursing Implications

> Monitor client related to activities and exercise—optimize positive effects but decrease stress on heart

> Teach client about medications and management strategies

> Often care is palliative and requires support and sensitivity to maximize quality of life and contentment

Priority Medications

> metoprolol
  - Beta-blocker (-ol)
  - Assess pulse
  - Cautious use with asthma, kidney disease, and COPD

> digitalis
  - Cardiac glycocide
  - Watch for toxicity
  - Hold for apical heart rate less than 60 bpm, take apical heart rate one full minute

> nifedipine, verapamil
  - Calcium channel blockers
  - Assess blood pressure and pulse

> lisinopril
  - Angiotensin-converting enzyme (ACE) inhibitors
  - Assess for benign, but nagging, cough

Priority Education/Discharge Issues

> Teach client to monitor for signs of heart failure including dyspnea, pedal edema, orthopnea, fatigue, weight gain

> Encourage adequate hydration (unless fluid restricted) and a low sodium diet, avoid large meals

> Avoid alcohol, caffeine, and other stimulants

> Encourage light exercise, avoiding heavy lifting or isometric exercises, and adequate rest

> Teach caregivers CPR

> May be at risk for infective endocarditis—prophylactic antibiotics

Coronary artery disease (CAD)

Pathophysiology/Description

> Deposits of lipids, endothelial injury, and inflammation within the intima of an artery

> Although known by many names, most symptomatic is atherosclerosis of the coronary arteries

> Progressive disease that develops in stages with fatty streaks (lipid deposits), fibrous plaques (changes in endothelium and reduction in blood flow), and complicated lesions (plaque ulceration and rupture, thrombus formation)

> Characterized by modifiable (elevated serum lipids, hypertension, tobacco use, physical inactivity, obesity), contributing/modifiable (diabetes mellitus, metabolic syndrome, stress/anger, high homocysteine levels, and substance abuse) and non-modifiable risk factors (age, gender, ethnicity, family history)

Priority Assessments or Cues

> Assess family history and for nonmodifiable risk factors

> Assess for symptoms of occlusion of a vessel (angina/MI) or poor perfusion

> Ask clients about modifiable risk factors and lifestyle

Priority Laboratory Tests/Diagnostics

> C-reactive protein is elevated with inflammation

> Serum cholesterol levels (Risk associated with total cholesterol >200 mg/dL; triglycerides >150 mg/dL; LDL >160 mg/dL; HDL <40 mg/dL in men; HDL <50 mg/dL in women)

> Fasting blood glucose >100 mg/dL increases risk

Priority Interventions or Actions

> Promote physical activity, optimal nutrition

> Smoking and substance use cessation

> Frequent monitoring of blood levels and risk assessment

Priority Potential & Actual Complications

> Acute coronary syndrome-unstable angina, MI

> Sudden cardiac may be fatal

Priority Nursing Implications

> Role in screening and assisting clients to manage modifiable and contributing modifiable risk factors

> Omega-3 fatty acids, niacin, psyllium and soy have been associated with reductions in serum cholesterol levels

> Lifestyle changes may be difficult for clients and require information, goal setting, enhanced motivation, and ongoing support

Priority Medications

> simvastatin
  - Antilipemic (statin)
  - Take at night to increase destruction of LDLs
  - May cause GI upset; avoid grapefruit and grapefruit juice
  - Watch for rhabdomyolysis which are extreme muscle aches (adverse reaction)

> niacin
  - Antilipemic
  - May cause significant flushing (may premedicate with NSAIDs or ASA)
  - May also cause GI side effects or orthostatic hypotension

> low dose aspirin
  - Antiplatelet
  - Assess for bleeding
  - Take with meals and assess for GI upset, potential ulcerative
  - Clients who don't tolerate ASA may consider clopidogrel

> ezetimibe
  - Inhibit cholesterol absorption
  - Should be taken along with dietary revision
  - May be combined with statin medications
  - Considered a lifetime medication choice

Priority Education/Discharge Issues

> Teach assets of moderate exercise (30 minutes/day on most days)

> Encourage ongoing attention to modifying lifestyle, regular blood work, and return to HCP for evaluation

> Teach about diet with decreased saturated fats (animal-based) and adequate amount of plant-based polyunsaturated fats

_____

_____

_____

_____

_____

_____

_____

Myocardial infarction (MI)/acute coronary syndrome

📋 Pathophysiology/Description

> MI is Ischemia and necrosis of myocardial tissue, often related to thrombus blockage of a coronary vessel, described based on vessel/location of damage dictates severity, severity also impacted by extent of collateral circulation

> Acute coronary syndrome includes unstable angina, non-ST segment elevation MI, and ST elevation MI

> Unstable angina is a medical emergency when there is a change from previous, chronic angina, and significant chest pain with little exertion and fatigue

✏️ Priority Assessments or Cues

> Assess vital signs and observe for elevated HR/RR, decreased or increased BP, decreased oxygen saturation

> Assess for chest pain. Assess for severe pain that is not relieved by rest, position change or nitrates, pain is described as heavy pressure on the chest or upper abdomen

> May include atypical presentations, for example, women may present with jaw or chin pain, fatigue, arm and chest pain, shortness of breath-leading to delays in treatment

> Observe end-organ perfusion in extremities, level of consciousness, urine output

> Ask about nausea/vomiting

> Observe for fever, diaphoresis, ashen/pale skin color, anxious appearance

🧪 Priority Laboratory Tests/Diagnostics

> ECG may show ST elevation, T wave inversion, abnormal Q waves

> Serum cardiac markers include cardiac specific troponin T/cardiac specific troponin I (increase 4-6 hours after MI, peak 10-24 hours, baseline 10-14 days), creatine kinase/creatine kinase MB (rise 6 hours after MI, peak at 18 hours, baseline 10-14 days), Myoglobin (rise 2 hours after MI and peak 3-15 hours)

> Coronary angiography

⚠️ Priority Interventions or Actions

> Bedrest with HOB elevated, establish IV access, progressive activity

> MONA (Morphine IV, Oxygen, Nitroglycerine SL, chewable Aspirin)

> Unstable angina with negative cardiac markers: Antiplatelets and heparin

> Reperfusion therapy
> • Interventional cardiac catheterization/percutaneous coronary intervention
> • Thrombolytics for MI (within 30 minutes of presentation--maximum 6 hours after symptoms)
> • Surgical revascularization (coronary artery bypass graft)

🚩 Priority Potential & Actual Complications

> Dysrhythmias, heart failure, or cardiogenic shock

> Papillary muscle dysfunction (leading to mitral valve dysfunction), ventricular aneurysm, pericarditis, Dressler syndrome (antibody-antigen response post-MI- includes pericarditis with fluid/effusion and fever)

> May be fatal

🤚 Priority Nursing Implications

> Have client rate pain and describe location, radiation, relieving and precipitating factors

> Monitor pulse oximetry and vital signs closely

> Relieve client stress and provide analgesics as needed

> Lower head of bed with hypotension

💧 Priority Medications

> nitroglycerine
> • (NTG)-IV or SL
> • Watch for hypotension
> • May become tolerant

> morphine
> • For chest pain unrelieved by NTG
> • Decrease chest pain and anxiety
> • Watch for respiratory depression or hypotension

> docusate sodium
> • Stool softeners
> • Bed rest and opioids
> • Prevent straining-Valsalva induced bradycardia

> Other medications may include antiplatelets, anticoagulants, beta blockers, angiotensin-converting enzyme inhibitors, thrombolytics, and aspirin

👤 Priority Education/Discharge Issues

> Cardiac rehabilitation including progressive exercise, recommendations on sexual activity, and diet low in cholesterol and sodium, high in fiber

> Teach to avoid stressful situations, abrupt changes in environmental temperature and heavy meals

> Instruct on management of angina and emergency care

> Teach about home use and safe storage of NTG

> Teach client about risk factors and the benefits of cessation of smoking, weight management, moderation in alcohol, and a diet low in fat/sodium/cholesterol and high in fiber

Peripheral artery disease (PAD)

Pathophysiology/Description

> The peripheral arteries become narrowed and thickened in the upper and lower extremities, causing changes in perfusion

> Changes occur distal to the level of the obstruction

> Related to diabetes, other cardiovascular disease (atherosclerosis), and lifestyle choices

> May be acute or chronic

Priority Assessments or Cues

> Ask about risk factors include tobacco use, diabetes, hyperlipidemia, and hypertension

> Consider family history, lifestyle (increased when sedentary), and levels of stress

> Assess for effected extremities including intermittent claudication, paresthesias, skin may be shiny, tight, with loss of hair, thickening of toenails, pulses decreased or absent, elevation pallor/dependent rubor, prolonged capillary refill, rest pain, and cool extremities

> Assess segmental blood pressures and note discrepancies

Priority Laboratory Tests/Diagnostics

> Assess for elevated C-reactive protein, serum lipid levels

> Duplex doppler imaging and doppler pulse readings

> Serum blood glucose levels and glycosylated hemoglobin (HgbA1c)

> Arteriogram or ankle-brachial index to determine severity of PAD

Priority Interventions or Actions

> Risk modification including smoking cessation, management of diabetes and hypertension

> Control of serum lipid levels including diet and medications

> Exercise, weight reduction, and dietary modification-walking programs

> Skin care-clean and inspect feet regularly, do not soak feet

> Keep feet dependent and without constriction to increase blood flow

> Ulcerations may require surgical or radiological revascularization-peripheral artery bypass graft or percutaneous transluminal angioplasty with or without a stent

> An acute occlusion requires revascularization or infarction/necrosis may result

Priority Potential & Actual Complications

> May progress to rest pain, ulceration, sepsis and/or gangrene, indicative of critical limb ischemia

> Gangrene and infection leading to potential amputation

> Acute arterial ischemia (sudden obstruction of blood flow caused by embolism, thrombosis, trauma, or atherosclerosis of artery)

Priority Nursing Implications

> Nurses should assess extremities thoroughly and frequently to detect changes early

> Provide skin care and refrain from soaking feet or hands to avoid maceration

> Position clients to avoid constriction; do not bend knees, use knee gatch, or cross legs

> Assess for and manage pain associated with obstruction and claudication

Priority Medications

> aspirin (ASA)
  - Antiplatelet
  - Doses of 75-325 mg/day
  - Watch for bleeding
  - Assess for GI upset

> clopidogrel
  - Antiplatelet
  - Watch for bleeding
  - Clients may receive clopidogrel with ASA following revascularization

> cilostazol
  - Inhibits platelet aggregation and is a vasodilator
  - Used for intermittent claudication
  - May require additional antiplatelet therapy (clopidogrel, dipyridamole)

Priority Education/Discharge Issues

> Teach about vigilant foot care, to wear white, all-cotton socks and to avoid extremes in temperature

> Provide client with a complete list of changes to watch for in circulation—appearance of feet and for changes in sensation or function

> Teach clients about optimal diet, to include: High fiber, high protein, low-fat, low refined sugars, reduce sodium intake and drink plenty of water; avoid caffeine

> Teach client to relieve extremity pain by placing limb dependent; if edema exists, legs may be elevated but not above level of the heart

Buerger's Disease and Raynaud's Phenomenon

Pathophysiology/Description

> Thromboangiitis obliterans (Buerger's Disease)
  - Recurrent arterial inflammation in arms and legs when thrombus blocks the vessel—causes thrombosis, fibrosis, and ischemia
  - More in men with histories of smoking tobacco or marijuana
  - Associated with chronic periodontal infections

> Raynaud's Phenomenon
  - Spastic, episodic inflammation of small, cutaneous arteries
  - More common in women
  - May occur alone or with arthritis or systemic lupus erythematosus
  - Increased with chronic exposure to cold, vibrating machinery, or heavy metals

Priority Assessments or Cues

> Thromboangiitis obliterans (Buerger's Disease)
  - Ask about intermittent claudication, pain at rest/aching pain most severe at night, paresthesias, cold sensitivity, and skin ulcerations
  - Assess changes in perfusion, pulses, skin temperature, lesions, and color--may be cool and red in dependent position

> Raynaud's Phenomenon
  - Assess perfusion in fingers, toes, nose, ears and cheeks-for temperature and color-pale to blue to purple
  - Assess recirculation after spasm for redness (rubor)
  - Client description of coldness and numbness/tingling followed by throbbing, aching pain, and swelling
  - Assess changes in skin and nails, assess for ulcers and lesions

Priority Laboratory Tests/Diagnostics

> Both conditions diagnosed based on symptoms, skin changes, and risk behaviors

Priority Interventions or Actions

> Thromboangiitis obliterans (Buerger's Disease)
  - Smoking cessation of tobacco and marijuana (nicotine replacement not an option)
  - Avoid triggers (tobacco, marijuana) progressive exercise, symptom management of skin lesions, and pain management

> Raynaud's Phenomenon
  - Avoid precipitating factors
  - Warm water soaks during vasoconstriction

Priority Potential & Actual Complications

> Thromboangiitis obliterans (Buerger's Disease)
  - Vascular occlusion, gangrene, and amputation

> Raynaud's Phenomenon
  - Ischemia requiring surgical debridement
  - In advanced cases of both sympathectomy done to transect the sympathetic nerve and relieve vasoconstriction

Priority Nursing Implications

> Assess skin breakdown and infections in clients at high-risk for peripheral vascular conditions
> Assist clients with smoking cessation or participation in vasoconstrictive activities

Priority Medications

> cilostazol
  - antiplatelet and vasodilator improve circulation (more effective with vasospasm than vessel occlusion)
  - Causes orthostatic hypotension
  - Not with alcohol-increases hypotension

> pentoxifylline
  - decreases viscosity of blood

> nifedipine
  - relax smooth muscles of the arterioles
  - calcium channel blockers

Priority Education/Discharge Issues

> Thromboangiitis obliterans (Buerger's Disease)
  - Permanent cessation of vasoconstrictive chemicals
  - Avoid trauma/infection

> Raynaud's Phenomenon
  - Teaching about triggers for episodes including avoiding emotional upset, exposure to cold, caffeine, cocaine, and tobacco
  - Teach to avoid restrictive clothing, extreme changes in exposure, and vasoconstrictive chemicals, to wear warm clothes when exposed to cold
  - Teach to soak toes and fingers in warm water during "attacks"
  - Stress management strategies

Next Gen Clinical Judgment

A nurse is teaching a client who is newly diagnosed with Raynaud's disease. In planning the teaching:

1. Which symptoms of this disease would the nurse emphasize in the instruction?

2. Which would the nurse teach the client that may relieve the symptoms of this disease?

3. How would the nurse evaluate effective teaching?

Hypertension

Pathophysiology/Description

> High blood pressure associated with genetic, physiological, and lifestyle factors
> May be primary or secondary
> Related to water and sodium retention, altered renin-angiotensin-aldosterone mechanism, stress and increased sympathetic nervous system activity, insulin resistance and hyperinsulinemia, and endothelium dysfunction

Priority Assessments or Cues

> Assess blood pressure in both arms and note differences, assess for orthostatic changes in blood pressure and may be diagnosed after two or more readings
> Use the correct size cuff, allow one minute between readings, and ensure that the arm is at the level of the heart for assessments
> Although associated with few symptoms, ask client about headaches, epistaxis, fatigue, angina, dizziness, anxiety, visual disturbances, or dyspnea
> Determine client's age and ethnicity, ask about family history, stress, and related medical history (diabetes, hypercholesterolemia)
> Determine weight and BMI (Body mass index)
> Discuss lifestyle including cigarette smoking, sodium intake, alcohol intake, level of activity and exercise, sedentary habits, and usual diet

Priority Laboratory Tests/Diagnostics

> Routine urinalysis, BUN and creatinine/creatinine clearance
> Basic metabolic panel/CBC
> Lipid profile
> ECG

Priority Interventions or Actions

> Weight reduction, low sodium diet, DASH diet (high in fruits and vegetables, low-fat meats and milk products, few sweets and added sugars)
> Smoking cessation and reduction in alcohol and caffeine intake
> Physical activity and stress management
> Antihypertensive medications

Priority Potential & Actual Complications

> Coronary artery disease, left ventricular hypertrophy, and heart failure
> Cerebrovascular disease and CVA (stroke)
> Peripheral vascular disease, nephrosclerosis, and retinal damage
> Hypertensive crisis

Priority Nursing Implications

> Assist with major lifestyle changes
> Reinforce need for treatment despite absence of symptoms

Priority Medications

> hydrochlorothiazide
  • Diuretics
  • Potassium-wasting-take potassium in diet or supplement
  • Orthostatic hypotension
> atenolol
  • Beta Blockers (end in -OL)
  • Monitor pulse and blood pressure
  • Contraindicated with asthma or COPD-bronchoconstriction
> lisinopril
  • ACE inhibitors (end in -pril)
  • Dry, hacking cough-benign side effect
  • NSAIDS and ASA may reduce effectiveness
  • Not with K sparing diuretics
> nifedipine, verapamil
  • Calcium channel blockers
  • Assess for headache, edema, and hypotension

Priority Education/Discharge Issues

> Watch for orthostatic hypotension and risk for falls
> Monitoring of blood pressure with phone apps, home monitoring
> Life-long treatment, adherence to medication regimen, and life style changes
> Explore use of fish oils and Omega-3 fatty acids
> Contact HCP before using OTC medications

Current Hypertension Guidelines in the Adult		
	SYSTOLIC	DIASTOLIC
Normal		
Elevated		
Stage 1		
Stage 2		
Crisis		

Table 6-1: Search the internet (www.heart.org) and complete this table.

Stroke-cerebrovascular accident (CVA)

Pathophysiology/Description

> Also called brain attack (conveys message of medical emergency), causes brain cell necrosis/infarction
> Effects and prognosis depends upon location and extent of brain damage
> Increasing incidence with aging population
> Risk factors
  • Non-modifiable include age, gender, race/ethnicity, and family history/heredity
  • Modifiable include hypertension, heart disease, diabetes, hypercholesterolemia, smoking, alcohol abuse, cocaine, abdominal obesity, physical activity, high estrogen/progestin oral contraceptives, sickle cell disease, dysrhythmias (atrial fibrillation)
> Types:
  • Ischemic stroke
    - Thrombotic occlusion of a vessel-related to hypertension and diabetes, often preceded by a TIA (transient ischemic attack)
    - Embolic in which thrombus from heart or elsewhere travels to cerebral vessel and lodges, rapid progression
  • Hemorrhagic is bleeding into the brain tissues, intracerebral, subarachnoid, cerebral aneurysm—related to hypertension, poor prognosis

Priority Assessments or Cues

> Assess vital signs and neurological status by checking pupils (dilation), blood pressure
> Assess for motor changes contralateral to site of brain cell death, visual changes, weakness, hemiparesis, numbness, loss of sensation, facial drooping, tinnitus, vertigo, darkened or blurred vision, diplopia, ptosis, dysphagia, dysarthria, ataxia, aphasia, headache ("the worst of my life"), nausea/vomiting, loss of bowel/bladder function, change in level of consciousness/cognitive abilities/changes in affect/memory limitations, spatial/perceptual alterations (homonymous hemianopsia)
> Assess for transient ischemic attacks (TIA) which are short-term changes in neurological function without brain infarction (1/3 TIA victims have a stroke, 1/3 have additional TIAs, 1/3 have no further effects)

Priority Laboratory Tests/Diagnostics

> CT Scan or MRI (serial CT scans for progress)
> CT angiography or MR angiography/Intraarterial digital subtraction angiography
> Cardiac, carotid angiography
> Transcranial doppler, lumbar puncture (avoid with increased intracranial pressure [ICP])

Priority Interventions or Actions

> Prevention such as lifestyle changes and routine antiplatelet therapy
> Acute management with oxygenation and ventilation, stabilize blood pressure, balance hydration: Maintain perfusion without increasing ICP (maintain normal ICP), assess sodium and glucose levels
> Ischemic treated with fibrinolytic treatment. Must have BP < or equal to 180/105; surgery: Carotid endarterectomy, transluminal angioplasty, stenting, mechanical embolus removal
> Hemorrhagic stroke is managed by controlling hypertension and surgical evacuation of hemorrhage
> Rehabilitation includes the transdisciplinary team-physical/occupational/speech therapy for swallow therapy and speech therapy

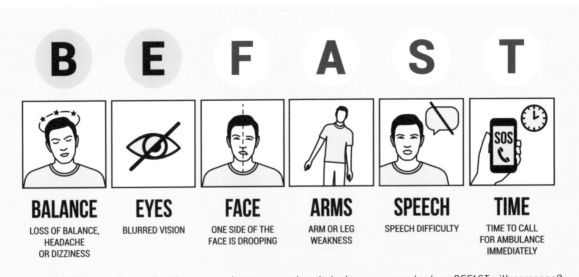

Image 6-2: What are 3 opportunities you may have as a nursing student or new nurse to share BEFAST with someone?

⚑ Priority Potential & Actual Complications

> About one-third of stroke victims have permanent disability, about one-fourth require long-term care

> Strokes are the 4th leading cause of death in adults

> Long-term consequences include hemiparesis, inability to walk, aphasia, lack of independence in personal care, and depression

> Other complications related to immobility, disuse, and treatment/lack of treatment (hemorrhage, neurological compromise, cerebral edema, urinary tract infection)

☬ Priority Nursing Implications

> Significant role of nursing is prevention such as assessing and managing modifiable risk factors-healthy diet, smoking cessation, regular exercise, weight control, limitation of alcohol, and routine screening

> Use evidence-based stroke assessment scales

> During acute treatment nurses maintain client safety-seizure precautions, pain management, watch hydration status closely, prevent constipation, aspiration, venous thromboembolism, skin breakdown, and avoid neck and leg flexion to avoid increased ICP

> For clients on ventilator should receive oral care every two hours to prevent VAP (ventilator-associated pneumonia)

> Provide strategies to prevent pneumonia (coughing, deep breathing, turning) and contractures/skin breakdown (positioning, splinting, passive and active ROM exercises)

> Provide support in communication, dealing with visual and functional changes (bowel and bladder retraining), unilateral neglect causes by visual field changes

♦ Priority Medications

> tissue plasminogen activator (tPA)
  • Thrombolytic
  • With ischemic strokes
  • 3-4.5 hours from onset of symptoms
  • Monitor closely for bleeding
  • Administered intravenously or intraarterially

> aspirin
  • Antiplatelet
  • Prevention 81-325 mg/day
  • Monitor for gastric bleeding

> clopidogrel
  • Antiplatelet
  • Hold prior to surgery or dental procedures

> simvastatin
  • Antilipemic
  • Control cholesterol
  • Take at bedtime
  • Watch for rhabdomyolysis

> labetalol
  • Beta-blocker
  • To control blood pressure
  • Given prior to tPA administration

👤 Priority Education/Discharge Issues

> Provide client/family support and education related to changes in function

> Explore strategies to enhance self-esteem -self-care in all activities of daily living, dealing with frustration, fear, and emotional lability

> Provide referrals for rehabilitation-access adapted devices to promote self-care

> Assess community resources and supports for client and family

List 5 symptoms for each followed by priority Nursing Concerns

LEFT-BRAIN STROKE

Symptoms:
1. _____
2. _____
3. _____
4. _____
5. _____

Priority Nursing Concerns:
1. _____
2. _____
3. _____
4. _____
5. _____

RIGHT-BRAIN STROKE

Symptoms:
1. _____
2. _____
3. _____
4. _____
5. _____

Priority Nursing Concerns:
1. _____
2. _____
3. _____
4. _____
5. _____

Table 6-2: Left-brain and Right-brain stroke

Valvular heart disease

Pathophysiology/Description

> Determined on which valve is affected (mitral, pulmonic, aortic, or tricuspid) and alteration (stenosis [constriction] or regurgitation [insufficiency]), or prolapse

> Occurs in children and teens from congenital heart defects or rheumatic heart disease; older adults from cardiovascular disease (previous MI, cardiomyopathy)

> Rheumatic heart disease from untreated streptococcal infections-represents key prevention strategy

Priority Assessments or Cues

> Assess heart sounds, be alert for murmurs, S3, S4, premature ventricular contractions (PVCs), pulse irregularities

> Assess end organ perfusion in extremities (peripheral pulses, skin color, skin temperature), level of consciousness, urine output, water hammer pulse (aortic stenosis)

> Ask about history of chest pain, hemoptysis, shortness of breath, fatigue, palpitations, weakness, orthopnea, paroxysmal nocturnal dyspnea, peripheral edema, dizziness

Priority Laboratory Tests/Diagnostics

> Chest X-ray-may indicate cardiomegaly

> CT of chest

> CBC

> ECG-with changes specific to the involved valve

> Cardiac ultrasound-transesophageal echocardiography/catheterization

Priority Interventions or Actions

> Medications to prevent or treat heart failure, anticoagulants, antidysrhythmia agents

> Percutaneous valve replacement or percutaneous transluminal balloon valvuloplasty

> Potential for surgical intervention (valve repair or replacement) requires client teaching, assessment, and pre/post-op care

> Sodium restricted diet, sometimes limit caffeine

> Anticoagulation therapy with valve replacement (for life with mechanical value, 3-6 months for bioprosthetic valve)

Priority Potential & Actual Complications

> Mitral stenosis-atrial fibrillation, emboli (stroke)

> Mitral regurgitation-left ventricular hypertrophy, pulmonary hypertension/edema

> Aortic stenosis-aortic dissection, sudden cardiovascular collapse

> Infective endocarditis

> Balloon Valvuloplasty-bleeding, pulmonary emboli,

Priority Nursing Implications

> Monitor client safety with medications, especially bleeding precautions for anticoagulants, fall precautions, and for symptoms of heart failure

> Provide pre-procedural or preoperative teaching

> Encourage communication and provide support to clients suffering chronic illness

Priority Medications

> nitroglycerine
  - Vasodilator
  - For angina
  - Watch for hypotension-risk for syncope, falls
> antibiotics
  - To prevent subacute bacterial endocarditis
  - Prior to each dental or surgical procedure (new research may question this as a routine practice)
> atenolol
  - Beta blocker
  - Assess pulse and blood pressure
  - Avoid use with asthma or COPD (bronchoconstriction)
> warfarin
  - Oral anticoagulant
  - Monitor bleeding times
  - Limit intake of Vitamin K rich foods

Priority Education/Discharge Issues

> Encourage smoking cessation and moderate exercise regimens

> Follow healthcare providers' recommendations for antibiotic prophylaxis for dental and surgical procedures and for clients with history of rheumatic heart disease, congenital heart disease, or infective endocarditis. Prophylactic treatment for low risk clients is no longer recommended

> Encourage adequate hydration and, in some cases, limit caffeine

> Teach client to monitor for signs of heart failure: Shortness of breath, pedal edema, orthopnea, fatigue

> If discharged on warfarin, teach client to monitor for bleeding and have INR levels monitored

Venous thromboembolism (VTE)

Pathophysiology/Description

> Forming of a thrombus (clot) with inflammation of the vein

> May be superficial (SVT) or deep (VTE)

> Occur as the result of venous stasis, damage to the internal lining of the vein, and increased coagulability of the blood

> May become an embolus when it breaks off and goes through the bloodstream

Priority Assessments or Cues

> Note calf, thigh, or groin pain with or without swelling, warmth and tenderness superficial to the area of pain

> Measure calves and thighs for comparison and baseline

> Homan's sign is controversial and may yield false positives and may mobilize the clot, not recommended in at risk clients

> With SVT, vein may be itchy, swollen, red or warm

> With VTE, symptoms of SVT plus paresthesias, may be febrile, marked edema or cyanosis of extremity

Priority Laboratory Tests/Diagnostics

> Venous compression/Duplex ultrasound

> D-Dimer-elevated results suggest VTE (normal <250 ng/mL)

> Fibrin monomer complex-thrombin>antithrombin (normal < 6.1 mg/L)

> CT/MRI

> aPTT, INR, Hgb, Hct

Priority Interventions or Actions

> With SVT, larger may require anticoagulants, smaller clots may be treated with oral and topical NSAIDs, anti-embolic stockings, and light ambulation

> With Acute VTE, bedrest with elevation of extremity, promote deep vein circulation with anti-embolic stockings, pneumatic compression boots, and progressive activity

> May warrant thrombolytic therapy to dissolve clot

> Anticoagulation therapy to prevent enlargement of clot or new clot formation

> Provide warm, moist compresses

Priority Potential & Actual Complications

> If superficial thrombi are not managed, may progress to VTE

> Pulmonary embolism

> Post-thrombotic syndrome-20-50% of clients with VTE-venous stiffening, hypertension, and scarring-symptoms include pain, swelling, tingling, venous ulceration

> Phlegmasia cerulea dolens-rare, may occur with cancer, swollen, blue, and painful leg (may progress to gangrene)

Priority Nursing Implications

> Assess clients at risk and provide preventive teaching and care-exercise, refraining from constrictive clothing

> Assess for risk for bleeding on hemorrhage in clients on anticoagulant therapy (bleeding precautions)

> Avoid massaging of clot site and avoid pneumatic compression devices with actual VTE -may mobilize clot

> Avoid antiplatelets or NSAIDs with anticoagulants

> Encourage clients on bed rest to turn

> Change position every two hours and perform leg exercises every two hours while awake

Priority Medications

> heparin
  - Anticoagulant
  - Subcutaneously or continuous IV infusion
  - Monitor aPTT (normal 25-35 seconds, on heparin-1.5-2.5 times the normal)
  - Antidote is protamine sulfate
  - With subcutaneous injection, deep into the tissue, do not aspirate or rub site
  - Watch for heparin-induced thrombocytopenia
  - Monitor for osteoporosis

> warfarin
  - Anticoagulant
  - Monitor INR (International normalized ratio) (0.9-1.1 not on anticoagulants, 2-3 on warfarin, 2.5-3.5 for high-risk clients)
  - Vitamin K is antidote

> enoxaparin
  - Anticoagulant
  - Low molecular weight heparin
  - Monitor CBC at regular intervals
  - Clients may be taught self-administration
  - Rotate injection sites

> Increasing use of NOACs (novel oral anticoagulants)

Priority Education/Discharge Issues

> Teach women about risk of VTE with oral contraceptives or hormone replacement, especially when combined with smoking

> Teach about prevention for those at risk including leg exercises, increased activity, early ambulation, elastic stockings (must be fitted and worn correctly), sequential compression boots (while in hospital), avoid restrictive clothing or crossing legs when sitting

> Instruct clients that some herbs (ginger, garlic, ginseng, gingko) increase bleeding

> Clients should avoid smoking or vasoconstrictive activities

Pulmonary embolism (PE)

Pathophysiology/Description

> Occlusion of the pulmonary arteries by a thrombus, fat, or air embolus, or tumor

> Emboli are frequently mobilized from DVTs in the lower extremities, large emboli from the iliac and femoral veins are most lethal. May also originate in the heart secondary to atrial fibrillation

> Fat emboli are from long bone fractures and air emboli from intravenous administration

> Emboli may travel through the circulatory system until they become wedged in a vessel, obliterating blood flow to the area

> With PE, the embolus travels through venous systems and into the pulmonary circulation and cuts off the blood supply to the alveoli, most often in the lower lobes

Priority Assessments or Cues

> Ask client about risk factors including advanced age, pregnancy, oral contraceptives/hormone therapy, prolonged air travel, surgery, reduced activity, or immobility, tobacco use, heart failure, clotting disorders, DVTs, cancer, obesity, and trauma

> Assess respiratory status including dyspnea (may be associated with angina, increased on inspiration), hypoxemia, cyanosis, tachypnea, chest pain, cough, crackles, hemoptysis, wheezing, shallow respirations

> Assess vital signs such as accentuated pulmonic heart sound, tachycardia, hypotension, pulse oximetry, and low-grade fever

> Assess level of consciousness and for syncope, assess for pain and anxiety, restlessness, or apprehension

> Assess for petechiae in axillae or chest

Priority Laboratory Tests/Diagnostics

> D-Dimer-fibrin fragments-may not be specific nor sensitive to PEs
> Spiral CT scan with contrast
> Ventilation perfusion (V/Q) scan-perfusion/ventilation scanning
> Pulmonary angiography
> Arterial blood gases, CXR, ECG

Priority Interventions or Actions

> Prophylaxis including pneumatic compression boots, early ambulation, anticoagulant medications

> Provide oxygen and ventilation, prevent atelectasis

> Anticoagulant therapy

> Surgical intervention if unstable or fibrinolytic therapy contraindicated, is high mortality rate

> Inferior vena cava filter is for those at risk, threaded via femoral artery

Priority Nursing Implications

> Nurses have a significant role in identifying those at risk and in the prevention of DVT

> Prognosis is better with early intervention

> When PE is a medical emergency, contact the Rapid Response Team as per agency protocol

> Elevate head of bed to ease respirations

> Ensure intravenous access

> Provide care to allay effects of immobility including turning, positioning, pad pressure areas, frequent assessments

> Place appropriate clients on fall precautions

> Provide emotional support, clients may feel a sense of doom or anxiety

Priority Medications

> enoxaparin
  • Anticoagulant
  • Low-molecular weight heparin
  • Administered subcutaneously
  • Assess for bleeding, hematomas, other sources of bleeding
> heparin
  • Anticoagulant
  • Monitor aPTT (normal 25-35 seconds, on heparin-1.5-2.5 times the normal)
  • Bleeding precautions
  • IV administration in emergency situations
  • Antidote-protamine sulfate
> warfarin
  • Anticoagulant
  • Overlap with intravenous heparin
  • Warfarin for 3-6 months
  • Monitor INR (0.9-1.1 not on anticoagulants, 2-3 on warfarin, 2.5-3.5 for high-risk clients)
  • Antidote-Vitamin K
> tissue plasminogen activator (tPA)
  • Thrombolytic to dissolve current thrombi/emboli
  • Within 3 hours of event
> rivaroxaban
  • Novel oral anticoagulant
  • No lab monitoring needed
  • Observe for bleeding

Priority Education/Discharge Issues

> Provide education and support for clients on anticoagulants

> Ensure that client and support systems understand the risk for and means to prevent DVTs and future PEs

> Educate client on means and frequency of monitoring anticoagulants

> Counsel client on progressive activity and exercise program

> Teach client to limit Vitamin K foods while on warfarin

Disseminated intravascular coagulation (DIC)

Pathophysiology/Description

> Uncontrolled bleeding/hemorrhage from disturbances in bleeding (hemorrhagic manifestations), coagulation, and thrombosis (thrombotic manifestations)

> Caused by systemic clot formation with depletion of coagulation factors and platelets

> Many risk factors including shock, septicemia, transfusion of incorrect blood type, obstetric procedures (abruptio placentae, HELLP syndrome), malignancies, burns or severe injury, liver disease, and lupus

Priority Assessments or Cues

> Monitor vital signs for tachycardia, hypotension, and for deteriorating neurological status including restlessness, headache, irritability, visual changes, confusion

> Assess for profuse bleeding including petechiae, purpura, pallor, hematomas, occult blood, and bleeding not responding to pressure, abdominal distension, blood in urine

> Assess respiratory status including hemoptysis, tachypnea, orthopnea

> Assess skin for cyanosis, ischemic tissue necrosis, reductions in kidney function, paralytic ileus, and abdominal pain

Priority Laboratory Tests/Diagnostics

> Complete blood count

> Bleeding times prolonged (prothrombin time, partial thromboplastin time, activated partial thromboplastin time, thrombin time), reduced platelets and fibrinogen

> Elevated D-dimer levels (normal < 250 ng/dl)

Priority Interventions or Actions

> Stabilize the client with oxygenation, ventilation, fluids

> Treat underlying cause

> With bleeding, administer blood products-platelets, cryoprecipitate, fresh frozen plasma

> With thrombosis, administer heparin or enoxaparin, and, less commonly, antithrombin III

Priority Potential & Actual Complications

> Hemorrhage

> Renal failure/multiorgan system failure

Priority Nursing Implications

> Be aware of conditions that may lead to DIC

> Ensure intravenous access with a large bore needle

> Conduct frequent assessments of bleeding and skin changes associated with thrombosis

> Follow evidence-based practices and agency policies when administering blood products

Priority Medications

> heparin
  • Anticoagulant
  • Subcutaneous or IV infusion
  • Monitor bleeding times
  • Antidote: Protamine sulfate

> enoxaparin
  • Low-molecular weight heparin
  • Administered subcutaneously

Priority Education/Discharge Issues

> Assist clients and family to cope with and rehabilitate from critical illness

> Provide information about the disorder and underlying conditions that precipitate DIC

List 5 causes of:
DIC IN PREGNANCY

1. _____

_____

2. _____

_____

3. _____

_____

4. _____

_____

5. _____

_____

Table 6-3: Research the causes of DIC in pregnancy and list 5 causes. Make a note card for each of the 5 causes you list. For each card, list 3 priority assessments related to that cause.

1. The nurse is caring for a client with Buerger's Disease. What statement by the client requires immediate follow-up by the nurse?
   1. "I stopped smoking marijuana two weeks ago."
   2. "My mouth hurts when I chew food."
   3. "I wear an extra layer of socks when I'm outside in the cold."
   4. "The wound on my leg is draining pink-tinged watery fluid."

2. The nurse is caring for a client with Raynaud's phenomenon. When arriving at the clinical, the client reports that her fingers are white in color and very painful after coming in from the cold weather. What action should the nurse take first?
   1. Immerse the client's hands in warm water.
   2. Ask the client if they use tobacco products.
   3. Instruct client to wear loose, warm clothing and gloves when outside.
   4. Administer prescribed pain medication.

3. The nurse is planning discharge education for a client who is at the clinic for a blood pressure check. Which instruction will guide the client to reduce risk of arteriosclerosis?
   1. Return to the clinic if you develop a wound on your lower leg.
   2. Begin a smoking cessation program.
   3. Have eyes and vision evaluated annually.
   4. Monitor for cramping pain in the legs when walking.

4. The nurse is caring for the postpartum client who is experiencing disseminated intravascular coagulation (DIC). The client's condition is deteriorating, and family members are at the bedside. What is the priority action for the nurse when caring for the family unit?
   1. Show the family to waiting room until crisis resolved.
   2. Provide reassurance to family that they will see improvement with treatment.
   3. Ask family if they have a desire for religious or spiritual counsel.
   4. Obtain additional client history data from family members.

5. When providing nutrition to the client who is recovering from an embolic stroke, what is the nurse's priority intervention?
   1. Provide client with liquid diet only for first 24 hours.
   2. Administer nutrition through peripheral intravenous line.
   3. Consult speech therapist to perform swallowing evaluation.
   4. Provide pureed food choices.

6. The nurse is preparing to administer medication to a client with acute hemorrhagic stroke. Which prescription requires immediate follow-up by the nurse?
   1. Administer intravenous anti-hypertensive medication.
   2. Administer intravenous anti-seizure medication.
   3. Administer oral platelet inhibitor medication.
   4. Administer intravenous fluids using 0.9% sodium chloride solution.

7. The nurse is caring for a client who experienced an embolic stroke. Which assessment finding would cause the nurse to be concerned about the client's respiratory function?
   1. Dysphagia.
   2. Hemiparesis.
   3. Unequal pupil responses to light.
   4. Limb ataxia.

8. The nurse is completing an assessment of the client being treated for a pulmonary embolism. The nurse notes mild bleeding from the gums following oral care. What action would be priority for the nurse?
   1. Decrease the rate of anticoagulant infusion.
   2. Provide client education on prevention of bleeding while on anticoagulation therapy.
   3. Notify the healthcare provider of the bleeding gums.
   4. Evaluate International Normalized Ratio or a PTT results.

9. The nurse is caring for a client recently admitted with acute coronary syndrome. The client states that he is experiencing an increase in chest pain. What action should the nurse implement first?
   1. Obtain a 12-lead electrocardiogram.
   2. Administer prescribed pain medication.
   3. Ensure client is receiving supplemental oxygen.
   4. Notify the healthcare provider of the increase in pain.

10. The nurse has completed the admission assessment on a client who reports that their mother is incapacitated by a stroke and father died from a ruptured aortic aneurysm. Which statement by the client best indicates understanding of personal risk?
    1. "I check food labels for the amount of fat per serving."
    2. "I eat lean meats and lots of vegetables."
    3. "I monitor my blood glucose daily."
    4. "I have labs drawn every month to assess kidney function."

11. The nurse is providing discharge teaching to a client with dilated cardiomyopathy. Which statement by the client indicates the need for further education?
    1. "I will take the ACE inhibitor every day so my heart doesn't work as hard."
    2. "I am at risk for blood clots because I have atrial fibrillation."
    3. "I need to take the diuretic on the days my feet are swollen."
    4. "Going to cardiac rehabilitation may help me manage my activities better."

12. The nurse is providing discharge instructions for the client with newly diagnosed heart failure. Which statement by the client indicates further planning is required?
    1. "My daughter will help make sure I take my medications correctly."
    2. "I should increase my activity until I can walk to the mailbox."
    3. "I will schedule my doctor's appointments around my weekly card club."
    4. "I will need to plan ahead when I leave the house because of the diuretic effects."

13. The nurse is providing education to clients in a local support group who have been diagnosed with heart failure. Which goal should the nurse stress in the education plan?
    1. Clients should be self-sufficient in caring for their disease.
    2. Clients should report weight gain of 2 pounds in a week.
    3. Clients can eat their normal diet as long as they do not add salt.
    4. Clients should increase activities gradually, avoiding fatigue.

14. Metoprolol 25 mg twice daily by mouth has been prescribed. Which vital signs listed would require the nurse to hold the medication?
    1. T 98.1°F, RR 18, Apical Pulse 88, BP 100/68.
    2. T 98.5°F, RR 16, Apical Pulse 50, BP 98/64.
    3. T 100.4°F, RR 20, Apical Pulse 100, BP 148/88.
    4. T 99.2°F, RR 16, Apical Pulse 80, BP 96/76.

15. The nurse is caring for a client in septic shock. Which assessment finding would indicate worsening of the client's condition?
    1. Increase in mean arterial pressure (MAP).
    2. Urinary output greater than 30 mL in one hour.
    3. Blood culture report indicates Escherichia coli.
    4. Responding inappropriately to the nurse's questions.

16. The nurse is caring for a client with chest pain. Which intervention by the nurse will decrease the client's risk of experiencing a myocardial infarction?
    1. Lie client supine on bed.
    2. Obtain a 12-lead electrocardiogram.
    3. Administer aspirin.
    4. Obtain baseline vital signs.

17. The nurse is caring for a client who is being seen in the clinic for pneumonia. The nurse notes an irregular pulse and obtains an ECG, which shows atrial fibrillation at a rate of 148. The client reports experiencing an irregular heartbeat for several days. Which intervention does the nurse perform first?
    1. Auscultate heart sounds for murmur/adventitious sounds.
    2. Electrical cardioversion with 50 joules.
    3. Administration of anticoagulant medication.
    4. Administration of β-blocker medication.

18. The nurse is implementing an educational plan for the client who is on bedrest. Which statement by the client requires follow-up by the nurse?
    1. "I am at risk for blood clots in my legs."
    2. "I am going to receive an injection in my abdomen every day."
    3. "I need to change position at least every two hours."
    4. "I need to wear compression hose when I sleep at night."

19. The nurse is caring for a client in cardiogenic shock. Which assessment finding indicates that treatment with pharmacological measures is effective?
    1. Narrow pulse pressure.
    2. Toes and fingers are warm to the touch.
    3. Crackles bilaterally in the bases of the lungs.
    4. Decreased peripheral pulses.

20. The nurse is conducting an initial postoperative assessment of a client who has undergone abdominal surgery. The findings include heart rate of 124 bpm, thready pulse, and clammy pale skin. The client complains of feeling lightheaded and anxious. Which statement by the nurse will best help to decrease the client's anxiety?
    1. "I'm going to call the surgeon to come see you right away."
    2. "These are common postoperative findings and will pass soon."
    3. "I am going to stay with you until you are feeling better."
    4. "I will be sure to let your family know what is going on so they don't worry."

21. The nurse is implementing discharge education for a postoperative client with history of hypertension. What information should the nurse include in the teaching plan? Select all that apply.
    1. Inadequate sleep can elevate the blood pressure.
    2. Do not take blood pressure medication if taking pain medication.
    3. Sit down if experiencing dizziness or lightheadedness.
    4. Taking pain medication sparingly helps to maintain normal blood pressure.
    5. Rise slowly when getting out of bed in the morning.
    6. Smoking will increase blood pressure and slow wound healing.

22. The nurse is caring for a client experiencing chronic heart failure. Which diagnostic test results require immediate follow-up by the nurse? Select all that apply.
    1. Magnesium 1.3 mEq/L.
    2. Sodium 122 mEq/L.
    3. Digoxin level 0.8 ng/mL.
    4. Potassium 3.3 mEq/L.
    5. Second-degree heart block on electrocardiogram.
    6. BUN 25 mg/dL.

23. The nurse is caring for a client who has sustained significant blood loss following a motor vehicle crash resulting in abdominal trauma. When implementing the plan of care, which interventions are most important to decrease risk of hypovolemic shock? Select all that apply.
    1. Initiate crystalloid intravenous infusion.
    2. Monitor urinary output.
    3. Measure girth of abdomen at regular intervals.
    4. Administer pain medication intravenously.
    5. Assess for blood in urine and stool.
    6. Control bleeding from external injuries.

24. The nurse is conducting a neurologic assessment on a client who is recovering from a mild embolic stroke. Which risk factors should the nurse teach the client to modify? Select all that apply.
    1. Hypertension.
    2. Family history of stroke.
    3. Obesity.
    4. Lack of exercise.
    5. Age.
    6. Smoking.

25. The outpatient clinic nurse is assessing a new client who is being evaluated for left leg pain. The assessment reveals an irregularly shaped superficial ulcer on the lateral lower leg near the ankle. The client's sock is saturated with yellow drainage, the surrounding skin is red, and the ulcer is painful to touch. The peripheral pulses are present and capillary refill is less than 3 seconds. There is a moderate amount of lower leg edema bilaterally. When implementing the teaching plan, which statements by the client indicate a good understanding of teaching? Select all that apply.
    1. "I need to elevate the footrest on my recliner when watching television."
    2. "I'm glad my skin will look normal when it is shorts season in two months."
    3. "I should change the dressing using dry gauze every day."
    4. "I need to avoid meat and cheese until this wound heals."
    5. "If the drainage changes color, I should return to the clinic."
    6. "I will wear the compression stockings I had during my last hospitalization."

26. The nurse is conducting a physical assessment on a client receiving follow-up care at the outpatient heart failure clinic. When obtaining vital signs, the nurse notes that the radial pulse is weak and disappears when pressure is applied. In what order should the nurse proceed in the cardiovascular assessment? Rank order the responses.
    1. Inspect the precordium for heaves.
    2. Auscultate heart sound in tricuspid area.
    3. Take the radial pulse for a full minute.
    4. Auscultate heart sound in pulmonic area.
    5. Auscultate heart sound in aortic area.
    6. Palpate over heart valves for thrills.

27. The client being treated for deep vein thrombosis reports that he cut himself shaving and is bleeding profusely. In what order should the nurse respond?
    1. Assess vital signs.
    2. Assess for other signs of bleeding.
    3. Notify healthcare provider of any abnormalities.
    4. Control bleeding.
    5. Educate client on safe practices while taking medication for DVT.
    6. Evaluate laboratory results.

28. The nurse is planning care for the client with systemic lupus erythematosus and chronic disseminated intravascular coagulation. Which assessment findings require immediate follow-up? Select all that apply.
    1. Petechiae on lower arms.
    2. Oozing from intravenous site.
    3. Decreased heart rate.
    4. Increased urinary output.
    5. Altered mental status.
    6. Abdominal distention.

29. The nurse is to weigh the client in heart failure each morning. The nurse has an order to administer furosemide 40 mg intravenously for weight gain greater than 2 kg. Today's weight is 243 pounds; yesterday's weight was 239 pounds. How much furosemide should the nurse administer?

    _____

30. The nurse is caring for a client who is experiencing a ST-elevation myocardial infarction (STEMI). A nitroglycerin infusion is running at 10 mcg/minute. The client is complaining of severe chest pain and rates it a 7/10. The order protocol states the infusion can be increased 10-20 mcg/minute every 5 minutes, titrating for pain with a maximum infusion rate of 200 mcg/minute. The bottle of 250 mL normal saline label reads: 50 mg nitroglycerin. To increase the nitroglycerin infusion 10 mcg/minute, the nurse should set the pump at what rate?

    _____

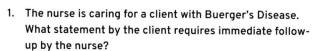

1. The nurse is caring for a client with Buerger's Disease. What statement by the client requires immediate follow-up by the nurse?
   1. "I stopped smoking marijuana two weeks ago." *The client has stopped smoking marijuana so this is no longer a contributing factor.*
   2. 🔘 "My mouth hurts when I chew food."
   3. "I wear an extra layer of socks when I'm outside in the cold." *This is an appropriate adaptation to the symptom of cold sensitivity.*
   4. "The wound on my leg is draining pink-tinged watery fluid." *Serosanguinous fluid would not be a concern, as it does not indicate an infection.*

   Rationale: Buerger's disease occurs most commonly in young men (<45 years old), with long history of tobacco and/or marijuana use, chronic periodontal infection but without other cardiac risk factors. Nurse should follow-up to inquire about dental care and assess the mouth for evidence of periodontal infection. The client has stopped marijuana use which requires encouragement. A symptom is cold sensitivity, which he is managing by wearing an extra layer of socks. His leg ulcer is draining serosanguinous fluid indicating that infection is not present.

   THIN Thinking: Top Three – *Knowing that periodontal infection is a concern, inspection of the oral mucosa is a priority. Additional concerns are with circulation to the extremities, not an issue with this scenario.* **NCLEX®:** Reduction of Risk Potential **QSEN:** Patient-centered Care

2. The nurse is caring for a client with Raynaud's phenomenon. When arriving at the clinical, the client reports that her fingers are white in color and very painful after coming in from the cold weather. What action should the nurse take first?
   1. 🔘 Immerse the client's hands in warm water.
   2. Ask the client if they use tobacco products. *Although smoking can contribute to vasospasms, the priority would be pain relief and circulation promotion.*
   3. Instruct client to wear loose, warm clothing and gloves when outside. *This is a good intervention to help prevent future attacks but will do nothing to help the client right now.*
   4. Administer prescribed pain medication. *Nurses should try the least involved treatment first. Immersing the hands in warm water should offer immediate relief and pain medication might not be needed.*

   Rationale: The client's immediate concern is pain. Relief may be obtained quickly by immersing hands in warm water, eliminating the need for pain medication. Quickly alleviating the vasospasms helps slow progression of the disease, which can lead to ulcerations, punctate lesions, and gangrenous infections. Assessment of tobacco use and education are important but can be better done after pain controlled.

   THIN Thinking: Help Quick – *Immersion in warm water can relieve the spasms and improve circulation with vasodilation. This intervention works more quickly than pain medicine in most cases.* **NCLEX®:** Basic Care and Comfort **QSEN:** Patient-centered Care

3. The nurse is planning discharge education for a client who is at the clinic for a blood pressure check. Which instruction will guide the client to reduce risk of arteriosclerosis?
   1. Return to the clinic if you develop a wound on your lower leg. *This would not reduce the risk of the disease.*
   2. 🔘 Begin a smoking cessation program.
   3. Have eyes and vision evaluated annually. *This is a good health maintenance but won't help prevent the disease.*
   4. Monitor for cramping pain in the legs when walking. *Cramping in the legs can be a symptom of this disease, not a method for reducing risk.*

   Rationale: Smoking creates risk for a multitude of cardiovascular disease processes. The remaining items are important to teach the client; however, they are the result of arteriosclerosis and atherosclerosis and not creating the risk.

   THIN Thinking: Nursing Process –*When creating a plan of care, the nurse should identify the goals of care and focus instruction on the risks that the client presents with.* **NCLEX®:** Health Promotion and Maintenance **QSEN:** Patient-centered Care

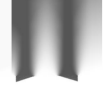

4. The nurse is caring for the postpartum client who is experiencing disseminated intravascular coagulation (DIC). The client's condition is deteriorating, and family members are at the bedside. What is the priority action for the nurse when caring for the family unit?
   1. Show the family to waiting room until crisis resolved. *In this critical situation, the client might not survive, so it would be wrong to prevent family members from being with each other.*
   2. Provide reassurance to family that they will see improvement with treatment. *The nurse should not give false assurances.*
   3. 🔘 Ask family if they have a desire for religious or spiritual counsel.
   4. Obtain additional client history data from family members. *Additional family history would not be pertinent in a crisis situation.*

   Rationale: DIC can occur as an acute, catastrophic condition.' Risk factors for DIC include several obstetric conditions. The focus of this question is psychosocial care; hence the focus is not on physical care of the client. The nurse needs to ensure that the family is cared for by meeting their psychosocial needs--one of which is spiritual care. There is no need to remove the family and it is not the time to be obtaining additional history information. The client is deteriorating with a condition that has a high mortality rate. Telling the family that they will see improvement is giving them false hope.

   THIN Thinking: Top Three – *It is important to meet the needs of both the client and family during this difficult time. Offering additional support systems can help.* **NCLEX®:** Psychosocial Integrity **QSEN:** Patient-centered Care

5. When providing nutrition to the client who is recovering from an embolic stroke, what is the nurse's priority intervention?
   1. Provide client with liquid diet only for first 24 hours. *Need to be evaluated for swallowing first.*
   2. Administer nutrition through peripheral intravenous line. *Oral feeding preferred if safe and intestinal track is working.*
   3. 🔘 Consult speech therapist to perform swallowing evaluation.
   4. Provide pureed food choices. *Pureed foods are not recommended due to texture and taste but may be required after swallowing evaluation.*

   Rationale: A speech therapist or occupational therapist should perform a swallowing evaluation prior to initiating any oral intake. Further determination about short- and long-term nutritional needs will then be addressed. Pureed food is not recommended because they are bland and too smooth.

THIN Thinking: Identify Risk to Safety – *Oral feeding cannot begin until it is deemed safe. A collaborative consultation with a speech therapist is needed to perform this.* **NCLEX®:** Reduction of Risk Potential **QSEN:** Teamwork and Collaboration

6. The nurse is preparing to administer medication to a client with acute hemorrhagic stroke. Which prescription requires immediate follow-up by the nurse?
   1. Administer intravenous anti-hypertensive medication. *BP medications are important to control blood pressure and prevent hypo and hypertensive episodes.*
   2. Administer intravenous anti-seizure medication. *The client is at risk, depending on what part of the brain is affected. Medication should be delivered.*
   3. 🔘 Administer oral platelet inhibitor medication.
   4. Administer intravenous fluids using 0.9% sodium chloride solution. *The nurse should always monitor clients who are receiving IV fluids, but this would not be the priority.*

   Rationale: Oral platelet inhibitors are contraindicated when active bleeding is occurring. Anti-hypertensive drugs are the main therapy, while anti-seizure medication is situation-specific. Other medications are not suggested for the acute period; however, the client needs to be hydrated. Use of glucose in IV fluids are hypotonic and may increase intracranial pressure.

   THIN Thinking: Identify Risk to Safety – *The delivery of a platelet inhibitor or blood thinner is contraindicated after a hemorrhagic stroke as it can cause additional bleeding.* **NCLEX®:** Pharmacological and Parenteral Therapies **QSEN:** Safety

7. The nurse is caring for a client who experienced an embolic stroke. Which assessment finding would cause the nurse to be concerned about the client's respiratory function?
   1. 🔘 Dysphagia.
   2. Hemiparesis. *Inability to move one side of the body is concerning, but wouldn't have a huge impact on respiratory function.*
   3. Unequal pupil responses to light. *Unequal pupil responses could indicate brain damage but wouldn't be as much of a risk factor for respiratory function as dysphagia.*
   4. Limb ataxia. *This would be concerning, but not an immediate threat to respiratory function.*

   Rationale: Each assessment finding will concern the nurse and require further assessment and intervention; however, dysphagia is the only one that impacts respiratory status as aspiration pneumonia is a high-risk.

   THIN Thinking: Safety – *Dysphagia is a common concern with strokes and increase the risk of aspiration. A thorough assessment is needed before fluids can safely be given.* **NCLEX®:** Reduction of Risk Potential **QSEN:** Safety

8. The nurse is completing an assessment of the client being treated for a pulmonary embolism. The nurse notes mild bleeding from the gums following oral care. What action would be priority for the nurse?
   1. Decrease the rate of anticoagulant infusion. *This action requires an order from the healthcare provider.*
   2. Provide client education on prevention of bleeding while on anticoagulation therapy. *This would not address the current bleeding problem.*
   3. Notify the healthcare provider of the bleeding gums. *The HCP does need to be notified, but it would be most helpful to have the latest lab results prior to calling.*
   4. 🎯 Evaluate International Normalized Ratio or a PTT results.

   Rationale: The bleeding is mild; therefore, not a crisis to manage. While the healthcare provider needs to be notified, they will first ask what the latest INR/aPTT result was to determine how best to proceed. The nurse should be prepared with that information prior to placing the call. The healthcare provider may order a decreased rate of infusion based on the result. The client education is necessary but not the priority for this situation.

   THIN Thinking: Nursing Process – *Further assessment of the lab work is a priority before the intervention of calling the HCP.* **NCLEX®:** Reduction of Risk Potential **QSEN:** Patient-centered Care

9. The nurse is caring for a client recently admitted with acute coronary syndrome. The client states that he is experiencing an increase in chest pain. What action should the nurse implement first?
   1. Obtain a 12-lead electrocardiogram. *The nurse would do this after obtaining an order, and first should apply oxygen.*
   2. Administer prescribed pain medication. *The nurse would do this if the pain is not relieved by oxygen.*
   3. 🎯 Ensure client is receiving supplemental oxygen.
   4. Notify the healthcare provider of the increase in pain. *This would be done if the client did not find relief from oxygen and medications.*

   Rationale: Priorities for nursing interventions include pain relief, monitoring, rest and comfort, alleviation of anxiety and understanding the client's emotional response. Pain can be managed by medication and oxygen. Since oxygen can have an immediate effect and hypoxia is detrimental to the client, ensuring adequate oxygen is priority followed by administering pain medication such as nitroglycerin or morphine. An ECG requires an order, which can be obtained when the healthcare provider is notified, if pain not resolved with prescribed treatments.

   THIN Thinking: Top Three – *Chest pain in a client with ACS is a sign of tissue hypoxia. Increasing oxygen in the blood can improve the situation and should be applied first.* **NCLEX®:** Physiological Adaptation **QSEN:** Patient-centered Care

10. The nurse has completed the admission assessment on a client who reports that their mother is incapacitated by a stroke and father died from a ruptured aortic aneurysm. Which statement by the client best indicates understanding of personal risk?
    1. "I check food labels for the amount of fat per serving." *Checking food labels doesn't mean the client is following a proper diet.*
    2. 🎯 "I eat lean meats and lots of vegetables."
    3. "I monitor my blood glucose daily." *If the client is diabetic, daily blood glucose monitoring would be insufficient to control blood glucose levels.*
    4. "I have labs drawn every month to assess kidney function." *There would be no need for this client to have labs drawn that frequently.*

    Rationale: Checking food labels does not equate with making good food choices; however, eating lean meats and vegetables demonstrates application rather than intent. While diabetes plays a role, it is not the best response as the question deals with consequences of atherosclerosis and hypertension. Monthly labs for kidney function is too frequent for this client.

    THIN Thinking: Nursing Process – Evaluating the client's understanding of risk is important in determining additional educational needs. **NCLEX®:** Reduction of Risk Potential **QSEN:** Evidence-based Practice

11. The nurse is providing discharge teaching to a client with dilated cardiomyopathy. Which statement by the client indicates the need for further education?
    1. "I will take the ACE inhibitor every day so my heart doesn't work as hard." *This is an accurate response. An ACE dilates and decreases blood pressure and workload.*
    2. "I am at risk for blood clots because I have atrial fibrillation." *This is an accurate response. Often clients with a-fib require anticoagulants.*
    3. 🎯 "I need to take the diuretic on the days my feet are swollen."
    4. "Going to cardiac rehabilitation may help me manage my activities better." *This is an accurate response. Cardiac rehabilitation allows strengthening of the heart with close medical monitoring.*

    Rationale: Diuretics are taken routinely, usually daily, with dilated cardiomyopathy to decrease preload on the heart. The other three responses are correct interpretations by the client of his condition.

    THIN Thinking: Identify Risk to Safety – *It is important to recognize and re-educate that diuretics should be taken every day.* **NCLEX®:** Health Promotion and Maintenance **QSEN:** Patient-centered Care

12. The nurse is providing discharge instructions for the client with newly diagnosed heart failure. Which statement by the client indicates further planning is required?
    1. "My daughter will help make sure I take my medications correctly." *This could be helpful in monitor medication compliance.*
    2. 🔦 "I should increase my activity until I can walk to the mailbox."
    3. "I will schedule my doctor's appointments around my weekly card club." *This indicates the client is willing to schedule and keep appointments.*
    4. "I will need to plan ahead when I leave the house because of the diuretic effects." *This indicates and understanding of the effects of a diuretic.*

    Rationale: This question addresses discharge planning. The client has a support system, desires to maintain normal non-exerting activities, and will plan around the effects of her diuretic. The client should increase activities to tolerance but be guided by dyspnea and fatigue rather than length of the walk.

    THIN Thinking: Identify Risk to Safety – *The client needs to recognize the signs and symptoms of over exertion and plan their activity accordingly.* **NCLEX®:** Reduction of Risk Potential **QSEN:** Patient-centered Care

13. The nurse is providing education to clients in a local support group who have been diagnosed with heart failure. Which goal should the nurse stress in the education plan?
    1. Clients should be self-sufficient in caring for their disease. *Having a support system is important in managing this disease.*
    2. Clients should report weight gain of 2 pounds in a week. *Weight gain of more than 3-5 pounds should be reported.*
    3. Clients can eat their normal diet as long as they do not add salt. *Clients need to avoid hidden salt found in processed foods.*
    4. 🔦 Clients should increase activities gradually, avoiding fatigue.

    Rationale: Gradual increase in walking and activities will promote improved tolerance and the client should not push to the point of fatigue or dyspnea. Having a support system is important to long-term management of the disease; weight gain should be reported if it is more than 3-5 pounds in a week. Sodium intake must be limited and monitored for all food intake.

    THIN Thinking: Nursing Process – *Realistic, safe, and obtainable goals are important to establish when planning care.* **NCLEX®:** Reduction of Risk Potential **QSEN:** Patient-centered Care

14. Metoprolol 25 mg twice daily by mouth has been prescribed. Which vital signs listed would require the nurse to hold the medication?
    1. T 98.1°F, RR 18, Apical Pulse 88, BP 100/68. *The heart rate is above 50.*
    2. 🔦 T 98.5°F, RR 16, Apical Pulse 50, BP 98/64.
    3. T 100.4°F, RR 20, Apical Pulse 100, BP 148/88. *The heart rate is above 50.*
    4. T 99.2°F, RR 16, Apical Pulse 80, BP 96/76. *The heart rate is above 50.*

    Rationale: Metoprolol is a beta blocker, which blocks the beta response in the heart receptors, slowing the heart rate. Metoprolol should be held whenever the heart rate is 50 or below as demonstrated by bradycardia.

    THIN Thinking: Identify Risk for Safety – *Administration of a beta blocker to someone with a low heart rate can cause a drop of blood pressure and cardiac output. It is important to assess vital signs before delivery.* **NCLEX®:** Pharmacological and Parenteral Therapies **QSEN:** Evidence-based Practice

15. The nurse is caring for a client in septic shock. Which assessment finding would indicate worsening of the client's condition?
    1. Increase in mean arterial pressure (MAP). *This would indicate an improvement in condition. The MAP is considered the perfusion pressure and should be >65.*
    2. Urinary output greater than 30 mL in one hour. *This indicates adequate perfusion of kidneys.*
    3. Blood culture report indicates Escherichia coli. *This is a common organism that might be the cause of the sepsis.*
    4. 🔦 Responding inappropriately to the nurse's questions.

    Rationale: Increased MAP and urinary output are treatment goals as they indicate an increase of perfusion. The blood culture report is expected to be positive for at least one organism. E-coli is commonly found with UTIs; commonly lead to sepsis, especially with the older adult. Responding to the nurse's questions with confusion indicates altered mental status, a sign of decompensation.

    THIN Thinking: Nursing Process – *Priority assessment is one that shows a deterioration of the client's condition. A change in LOC is a priority.* **NCLEX®:** Physiological Adaptation **QSEN:** Patient-centered Care

16. The nurse is caring for a client with chest pain. Which intervention by the nurse will decrease the client's risk of experiencing a myocardial infarction?
    1. Lie client supine on bed. *Elevated head of bed will make breathing easier.*
    2. Obtain a 12-lead electrocardiogram. *This would not decrease the risk for MI.*
    3. 💡 Administer aspirin.
    4. Obtain baseline vital signs. *This will help obtain data, but not decrease risk.*

    Rationale: Administering aspirin is the only action that will potentially affect an outcome. The client should be positioned upright, unless contraindicated. Responses 2 and 4 will provide additional diagnostic data but not decrease risk of MI.

    THIN Thinking: Top Three – *When a person experiences chest pain, treatment should include oxygen, aspirin administration, nitroglycerine and morphine. The aspirin will decrease platelet aggregation and prevent further clot formation.* **NCLEX®:** Reduction of Risk Potential **QSEN:** Patient-centered Care

17. The nurse is caring for a client who is being seen in the clinic for pneumonia. The nurse notes an irregular pulse and obtains an ECG, which shows atrial fibrillation at a rate of 148. The client reports experiencing an irregular heartbeat for several days. Which intervention does the nurse perform first?
    1. 💡 Auscultate heart sounds for murmur/adventitious sounds.
    2. Electrical cardioversion with 50 joules. *This would not be the first line of treatment for atrial fibrillation.*
    3. Administration of anticoagulant medication. *This may be ordered, but more information is needed to clarify the diagnosis.*
    4. Administration of β-blocker medication. *This may be ordered after further assessment has been completed.*

    Rationale: Assessment of heart sounds first will provide immediate baseline knowledge if heart murmur exists. B-blocker may be indicated if atrial fibrillation is sustained. Once the b-blocker has been administered and takes effect, the murmur may be less difficult to detect. Cardioversion is not indicated as the client is tolerating the symptoms and able to speak. No data is provided to indicate the client is deteriorating. Anticoagulants may be indicated based on further assessment.

    THIN Thinking: Nursing Process – *Assessment is a priority over implementation. Further assessment is needed before medical interventions.* **NCLEX®:** Physiological Adaptation **QSEN:** Patient-centered Care

18. The nurse is implementing an educational plan for the client who is on bedrest. Which statement by the client requires follow-up by the nurse?
    1. "I am at risk for blood clots in my legs." *There is an increased risk of clots with bedrest.*
    2. "I am going to receive an injection in my abdomen every day." *The delivery of low molecular weight heparin is common for bedridden clients to prevent clot formation.*
    3. "I need to change position at least every two hours." *Movement will decrease clot formation.*
    4. 💡 "I need to wear compression hose when I sleep at night."

    Rationale: The client is at risk for deep vein thrombosis. Venous thrombotic embolism prophylaxis measures include position change, anticoagulant therapy, and compression stockings. Compression stockings are to be worn at all times except during bathing, sleeping, or assessments of underlying skin integrity.

    THIN Thinking: Identify Risk to Safety –*If compression hose is not worn, they cannot work. Education needs to include when, where, and how to use them.* **NCLEX®:** Safety and Infection Control **QSEN:** Safety

19. The nurse is caring for a client in cardiogenic shock. Which assessment finding indicates that treatment with pharmacological measures is effective?
    1. Narrow pulse pressure. *This is a sign of inadequate perfusion.*
    2. 💡 Toes and fingers are warm to the touch.
    3. Crackles bilaterally in the bases of the lungs. *This can be a sign of worsening heart failure.*
    4. Decreased peripheral pulses. *This is a sign of inadequate perfusion.*

    Rationale: Crackles, narrow pulse pressure, and decreased pulses are not positive signs of reperfusion. Warm toes and fingers indicate increased peripheral perfusion.

    THIN Thinking: Nursing Process – *Assessment of improvement of perfusion is important in determining the effectiveness of the plan of care.* **NCLEX®:** Physiological Adaptation **QSEN:** Patient-centered Care

20. The nurse is conducting an initial postoperative assessment of a client who has undergone abdominal surgery. The findings include heart rate of 124 bpm, thready pulse, and clammy pale skin. The client complains of feeling lightheaded and anxious. Which statement by the nurse will best help to decrease the client's anxiety?
    1. "I'm going to call the surgeon to come see you right away." *This statement will not relieve the client's anxiety.*
    2. "These are common postoperative findings and will pass soon." *This statement demonstrates not taking the client's concerns seriously.*
    3. ⚈ "I am going to stay with you until you are feeling better."
    4. "I will be sure to let your family know what is going on so they don't worry." *This would not reassure the client or address their concerns.*

    Rationale: The focus of this question is psychosocial care of the client and the need to minimize the client's anxiety. The nurse should explain that the client will not be left alone and offer reassurance. Although the surgeon will be called to come immediately, this statement will likely increase anxiety and concern for self. The symptoms indicate hypovolemic condition and will not pass without intervention. While important to inform the family.

    THIN Thinking: Help Quick – *Psychosocial assessments indicate anxiety. Reassurance assurance is important to allow for calmness. The nurse should stay with the client while additional assistance is summoned to care for the client.* **NCLEX®:** Psychosocial Integrity **QSEN:** Patient-centered Care

21. The nurse is implementing discharge education for a postoperative client with history of hypertension. What information should the nurse include in the teaching plan? Select all that apply.
    1. ⚈ Inadequate sleep can elevate the blood pressure.
    2. Do not take blood pressure medication if taking pain medication. *Prescribed BP medications should be taken even with pain medication.*
    3. ⚈ Sit down if experiencing dizziness or lightheadedness.
    4. Taking pain medication sparingly helps to maintain normal blood pressure. *Pain can increase the client's BP.*
    5. ⚈ Rise slowly when getting out of bed in the morning.
    6. ⚈ Smoking will increase blood pressure and slow wound healing.

    Rationale: Sleep is often affected after surgery and a hospitalization resulting in risk for hypertension. Managing pain will help to control blood pressure but the client should not hold blood pressure medication unless instructed by the physician. Antihypertensive dosage may need to be adjusted short-term to prevent hypotension. Cautioning the client to sit down if dizzy or lightheaded impacts safety, as does rising slowly to prevent orthostatic hypotension that may result from combination of post-op physiological changes, pain medication, and antihypertensive agents. Smoking increases blood pressure. Unrelieved acute pain can lead to increased heart rate and blood pressure.

    THIN Thinking: Nursing Process – *Planning for discharge teaching needs to be comprehensive and specific to the client's medication and medical situation.* **NCLEX®:** Physiological Adaptation **QSEN:** Patient-centered Care

22. The nurse is caring for a client experiencing chronic heart failure. Which diagnostic test results require immediate follow-up by the nurse? Select all that apply.
    1. Magnesium 1.3 mEq/L. *This is in the normal range.*
    2. ⚈ Sodium 122 mEq/L.
    3. Digoxin level 0.8 ng/mL. *This is in the normal range.*
    4. ⚈ Potassium 3.3 mEq/L.
    5. ⚈ Second-degree heart block on electrocardiogram.
    6. ⚈ BUN 25 mg/dL.

    Rationale: The correct answers are outside the normal range/findings and result from diuresis and effects of heart failure. Hyponatremia can result in fluid imbalance, hypokalemia can cause dysrhythmias, heart block can cause a decreased cardiac output, and a high BUN can indicate dehydration, kidney impairment or other concerns.

    THIN Thinking: Help Quick – The nurse needs to identify abnormal labs and diagnostic findings in order to report to the HCP and prevent further complications. **NCLEX®:** Reduction of Risk Potential **QSEN:** Patient-centered Care

23. The nurse is caring for a client who has sustained significant blood loss following a motor vehicle crash resulting in abdominal trauma. When implementing the plan of care, which interventions are most important to decrease risk of hypovolemic shock? Select all that apply.
    1. ⚈ Initiate crystalloid intravenous infusion.
    2. Monitor urinary output. *This would help with early detection in decreased perfusion, but not decrease the risk for hypovolemic shock.*
    3. Measure girth of abdomen at regular intervals. *This will determine if there is internal bleeding.*
    4. Administer pain medication intravenously. *This would have no effect on the development of shock.*
    5. Assess for blood in urine and stool. *This could help detect shock but wouldn't decrease the risk.*
    6. ⚈ Control bleeding from external injuries.

Rationale: Decreasing risk requires taking action. Infusing crystalloids will replace fluid loss from traumatic bleeding, measuring girth will recognize distention from internal bleeding, and controlling bleeding will decrease blood loss leading to hypovolemic shock. Pain medication will not affect bleeding. Monitoring urine output and assessing for blood in urine and stool are important but will recognize a problem--not decrease risk until something is done to mitigate that problem.

THIN Thinking: Top Three – *Priorities for prevention of risk is to control bleeding and replace fluids/blood.* **NCLEX®:** Physiological Adaptation **QSEN:** Patient-centered Care

24. The nurse is conducting a neurologic assessment on a client who is recovering from a mild embolic stroke. Which risk factors should the nurse teach the client to modify? Select all that apply.
    1. 💡 Hypertension.
    2. Family history of stroke. *This is a non-modifiable risk factor.*
    3. 💡 Obesity.
    4. 💡 Lack of exercise.
    5. Age. *This is a non-modifiable risk factor.*
    6. 💡 Smoking.

Rationale: #2 and #5 are non-modifiable risk factors that the client cannot change. The nurse can provide education to help the client decrease risks related to hypertension, obesity, exercise, and smoking.

THIN Thinking: Nursing Process – *Recognition of modifiable risk factors are important to include as part of the teaching plan.* **NCLEX®:** Reduction of Risk Potential **QSEN:** Patient-centered Care

25. The outpatient clinic nurse is assessing a new client who is being evaluated for left leg pain. The assessment reveals an irregularly shaped superficial ulcer on the lateral lower leg near the ankle. The client's sock is saturated with yellow drainage, the surrounding skin is red, and the ulcer is painful to touch. The peripheral pulses are present and capillary refill is less than 3 seconds. There is a moderate amount of lower leg edema bilaterally. When implementing the teaching plan, which statements by the client indicate a good understanding of teaching? Select all that apply.
    1. 💡 "I need to elevate the footrest on my recliner when watching television."
    2. "I'm glad my skin will look normal when it is shorts season in two months." *This type of wound may take longer to heal. Skin discoloration will not go away.*

3. "I should change the dressing using dry gauze every day." *Dressings are moist, not dry.*
4. "I need to avoid meat and cheese until this wound heals." *Protein will help with healing process.*
5. 💡 "If the drainage changes color, I should return to the clinic."
6. "I will wear the compression stockings I had during my last hospitalization." *Stockings must be properly fitted.*

Rationale: Legs should be elevated to decrease edema and change in drainage color is one indication of possible infection. The condition is chronic and the skin color will not return to normal; dressings are usually wet or moist; and protein (meat and cheese) will aid in healing process. Compression stockings must be fitted by measurement and snugly provide pressure. Previously worn stockings may be stretched out.

THIN Thinking: Nursing Process –*It is important for the nurse to understand the assessment differences between arterial and venous circulation and provide appropriate interventions.* **NCLEX®:** Safety and Infection Control **QSEN:** Patient-centered Care

26. The nurse is conducting a physical assessment on a client receiving follow-up care at the outpatient heart failure clinic. When obtaining vital signs, the nurse notes that the radial pulse is weak and disappears when pressure is applied. In what order should the nurse proceed in the cardiovascular assessment? Rank order the responses.
    1. Take the radial pulse for a full minute.
    2. Inspect the precordium for heaves.
    3. Palpate over heart valves for thrills.
    4. Auscultate heart sound in pulmonic area.
    5. Auscultate heart sound in aortic area.
    6. Auscultate heart sound in tricuspid area.

Rationale: The nurse is already assessing the radial pulse and should finish that assessment. There is no indication in the stem of the question that the client is in extremis. The remaining answers follow the established assessment routine of inspection and palpation as well as the established order of listening to heart sounds.

THIN Thinking: Nursing Process – *When performing a focused cardiovascular assessment, the nurse must proceed in the proper order.* **NCLEX®:** Health Promotion and Maintenance **QSEN:** Patient-centered Care

27. **The client being treated for deep vein thrombosis reports that he cut himself shaving and is bleeding profusely. In what order should the nurse respond?**
   1. Control bleeding.
   2. Assess for other signs of bleeding.
   3. Assess vital signs.
   4. Evaluate laboratory results.
   5. Notify healthcare provider of any abnormalities.
   6. Educate client on safe practices while taking medication for DVT.

   Rationale: The client on anticoagulation therapy has active bleeding. Controlling active bleeding is a priority since this client has airway and breathing are not affected. The nurse should assess for additional bleeding sites, including bruising. This should be done before obtaining vital signs to ensure active bleeding discovered elsewhere is controlled. Vital signs should then be assessed to determine if blood loss has altered blood pressure or heart rate. Lab results (aPTT or INR) should be checked prior to contacting the healthcare provider so the nurse has all necessary information. Client education should occur once other priority interventions have been completed.

   THIN Thinking: Help Quick – *Control of bleeding first needs to take place so there is not further loss of blood. Once it is controlled, the vital signs can be determined.* **NCLEX®:** Physiological Adaptation **QSEN:** Patient-centered Care

28. **The nurse is planning care for the client with systemic lupus erythematosus and chronic disseminated intravascular coagulation. Which assessment findings require immediate follow-up? Select all that apply.**
   1. 🔘 Petechiae on lower arms.
   2. 🔘 Oozing from intravenous site.
   3. Decreased heart rate. *Signs of hemorrhage would include tachycardia, not bradycardia.*
   4. Increased urinary output. *Poor circulation and bleeding would decrease urine output.*
   5. 🔘 Altered mental status.
   6. 🔘 Abdominal distention.

   Rationale: Petechiae and oozing are external signs of external signs of bleeding, while altered mental status and increased abdominal girth are signs of possible internal bleeding. Increased heart rate and decreased urinary output would be expected.

   THIN Thinking: Nursing Process – *The nurse must recognize the assessment changes of hemorrhage as to determine the urgency of care.* **NCLEX®:** Physiological Adaptation **QSEN:** Patient-centered Care

29. **The nurse is to weigh the client in heart failure each morning. The nurse has an order to administer furosemide 40 mg intravenously for weight gain greater than 2 kg. Today's weight is 243 pounds; yesterday's weight was 239 pounds. How much furosemide should the nurse administer?**

   Answer: 0 mg

   Rationale: Daily weights are an accurate measure of volume status. This item addresses conversion of pounds to kilograms so the nurse can analyze whether to administer a medication.

   243 pounds = 110.45 kg
   239 pounds = 108.63 kg

   The difference is 1.82 kg so the nurse should not administer the furosemide.

   THIN Thinking: Identify Risk to Safety – *Accurate medication calculations are important to client safety.* **NCLEX®:** Pharmacological and Parenteral Therapies **QSEN:** Patient-centered Care

30. **The nurse is caring for a client who is experiencing a ST-elevation myocardial infarction (STEMI). A nitroglycerin infusion is running at 10 mcg/minute. The client is complaining of severe chest pain and rates it a 7/10. The order protocol states the infusion can be increased 10-20 mcg/minute every 5 minutes, titrating for pain with a maximum infusion rate of 200 mcg/minute. The bottle of 250 mL normal saline label reads: 50 mg nitroglycerin. To increase the nitroglycerin infusion 10 mcg/minute, the nurse should set the pump at what rate?**

   Answer: 6 mL/hour

   Rationale:
   $$\frac{20 \text{ mcg}}{1 \text{ min}} \times \frac{1 \text{ mL}}{200 \text{ mcg/mL}} \times \frac{60 \text{ min}}{1 \text{ hour}} = 6 \text{ mL/hour}$$

   THIN Thinking: Identify Risk to Safety – *Safe medication calculations are critical to client safety.* **NCLEX®:** Pharmacological and Parenteral Therapies **QSEN:** Safety

Protection

Immunity / Inflammation / Infection

The immune system is the body's first line of defense. When functioning properly, the immune system prevents or limits the risk of infections in our bodies. Through intricate processes, it recognizes and disposes of substances that it identifies as foreign and potentially detrimental to the body's health. However, when there are problems with the immune system and it does not function as it should there is the risk of diseases occurring in the body.

When there is injury of any type in the body inflammation is likely to occur. This is the body's way of attempting to defend itself against the cause of the injury and restore the tissue to functionality. However, pathogens often pose challenges to the immune system and invade our bodies causing a myriad of infections. Nurses must be knowledgeable about the role immunity plays in the body and skilled when caring for clients with all types of infections, as new strains of bacteria are emerging constantly.

Priority Exemplars:

> Meningitis
> Pancreatitis
> Appendicitis/peritonitis
> Cellulitis/wound infection/septicemia
> Gout
> Systemic lupus erythematosus
> Rheumatoid arthritis
> HIV/AIDS
> Hypersensitivity reactions
> Influenza
> Polycystic kidney
> Urinary tract infection
> Pyelonephritis
> Methicillin-resistant Staphylococcus Aureus/ vancomycin resistant Enterococcus

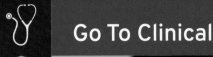
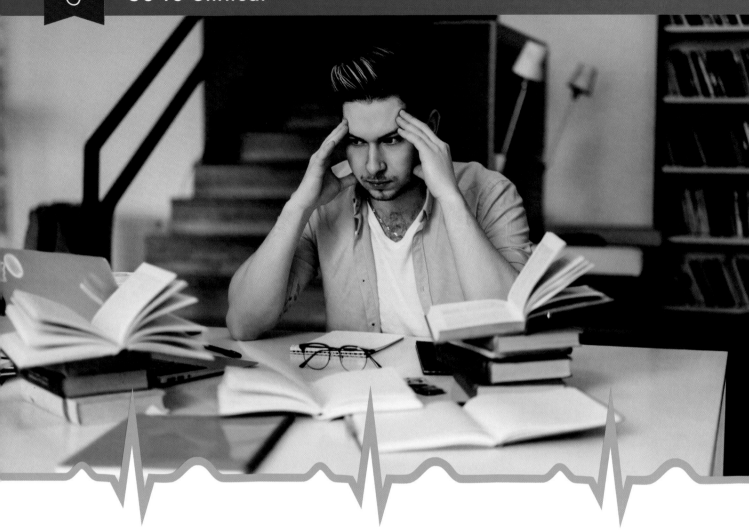

Go To Clinical Case 1

J.S. is a 22-year-old college student who presents to the clinic because of red spots that have appeared all over his body and a bad headache. He has just come home from college for summer break and admits that before he left campus, he vomited a few times and just "didn't feel well." His parents are worried because along with the other symptoms, J.S. now says his neck is stiff and yesterday when he went outside in the sun, he had difficulty tolerating the sunlight.

Vital signs are: Blood pressure 128/82, heart rate 90, respirations 18, temperature 100.2. Further assessment reveals a positive Brudzinski's and Kernig's sign. Meningitis is suspected and J.S. is sent immediately to the local hospital as a direct admission. You are the nurse caring for J.S.

NurseThink® Time

Using the NurseThink® system, complete the priorities. Check your answers designated by 💡 in the Meningitis Priority Exemplar.

Clinical Hint

Any change in a client's neurological function, level of consciousness, or behavior may be an early sign of an impending status change! Consider it carefully!

✏ Priority Assessments or Cues

1.

2.

3.

⚗ Priority Laboratory Tests/Diagnostics

1.

2.

3.

⚠ Priority Interventions or Actions

1.

2.

3.

⚑ Priority Potential & Actual Complications

1.

2.

3.

⚕ Priority Nursing Implications

1.

2.

3.

◔ Priority Medications

1.

2.

3.

☻ Priority Education/Discharge Issues

1.

2.

3.

Meningitis

Pathophysiology/Description

> Inflammation of the membranes surrounding the brain and spinal cord

> Cause is often times related to a viral infection but can be caused by viral or bacterial infections

> Viral meningitis is caused by enteroviruses and usually resolves without requiring treatment

> Bacterial meningitis is serious and can be fatal in a few days if not treated early

> Bacterial meningitis travels via the bloodstream to the brain and spinal cord. Bacteria can also invade the meninges of the brain directly because of sinus and ear infections, as well as skull fracture

> Risk factors for meningitis include
> - Community environments where large groups of people gather
> - Individuals who work with bacteria that cause meningitis
> - Travelers to certain parts of the world where conditions are ideal for the disease, like sub-Saharan Africa
> - Pregnant women who contract listeriosis, a condition caused by the bacteria Listeria Monocytogenes

> The disease is spread from person to person in several ways
> - Breathing in the bacteria when a carrier coughs or sneezes
> - Sharing respiratory secretions, as in kissing
> - Eating food contaminated from infected persons who did not wash their hands properly
> - Mothers passing the bacteria to their infants during birth

> Bacteria commonly associated with meningitis
> - Streptococcus pneumoniae (most common cause)
> - Neisseria meningitidis
> - Haemophilus influenzae
> - Group B Streptococcus
> - Listeria monocytogenes

> Encephalitis
> - Acute inflammation of the brain that affects the cerebellum, brainstem and cerebrum
> - Causes
>   - Viruses
>   - Epidemic encephalitis is usually transmitted by mosquitoes and ticks
>   - Nonepidemic cases usually occur because of complications from certain diseases, such as mumps, chickenpox, measles, herpes simplex 1 virus
> - Clinical manifestations
>   - Nausea, vomiting, headache, fever
>   - Alteration in mental status, usually occurs 2 to 3 days after initial symptoms
>   - Other neurological symptoms can occur, such as tremors, amnesia, dysphagia, hemiparesis and seizures
> - For the best outcome, encephalitis must be identified and treated early

Priority Assessments or Cues

> Complete history and physical. Assess for nuchal rigidity, severe headache, vomiting and fever, all key indicators of meningitis

> Assess for positive Brudzinski's sign, which is involuntary flexion of the hip and knee when the neck is bent forward and positive Kernig's sign, which is the inability to extend the leg while the hip is flexed to 90 degrees

> Assess neurologic status, looking for decreased level of consciousness, signs of increased intracranial pressure and seizures

> Ask about intolerance to light, called photophobia

> Monitor vital signs

> Assess intake and output. Look for dehydration that can be caused by insensible fluid loss due to high fever

> Assess nutritional status and ensure supplemental feeding as needed, to maintain nutritional status

> Additional assessments in a newborn
> - Excessive sleepiness, fussiness, sluggishness, constant crying, difficult to comfort
> - Stiffness not just in the neck as with adults, but in the body as well, a bulging fontanel

> Additional assessments specific to encephalitis
> - Ask client about insect bites, exposure to infectious agents, swimming or bathing in fresh water or travel to encephalitis prevalent areas. A causative virus for encephalitis lives in warm fresh water and can enter the body via the nasal mucosa
> - Assess for presence of oral ulcerations or cold sores. Herpes simplex virus is a causative agent for encephalitis
> - Assess need for rehabilitation due to deficits in neurologic system or physical function

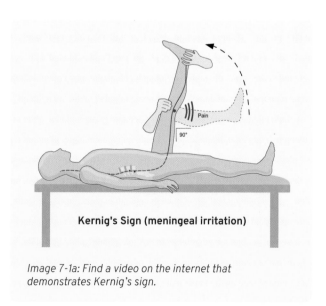

Kernig's Sign (meningeal irritation)

Image 7-1a: Find a video on the internet that demonstrates Kernig's sign.

🧪 Priority Laboratory Tests/Diagnostics

💡 Blood culture shows the causative bacteria

💡 Lumbar puncture shows cerebrospinal fluid (CSF) with low glucose level, increased protein, increased white blood cells and a cloudy color. For encephalitis, CSF color is clear and no glucose is present

💡 Computed tomography and magnetic resonance show inflammation and swelling and rule out an obstruction in the foramen magnum

➤ Xpert EV test is used to test for viral meningitis. CSF is placed on a single-use disposable cartridge, which is then loaded into an instrument that provides quick results

➤ With viral meningitis, the CSF usually appears cloudy or clear and is positive for white blood cells

➤ Additional diagnostics specific to encephalitis
  • Magnetic resonance imaging (MRI) and positron emission testing (PET) provide imaging of the brain
  • Electroencephalogram (EEG), to determine seizure activity
  • Polymerase chain reaction (PCR) testing to determine if encephalitis is West Nile or herpes simplex related

⚠️ Priority Interventions or Actions

💡 Immediate interventions
  • Place client on isolation for bacterial meningitis
  • Prepare client for lumbar puncture procedure
  • Administer antibiotics and intravenous fluid
  • Administer antipyretics for fever
  • Initiate seizure precautions and administer antiseizure drugs, if needed
  • Maintain ongoing monitoring of neurologic status

Brudzinski's Sign (meningeal irritation)

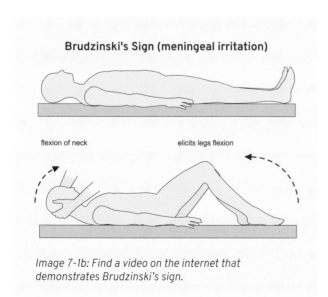

flexion of neck   elicits legs flexion

Image 7-1b: Find a video on the internet that demonstrates Brudzinski's sign.

💡 Maintain safety as client will likely experience mental distortion

💡 Decrease environmental stimuli. Keep client in a darkened room and cover eyes with a cool cloth to relieve the effects of photophobia and to keep client calm

➤ Keep head of bed elevated to 30 degrees to increase comfort for the patient. Avoid flexion of the hip and neck

➤ Use cooling blanket or a tepid sponge bath if fever persists after use of antipyretics

➤ Monitor client for adverse effects of antibiotics and manage accordingly. For vancomycin, slow the rate of infusion if flushing and itching occurs

➤ Additional interventions specific to encephalitis
  • Perform ongoing focused assessment on neurologic status to include use of the Glasgow Coma Scale. Assess for signs of increased intracranial pressure
  • Administer acyclovir as prescribed
  • Start a plan to incorporate physical, occupational and speech therapy into care, as needed

🚩 Priority Potential & Actual Complications

💡 Seizures, brain damage
💡 Hearing loss, memory difficulty, learning disabilities
💡 May be fatal

℞ Priority Nursing Implications

💡 It is important to note that a lumbar puncture is done only after a CT scan rules out a foramen magnum obstruction. If lumbar puncture is done in the presence of a foramen magnum obstruction, a fluid shift can occur, causing herniation

💡 Viral meningitis cannot be treated with antibiotics. It is resolved with fluids, rest and over-the-counter medications for aches and pain

💡 Allow someone who is familiar to the client to be in the client's hospital room. A familiar person may help to calm and soothe the client who is frightened and experiencing hallucinations, that often occur with meningitis

➤ Be careful when administering penicillin drugs that are referred to by their trade names and do not have the penicillin identifying "cillin." Augmentin and Zosyn are examples

➤ If allergic to penicillin, client will likely be allergic to cephalosporins

➤ The blood levels of vancomycin must be monitored to maintain a safe level in the body. Levels greater than 50 mcg/dL may cause toxicity, resulting in hearing loss and kidney damage. Itching and flushing to trunk, neck, head and face (red man syndrome) is another adverse effect of vancomycin

➤ Phenytoin may cause urine to be red, reddish brown or pink. May cause gingival hyperplasia so good dental care is essential

🜄 Priority Medications

💡 Antibiotics

- penicillin, ampicillin. Tricyclic glycopeptide like vancomycin

- cephalosporins such as cefuroxime, ceftriaxone, ceftazidime, cefotaxime, ceftizoxime

- Administered oral, intravenous or intramuscular. Dosages vary based on route being administered and the specific antibiotic used

💡 Corticosteroids

- dexamethasone

- Given to prevent neurological complications, like cerebral edema

- Initial dose is 10 mg IV once, followed by 4 mg intramuscular every 6 hours until maximal response is noted. Reduce dose after 2-4 days then gradually discontinued over a period of 5-7 days

❯ Anti-seizure medications

- phenytoin, levetiracetam, used to treat seizures that can occur with meningitis

- phenytoin is administered as oral chewable tablets, oral suspension, extended-release capsules, intravenous, intramuscular

- levetiracetam is administered oral and intravenous and dosage is dependent on the type of seizure suspected

💡 Antipyretics

- aspirin, acetaminophen common ones used

- Used to treat pain. Administered oral, rectal and now intravenous (new medication)

- Maximum daily dosage should not exceed 4 grams. Antidote for overdose of acetaminophen is acetylcysteine

❯ Medications specific to encephalitis

- acyclovir is an antiviral agent used to treat encephalitis when herpes simplex virus is the cause

- Administered oral or intravenous

- Oral dosage is 200-800 mg 5 times daily; intravenous dose is 5-10 mg/kg every 8 hours. Both oral and intravenous are administered for 7-10 days

👤 Priority Education/Discharge Issues

❯ Educate on types of meningococcal vaccines currently available

💡 Teach that once discharged from acute care, it may take several weeks before client feels well enough to resume normal activities

❯ Teach client to increase exercise gradually but take rest breaks as needed

💡 Teach the importance of proper nutrition, consuming a high-calorie and high-protein diet

💡 Teach that client may still experience rigidity in the neck and that taking warm baths and doing range of motion exercises will relieve the stiffness

❯ Educate on complications of meningitis and when to call the healthcare provider

❯ Teach the importance of keeping all follow-up healthcare provider appointments

❯ Additional teaching specific to encephalitis

- Educate on the importance of mosquito control. This includes removing old containers in the yard that hold water and cleaning gutters to prevent mosquitoes from breeding

- Teach importance of taking prescribed medications, such as acyclovir. Teach side effects and when to contact the healthcare provider

- Assist caregivers to locate community resources if needed, based on severity of client's condition. These may include rehabilitation or a long-term care facility

- Educate caregiver on modification of the home to care for client if severe brain damage occurs

Go To Clinical Answers

Text designated by 💡 are the top answers for the Go To Clinical related to Meningitis.

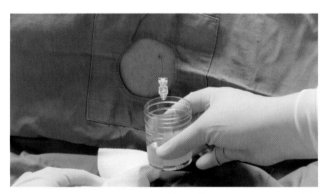

Image 7-2: Lumbar punctures (LP) help diagnose meningitis. List 3 statements by a client undergoing an LP that would indicate they understand what to expect.

1. _____

_____

2. _____

_____

3. _____

_____

LUMBAR PUNCTURE
Priority nursing concerns

Before:

1. _____

_____

2. _____

_____

3. _____

_____

During:

1. _____

_____

2. _____

_____

3. _____

_____

After:

1. _____

_____

2. _____

_____

3. _____

_____

Table 7-1: Priority nursing concerns for a client needing a lumbar puncture.

Meningitis

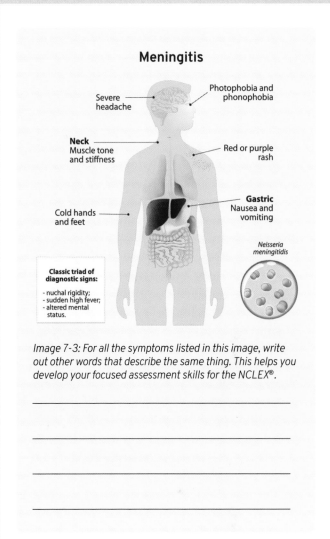

Severe headache

Photophobia and phonophobia

Neck
Muscle tone and stiffness

Red or purple rash

Cold hands and feet

Gastric
Nausea and vomiting

Neisseria meningitidis

Classic triad of diagnostic signs:
- nuchal rigidity;
- sudden high fever;
- altered mental status.

Image 7-3: For all the symptoms listed in this image, write out other words that describe the same thing. This helps you develop your focused assessment skills for the NCLEX®.

_____

_____

_____

_____

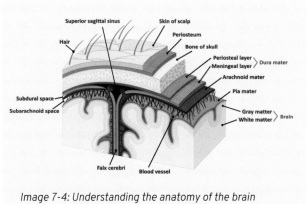

Image 7-4: Understanding the anatomy of the brain explains the manifestations of meningitis.

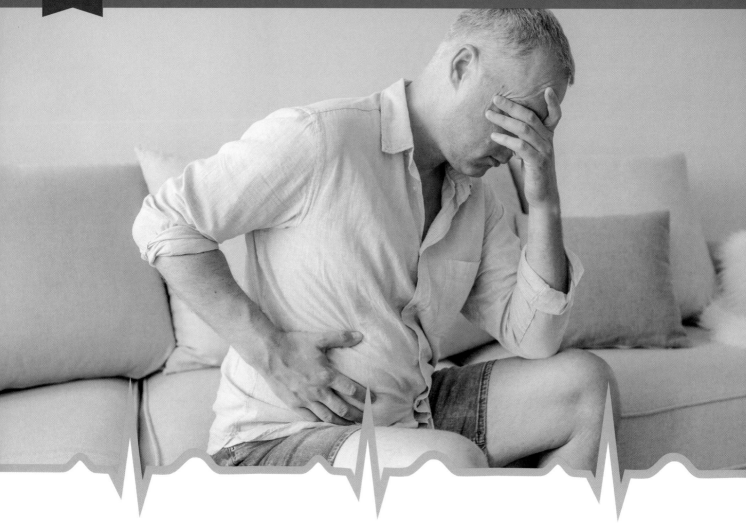

Go To Clinical Case 2

E.S. presents to the emergency department in excruciating pain to the abdomen, which he states is now in his back. He says that he was okay this morning but while at the bar this evening drinking with his buddies, he felt "bad" and the pain seemed to have "hit me suddenly." As he is speaking with the nurse he becomes nauseated and vomits.

Vital signs are: Blood pressure 98/66 mmHg, heart rate 120, respirations 24, temperature 99.9°F. Upon assessment, bluish colored bruising is observed on his flanks and around his umbilicus. Pancreatitis is suspected and E.S is admitted to the medical-surgical unit. You are the nurse caring for E.S.

NurseThink® Time

Using the NurseThink® system, complete the priorities. Check your answers designated by 💡 in the Pancreatitis Priority Exemplar.

Clinical Hint

Make sure you auscultate bowel sounds prior to palpating. Touching and manipulating the abdomen may change the sounds and lead to incorrect findings.

✎ Priority Assessments or Cues

1.

2.

3.

⚗ Priority Laboratory Tests/Diagnostics

1.

2.

3.

⚠ Priority Interventions or Actions

1.

2.

3.

⚑ Priority Potential & Actual Complications

1.

2.

3.

℧ Priority Nursing Implications

1.

2.

3.

◦ Priority Medications

1.

2.

3.

⬤ Priority Education/Discharge Issues

1.

2.

3.

Pancreatitis

Pathophysiology/Description

> Inflammation of the pancreas

> Two categories of pancreatitis
> - Acute, occurring suddenly and usually lasts for days
> - Chronic, occurring over months to years

> If pancreatitis is mild, it may not require treatment but when severe, it can cause serious complications

> Main presenting symptoms for acute pancreatitis
> - Severe pain is the main symptom. It is sudden abdominal pain that usually radiates to the back and worsens with food
> - Fever, nausea, vomiting,
> - Tenderness to abdomen. Client will guard the abdomen

> Symptoms for chronic pancreatitis
> - Weight loss that occurs without trying to lose weight
> - Stools that are foul smelling and oily, termed steatorrhea
> - Pain in upper abdomen

> Recurring acute pancreatitis can result in scar tissue formation in the pancreas. This can cause the pancreas to function poorly, leading to diabetes and digestion problems

> Common causes of pancreatitis
> - Gallstones
> - Alcoholism
> - Abdominal surgery
> - Biliary sludge comprised of calcium salts and cholesterol crystals
> - Cigarette smoking
> - High triglycerides, usually levels greater than 100 mg/dL
> - Pancreatic cancer

Priority Assessments or Cues

> Complete full system assessment as well as focused assessment

> Ask about abdominal pain. Pain usually occurs suddenly in the left upper quadrant and radiates to the back. Ask for a description of the pain. Pain with acute pancreatitis is often described as piercing, deep and severe

> Ask about alcohol intake and type of meal last consumed. Alcohol and fatty foods can increase the pain

> Assess for fever, nausea and vomiting, decreased or absent bowel sounds. Observe for guarding of the abdominal area. Assess for bowel distention, caused by paralytic ileus.

> Assess for Cullen's sign (bluish discoloration around the umbilicus) and Grey Turner's sign (bluish discoloration on the flanks), caused by bloody exudate seeping from the pancreas

> Measure vital signs, client is usually tachycardic and hypotensive

> In severe pancreatitis, assess respiratory system for complications such as pleural effusion, atelectasis or acute respiratory distress syndrome

> If surgery was done, assess site for bleeding and infection

> Assess for foul smelling, fatty stools in chronic pancreatitis

Priority Laboratory Tests/Diagnostics

> Blood test
> - Serum amylase and lipase, urinary amylase, glucose, triglycerides will be elevated
> - Serum calcium will be decreased

> Computed tomography (CT) scan will show gallstones, abscess or pseudocyst

> Stool test will show fat, indicating poor absorption of nutrients (mostly for chronic pancreatitis)

> Abdominal ultrasound will show pancreatic inflammation and gallstones

> Magnetic resonance imaging (MRI) reveals gallbladder, pancreatic and pancreatic duct abnormalities

Priority Interventions or Actions

> Withhold oral intake and initiate intravenous fluids. Insert nasogastric tube to prevent vomiting and gastric distention. Administer parenteral nutrition to supplement nutrition

> Administer oxygen to keep oxygen saturation greater than 95%

> Manage pain with intravenous morphine. Encourage client to lie on the side with head up to 45 degrees. This helps to ease the pain by decreasing abdominal tension

> Monitor glucose levels

> Administer medications that decrease production of hydrochloric acid to prevent pancreatic enzymes from being activated

> Ongoing monitoring of vital signs as fever, tachypnea and hypotension can cause compromise in hemodynamic stability

> Monitor fluid and electrolytes

> In severe acute pancreatitis, vasoactive medications may be administered to correct hypotension

> Monitor client for pancreatic necrosis and administer antibiotic as prescribed

> Prepare client for surgery if pancreatitis is caused by gallstones that must be removed
> - An endoscopic retrograde cholangiopancreatography (ERCP) is done using general anesthesia or sedative to examine internal structures and confirm gallstones and may include a sphincterotomy
> - Cholecystectomy may be performed to prevent recurrence

- Monitor surgical site for bleeding and infection. Manage drainage tube
> When client can eat, provide meals in small amounts and at frequent intervals

Priority Potential & Actual Complications

- Pseudocyst, the formation of a pocket in the pancreas that is filled with debris and fluid. If the cyst ruptures, bleeding and infection can occur
> Kidney failure
- Diabetes
> Pancreatic cancer
- Respiratory problems such as acute respiratory distress syndrome (ARDS), pleural effusion and atelectasis

Priority Nursing Implications

- For the client who has alcohol use disorder, assistance may be needed to get support for the client to quit drinking, to minimize the likelihood of a future pancreatitis exacerbation from alcohol intake
- Remember that pain is excruciating with acute pancreatitis, so pain management must be a priority
- With acute pancreatitis, it is crucial to prevent all actions that can stimulate the pancreas as this will only aggravate the condition. Patients must not be fed any foods by mouth until the acute condition is resolved

Priority Medications

- pancrelipase
  - Pancreatic enzyme replacement
  - Used for chronic pancreatitis
  - Usual dose is 8,000 to 36,000 units taken orally with each meal
- morphine
  - Administered intravenously for pain
  - Usual dose is 2 to 10 mg every 4 hours. Administered over 4 to 5 minutes
  - 5 to 15 mg is the dose range
- Proton pump inhibitors
  - Used to decrease acid secretion, which acts as a stimulus for pancreatic activity
  - omeprazole is given 60 mg PO daily initially, then administered in multiple or single daily does to a maximum of 120 mg PO three times daily
  - pantoprazole administered via oral or intravenous routes. Usual dose is 20-80 mg daily

> Antispasmodics
  - dicyclomine (common one used in the class), used to decrease motility and pancreatic outflow
  - Administered orally
  - Usual dosage is 80-160 mg daily, divided in in 4 doses

Priority Education/Discharge Issues

- Teach client to avoid the triggers of pancreatitis, such as alcohol intake and cigarette smoking
> Teach client that the condition may cause weakness and loss of strength so physical therapy to increase muscle strength may be needed when discharged
- Teach client to avoid fatty foods as they stimulate the pancreas and can cause an attack of pancreatitis
> Teach client to monitor the quality of stools and report increased foul-smelling stools that contain fat (steatorrhea) to the healthcare provider
> Teach the signs and symptoms of diabetes
- For client with chronic pancreatitis, instruct on intake of pancreatic enzymes with meals
> Educate on the importance to keeping all follow-up medical appointments

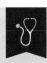

Go To Clinical Answers

Text designated by 💡 are the top answers for the Go To Clinical related to Pancreatitis.

Next Gen Clinical Judgment

You are caring for a client with pancreatitis. The client is recommended to abstain from alcohol. The client tells you "I don't think I will be able to stop drinking. My entire social life revolves around the local bar. All my friends are there. I drink every night-about 6-10 beers and a few shots a night. I still get up every day for work. Why do I have to quit drinking? Can I just cut down?"

Develop 5 recommendations for this client to facilitate this behavior change:

1. _____

2. _____

3. _____

4. _____

5. _____

Appendicitis/peritonitis

📋 Pathophysiology/Description

> Appendicitis is inflammation of the narrow tube of tissue that extends from the cecum, called the appendix

> Appendicitis accounts for many emergency visits and is the most common reason for abdominal surgery

> The goal is to remove the inflamed appendix before it ruptures but rupture often occurs, causing peritonitis. Appendicitis is a medical emergency

> The condition is commonly seen in ages 10-30

> Common cause of appendicitis is accumulated fecal deposits causing obstruction

> Clinical manifestations
  - Dull, persistent pain around the umbilicus that frequently moves to the right lower quadrant
  - The pain usually localizes between the right iliac crest and the umbilicus, known as McBurney's point
  - Nausea, vomiting and low-grade fever
  - Rebound tenderness (when pressure is applied to the abdomen and released, the pain is more intense) and client guards the abdomen
  - Client often lies on side with legs flexed to guard abdomen

✏️ Priority Assessments or Cues

> Assess for abdominal pain to umbilical area and right lower quadrant

> Assess for nausea and vomiting

> Asses if client can deep breathe, cough or sneeze without increase in pain. With appendicitis, these actions will worsen that pain

> Assess for rebound tenderness, which is indicative of appendicitis

> Monitor vital signs

> Assess for abdominal distention, tachycardia and fever if peritonitis is suspected

> Assess nasogastric tube to ensure proper functioning

> Assess surgical site for bleeding post and signs of infection

> Assess vital signs, if losing of blood from peritonitis, client may be hypotensive with tachycardia trying to compensate for hypotension

Next Gen Clinical Judgment

List 3 statements by a client suffering from an appendicitis.

_____

_____

_____

🧪 Priority Laboratory Tests/Diagnostics

> White blood cell count is expected to be elevated

> Computed tomography (CT) scan, magnetic resonance imaging and ultrasound used for appendicitis and peritonitis to examine the degree of damage as well as determine cause of either condition

> Urinalysis, to determine if appendicitis is being mimicked by a genitourinary condition

> Abdominal X-ray may show loops of dilated bowels, indicating conditions such as obstruction or paralytic ileus. Used when peritonitis is suspected

> Peritoneoscopy can allow direct view of the peritoneum. Used when peritonitis is suspected

⚠️ Priority Interventions or Actions

> Keep the client NPO (nothing by mouth) until a decision regarding surgery is made

> Monitor for signs that indicate appendix has ruptured

> Monitor bowel sounds

> Ongoing monitoring of status and vital signs to determine change in condition

> Prepare client for emergency appendectomy

> Administer pain medications

> Administer medications for nausea and vomiting

> Administer antibiotic therapy and monitor for side effects

> Provide comfort measures, such as positioning client in a right side-lying position

> Administer antibiotics for peritonitis

> With peritonitis, insert nasogastric tube and connect to low-intermittent suction to decrease gastric distention

> With peritonitis, monitor intake, output and electrolytes level to guide fluid replacement

> Manage surgical drain if one was used

🚩 Priority Potential & Actual Complications

> Complication of appendicitis
  - Perforation, with resulting peritonitis

> Complications of peritonitis
  - Hypovolemic shock
  - Paralytic ileus
  - Sepsis
  - Abscess formation in the abdomen
  - Acute respiratory distress syndrome

Priority Nursing Implications

> Note that with appendicitis, peritonitis is a significant complication. However, peritonitis can be caused by other factors as well, such as perforated duodenal or gastric ulcers, abdominal trauma, liver cirrhosis and ascites, infections of the genital tract or blood-borne pathogens.

> When there is peritonitis from a ruptured appendix, intravenous fluids given for 6-8 hours prior to an appendectomy aids in the prevention of dehydration and sepsis

> With appendicitis, do not apply heat of any type to the abdomen as heat can cause the appendix to rupture

Priority Medications

> Analgesics
> - Used to manage pain
> - There are numerous analgesic medications from which to choose
> - Available via all routes. The choice of route and medication is dependent on the healthcare provider's assessment of the client and the severity of the pain. There is no one specific analgesic that is used in appendicitis and/or peritonitis

> Antiemetic medications
> - Used to treat nausea and vomiting
> - There are many in this class of drugs from which a prescriber can choose. Some common ones are ondansetron, prochlorperazine and dolasetron
> - Available oral, intravenous, intramuscular and rectal. For the client with appendicitis and or peritonitis it will most likely not be administered via the intravenous route

> Antibiotics
> - Cephalosporins most commonly used. Treat infection from a ruptured appendix, peritonitis or as prophylaxis
> - Several in the class of cephalosporins. Few common ones are cefuroxime, ceftriaxone, ceftazidime
> - Dosage varies, based on route and severity of the condition

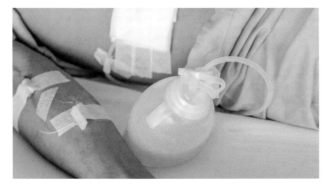

Image 7-5: Surgical drains are sometimes needed after an appendectomy.

Priority Education/Discharge Issues

> Teach client that discharge expectation after an appendectomy is 24 hours and that after 2-3 weeks they should be able to resume normal activities

> If discharged with antibiotics, teach the importance of, and rationale for taking all the medication and not stopping when they feel better

> Teach signs and symptoms of a wound infection and when to notify the healthcare provider

> Educate on importance of keeping follow-up medical appointments

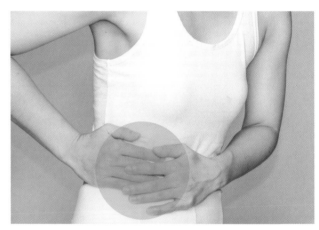

Image 7-6: Place your hand in the area described in the question. Try it, place your hand over your spleen, then your stomach, then your bladder, then your appendix.

Next Gen Clinical Judgment

Consider these questions:

1. Why is it critical to manage appendicitis prior to the appendix rupturing?

2. How is the management of a client with a ruptured appendix different from a client with appendicitis without rupture?

_____

_____

_____

_____

Cellulitis/wound infection/septicemia

📋 Pathophysiology/Description

> A wound infection occurs when bacteria invades an open wound

> Causes
  - Surgical complication
  - Poor aseptic technique
  - Certain medical conditions predispose to infections, such as diabetes mellitus

> Wound infections must be treated timely and appropriately to foster healing and prevent complications. One of the more serious complications is septicemia, which is bacteria in the bloodstream

✏️ Priority Assessments or Cues

> Assess client for fever and chills, indicative of an infection

> Assess wound for tenderness, swelling, warmth, malodorous and purulent drainage

> Assess pain level. There is usually pain with an infected wound and with cellulitis

> Assess size of wound. Examine wound for dead tissue as necrotic tissue is often present in infected wounds

> Assess complete blood count, expect increase in white blood cells due to infection and fever

> Assess vital signs, expect temperature elevation.

> Assess for cellulitis, manifested as inflammation to surrounding skin and soft tissues under the skin, and red streaking to the skin

> If there is cellulitis, perform ongoing assessments to determine if fever, tachycardia and tachypnea are resolving with treatment

> Assess for septicemia, manifested as chills, fever, tachycardia and tachypnea. Confusion, reduced urine output and shock are likely if septicemia progresses without treatment

> Perform a complete physical assessment

> Complete a detailed health history

🧪 Priority Laboratory Tests/Diagnostics

> Complete blood count will show elevated white blood cell count

> Wound culture will show the causative bacteria

> X-ray or computed tomography (CT) scan to look for foreign objects in wound (as in an object left in a surgical wound) or examine deep tissues for signs of infection

⚠️ Priority Interventions or Actions

> Collect wound samples for culture and sensitivity and send to the lab promptly

> Administer prompt treatment of septicemia. If present, to prevent progression to sepsis and septic shock.

> Administer antibiotics promptly as prescribed and monitor for effectiveness

> Administer wound treatment as prescribed

> Monitor wound to determine effectiveness of treatment

> Monitor blood test to determine decrease in white blood cell count

> Monitor skin with cellulitis to determine if inflammation is resolving

> Administer analgesics for pain, especially before performing wound care

> Assist with wound debridement procedure to remove dead tissue from wound

> If foreign body in wound, prepare client for procedure to remove the object

> Apply wound vacuum to assist with wound healing, if prescribed and monitor wound drainage

🚩 Priority Potential & Actual Complications

> Chronic infection

> Loss of limb as a result of untreated infected wound

> Septicemia, which is bacteria in the blood that can result in sepsis. Some still refer to septicemia as blood poisoning or bacteremia. Septicemia occurs when bacteria gets into the bloodstream from another part of the body, as in an infected wound. Client can have chills, fever, fast heart rate and respirations, confusion, reduced urine output and shock

> Sepsis is a widespread and potentially fatal inflammation of the body in response to bacteria in the bloodstream. Both septicemia and sepsis must be treated promptly

> May be fatal

🖐 Priority Nursing Implications

> Cellulitis can occur as a result of a wound infection, but it can also be seen in other conditions such as a foreign body in the skin, a tear to the skin, or chronic conditions such as eczema. Cellulitis must be treated promptly

Priority Medications

- cephalexin
  - Antibiotic
  - First generation cephalosporin that is commonly used to treat bacterial and skin infections
  - Dose is 250-500 mg every 6 hours
- amoxicillin
  - Antibiotic in the penicillin family
  - Commonly prescribed for skin infections
  - Dose is 250-500 mg every 8 hours
- augmentin
  - Antibiotic
  - Used when amoxicillin and cephalexin are not effective
  - Dose is 250 mg every 8 hours or 500 mg every 12 hours. For infections that are more severe, dose is 875 mg every 12 hours or 500 mg every 8 hours.
- Analgesics
  - Used to manage pain
  - There are numerous analgesic medications from which to choose
  - Available via all routes. The choice of route and medication is dependent on the healthcare provider's assessment of the client and the severity of the pain. There is no one specific analgesic that is used for the client with a wound infection, septicemia or cellulitis

Priority Education/Discharge Issues

- Instruct client to finish all the antibiotics prescribed
- Teach client how to care for wound at home to prevent re-infection
- Teach client the signs and symptoms of septicemia
- Teach signs and symptoms of wound infection and when to contact the healthcare provider
- Educate on the importance of follow-up medical care
- Teach client about healthy nutrition to promote wound healing
- Teach about management of other health conditions the client has, especially those associated with poor wound healing, like diabetes
- Educate client about the effects of smoking on wound healing. It causes poor wound healing
- Assist client to schedule visits to a wound care clinic if client is unable to care for wound

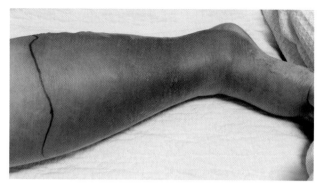

Image 7-7: This client has cellulitis and a deep vein thrombosis. What are the priority diagnostics that can confirm this diagnosis? What are priority interventions by the nurse?

Complete this MNEMONIC
SEPSIS Symptoms

S _____

E _____

P _____

S _____

I _____

S _____

Table 7-2: Feel free to search the Internet or create your own.

_____

_____

_____

_____

_____

_____

Gout

Pathophysiology/Description

> Gout is a systemic condition characterized by high levels of uric acid (called hyperuricemia) and deposits of uric acid crystals in joints

> Gout is not a continuous condition but one that presents with long intervals of remission and periods of exacerbation

> There are two forms of gout
> • Primary, which occurs as a result of a problem with purine metabolism in the body. This is the most common type of gout
> • Secondary, which results from some other condition in the body, such as renal insufficiency sickle cell anemia, hyperlipidemia, medications

> Causes of primary gout
> • Kidney reduced capacity to excrete uric acid
> • Increased production of uric acid
> • Dietary increase in purine rich foods, such as shellfish, red meat, drinks with fructose

> There are 4 phases to gout
> • Asymptomatic phase, where there is hyperuricemia, but the individual has no symptoms
> • Acute phase, where one or more small joints is inflamed, causing excruciating pain. Pain is usually in the great toe
> • Intermittent phase, where the individual experiences intermittent periods with no symptoms between acute exacerbations or attacks
> • Chronic phase that is characterized by repeated attacks. With chronic gout, there can be deposit of urate crystal in major organs

Priority Assessments or Cues

> Assess for swelling and inflammation of joints, expect joints to be very tender and painful. Clients usually state that the affected area is very sensitive when touched lightly

> Examine great toe as this is the most common location where gout first manifests

> Assess color of affected joints (maybe cyanotic and dusky in color)

> Assess range of motion limitation

> Ask client about family history. Complete a thorough health history

> Ask about risk factors for gout. This will help with client education on prevention of exacerbations

> Ask about onset of pain. Gout typically starts at night with swelling that occurs suddenly, followed by excruciating pain

> Assess vital signs, a low-grade temperature is usually present

> Examine joint for presence of tophi which appear as hard nodules in the skin. Tophi occur from deposits of sodium urate crystals

> Ask client about itching (pruritus) to skin. Urate crystals in skin causes itching

Priority Laboratory Tests/Diagnostics

> Serum uric acid will usually be elevated above 6 mg/dL

> 24-hour urine uric acid. This determines if gout is related to overproduction of uric acid or decreased excretion of uric acid from the kidneys

> Synovial fluid aspiration. This is the gold standard for diagnosis and will show urate crystals.

> X-ray of the affected area will show tophi in chronic gout but may be normal in the early stages of gout

Priority Interventions or Actions

> Use a bed cradle to prevent the bed linens from touching the affected lower extremity. Handle extremity carefully to avoid direct touching of the affected area

> Administer anti-inflammatory, uricosuric drugs and analgesic medications as prescribed, to treat the condition. Monitor for desired, and side effects

> Monitor intake and output to ensure uric acid is not being precipitated in the renal tubules. Encourage fluid intake of 2000 mL/day

> Ensure client has a diet low in purine. Encourage client to eat foods that help to increase the pH of urine (above 6), called alkaline ash foods. Most vegetables and fruits fall in this category

> Encourage bedrest initially to immobilize affected joint, until condition has started to resolve

> Monitor for common adverse effect of NSAIDs, gastrointestinal bleeding

Priority Potential & Actual Complications

> Deformity to joints
> Urate deposits in organs causing organ dysfunction
> Renal calculi

Priority Nursing Implications

> Bedrest may be needed in initial stage of acute gout when it is most painful. However, be mindful of problems that can occur when clients are immobilized, such as pressure ulcers and use strategies to prevent complications

> Note that even though the gold standard for diagnosing gout is synovial fluid aspiration, it is only done in a small percentage of clients. This is because clinical symptoms alone can usually diagnose gout

Priority Medications

> colchicine

- The oldest drug used to treat acute gout

- Reduces the inflammatory response. Provides excellent pain relief in 12 -24 hours

- Usual initial oral dose is 0.6 mg to 1.2 mg, then 0.6 mg every 1 to 2 hours until the client's pain is relieved

> Non-steroidal anti-inflammatory drugs (NSAIDs)

- For acute treatment of inflammatory process

- There are several that can be used but indomethacin, naproxen and sulindac are quite often used for gout. Dosages vary

- Most significant adverse effect of NSAIDs is gastrointestinal bleeding

> allopurinol

- Used as maintenance therapy

- Prevents uric acid production

- Usual dose is 200 to 600 mg daily administered orally

> probenecid

- Used to increase the kidney's excretion of uric acid in urine

- Usual dosage is 250 mg twice daily for one week, then 500 mg twice daily

- Probenecid is ineffective if client has renal impairment

> febuxostat

- This is the first new drug for gout in recent years

- Used for chronic gout to manage high levels of uric acid in the blood

- Usual dosage is 40 to 80 mg daily

> pegloticase

- Used when clients do not respond to other drugs that decrease uric acid level in the blood

- Usual dosage is 8 mg via intravenous infusion every 2 weeks. Must be administered over no less than 120 minutes

- Pre-medicate client with corticosteroids or antihistamines before pegloticase to prevent infusion reactions

> Corticosteroids

- Can be used to treat attacks, especially for clients who cannot take NSAIDs and/or colchicine

- Administered oral or intraarticular (into the joints)

- Several used at various dosages, but most common are dexamethasone, prednisone, triamcinolone, hydrocortisone, methylprednisolone

Priority Education/Discharge Issues

> Teach the importance of adhering to the treatment plan. Take medications as prescribed

> Educate on the importance of getting uric acid in the blood checked periodically

> Teach the importance of keeping follow-up medical appointments

> Teach signs and symptoms of gout attack

> Educate on factors that can precipitate a gout attack such as overeating foods that are rich in purine These include organ meat, anchovies, shellfish

> Educate on avoidance of alcoholic drinks as alcohol precipitates gout attacks

> Teach about adverse effects of maintenance drugs such as allopurinol. Allopurinol has the following serious adverse effects

- Aplastic anemia

- Toxic epidermal necrolysis

- Agranulocytosis

- Stevens-Johnson syndrome

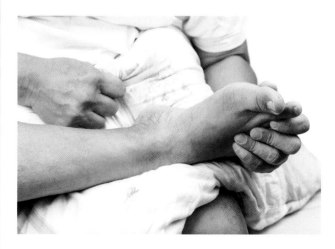

Image 7-8: What would the nurse feel when palpating this client's toe if gout is present?

_____

_____

_____

_____

_____

Systemic lupus erythematosus

Pathophysiology/Description

> Systemic lupus erythematosus is a chronic, autoimmune, progressive multisystem disease that causes failure to major organ systems of the body

> Occurs most frequently in women of child-bearing age and generally seen most often in Hispanics, Native Americans, African Americans and Asian Americans

> The disease is characterized by exacerbations and remissions

> Cause
> • Even though the etiology is unknown, it is observed that SLE usually runs in families, so genetics is suspected as a causative factor
> • Hormonal involvement. Observed that the disease worsens with menstruation, during and immediately after pregnancy and when oral contraceptives are used
> • Environmental factors such as sunlight, chemical exposure and stress have been known to exacerbate SLE.
> • Several medications have been identified as triggers for SLE

> With SLE, instead of protecting the body as it normally does, the immune system attacks the body's own tissues causing major damage to many organs. Fibrin deposits and connective tissue collect on collagen fibers and inside the blood vessels, causing widespread inflammation and necrosis

> All body systems are affected with SLE

> There is no cure for SLE but clients experience periods of remission

Priority Assessments or Cues

> Assess for joint pain

> Ask about excessive fatigue, weight loss and fever as these symptoms usually occur before SLE activity worsens

> Assess skin for redness to face with classic "butterfly" rash over cheeks and bridge of nose, scaly rash to face and upper torso. Assess palms for erythema

> Assess for general feeling of malaise, weakness and anorexia

> Assess for ulcers to mouth and nose, these are common with SLE

> Assess hair for balding and lesions to scalp

> Assess for infections due to increased susceptibility to infections

> Assess for cough and difficulty breathing, suggestive of lung involvement

> Assess for cardiac dysrhythmias due to fibrosis of atrioventricular nodes

> Assess for polyarthralgia (pain in many joints) and stiffness in the morning (this is a common complaint). Look for stiffness to joints

> Assess for renal involvement, shows SLE impact on renal system

> Assess for neurological involvement such as seizures, disordered thinking, impaired memory and peripheral neuropathy. Assess for photosensitivity

> Assess for anxiety, depression and psychosis due to the stress of a major life-altering illness

> Assess labs, looking for hematologic conditions such as thrombocytopenia, anemia, leukopenia and clotting issues

> Complete history and physical and physical assessment

Priority Laboratory Tests/Diagnostics

> Antinuclear antibody (ANA), a type of antibody directed against the nuclei of the cell: will be positive in about 97% of clients with SLE

> Antiphospholipid Antibodies (ALPs), antibodies that are directed at phospholipids: will be positive in about 30% of clients with SLE

> anti-Smith antibody, a protein found in cell nucleus called Sm, will be positive in about 30% of clients with SLE

> C-Reactive Protein (CRP), a protein in body that can suggest inflammation, will be elevated: not used to diagnose the disease but is used to determine therapy effectiveness and activity of the disease

> Erythrocyte sedimentation rate is elevated in SLE and is used to monitor SLE activity and effectiveness of therapy

Priority Interventions or Actions

> Monitor for signs of organ involvement, such as peritonitis, hypertension, arrhythmias, nephritis, pericarditis, anemia and coronary artery disease (this is not an exhaustive list since all systems are impacted)

> Monitor skin integrity and provide meticulous skin care

> Apply creams and ointments for skin rash, as prescribed

> Administer medication as prescribed to manage pain and decrease the inflammatory response

> Perform patient care activities, to include rest periods due to fatigue

> Ensure client is provided with proper nutrients due to weight loss

> Provide appropriate respiratory care if respiratory system involvement, such as oxygen

> Measure intake and output, primarily if the client is receiving corticosteroids. Corticosteroids can cause fluid retention

> Monitor neurologic functioning to determine change in neurologic symptoms, such as memory deficits, personality changes and seizures. Administer anti-seizure medications if seizure involvement

> Monitor for bleeding or bruising due to hematologic involvement

> Monitor hands and feet to determine improvement in numbness, tingling and weakness. Peripheral neuropathy is an issue in SLE

> Provide diet high in iron, protein, folic acid and vitamins, if there are no contraindications to any of these, such as kidney disease that would prevent intake of a high-protein diet

> Provide emotional support for client and family

> Provide supportive environment for client to verbalize feelings about the disease

Priority Potential & Actual Complications

> Complications of SLE are many and affect all systems. This is not an all-inclusive list of possible complications
  - Stroke, seizure, memory impairment
  - Psychological problems, usually from coping with the myriad of complications
  - Heart attack, dysrhythmias, pericarditis, cardiac failure
  - Pleurisy, difficulty breathing
  - Kidney failure
  - Severe arthralgia, impaired mobility, paralysis, may be fatal

Priority Nursing Implications

> It is important to remember that SLE is a multisystem disorder that impacts every system in the client's body so focus of care will be on all body systems

> Managing and dealing with the myriad of system complications that SLE presents, some clients will likely suffer depression. It is important to assess for this and ensure appropriate referrals to address the issue

> Hydroxychloroquine causes retinopathy so client taking the drug should have an eye examination every 6-12 months

> Methotrexate has serious side effects of hepatoxicity and bone marrow suppression, so CBC must be monitored frequently

Priority Medications

> Non-steroidal anti-inflammatory drugs (NSAIDs)
  - NSAIDs are frequently used interventions for arthralgia and arthritis seen with SLE
  - There are several that can be used but indomethacin, naproxen and sulindac are quite often used for systemic lupus erythematosus. Dosages vary based on the drug used
  - Most significant adverse effect of NSAIDs is gastrointestinal bleeding

> hydroxychloroquine
  - Antimalarial drugs
  - Used to treat fatigue and joint and skin problems
  - Initial dose: 400 mg orally 1 to 2 times daily. Can be continued for several weeks or months, based on response of the client. Maintenance dose is 200 to 400 mg oral daily

> dapsone
  - Antileprosy drug
  - Administered if client cannot tolerate an antimalarial drug
  - Dose range is 25 to over 200 mg daily. The patient's condition dictates the exact dose

> Corticosteroids (several in the class)
  - Corticosteroids use should be limited
  - methylprednisolone used intravenously and in tapering doses may be effective in managing the flare-up from polyarthritis
  - High doses of corticosteroids are effective in treating severe cutaneous problems from SLE

> methotrexate
  - Steroid-sparing immunosuppressant. Considered a standard treatment
  - Used as an alternate to corticosteroids

> azathioprine, cyclophosphamide
  - Immunosuppressants, used to treat severe organ involvement with SLE
  - Prevents the need for long-term corticosteroid therapy
  - Both drugs given oral or intravenous

> warfarin
  - Anticoagulant
  - Used to thin the blood and prevent blood clotting, which is a complication of SLE
  - Dosage is dependent on desired therapeutic range of the drug. Labs must be drawn to determine the international normalized ratio (INR)

> tacrolimus, pimecrolimus
  - Topical immunomodulators that suppress immune activity of the skin
  - Used instead of corticosteroids to manage skin rashes
  - Dosage of these creams depend on the severity of the rash. Results are usually seen in 8-15 days

> belimumab
  - First approved immunosuppressant drug for specific treatment of systemic lupus
  - Works by specifically targeting immune cells

Priority Education/Discharge Issues

> Teach client about the disease and long-term expectations

> Explain the triggers for SLE and how the client can avoid these triggers

> Teach proper skin care at home, wash with mild soap and do not apply perfumed or harsh emollients to skin

> Instruct client to avoid sun or ultraviolet light

> Provide client with information for SLE support groups

> Provide client with a list of community resources

> Educate client about medication therapy, to include why the drugs are being used, how to use them and the side effects

> Teach client about foods to eat that will provide essential nutrients needed

Rheumatoid arthritis

📋 Pathophysiology/Description

> Rheumatoid arthritis is a chronic systemic immune disease

> It is characterized by inflammation and destruction of connective tissue and membranes within the synovial joints

> The disease is characterized by exacerbations and remissions and can occur at any point in an individual's life. However, incidence of RA peaks between 30 and 50 years and affect women more than men

> Even though the etiology is unknown, it is thought to result from genetic as well as environmental factors

> The condition is life-altering and without treatment, many with the condition will have significant functional impairment, such as required replacement of joints, use of mobility aids and loss of ability to perform activities of daily living without assistance

> There are 4 stages to RA. Stage 1 is characterized by mild symptoms, such as swelling of synovial membrane and soft tissue, and elevated white blood cell count in the synovial fluid. As the client progresses to the final stage (end-stage), there will be loss of joint function and formation of nodules in subcutaneous tissue.

> Definitive diagnostic criteria for RA is based upon scores the client receives from four specific categories: joint involvement, serology, acute phase reactants and duration of symptoms. Possible scores range from 0-10. A score greater than or equal to 6 is definitive for RA

✏️ Priority Assessments or Cues

> Assess for joint pain, warmth, limited range of motion, deformity, nodules at joints and muscle atrophy. Focus assessment on small and large joints as large peripheral joints may also be involved

> Assess for signs of inflammation manifested as heat, swelling and tenderness to area

> Ask about excessive fatigue, weight loss, anorexia and generalized stiffness as these usually signify the start of joint symptoms

> Ask about severity and duration of pain in the morning. Pain and stiffness usually occur in the morning and last for more than 30 minutes, sometimes all day`

> Assess vital signs, expect a low-grade temperature, because of the inflammatory process

> Ask client to grasp objects. RA may affect the extensor and flexor tendons in the wrist, making grasping objects difficult

> Assess for specific deformities of RA
> - swan neck deformity: the middle joint of a finger is extended (bent back) more than normal. The end joint is flexed (bent down)
> - ulnar drift: a hand deformity where swelling of the metacarpophalangeal joints (the knuckles at the base of the fingers) causes the fingers to become displaced towards the little finger
> - hallux valgus (bunion): lateral deviation of the hallux (great toe) on the first metatarsal

- Boutonniere deformity: the finger permanently bends down at the middle joint and the end joint bends backwards

> Assess all body systems as RA can impact all systems

> Assess for Sjogren's syndrome manifested by decreased secretion of saliva and tears, resulting in dry eyes, photosensitivity and mouth

> Assess for felty syndrome, especially if client's RA is long-standing, manifested by low white blood cell count and splenomegaly.

> Assess for signs of infection as felty syndrome predisposes client to infection

> Assess client and family's psychosocial needs

🧪 Priority Laboratory Tests/Diagnostics

> White blood cell count (WBC) in synovial fluid will be elevated with decreased viscosity

> X-ray will show erosion and narrowing of joint space, bony growths and osteoporosis because of corticosteroid usage

> Rheumatoid Factor (RH) will be positive in up to 90% of clients with RA

> Antinuclear antibody (ANA), a type of antibody directed against the nuclei of the cell, will be positive in up to 30% of clients with RA

> C-Reactive Protein (CRP), a protein in body that can suggest inflammation, will be elevated, showing active inflammation

> Erythrocyte sedimentation rate will be elevated showing active inflammation

> anti-cyclic citrullinated peptide (ant-CCP), autoantibodies that are directed against certain peptides and proteins, will be positive in more than 80% of clients with RA

⚠️ Priority Interventions or Actions

> Administer drug therapy as prescribed

> Assist with completion of activities of daily living, being mindful of morning stiffness

> Provide range of motion exercises to client's tolerance to maintain functioning of joint

> Monitor skin integrity and provide meticulous skin care

> Avoid weight bearing to inflamed extremity

> Apply cold and heat applications to joints as prescribed

> Administer medication as prescribed to manage pain and decrease the inflammatory response

> Perform patient care activities, to include rest periods due to fatigue and joint discomfort

> Ensure client is provided with proper nutrients due to loss of appetite from pain and fatigue

> Ensure client gets assistance from physical and occupational therapies, if needed

> Use splints on affected extremities to prevent contractures

> Measure intake and output, primarily if the client is receiving corticosteroids. Corticosteroids can cause fluid retention

> Provide supportive environment for client to verbalize feelings about the disease

Priority Potential & Actual Complications

> Complications mostly relate to rheumatoid nodules forming in body parts
  - Scleritis
  - Sjögren's Syndrome
  - Heart complications such as pericarditis and myocarditis
  - Lung problems such as pleural effusion, collapsed lung
> Physical immobility due to deformity of extremities

Priority Nursing Implications

> Hydroxychloroquine causes retinopathy so client taking the drug should have an eye examination every 6-12 months
> Leflunomide is teratogenic so must not be administered to women of child-bearing age unless pregnancy is ruled out
> For clients who are administered aspirin, serum salicylate levels must be checked if dosage is more than 3600 mg daily to avoid the complications of aspirin toxicity
> RA is common in older adults and they often use several medications to treat their health conditions. It is important that polypharmacy be considered and addressed with the older client
> Methotrexate has the serious side effects of hepatoxicity and bone marrow suppression so CBC must be monitored frequently

Priority Medications

> Non-steroidal anti-inflammatory drugs (NSAIDs)
  - There are several NSAIDs that can be used. celecoxib and aspirin are ones commonly used
  - Most significant adverse effect of NSAIDs is gastrointestinal bleeding
> hydroxychloroquine
  - Antimalarial drug
  - Used to treat fatigue and joint problems
> leflunomide, sulfasalazine
  - Antirheumatic drugs
  - Doses vary depending on drug used and severity of symptoms
  - leflunomide blocks immune cell overproduction and sulfasalazine decreases the pain and swelling of inflammatory arthritis, but may also prevent damage to joints
> Corticosteroids (several in the class)
  - Low-dose corticosteroids are usually administered until the antirheumatic drugs can start to take effect

  - Used to manage symptoms during acute RA flare-up
  - When administered as intraarticular injections, may decrease pain and inflammation
> methotrexate
  - Steroid-sparing immunosuppressant
  - Used as an alternate to corticosteroids
> tofacitinib
  - Antirheumatic drug
  - Interferes with certain enzymes (JAK enzymes) that cause joint inflammation
  - Usual oral dose is 5 mg twice daily and 11 mg daily for the extended-release tablet
> Tumor necrosis factor inhibitors
  - Used in clients who have not responded to the antirheumatic drugs
  - Decrease immune and inflammatory response
  - Several in this class and dosage is dependent on the drug used
> Interleukin-1 receptor antagonists
  - Interleukin inhibitor. There are several in the class
  - Mostly used to treat clients who have not responded to, or cannot tolerate other drugs used for RA
  - Administered via various routes

Priority Education/Discharge Issues

> Teach client about the disease and long-term expectations
> Provide instruction on protection of small joints such as avoiding repetitive movements, using strongest joint for tasks and modifying activities to decrease stress on joints
> Provide client with information for RA support groups and a list of community resources
> Educate client about medication therapy, to include why the drugs are being used, how to use them and the side effects
> Teach client about foods to eat that will provide essential nutrition needed
> Instruct client and/or caregiver about modifications that may need to be made to the home to maintain a safe environment, if client has functional deficits from RA
> Instruct client on safe use of assistive devices
> Explain the effects of corticosteroid therapy to client, the fact that it causes weight gain. Encourage a weight loss program and tolerable exercise regimen. Teach to minimize overexertion, which may worsen RA
> Instruct client to engage in aquatic exercises in warm water, this will make the joints move easier
> Teach use of cold and heat therapy to relieve stiffness, muscle spasms and pain
> Stress the importance for client to keep follow-up appointments

HIV/AIDS

Pathophysiology/Description

> Human immunodeficiency (HIV) is a retrovirus that damages the immune system and renders the host susceptible to infections that would otherwise be prevented because of the body's immune response

> Even though the infection is seen in both men and women, in the United States, it is more prevalent in men who are sexually active with other men

> Transmission
> • Can occur when contact is made with infected vaginal secretions, blood, semen, breast milk, sexual intercourse
> • Exposure to HIV infected blood or blood products
> • Sexual intercourse with infected partner
> • Through birth or breastfeeding

> The target cell for HIV in the body is the CD4 T cell. HIV binds with receptors on the outside of the cell and RNA from HIV enters the cell. Several processes occur ending in destruction of the CD4 T cell. The rate that HIV kills CD4 T cells exceeds the rate at which CD4 T cells can replicate.

> With inadequate CD4 T cells, immune function is impaired. Problems with immune function starts to occur when CD4 T cell count drops below 500 CD4 T cells/uL. With CD4 T cell count below 200 CD4 T cells/uL, severe immune function problems occur. When CD 4 T cells are destroyed to a point where not enough are left to maintain immune function, the host becomes susceptible to opportunistic infections

> When HIV progresses, and the individual meets at least one of the diagnostic conditions delineated by the following criteria, acquired immune deficiency syndrome (AIDS) is diagnosed
> • One significant opportunist infection, whether bacterial, fungal, viral or protozoal
> • CD 4 T cell count below 200 cells/uL
> • Wasting syndrome, an ideal body mass loss of more than 10%
> • An opportunistic cancer such as immunoblastic lymphoma, Burkitt's lymphoma (and others)

Priority Assessments or Cues

> Determine engagement in risky behaviors

> Assess for symptoms that resemble mononucleosis, such as nausea, headache, malaise, swollen lymph nodes, sore throat, fever, joint pain, rash. These symptoms usually present about 2-3 weeks after infection with HIV

> Assess eyes for papilledema and presence of exudates

> Assess cardiac problems such as pericardial friction rubs or murmurs

> Assess neuro status for neurological impairment such as memory loss, slurred speech, tremors, agitation, seizures, paralysis

> Assess breathing, may find dyspnea, tachypnea, wheezing, cough

> Assess gastrointestinal system, may see a myriad of impairments such as, candida patches, blisters and other lesions in mouth, tooth decay, gingivitis, white patches in throat, white lesions on sides of tongue, diarrhea, vomiting rectal lesions

> Complete a system assessment to detect presence of opportunistic infections

> Use diagnostic criteria to asses if HIV has progressed to AIDS

> Perform skin assessment, may find pallor, cyanotic areas, alopecia, poor skin turgor, lesions and other skin eruptions, bruises to mucous membranes

> Assess genitourinary system, may see lesions and discharge from genitals and excoriation to vagina or perianal area

> Assess client's access to social support

> Assess client's mindset regarding end-of-life care

Priority Laboratory Tests/Diagnostics

> Rapid HIV screening test: A device is placed in the mouth against the gum and fluid is drawn into the pad, the pad is placed in a solution and if client has the HIV antibodies, the corresponding change is noted. Results are available in 20 minutes. If positive, a follow-up blood test is needed

> In home testing for HIV: A drop of blood is placed on a test card and the card is mailed to a laboratory for testing. The card has a code number. Result is received when the client calls a special telephone number and enters the code

> P24 antigen assay detects the amount of HIV viral core protein in the client's blood. Blood is drawn in a lab. Can detect HIV about 2-3 weeks after infection occurs. Result is usually available hours to days

> CD 4 T cell count is used to monitor progression of HIV. Normal CD4 T cell count is 800-1200 cells/uL. The CD4 T cell count decreases as the disease progresses

> Viral load provides information on progression of HIV. Higher viral load indicates more disease activity

> Complete blood cell count (CBC) will likely show low white blood cell count due to opportunistic infections. Anemia and thrombocytopenia may be present due to effects of drug therapy or antiplatelet antibodies

Priority Interventions or Actions

> Administer ART therapy. Monitor for, and treat side effects

> Allow client time to process the news of being HIV positive, if new diagnosis

> Provide adequate oxygenation if client has pneumonia

> Provide other appropriate system care if client has AIDS

> Treat client with dignity and respect

> Provide safe care environment if client has neurological impairments from HIV/AIDS

> Provide gentle but meticulous skin care, as diarrhea and incontinence may be copious

> Be gentle when providing care as client may be emaciated

and hurting from muscle wasting
> Protect bony prominences to prevent pressure ulcer formation
> Support client through process of taking multiple medications several times daily
> Provide case management to client to manage social and post discharge plans
> Allow client time to verbalize emotions and end-of-life wishes

⚑ Priority Potential & Actual Complications

> Opportunistic infections
> Progression of HIV to AIDS
> Social isolation
> Severe depression
> Coma
> May be fatal

℧ Priority Nursing Implications

> The main cause of disability, disease and death of persons with HIV is opportunistic diseases
> It is important to note that ART interacts with many over-the-counter drugs and alternative therapies. Clients must understand that when on ART, they must seek advice from healthcare providers and pharmacists before taking OTC drugs and herbal remedies
> Think about the implication when older adults have HIV. They may be ashamed and not want to speak about it, which delays treatment. Nursing implication is that as nurses, a discussion about sexually transmitted diseases must be had when doing admissions of any client, regardless of age

◐ Priority Medications

> Non-nucleoside reverse transcriptase inhibitors (NNRTIs)
  • Stops the action of a protein needed by HIV to make copies of itself.
  • There are many drugs in this class
  • Example of dosage for a common drug in the class: nevirapine 200 mg daily for 14 days, administered orally, then twice daily
> Nucleoside or nucleotide reverse transcriptase inhibitors (NRTIs)
  • Stops the action of reverse transcriptase
  • There are many drugs in this class
  • Example of dosage for a common drug in the class: zidovudine 300 mg twice daily administered orally, or 1 mg/kg every 4 hours administered intravenously. This drug is also given in pregnancy orally until labor begins, then is administered intravenously until the umbilical cord is clamped

> Protease inhibitors (PIs)
  • Inactivate another protein that HIV needs to make copies of itself called HIV protease
  • There are many drugs in this class
  • Example of dosage for a common drug in the class: indinavir 800 mg every 8 hours administered orally
> Entry or fusion inhibitors
  • Block entry of HIV in CD4 T cells, thus decreasing replication
  • There are many drugs in this class
  • Example of dosage for a common drug in the class: enfuvirtide 90 mg twice daily administered via subcutaneous injection
> Integrase inhibitors
  • Disables a protein called integrase, which HIV uses to insert its genetic material into CD4 T cells.
  • There are many drugs in this class
  • Example of dosage for a common drug in the class: raltegravir 400 mg twice daily, administered orally
> Fixed dose combination drugs
  • These are more than one drug that may come from various classes that are combined into a single tablet

☻ Priority Education/Discharge Issues

> Teach preventative measures, in terms of not infecting future partners. Teach alternate safe sex activities, such as mutual masturbation
> Teach about HIV, the susceptibility to infection and treatment options
> Instruct client on signs and symptoms to report to healthcare team
> Provide community resources and support for psychosocial, financial and spiritual need
> Teach about slowing or preventing progression of HIV to AIDS
> Teach about not sharing drug equipment, such as needles, syringes and cookers, as they may be contaminated with blood
> Teach about use of a needle and syringe exchange program, if the client's community has one
> Teach about proper nutrition to ensure adequate intake of nutrients
> Teach client how to reduce risk of getting opportunistic infections
> Teach client to stay current with vaccines
> Teach about the preexposure prophylaxis drug therapy (tenofovir and emtricitabine) in event client may want to provide this information to loved ones.
> Instruct on how to manage end-of-life issues, especially for the client with AIDS

Hypersensitivity reactions

Pathophysiology/Description

> Hypersensitivity reactions are undesirable reactions that occur as a result of the immune response acting against foreign antigens or against its own tissue.

> Hypersensitivity reactions are considered over-reaction of the body's immune system

> Can result in outcomes as simple as being uncomfortable, to as severe as death

> Classified based on the source of the antigen, whether the reaction is immediate or delayed and the way the injury is caused

> There are four types of hypersensitivity reactions

- Type I: IgE mediated reactions: an allergic reaction that occurs because of re-exposure to a specific type of antigen called an allergen. Includes allergic reactions such as anaphylaxis and atopic reactions, such as rashes

- Type II: Cytotoxic and cytolytic reactions: the antibodies produced by the immune response bind to antigens on the individual's own cell surfaces. Common antigens involved in type II reactions are Rh factor and the ABO blood group

- Type III: Immune-complex reactions: Antigen-antibody complexes cause tissue damage in immune complex reactions. Type III reactions may be immediate or delayed, localized or systemic. Type III reactions are seen in autoimmune conditions such as rheumatoid arthritis and systemic lupus erythematosus

- Type IV: Delayed hypersensitivity reactions: is referred to as delayed type hypersensitivity meaning that the reaction takes several days to develop. It is not an antibody-mediated reaction but a type of cell-mediated response. Example is transplant rejections, reaction to bacterial infections, contact dermatitis

Priority Assessments or Cues

> Assess for history of exposure to allergens

> Assess for a pale wheal on the skin that is edematous, contains fluid and is surrounded by a red flare (called wheal and flare reaction), indicating an anaphylactic reaction that is localized. A mosquito bite is an example of such a reaction

> Assess for cause of hypersensitivity reaction

> Assess for systemic anaphylactic reaction, manifested by initial edema and pruritus to exposure site, followed by respiratory and cardiac involvement such as, constriction of bronchioles, airway obstruction and shock

> Assess for symptoms indicating atopic reactions such as angioedema, asthma, atopic dermatitis, hay fever and hives

> Assess for sneezing, nasal drainage, swelling of mucosa that obstructs airway, itching around the eyes and throat and excessive tearing from eyes, indicating hay fever

> Assess for wheezing, tightness in chest, thick sputum production and dyspnea, indicating asthma reaction

> Examine skin for lesions that are edematous and contain vesicle formation, indicating atopic dermatitis

> Ask client about swelling that started in the face and then progressed to other parts of the body and assess for lesions on the body that client describes as itching, burning or stinging, indicating angioedema reaction

> Assess for areas on the body that are raised, edematous, pink in color and described by client as itching, which may indicate urticaria reaction

> Assess for signs and symptoms of Type II hypersensitivity reaction as in Goodpasture's Syndrome and hemolytic blood transfusion reaction. Manifestations relate to kidney injury, pulmonary hemorrhage

> Assess for reaction to immunotherapy, if injection was initiated

Priority Laboratory Tests/Diagnostics

> Sputum, nasal and bronchial secretions: will show presence of eosinophils

> Pulmonary function test: if asthma reaction, will show poor pulmonary functioning

> Complete blood count with white blood cell differential, shows immunodeficiency if lymphocyte count is below 1200/µL

> Skin test for allergens (the preferred test) is done via different methods

- A patch test, where allergen is put on a patch that is then placed on skin. Reaction is delayed because the patch must be worn for 48-72 hours

- A scratch or prick test, where allergen is placed on the skin and a pricking device allows the allergen to enter the skin. Reaction is seen in 5-10 minutes

- An intradermal test, where the allergen is injected under the skin. Reaction is seen in 10 minutes

- Positive reaction to the tests is indicated by the presence of a wheal-and-flare response

Clinical Hint

Hypersensitivity reactions can be potentially fatal. Nurses must act with urgency when these occur in clients, especially in cases of anaphylactic reactions which are potentially fatal.

Clinical Hint

Anaphylaxis occurs rapidly, and survival of the client is dependent on quick intervention. Ensuring a patent airway is the number one priority followed immediately by measures to prevent further spread of the allergen.

⚠ Priority Interventions or Actions

- Ensure a list of all client's allergies are on the health record
- Observe for allergy to latex, as many clients do not know they have this allergy
- Use latex free gloves and supplies when caring for clients with known latex allergy
- Administer antihistamines as prescribed
- Administer decongestants as prescribed
- Administer anti-itch medications as prescribed
- Administer corticosteroids as prescribed
- Administer leukotriene receptor agonists as prescribed
- Monitor for adverse effects of prescribed medications
- Treat skin rashes and lesions as prescribed
- Manage hypovolemic shock if severe anaphylaxis
- Administer immunotherapy injections
- Rotate site for allergen injections
- Monitor client for anaphylactic or other reaction to immunotherapy
- Observe client for 20-30 minutes after immunotherapy injections to ensure no adverse reaction

⚑ Priority Potential & Actual Complications

- Anaphylactic shock
- May be fatal

℧ Priority Nursing Implications

- When skin testing occurs to diagnose allergens, some clients may be highly sensitive and may develop an anaphylactic reaction to the skin tests. Do not leave the client alone during testing
- With an anaphylactic reaction, the key is to act quickly as death will occur if immediate care is not rendered

♦ Priority Medications

- Antihistamines
  - Several in the class so dosage is dependent on drug used
  - Most common drugs for treating urticaria and allergic rhinitis
  - Relieve acute symptoms of allergic response. Cause drowsiness
- Antipruritic(anti-itch) drugs
  - Applied to skin to relieve itching
  - Should not be used if skin is broken
  - Several in the class but common ones are coal tar solutions and calamine lotion

- Sympathomimetic drugs
  - Main drug of choice in class is epinephrine
  - Used to treat anaphylactic reaction
  - Do not use epinephrine if solution is cloudy or contains particles
- Decongestants
  - Used primarily to treat allergic rhinitis
  - Main one in class is pseudoephedrine
- Leukotriene receptor antagonists
  - Blocks leukotriene, a major mediator of allergic inflammatory process
  - Used to treat asthma an allergic rhinitis
  - Several in the class so dosage is dependent on drug used
- Mast cell stabilizer
  - Used to inhibit the release of histamine and leukotriene
  - Treat allergic rhinitis. Only one used in the class is cromolyn
  - Used as a nasal spray, 1 spray in each nostril every 4 to 6 hours
- Corticosteroids
  - Treat allergic rhinitis
  - Not for long-term use but for cases of severe reaction
  - Administered as nasal spray
- Immunotherapy
  - Used when usual drug therapy is ineffective or when the client cannot avoid the allergen
  - Injections with titrated amounts of allergen administered subcutaneously for 1-2 years to reach maximum effect
  - Allergen placed under the tongue, and administered by the client at home until hyposensitivity to the allergen is achieved

👤 Priority Education/Discharge Issues

- Teach importance of avoiding the allergen that caused the client's reaction
- Teach client the signs and symptoms of hypersensitivity reaction specific to the client's condition
- Teach proper administration of medications, such as nasal sprays
- Teach client about delayed reaction to immunotherapy injections and what to do if a reaction occurs
- Teach client to seek medical assistance at the first sign of anaphylaxis
- Teach client to report all allergies on medical visits, including allergy to latex

Influenza

Pathophysiology/Description

> Influenza is a highly contagious viral respiratory illness that may be caused by several different types of viruses

> Influenza (flu) is contracted by many individuals each year, resulting in many hours lost from work and school.

> Classified as types A, B and C
>   • A is the most common and virulent, affects humans and animals. Example is the swine flu (H1N1 influenza)
>   • B and C affect humans only

> Influenza is particularly troublesome because several strains exist, and the viruses can mutate. This is the reason the flu vaccine is administered every year

> Transmission by human to human via inhalation of infected particles or contact with infected droplets and from animals to humans when contact is made with animals that are infected

> There are two types of influenza that are common to animals but have impacted humans in recent years, swine influenza (H1N1) and avian influenza (H5N1)
>   • Swine influenza is a strain of influenza that originated in pigs but is spread from human to human. It emerged in 2009 as a pandemic
>   • Avian flu is a strain of influenza that affects birds, including chickens and turkeys. Swine influenza is common to humans but there have been sporadic human cases

Priority Assessments or Cues

> Ask client about onset of muscle aches and fever, onset of influenza symptoms is usually abrupt. Also, antiviral treatment should ideally begin within 2 days of onset of symptoms

> Assess for chills, headache, sore throat, cough, fatigue and malaise, expected with influenza

> Assess respiratory system, may find crackles and dyspnea if pulmonary involvement

> Assess for lethargy and weakness especially with the elderly

> Assess for complications of influenza, such as ear infections, pneumonia, dehydration

> Ask if client had an influenza vaccine

> Assess vital signs

Priority Laboratory Tests/Diagnostics

> Viral cultures done with swab from throat, nasopharyngeal, sputum or bronchial washing will identify the virus and the particular strain. Results can delay care as it takes 3-10 days so quite often diagnosis is made based on the client's clinical findings and history

> Rapid influenza test: Swab from nasal secretions gives result within minutes and will show influenza virus

Priority Interventions or Actions

> Perform viral culture or rapid influenza test

> Place client on droplet precautions, in acute care setting

> Treat complications of influenza, as prescribed

> Allow client to get adequate rest to relieve fatigue

> Administer antiviral medications as ordered

> Administer antitussives to alleviate cough

> Administer antipyretics to reduce fever

> Monitor lung sounds, to determine pulmonary compromise

> Encourage adequate fluids to liquefy secretions and prevent problems in pulmonary system

Priority Potential & Actual Complications

> Pneumonia, severe sinus and ear infections, and dehydration in older clients

Priority Nursing Implications

> For maximum effectiveness of antiviral therapy for influenza, treatment should start within 2 days of the onset of influenza symptoms

> There is a higher dose influenza vaccine for older adults to compensate for their weaker immune systems, caused by the aging process

Priority Medications

> zanamivir
>   • Reduce the duration of influenza by several days
>   • Administered as inhalation therapy
>   • Dose is 10 mg twice daily

> oseltamivir
>   • Reduce the duration of influenza by several days
>   • Administered orally
>   • Usual dose is 75 mg twice daily for 5 days

> peramivir
>   • New drug for treating influenza
>   • Administered intravenous with a single use dosage of 600 mg

> Influenza vaccines
>   • Must be administered yearly
>   • Administered as an intramuscular injection that contains killed influenza virus. Dose is 0.5 mL
>   • Administered intranasally and contains weakened live influenza virus

Priority Education/Discharge Issues

> Teach importance of taking the influenza vaccine each year

> Teach that the best time to take the influenza vaccine is before exposure to the virus, which is usually in September

> Dispel the common myth that the influenza vaccine causes influenza

> Teach client to expect soreness at vaccination site

> Teach client preventive measures such as covering cough, washing hands

Polycystic kidney

📋 Pathophysiology/Description

> Polycystic kidney disease is formation of cysts and hypertrophy of the kidneys. It is considered a very common genetic condition worldwide.

> The sequelae of the condition start with many tiny cysts in the medulla and cortex of the kidney. The cysts contain pus and fluid. They grow large and compress the surrounding tissue. These cysts usually rupture causing scar formation, infection, and nephrons that cannot function because of damage

> Forms of polycystic kidneys

- Genetic in childhood, which is a rare inherited autosomal recessive disorder. The infant usually does not survive and dies within months

- Adult onset, which is an autosomal dominant disorder, manifested in the third to fourth decade of life

> Both kidneys are usually involved. The condition is not gender specific

> Polycystic kidney disease can also affect other organs in the body

> By age 60, about half of clients with PKD have end-stage renal disease, needing either dialysis or transplant

✏️ Priority Assessments or Cues

> Ask client about recurrent urinary tract infections

> Ask about feelings of heaviness in the side, abdomen or back, from enlarged cysts

> Assess for proteinuria, pyuria and hematuria, which occur from ruptured cysts

> Asses for chronic pain, usually described as a constant pain

> Assess for headaches and hypertension

> Assess for fever and chills, which might indicate infection

> Palpate kidneys usually felt as enlarged on both sides

> Assess abdominal girth, usually enlarged

> Assess all body systems to determine signs and symptoms of PKD's impact on other organs, such as cysts in liver or diverticulosis in the intestines

🧪 Priority Laboratory Tests/Diagnostics

> Ultrasound and computed tomography (CT) scan of the kidneys and surrounding structures show evidence of the disease

⚠️ Priority Interventions or Actions

> Monitor for signs of urinary tract infection and treat as prescribed, if present

> Prevent urinary tract infection, if client does not already have an infection

> Monitor for hematuria

> Encourage bedrest if bleeding occurs from ruptured cysts

> Administer medications to treat fever

> Use dry heat to abdomen and flanks for comfort when cysts are infected

> Increase fluid and sodium intake as sodium is usually lost with PKD

> Administer pain medications as needed

> Administer antihypertensive medications, if client is hypertensive

> Prepare client for procedure to drain cyst if obstruction or abscess is present

> Prepare client for dialysis or renal transplantation, if client is at that stage of the disease

🚩 Priority Potential & Actual Complications

> Diverticulosis

> Cerebral aneurysm

> Liver cysts

> Abnormal heart valves

> Dialysis

> Renal transplantation

Priority Nursing Implications

> Do not use non-steroidal anti-inflammatory drugs to treat pain with PKD because of the risk of bleeding if cysts rupture

> A cyst may need to be punctured and drained if it is abscessed or if there is obstruction

💧 Priority Medications

> There are no medications to treat PKD. Medications are used to treat symptoms that may arise from complications

👤 Priority Education/Discharge Issues

> Explain the progression of PKD to client

> Educate on future treatment options

> Explain to client and family the importance of seeking genetic counseling

> Teach strategies to prevent infection

> Teach signs and symptoms of urinary tract infection and ruptured cyst

> Teach signs and symptoms of worsening PKD and when to notify healthcare provider

Urinary tract infection

Pathophysiology/Description

> A urinary tract infection is an inflammation of the bladder that results from bacteria, obstruction of the urethra or other factors.

> Of all possible causes of a UTI, bacterial infection is the most prevalent

> By far, the most common bacteria related to urinary tract infections is Escherichia coli, commonly called E. coli.

> Urinary tract infections can also be caused by parasitic and fungal infections, but these causes are rare. When seen, they are usually in clients who are immunosuppressed

> Urinary tract infections are more common in women than men due to the close proximity of the urethra to the rectum

> Classification
  - Upper UTI: Occurring in the ureters, pelvic area or renal parenchyma
  - Lower UTI: Occurring in the urethra and bladder

> Types of UTI based on location
  - Urethritis inflammation occurring in the urethra
  - Cystitis inflammation occurring in the bladder
  - Pyelonephritis inflammation occurring in collecting system and renal parenchyma

> Urinary tract infection can be complicated or uncomplicated
  - With uncomplicated UTI, there are no other conditions complicating the infection
  - With complicated UTI, there are other co-existing conditions impacting the UTI, such as diabetes, renal stones among others

> Sexual intercourse and urinary catheterization increase the risk of getting a UTI because of possible introduction of bacteria

Priority Assessments or Cues

> Assess for fever, chills and flank pain, indicating upper UTI

> Assess for burning and pain with urination

> Ask client about difficulty starting urine stream or delay between start and beginning of the urine flow, may be because urethral sphincter has relaxed

> Ask about interruption of stream once started or voiding in small amounts

> Ask about incomplete emptying of bladder and dribbling of urine after voiding

> Assess color of urine, cloudiness may indicate UTI

> Assess for bladder spasms

> Ask about frequency of urinating, usually multiple times in a 24-hour period, with insignificant amounts each time (less than 200 mL)

> Ask about wetting the bed at nights (nocturnal enuresis)

Priority Laboratory Tests/Diagnostics

> Urine dipstick, shows nitrites, leukocyte esterase, white blood cells,

> Microscopic urinalysis shows elevated white blood cell count, usually greater than 11,000 mm^3 as well as pus in the urine (pyuria)

> Urine culture and sensitivity will show the causative bacteria and the most effective antibiotic to treat the bacteria

Priority Interventions or Actions

> Ask client to collect a clean-catch urine sample. Teach correct way to collect the sample to prevent contamination of the sample

> Refrigerate urine sample for culture immediately upon collection

> Send urine sample for culture to lab within 24 hours of collection

> Administer antibiotic as ordered and monitor for side effects

> Administer analgesic as ordered for pain

> If a urinary catheter must be inserted, ensure sterile technique is used

> Provide client with adequate fluids and encourage intake of up to 3000 mL/day, help to flush the urinary tract of the bacteria

> Allow client to use sitz bath or heat to abdomen if discomfort is unbearable

> Re-culture urine after completion of antibiotic therapy to determine resolution of the infection

Priority Potential & Actual Complications

> Urosepsis
> Septicemia
> Sepsis

Priority Nursing Implications

> Understand that older adults with a UTI may not present with the usual symptoms of the condition. Quite often a UTI is manifested as an alteration in mentation, such as agitation and confusion

Clinical Hint

Current practice dictates that urinary catheters are used with caution due to the incidence of catheter-associated urinary tract infections (CAUTIs).

Priority Medications

> There are several antibiotics from various classes that can be used to treat a UTI. The ones below are the first- choice drugs to treat uncomplicated and complicated UTI

> trimethoprim/sulfamethoxazole
> - First choice antibiotic to treat UTI
> - Usual oral dose 800 mg-160 mg every 12 hours for 10 to 14 days
> - Usual intravenous dose to treat severe urinary tract infection is 8 to 10 mg/kg/day in divided doses, given at set daily intervals, for up to 14 days

> nitrofurantoin
> - First choice antibiotic to treat UTI
> - Usual dose is 50-100 mg four times daily
> - When used for urinary tract prophylaxis the dose is 50 -100 mg daily at bedtime

> fosfomycin
> - First choice antibiotic to treat UTI
> - Administered as a single one-time dose
> - Dose is 3 grams (1 sachet)

> ciprofloxacin
> - Used to treat complicated UTI
> - Usual oral dose 250 to 500 mg orally every 12 hours for 7 to 14 days
> - Usual intravenous dose 200 to 400 mg IV every 8 to 12 hours for 7 to 14 days

> levofloxacin
> - For complicated urinary tract infection
> - Usual dose is 250 mg oral or intravenous every 24 hours for 10 days or 750 mg oral or intravenous every 24 hours for 5 days
> - Has a serious adverse effect of tearing or rupture of a tendon, primarily Achilles' tendon

> phenazopyridine
> - Urinary analgesic and anesthetic, so it anesthetizes and reduces pain and discomfort
> - Usual dose is 190 to 200 mg orally three times daily
> - Should not be used for more than 2 days

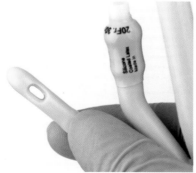

Image 7-9: When assessing a client for urinary retention or residual volume, what can be done instead of catheterization?

Priority Education/Discharge Issues

> Teach women to urinate after sexual intercourse to prevent possible infection from bacteria that may be on the genitals

> Teach women to wipe from front to back to prevent tracking bacteria from the rectum to the urethra

> Teach clients to keep the genital area clean to minimize the risk of bacterial growth

> Teach client to clean perineal area with warm water and soap after bowel movements, to decrease risk of bacterial growth and tracking into the urethra

> Teach women that cotton underwear and loose-fitting clothing help to keep the area around the urethra dry

> Teach signs and symptoms of urinary tract infection and when to contact a healthcare provider

> Teach client to complete the full course of antibiotics prescribed, even if the symptoms resolve, to ensure the infection is fully gone

> Teach client to empty bladder at least every 3-4 hours to prevent urinary stasis that can foster growth of bacteria

> Instruct client on foods that will help to maintain an acidic urine (pH of 5.5 or below), such as blueberries, prunes or cranberries. Drinking cranberry juice daily reduces the risk of a UTI

> Teach client to avoid or decrease intake of caffeinated beverages, such as coffee and cola, as both can cause bladder irritation

> Explain to client the importance of returning for follow-up urine culture once the course of antibiotic is finished

> Recognize clients at risk for a UTI and teach client how to minimize risk

Next Gen Clinical Judgment

You are caring for a 82-year-old man brought to the primary care provider's office because of new onset confusion and disorientation. The son that brought him stated "My dad is usually really with it. He woke up this morning not making any sense and rambling on about some pain in his belly. I can't get him to tell me what's wrong and it took me forever to get him dressed today. I don't know what is wrong with him."

The nurse practitioner orders a urine culture.

Consider these questions:

1. Why would a urine culture be indicated?

2. What additional treatments may be indicated?

3. What client/family teaching would be warranted about the current treatment and means to prevent future infections?

Pyelonephritis

Pathophysiology/Description

> Pyelonephritis is inflammation of the collecting ducts, renal parenchyma and pelvis

> Bacteria is the most common cause, but it can also be caused by parasitic and fungal infections

> The etiology of pyelonephritis is that it starts with bacteria and infection in the lower urinary tract or it occurs after invasive procedures. The renal medulla is usually first affected then it moves to the renal cortex

> Pyelonephritis usually occurs in the presence of a pre-existing condition such as diabetes, retrograde flow of urine or presence of urinary stones, catheter-associated urinary tract infections, to name a few

> As with lower urinary tract infection, Escherichia coli (E.coli) is the most common causative agent

> When pyelonephritis is recurrent in the presence of chronic conditions that cause obstruction, it ensues in chronic pyelonephritis

> Chronic pyelonephritis
> • Kidneys shrink in size
> • Ureter narrowed by strictures
> • Scarring occurs
> • End-stage renal disease occurs
> • Dialysis and/or transplantation is needed if both kidneys are affected

Priority Assessments or Cues

> Assess for flank pain on side that is affected, indicates inflamed kidney

> Assess for costovertebral angle tenderness, which indicates inflamed kidneys

> Assess for nausea, fever and chills, vomiting indicative of infection

> Assess for blood in urine.

> Ask about dysuria

> Assess color and smell of urine. Foul-smelling, cloudy urine is usually present with pyelonephritis

> Ask about frequency and urgency of urination

> Ask about recurring urinary tract infections, can help to determine chronic pyelonephritis

> Ask about usage of a urinary catheter, which is associated with chronic pyelonephritis

> Ongoing assessment of vital signs, primarily to determine decrease in temperature

Priority Laboratory Tests/Diagnostics

> Urinalysis shows elevated white blood cell count, hematuria, pyuria and bacteriuria in the urine. Proteinuria and azotemia may be present in the urine with chronic pyelonephritis, because the kidneys may not be able to filter protein properly or get rid of nitrogen waste

> With involvement of the renal parenchyma, WBC casts may be seen in urinalysis

> Urine culture and sensitivity will show the causative bacteria and the most effective antibiotic to treat the bacteria

> Complete blood count (CBC) shows immature neutrophils and leukocytes

> Blood cultures for clients who are severely ill is done to determine if infection is more systemic and may show septicemia

> Ultrasound to look for obstructions and/or other abnormalities of the urinary system

> Computed tomography (CT) scan to look for complications of the condition, such as renal abscess

> Renal biopsy may be used in chronic pyelonephritis to determine infiltration of the renal parenchyma and functionality of nephrons

Priority Interventions or Actions

> Ask client to collect a clean-catch urine sample. Teach correct way to collect the sample to prevent contamination of the sample

> Refrigerate urine sample for culture immediately upon collection

> Send urine sample for culture to lab within 24 hours of collection

> Administer antibiotic as ordered and monitor for side effects

> Administer analgesic as ordered for pain

> If a urinary catheter must be inserted, ensure sterile technique is used

> Administer intravenous fluids in acute setting until client can tolerate oral fluids

> Monitor intake and output

> Provide client with adequate oral fluids and encourage intake of up to 3000 mL/day, help to flush the urinary tract of the bacteria and prevent dehydration

> Monitor client for urosepsis and septicemia, complications of pyelonephritis

> Apply warm, moist heat to the client's flank area to minimize discomfort caused by pain

> Monitor for signs of progression of chronic pyelonephritis to chronic kidney disease

> Re-culture urine after completion of antibiotic therapy to determine resolution of the infection

Priority Potential & Actual Complications

> Urosepsis
> Septicemia
> Chronic kidney disease
> Dialysis
> Renal transplantation

Priority Nursing Implications

> Understand that for older adults living in long-term and skilled nursing facilities, a common cause of pyelonephritis is catheter-associated urinary tract infections (CAUTI)

> If vancomycin is administered too quickly itching of the head, face neck and upper torso, along with flushing (called red man syndrome), is likely to occur. The rate of infusion will need to be decreased if this syndrome occurs

Priority Medications

> ampicillin
  - Broad-spectrum antibiotic
  - Started immediately before result of urine culture is received
  - Usual dose is 500 mg oral, intramuscular or intravenous every 6 hours

> vancomycin
  - Combined with tobramycin or gentamycin
  - Started immediately before result of urine culture is received
  - Usual dose is 500 mg intravenous every 6 hours or 1 gram intravenous every 12 hours. Drug levels of vancomycin must be monitored for therapeutic range. Trough drug level should be 10-20 mcg/mL. Peak level is no longer monitored

> tobramycin
  - Combine with vancomycin
  - Start immediately before urine culture received
  - Usual dose is 1 mg/kg intravenous or intramuscular every 8 hours

> gentamycin
  - Combine with vancomycin
  - Start immediately before urine culture received
  - Dose is 2 mg/kg loading dose, followed by 1.7 mg/kg intravenous every 8 hours or 5 mg/kg intravenous every 24 hours

> trimethoprim/sulfamethoxazole
  - Switch to this drug once urine culture results are received
  - Usual oral dose 800 mg-160 mg every 12 hours for 10 to 14 days
  - Usual intravenous dose to treat severe urinary tract infection is 8 to 10 mg/kg/day in divided doses at set daily intervals, for up to 14 days

> ciprofloxacin
  - Switch to this drug once urine culture result is received
  - Usual oral dose 1000 mg orally every 12 hours for 7 to 14 days
  - Usual intravenous dose 200 to 400 mg intravenous every 8 to 12 hours for 7 to 14 days

> levofloxacin
  - Switch to this drug once urine culture result is received

- Usual dose is 250 mg oral or intravenous every 24 hours for 10 days, or 750 mg oral or intravenous every 24 hours for 5 days
- Has a serious adverse effect of tearing or rupture of a tendon, primarily Achilles' tendon

> ofloxacin
  - Switch to this drug once urine culture result is received
  - Usual dose is 200 to 400 mg orally every 12 hours for 7 to 14 days
  - Has a serious adverse effect of tearing or rupture of a tendon, primarily Achilles' tendon

> Non-steroidal anti-inflammatory drugs (NSAIDs)
  - For outpatient management of mild pain and discomfort
  - There are several that can be used but indomethacin, naproxen and sulindac are quite often used. Dosages vary
  - Most significant adverse effect of NSAIDs is gastrointestinal bleeding

Priority Education/Discharge Issues

> Teach women to urinate after sexual intercourse to prevent possible infection from bacteria that may be on the genitals

> Teach women to wipe from front to back to prevent tracking bacteria from the rectum to the urethra

> Teach clients to keep the genital area clean to minimize the risk of bacterial growth

> Teach client to clean perineal area with warm water and soap after bowel movements, to decrease risk of bacterial growth and tracking into the urethra

> Teach women that cotton underwear and loose-fitting clothing help to keep the area to the urethra dry.

> Teach clients to empty bladder at least every 3-4 hours to prevent urinary stasis that can foster growth of bacteria

> Teach signs and symptoms of pyelonephritis and when to contact a healthcare provider

> Teach clients with known urinary tract abnormalities to seek regular medical care

> Teach client to complete the full course of antibiotics prescribed, even if the symptoms resolve, to ensure the infection is fully gone

> Instruct client on foods that will help to maintain an acidic urine (pH of 5.5 or below), such as blueberries, prunes or cranberries. Drinking cranberry juice daily reduces the risk of a UTI that can progress to pyelonephritis

> Teach client to avoid or decrease intake of caffeinated beverages, such as coffee and cola, as both can cause bladder irritation

> Explain to client the importance of returning for follow-up urine culture once the course of antibiotic is finished

> Recognize clients at risk for pyelonephritis and teach client how to minimize risk

Methicillin-resistant Staphylococcus Aureus/vancomycin resistant Enterococcus

Pathophysiology/Description

> Resistance to antibiotics has become a major issue as more and more bacteria are becoming resistant to antibiotics normally used to treat them

> Pathogens have become smarter and have discovered that they can become adaptable and modify themselves to make it more difficult for drugs to kill them

> Methicillin-resistant Staphylococcus (MRSA) and vancomycin-resistant Enterococcus (VRE) are two strains of bacteria that have become resistant to many antibiotics and so when clients have infections where these are the causative agents, treatment modalities must be used that are effective in killing these resistant pathogens

> Even though both strains are serious and can cause serious complications, VRE can cause more serious disease and infection (more virulent) than MRSA

> These resistant strains were once only localized to the healthcare setting but in recent years, MRSA has been identified in community settings such as fitness centers and sports locker rooms

> Community-acquired methicillin-resistant Staphylococcus aureus (CA-MRSA) occurs in healthy individuals in the community and usually causes severe systemic diseases

> Some Risk factors for CA-MRSA
> - Prisoners
> - Athletes
> - Crowded living conditions
> - Individuals who get tattoos
> - Day care workers
> - Persons using shared items at fitness centers
> - Persons who abuse intravenous drugs
> - Persons who are immunocompromised

> The problem of medication over-use and misuse is thought to have contributed significantly to the emergence of resistant strains of bacteria

Priority Assessments or Cues

> Assess for nausea, fever and chills and vomiting which are suggestive of infection, regardless of where in the body the infection is located

> Perform focused system assessment based on location of infection to determine effectiveness of treatment

> Ask about onset of symptoms and history of recent activity to try and isolate where infection occurred, important information to have if infection is CA-MRSA

> Ongoing assessment of vital signs, primarily to determine decrease in temperature

> Assess client's understanding of disease and preventative measures while hospitalized and upon discharge

Priority Laboratory Tests/Diagnostics

> Culture and sensitivity of infected area will show the causative bacteria and the most effective antibiotic to treat the bacteria

> Complete blood count (CBC) shows immature neutrophils and leukocytes, indicating infection

> Blood cultures for clients who are severely ill is usually done to determine if infection is more systemic and may show blood involvement (septicemia)

Priority Interventions or Actions

> Collect and send culture of affected area to lab in a timely manner to facilitate early treatment

> Practice good hand hygiene

> Change gloves when moving from one task to another, even while caring for the same client, to minimize cross contamination

> Use standard, as well as transmission-based precautions for client admitted with MRSA and VRE and ensure use of the correct personal protective equipment (PPE)

> Ensure client is not removed off isolation until cleared of the infection

> Administer antibiotics as ordered

> Administer intravenous fluids in acute setting until client can tolerate oral fluids

> Monitor intake and output

> Provide client with adequate oral fluids and encourage intake of up to 3000 mL/day, help to flush the bacteria from the body and prevent dehydration

> Re-culture urine after completion of antibiotic therapy to determine resolution of the infection

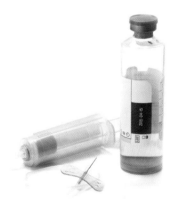

Image 7-10: What are the steps in collecting a sample for a blood culture?

▶ Priority Potential & Actual Complications

> Septicemia
> Sepsis
> May be fatal

↻ Priority Nursing Implications

> If vancomycin is administered too quickly itching of the head, face neck and upper torso, along with flushing (called red man syndrome), is likely to occur. The rate of infusion will need to be decreased if this syndrome occurs

> Because linezolid is a monoamine oxidase inhibitor (MAOI), it must not be taken within 14 days of a client taking an MAOI. If this precaution is not taken, the level of these compounds in the system may be increased, causing increased side effects

● Priority Medications

> ampicillin
  • Treat VRE
  • Dosages vary based on what part of the system the VRE is located
  • Usual dose is 250 to 500 mg intramuscular or intravenous every 6 hours

> vancomycin
  • Treat MRSA
  • Usual dose is 500 mg intravenous every 6 hours or 1 gram intravenous every 12 hours
  • Drug levels of vancomycin must be monitored for therapeutic range. Trough drug level should be 10-20 mcg/mL. Peak level is no longer monitored

> linezolid
  • Treat VRE
  • Usual dose is 600 mg intravenous or oral every 12 hours for 14 to 28 days
  • Should not be started if client used a Monoamine oxidase inhibitor (MAOI) in the past 14 days

● Priority Education/Discharge Issues

> Teach client to complete the full course of antibiotics prescribed, even if the symptoms resolve, to ensure the infection is fully gone

> Explain to client the importance of returning for follow-up culture once the course of antibiotic is finished

> Provide education to client about the infection (VRE or MRSA) and preventative measures while hospitalized

> Teach client that MRSA and VRE can be transmitted to family members in the community setting. Teach preventive measures, to include proper handwashing and personal hygiene practices

> Teach client to take all the prescribed antibiotics, even if symptoms seem to be gone, to ensure all the infection is cleared from the body

> Teach client to not save old antibiotics and reuse them as needed, as antibiotic overuse contributes to drug resistance

> Educate client to only take antibiotics that have been prescribed

> Teach client not to request antibiotics from healthcare providers to treat a cold or influenza

> Teach signs and symptoms of recurring infection and when to contact the healthcare provider

> Explain the importance of returning to the health care provider for a follow-up culture to ensure the infection is all gone

> For prevention of C-MRSA
  • Educate on not sharing towels or other personal items at home, at the gym or in the sports locker room.
  • Instruct on cleaning of gym and day care equipment before use
  • Teach to avoid crowded environments as best as possible
  • Teach clients who engage in intravenous drug use not to share drug paraphernalia

Next Gen Clinical Judgment

Consider these questions:

1. Why are antibiotic resistant strains such an important current health concern?

2. What behaviors enhance the potential for the development of resistant strains?

3. What can be done to prevent antibiotic resistance?

_____

_____

_____

_____

1. The nurse is admitting a confused older adult client with appendicitis who is combative and yelling at the staff. The surgeon is planning surgery in one hour. Which action is the highest priority?
   1. Explain to the client the need and urgency for surgery.
   2. Determine if there is family available.
   3. Assess pain level.
   4. Evaluate for rebound tenderness.

2. The nurse is caring for a client at home with a T-tube secondary to liver and gallbladder cancer. Assessment includes temperature 100.2°F (37.8°C), heart rate 110 beats/minute, respirations 22 breaths/minute, blood pressure 110/76 mmHg, and pain 3 on a 1-10 scale. What should be the nurse's next action?
   1. Ask the client when he last had something for pain.
   2. Assess the T-tube color and amount.
   3. Evaluate the insertion site of the T-tube.
   4. Determine if the client has jaundice.

3. The nurse manager in a care center has identified an increase in the cases of pyelonephritis of its female residents over the last month. What should be included in a training session for staff in the care of these clients?
   1. Reason for increased risk for pyelonephritis in older adult females.
   2. The importance of cleaning the perineum back to front.
   3. The need to provide a diet high in protein and vitamins.
   4. Early recognition of lower abdominal pain.

4. The nurse is caring for a client recently diagnosed with rheumatoid arthritis (RA). The 15-year-old is tearful and says to the nurse, "my girlfriend's mother has rheumatoid arthritis, and her hands make her look like a freak. I'll never be normal again." How should the nurse reply?
   1. "Each person's illness takes a different path, and there is no way of knowing how RA will affect you. Tell me more about what you think is normal."
   2. "Rheumatoid arthritis is curable. I'm sure with the proper treatment; you will not have extensive deformities."
   3. "Your girlfriend's mother is a rare situation, and I'm sure you don't have to worry."
   4. "I hope you are not having much pain. Can I get you something for discomfort?"

5. The nurse is completing a follow-up visit with an 8-year-old child with polycystic kidney disease. Which statement by the parent is most concerning?
   1. "My son seems to drink a lot of water during the day."
   2. "He doesn't seem to make friends very easily and would rather play alone."
   3. "His new shoes I just bought last week are already too tight."
   4. "My spouse is facing a job change, and we expect different insurance soon."

6. A client with candida cystitis is being treated with amphotericin B bladder irrigations. Which action should the nurse perform before delivery of the first dose?
   1. Evaluate BUN and Creatinine levels.
   2. Assess the lung sounds.
   3. Determine the level of consciousness.
   4. Assess code status.

7. The nurse is caring for a client receiving high dose doxycycline for vancomycin-resistant enterococci. The client has developed diarrhea secondary to the medication. What action should the nurse take?
   1. Stop the delivery of the IV antibiotics.
   2. Provide soothing wipes for excoriated skin around the rectum.
   3. Increase the fiber in the client's diet.
   4. Encourage fluid intake.

8. The nurse is caring for a female teenager with recurring urinary tract infections. Which observation made by the nurse is most concerning?
   1. Consumption of 32 ounces of soda.
   2. Eating a cranberry muffin.
   3. An unfinished prescription for antibiotics.
   4. A tampon among her items.

9. The nurse is delivering a handoff report for a client admitted during the night with meningococcal meningitis. What information is most important to share during handoff?
   1. The significant other's name and contact information.
   2. If the headache has resolved.
   3. The results of the lumbar puncture.
   4. The type of isolation precaution being used.

10. A nurse is working in an outpatient dialysis unit and notices a reddened, skin infection on the right arm of a client. The client shares that it was a bug bite but has gotten worse since discharge from the hospital two weeks ago. What action should the nurse take next?
    1. Apply gloves and explore the wound more closely.
    2. Encourage the client to apply antibiotic cream and keep it covered.
    3. Ask why the client was hospitalized.
    4. Culture the wound.

11. A pregnant nurse receives an accidental exposure from a needle stick of a client dying from acquired immune deficiency syndrome (AIDS). The nurse is very upset and afraid, wanting to give up nursing forever. How should the manager counsel the nurse?
    1. Suggest the nurse take an extended vacation.
    2. Encourage the nurse to become involved in an AIDS volunteer group.
    3. Determine if the nurse is religious or has other support groups.
    4. Suggest she discusses her concerns with her colleagues.

12. The nurse delivers a new sulfa medication to a client as prescribed. Although the client states having the medication a year ago, small raised bumps are noted on the client's chest and back six hours after the first dose. What should the nurse do next?
    1. Assess for other signs of a reaction.
    2. Apply hydrocortisone cream to the rash.
    3. Hold the second dose and notify the healthcare provider.
    4. Deliver the medication as prescribed.

13. A client has septicemia. The client's condition is noted to be deteriorating. The nurse begins to infuse the ordered intravenous albumin. Which change indicates the effectiveness of the treatment?
    1. An increase of fine bilateral crackles.
    2. An increase of mean arterial pressure (MAP) from 54 to 67.
    3. A decrease in urine output from 43 to 23 mL/hr.
    4. A decrease in temperature from 100.5°F (38.6°C) to 99.8°F (37.6°C).

14. A client presents to the emergency department with a 3-day history of nausea, headache and stiffness to the back of the neck. Nursing assessment reveals a rash on the client's lower extremities. Vital signs are blood pressure 142/88 mmHg, temperature 102.2°F, heart rate 100 and respirations 22. What is the nurse's priority action?
    1. Administer prescribed pain medication.
    2. Place the client on respiratory isolation.
    3. Apply prescribed ointment on the client's rash.
    4. Place the client in a darkened room to decrease stimuli.

15. The nurse is caring for a client in the clinic who was diagnosed with systemic lupus erythematosus four years ago. Which assessment change is most concerning?
    1. Drop in systolic blood pressure by 15 mmHg since the previous visit.
    2. Worsening butterfly mask on face.
    3. A temperature of 99.7°F (37.6°C) without other symptoms.
    4. Swollen left knee with 3/10 pain.

16. What is the best way to prevent the spread of the influenza infection during the peak winter season?
    1. Annual immunization.
    2. Balanced diet and rest.
    3. Limited exposure to the cold.
    4. Visit the health care provider for early symptoms.

17. Which actions should the nurse anticipate when caring for a client with an acute exacerbation of systemic lupus erythematosus? Select all that apply.
    1. Temperature assessment every 4 hours.
    2. Delivery of NSAIDs.
    3. Monitor intake and output.
    4. Observe for skin bruising.
    5. Delivery of corticosteroids.

18. The nurse is assessing a client for the risk of human immunodeficiency virus infection. What assessment questions will assist in determining the client's risk? Select all that apply.
    1. Do you ever share drug-using equipment with another person?
    2. Have you ever had a sexually transmitted infection?
    3. Do you ever use someone's toothbrush or drink from the same cup?
    4. Have you ever had a blood transfusion?
    5. Do you ever use public restrooms?

19. A client with type 2 diabetes with neuropathy is admitted for cellulitis of the right foot after stepping on a nail. What actions should the nurse include when planning care? Select all that apply.
    1. Educate about the importance of diabetic foot care.
    2. Assess for fall precautions.
    3. Apply hot compresses to the injured foot, twice a day.
    4. Check blood glucose levels every 6 hours.
    5. Monitor for warmth and redness at the site of the injury.

20. The nurse is performing routine care for a client admitted with gout. Place the nursing actions in order of priority.
    1. Assessment of vital signs.
    2. Assessment of pain.
    3. Evaluation of serum uric acid level.
    4. Education about low purine diet.
    5. Medicate with NSAIDS.
    6. Apply heat to swollen joints.

21. A client visits his school nurse presenting with moderate right-lower-quadrant pain, abdominal distension, and nausea. The client reports the pain began one to two hours prior to this visit. The nurse palpates the abdomen and notes rebound tenderness. Which is the next appropriate nursing action?
    1. Provide antacids and advice the client to return to class.
    2. Call his parents and advise them to immediately seek healthcare.
    3. Monitor the student's temperature and keep the client NPO in the office.
    4. Call for emergency transport for immediate surgical intervention.

22. The nurse receives handoff report on each of these clients experiencing complications from untreated cystitis. Which clients should be managed first? Rank order the responses.
    1. 81-year-old with nightly incontinence.
    2. 28-year-old at 38 weeks gestation in preterm labor.
    3. 54-year-old with flank pain and a temperature of 102°F (38.8°C).
    4. 67-year-old with a GFR of 25%.
    5. 32-year-old with cloudy yellow urine.

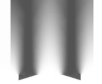

23. The nurse is caring for a client recovering from bacterial meningitis. The healthcare provider is expecting discharge the next day. The nurse reviews the collaborative note in the electronic health record. As a result of this information, what recommendation should the nurse make for discharge planning?

3/19/XX 0930 Physical Therapy	Ambulated to the door using a walker with 2-assist. States "legs feel like rubber" and knees beginning buckle. Placed in the recliner chair for two hours before returning to bed.

1. Intensive physical therapy is needed at home.
2. Discharge should be to an acute rehabilitation unit.
3. The client should remain hospitalized longer.
4. Physical therapy needs to work with the client 4-5 times each day until discharge.

24. The client is receiving ciprofloxacin 400 mg in 200 mL over 60 minutes IV every 12 hours for a catheter-associated urinary tract infection. The tubing drop factor is 10 gtts/mL. How many drops per minute will the nurse administer?_____ gtts/min

25. While completing an admission assessment on a client with a history of systemic lupus, the client states; "My husband and I have been trying to have a baby; however, I am not sure with my lupus. What are your thoughts?" Which is the best response by the nurse?
1. How long have you been in remission with your systemic lupus?
2. Longer gestations may be seen in women with a history of lupus.
3. In my opinion, it would be best if you tried to become pregnant within the first six months of being diagnosed with lupus.
4. Most women get relief of lupus symptoms when they are pregnant.

26. A child is to begin a treatment regimen for human immunodeficiency virus (HIV). Prior to initiating the treatment regimen, what is a priority nursing action?
1. Test for antiretroviral drug resistance.
2. Assess for adequate urine output.
3. Diagnose sexually transmitted infections.
4. Obtain baseline liver function tests.

27. An 11 kg child diagnosed with a severe infection is to receive ceftriaxone 75 mg/ kg every 12 hrs. The concentration of ceftriaxone is 1 gram per 10 mL. What volume of medication should the nurse administer for each dose? Go to the one decimal place.

_____

28. A child is admitted to the hospital with increasing pain that localized in the right lower quadrant. Upon arriving to the unit, the child's pain was initially improved, but over the next two hours, the pain has increased and he is nauseous and has a temperature of 102.6°F. What action does the nurse take?
1. Administer acetaminophen.
2. Increase the I.V. fluids.
3. Notify the primary care provide.
4. Provide an antiemetic.

29. A client with pancreatitis and a nasogastric (NG) tube in place complains of nausea. Which of the following nursing interventions is most appropriate?
1. Administer antiemetic medicine.
2. Remove NG tube and insert a new one.
3. Aspirate the gastric contents with a syringe.
4. Irrigate the NG tube with distilled water.

30. The healthcare provider placed an intracranial monitor device in a child with encephalitis and increased intracranial pressures. Which should the nurse most carefully monitor for?
1. Changes of breathing patterns due to the proximity to the device.
2. Tissue necrosis due to poor blood flow at the insertion site.
3. A rise in intracranial pressure due to insertion of the device.
4. Infection at the insertion site or in the brain.

1. **The nurse is admitting a confused older adult client with appendicitis who is combative and yelling at the staff. The surgeon is planning surgery in one hour. Which action is the highest priority?**
   1. Explain to the client the need and urgency for surgery. *Client is confused so reorientation is more important.*
   2. Determine if there is family available.
   3. Assess pain level. *Although important, having family available may make client less combative and easier to assess.*
   4. Evaluate for rebound tenderness. *Gaining surgical consent from family is the priority.*

   Rationale: Before surgery can be planned, consent must be obtained. Since this client is confused, he is not in a state to provide an informed decision for himself. The best option is to get consent from the family or power of attorney. If that is not an option, surgery may need to be delayed. "Treatment may need to be delayed while the client waits for significant family members to arrive before giving consent for a procedure or treatment." Since he is confused and combative, it is unlikely that explanation of the need and urgency for surgery will help. Assessment of pain and rebound tenderness is essential but gaining information about family is the priority since surgery consent is the priority.

   THIN Thinking: Top Three – *The priority is getting the client to surgery. Since the client is confused, family is needed to sign the consent.* **NCLEX®:** Management of Care **QSEN:** Patient-centered Care

2. **The nurse is caring for a client at home with a T-tube secondary to liver and gallbladder cancer. Assessment includes temperature 100.2°F (37.8°C), heart rate 110 beats/minute, respirations 22 breaths/minute, blood pressure 110/76 mmHg, and pain 3 on a 1-10 scale. What should be the nurse's next action?**
   1. Ask the client when he last had something for pain. *There is no indication that client is in pain.*
   2. Assess the T-tube color and amount. *This would not help evaluate possible infection.*
   3. Evaluate the insertion site of the T-tube.
   4. Determine if the client has jaundice. *Next action would be to check for infection.*

   Rationale: A T-tube is inserted into the common bile duct during surgery when a common bile duct exploration is part of the surgical procedure, under a sterile condition. The insertion site is as at risk for infection, and the skin should be cleaned daily using an antiseptic solution. It is appropriate to assess for pain, measure and monitor the amount and color and amount of the bile drainage and assess for jaundice. Given the information on the client and the fact that they have a fever, further infection evaluation needs to take place. Redness and swelling around the site could indicate infection and should be reported to the healthcare provider.

   THIN Thinking: Identify Risk to Safety – *With the identification of fever, further assessment is needed to determine the source.* **NCLEX®:** Safety and Infection Control **QSEN:** Safety

3. **The nurse manager in a care center has identified an increase in the cases of pyelonephritis of its female residents over the last month. What should be included in a training session for staff in the care of these clients?**
   1. Reason for increased risk for pyelonephritis in older adult females.
   2. The importance of cleaning the perineum back to front. *Cleaning should be front to back.*
   3. The need to provide a diet high in protein and vitamins. *This would not have an effect on increased infections.*
   4. Early recognition of lower abdominal pain. *This would not help prevent infections.*

   Rationale: Older adults, clients who are immunocompromised (e.g., cancer, human immunodeficiency virus [HIV], diabetes mellitus), and clients treated with immunosuppressive drugs or corticosteroids are at a higher risk for developing pyelonephritis. Health promotion activities, particularly for these individuals, can help decrease the frequency of infections and provide for early detection of infection. Health promotion activities include teaching preventive measures such as (1) emptying the bladder regularly and completely, (2) evacuating the bowel regularly, (3) wiping the perineal area from front to back after urination and defecation, and (4) drinking an adequate amount of liquid each day.

   THIN Thinking: Nursing Process – *Once a nurse recognizes an increase of infection rates it is important to create a plan for improvement.* **NCLEX®:** Health Promotion and Maintenance **QSEN:** Teamwork and Collaboration

4. **The nurse is caring for a client recently diagnosed with rheumatoid arthritis (RA). The 15-year-old is tearful and says to the nurse, "my girlfriend's mother has rheumatoid arthritis, and her hands make her look like a freak. I'll never be normal again." How should the nurse reply?**
   1. "Each person's illness takes a different path, and there is no way of knowing how RA will affect you. Tell me more about what you think is normal."
   2. "Rheumatoid arthritis is curable. I'm sure with the proper treatment; you will not have extensive deformities." *Inaccurate statement, RA is not curable.*
   3. "Your girlfriend's mother is a rare situation, and I'm sure you don't have to worry." *Offers false reassurance.*
   4. "I hope you are not having much pain. Can I get you something for discomfort?" *Does not address client's question and concern.*

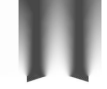

Rationale: Chronic, lifelong illness, such as rheumatoid arthritis can create strained family relationships, modifications in family activities, increased health care tasks, increased financial stress, the need for housing adaptation, social isolation, medical concerns, and grieving. The degree of disability and a client's perception of both the illness and the disability determine the extent to which lifestyle changes occur. As a teen, social isolation is a significant concern. It would be expected for a teenaged person to feel like they will be a "freak" from the physical changes they may be facing. Once the nurse can establish the feelings behind the statement, he/she can move towards increasing knowledge and control of the disease for the client and the family.

THIN Thinking: Nursing Process – *Therapeutic communication should be implemented to be empathetic and caring.* **NCLEX®**: Psychosocial Integrity **QSEN**: Patient-centered Care

5. **The nurse is completing a follow-up visit with an 8-year-old child with polycystic kidney disease. Which statement by the parent is most concerning?**
   1. "My son seems to drink a lot of water during the day." *Not a concern as long as child is also urinating.*
   2. "He doesn't seem to make friends very easily and would rather play alone." *This may be a concern, but not as important as potential fluid overload.*
   3. ☉ "His new shoes I just bought last week are already too tight."
   4. "My spouse is facing a job change, and we expect different insurance soon." *Not a priority concern.*

Rationale: Hereditary nephritis, congenital nephrotic syndrome, Alport syndrome, polycystic kidney, and several other hereditary disorders can result in renal failure in childhood. The development of chronic kidney disease (CKD) is often recognized after extensive kidney disease has occurred. As CKD progresses, clients have increasing difficulty with fluid retention and require diuretic therapy. Fluid retention can be measured by tight rings, clothing, and shoes.

THIN Thinking: Top Three – *Having tight shoes would indicate fluid retention and requires additional evaluations.* **NCLEX®**: Physiological Adaption **QSEN**: Patient-centered Care

6. **A client with candida cystitis is being treated with amphotericin B bladder irrigations. Which action should the nurse perform before delivery of the first dose?**
   1. ☉ Evaluate BUN and Creatinine levels.
   2. Assess the lung sounds. *Would not be a concern.*
   3. Determine the level of consciousness. *Would not be a concern.*
   4. Assess code status. *Would not be a concern.*

Rationale: Amphotericin B remains one of the drugs of choice for the treatment of severe systemic fungal infections. The medication has several adverse effects. These include headache, low blood pressure, increased heart rate, fever and chills. Also associated with amphotericin are nausea, vomiting, joint and muscle pain. It is also caustic to the kidneys and should be avoided in those with immune suppression, decreased renal function, and hypersensitivity. Candida cystitis and other fungal infections occurring in body cavities have benefited from the use of amphotericin when used as irrigation in these body cavities.

THIN Thinking: Identify Risk to Safety – *This medication is nephrotoxic. Delivery with impaired kidney function could cause renal failure.* **NCLEX®**: Pharmacological and Parenteral Therapies **QSEN**: Safety

7. **The nurse is caring for a client receiving high dose doxycycline for vancomycin-resistant enterococci. The client has developed diarrhea secondary to the medication. What action should the nurse take?**
   1. Stop the delivery of the IV antibiotics. *This would require a healthcare provider order.*
   2. ☉ Provide soothing wipes for excoriated skin around the rectum.
   3. Increase the fiber in the client's diet. *Increased fiber would increase GI motility.*
   4. Encourage fluid intake. *Although important to maintain fluid balance, it would not help diarrhea.*

Rationale: Diarrhea results in problems with skin breakdown from the constant irritation of the anus. "During the course of infection, support the client's body defense mechanisms. For example, if a client has diarrhea, maintain skin integrity by frequent cleansing, application of a skin-barrier cream, and frequent repositioning to prevent breakdown and the entrance of additional microorganisms. Other routine hygiene measures such as cleaning the oral cavity and bathing protect the skin and mucous membranes from invasion and overgrowth of organisms". Fluid and electrolyte imbalance can be a result of diarrhea, but nothing in this question indicates dehydration is a problem. The antibiotics cannot be discontinued without an order. Fiber will increase motility.

THIN Thinking: Help Quick – *Diarrhea is caustic to the skin and leads to breakdown which could lead to pain, discomfort and infection. Keeping the skin clean is important.* **NCLEX®**: Basic Care and Comfort **QSEN**: Patient-centered Care

8. The nurse is caring for a female teenager with recurring urinary tract infections. Which observation made by the nurse is most concerning?
   1. Consumption of 32 ounces of soda. *Although not a healthy habit, it is not the most concerning.*
   2. Eating a cranberry muffin. *There is not an issue with this.*
   3. 💡 An unfinished prescription for antibiotics.
   4. A tampon among her items. *This would not be of concern.*

   Rationale: Teaching prevention of a recurring urinary tract infection (UTI), includes: completion of all antibiotics as prescribed; practice of appropriate hygiene; emptying the bladder before and after sexual intercourse; urinating regularly; maintaining adequate fluid intake; avoidance of vaginal douches and harsh soaps, bubble baths, powders, and sprays in the perineal area; reporting of signs of recurrent UTI; and consideration of drinking unsweetened cranberry juice. The use of tampons is not a concern for recurring UTIs, but should be changed regularly.

   THIN Thinking: Identify Risk to Safety – *Stopping antibiotics prematurely can cause an over-growth infection that can lead to severe infections and septicemia.* **NCLEX®:** Reduction of Risk Potential **QSEN:** Patient-centered Care

9. The nurse is delivering a handoff report for a client admitted during the night with meningococcal meningitis. What information is most important to share during handoff?
   1. The significant other's name and contact information. *Important, but not as important as maintaining safety.*
   2. If the headache has resolved. *Important, but not as important as maintaining safety.*
   3. The results of the lumbar puncture. *Important, but not as important as maintaining safety.*
   4. 💡 The type of isolation precaution being used.

   Rationale: Handoff report should include information that is most critical to the client's needs and nurses plan of care. Protection of the nurse is also important and sharing infection control information can prevent the spread of illness. Meningitis requires respiratory isolation until the cultures are negative. Meningococcal meningitis is highly contagious, whereas other causes of meningitis may pose minimal to no infection risk with client contact. However, standard precautions are essential to protect the client and nurse. For this reason, isolation is more important for the protection of team members.

   THIN Thinking: Identify Risk to Safety – *Implementation of infection safety standards need to be clearly communicated to prevent injury to the client and staff.* **NCLEX®:** Management of Care **QSEN:** Safety

10. A nurse is working in an outpatient dialysis unit and notices a reddened, skin infection on the right arm of a client. The client shares that it was a bug bite but has gotten worse since discharge from the hospital two weeks ago. What action should the nurse take next?
    1. 💡 Apply gloves and explore the wound more closely.
    2. Encourage the client to apply antibiotic cream and keep it covered. *Nurse should first assess wound.*
    3. Ask why the client was hospitalized. *This would not provide pertinent information.*
    4. Culture the wound. *This would require an order from healthcare provider.*

    Rationale: Healthcare-associated infections (HAIs) are infections that are acquired as a result of exposure to microorganisms in a healthcare setting. Methicillin-resistant S. aureus (MRSA) is an example of emerging strains of antibiotic-resistant organisms that are transmitted in both the hospital and community settings. The compromised client is especially at risk of acquiring MRSA. MRSA has been known to cause rapidly forming skin infections and systemic diseases, including pneumonia and sepsis. Rates of MRSA infections appear to be on the rise, especially in the community setting. Since MRSA is spread through contact, the use of gloves is critical for the healthcare provider.

    THIN Thinking: Nursing Process – *Further assessment is needed before an intervention.* **NCLEX®:** Safety and Infection Control **QSEN:** Safety

11. A pregnant nurse receives an accidental exposure from a needle stick of a client dying from acquired immune deficiency syndrome (AIDS). The nurse is very upset and afraid, wanting to give up nursing forever. How should the manager counsel the nurse?
    1. Suggest the nurse take an extended vacation. *This does not address the nurse's concerns.*
    2. Encourage the nurse to become involved in an AIDS volunteer group. *This would not address the nurse's concerns.*
    3. 💡 Determine if the nurse is religious or has other support groups.
    4. Suggest she discusses her concerns with her colleagues. *Her colleagues may not be the best support system.*

    Rationale: The nurse is going though many emotional adjustments during this difficult time of unknown and needs outside resources that offer coping skills. It is understandable that she would want to give up on nursing considering the life change she may be facing. Affiliations, such as religious groups are excellent avenues for connections with others who may share the same beliefs and participate in similar rituals.

    THIN Thinking: Help Quick – *This stressful situation will require physical monitoring and emotional support. Identification of support systems can help.* **NCLEX®:** Psychosocial Integrity **QSEN:** Patient-centered Care

12. The nurse delivers a new sulfa medication to a client as prescribed. Although the client states having the medication a year ago, small raised bumps are noted on the client's chest and back six hours after the first dose. What should the nurse do next?

1. 💡 Assess for other signs of a reaction.
2. Apply hydrocortisone cream to the rash. *Need to determine if rash is from antibiotic prior to treating.*
3. Hold the second dose and notify the healthcare provider. *Need to further assess before jumping to the conclusion that it was caused by allergic reaction.*
4. Deliver the medication as prescribed. *Need to further assess.*

Rationale: Although the client has previously received this medication, it cannot be assumed they are not having a delayed hypersensitivity reaction. Further assessment for anaphylaxis symptoms would include the evaluation for breathing difficulties, itching, and hypotension. After completing the focused assessment, the medication should be held, and the health care provider notified. Topical hydrocortisone cream may be ordered if the rash causes itching.

THIN Thinking: Nursing Process – *Assessment is the priority, before interventions.* **NCLEX®:** Physiological Adaptation **QSEN:** Safety

13. A client has septicemia. The client's condition is noted to be deteriorating. The nurse begins to infuse the ordered intravenous albumin. Which change indicates the effectiveness of the treatment?

1. An increase of fine bilateral crackles *Indicates fluid overload.*
2. 💡 An increase of mean arterial pressure (MAP) from 54 to 67.
3. A decrease in urine output from 43 to 23 mL/hr. *Indicates insufficient fluid.*
4. A decrease in temperature from 100.5°F (38.6°C) to 99.8°F (37.6°C) *Temperature would not be an indicator of improved fluid status.*

Rationale: A client with septicemia that is deteriorating is often going into septic shock. If shock is present, blood volume replacements are used. Plasma or plasma volume expanders such as dextran or albumin may be given to improve perfusion. The mechanism of albumin moves fluid from the extravascular space into the blood vessels in an attempt to make it isotonic. As such, colloids increase the blood volume, and they are sometimes called plasma expanders. Moving fluid into the vascular space would decrease crackles, raise MAP, and increase urine output. There would not be an impact on the temperature.

THIN Thinking: Nursing Process – *Evaluation of the benefit of albumin would include signs of increasing intravascular fluid.* **NCLEX®:** Pharmacological and Parenteral Therapies **QSEN:** Safety

14. A client presents to the emergency department with a 3-day history of nausea, headache and stiffness to the back of the neck. Nursing assessment reveals a rash on the client's lower extremities. Vital signs are blood pressure 142/88 mmHg, temperature 102.2°F, heart rate 100 and respirations 22. What is the nurse's priority action?

1. Administer prescribed pain medication. *No, while this is needed to treat the headache, it is not priority over preventing the spread of a possible contagious infection.*
2. 💡 Place the client on respiratory isolation. *Correct, the client's symptoms are all indicative of meningococcal meningitis which is highly contagious. Priority is to prevent the spread by immediately placing the client on respiratory isolation.*
3. Apply prescribed ointment on the client's rash. *No, managing the meningococcal rash on the client's lower extremities will occur but it is not the priority.*
4. Place the client in a darkened room to decrease stimuli. *No, while this is needed to manage photophobia that often occurs with meningitis, it is not the priority.*

Rationale: Meningitis is highly contagious. Nurses must be astute to identifying presenting signs and symptoms of meningitis in clients so that spread of the infection might be prevented. The client's presenting symptoms are indicative of meningitis and the rash is common when the condition is caused by a meningococcus pathogen. The nurse must place the client on respiratory isolation until further testing can be done to make a definitive diagnosis. All the other interventions will be needed for the client but are not priority over preventing the likely spread of a highly contagious infection.

THIN Thinking: Top Three-Safe Practice – *Nurses must be astute in identifying assessment findings that require immediate implementation of safety measures to prevent the spread of contagious infections.* **NCLEX®:** Safety and Infection Control **QSEN:** Safety

15. The nurse is caring for a client in the clinic who was diagnosed with systemic lupus erythematosus four years ago. Which assessment change is most concerning?

1. Drop in systolic blood pressure by 15 mmHg since the previous visit. *One change in BP is not necessarily a concern.*
2. Worsening butterfly mask on face. *This is not a serious change.*
3. 💡 A temperature of 99.7°F (37.6°C) without other symptoms.
4. Swollen left knee with 3/10 pain. *This would be of concern, but not as concerning as possible infection.*

Rationale: Lupus symptoms include skin rashes and joint swelling. Blood pressure is typically not impacted, but not enough information is given to determine if it's a concern (no baseline). Clients with Lupus appear to have increased susceptibility to infection. Risk may be due to impaired ability to phagocytize invading bacteria, deficient production of antibodies, and immunosuppressive effects of many anti-inflammatory drugs. Infection is a major cause of death, and pneumonia is the most common infection. Fever may indicate an underlying infection rather than lupus activity alone.

THIN Thinking: Identify Risk to Safety – *The risk of infection is a concern for the client with lupus. A fever, even low-grade, could indicate a bigger issue.* **NCLEX®:** Reduction of Risk Potential **QSEN:** Safety

16. **What is the best way to prevent the spread of the influenza infection during the peak winter season?**
    1. ◉ Annual immunization.
    2. Balanced diet and rest. *This would be helpful, but is not the best way.*
    3. Limited exposure to the cold. *There is no scientific evidence that this would matter.*
    4. Visit the health care provider for early symptoms. *This would not prevent infection.*

    Rationale: There is a decreased incidence of infectious diseases (e.g., influenza, pneumonia) when more people are vaccinated against these diseases. Eating a balanced diet, providing for rest, and limiting stress on the body (with cold exposure and other things) can improve immunity but will not prevent spread. Visiting the HCP for early symptoms can shorten the length of illness if viral medicines are started with the early onset of symptoms.

    THIN Thinking: Identify Risk to Safety – *Immunizations allow for the development of antibodies and prevent the development of influenza.* **NCLEX®:** Health Promotion and Management **QSEN:** Evidence-based Practice

17. **Which actions should the nurse anticipate when caring for a client with an acute exacerbation of systemic lupus erythematosus? Select all that apply.**
    1. ◉ Temperature assessment every 4 hours.
    2. ◉ Delivery of NSAIDs.
    3. ◉ Monitor intake and output.
    4. ◉ Observe for skin bruising.
    5. ◉ Delivery of corticosteroids.

Rationale: During a disease exacerbation, the client may quickly become very ill. Nursing interventions include accurately recording the severity of symptoms and documenting the response to therapy. Specifically assess fever pattern, joint inflammation, limitation of motion, location and degree of discomfort, and fatigue. A 24-hour urine sample should be collected and tested for creatinine clearance and protein. The client's weight must be taken, and intake and output measured. These assessments are crucial if the client is being administered corticosteroids as this class of drugs can promote fluid retention which might result in failure of the renal system. Bleeding is also a concern with drug therapy and might manifest as tarry stools, pallor, bruising to the skin and petechiae.

THIN Thinking: Nursing Process – *The nurse should understand the anticipated assessment changes that occur with various illnesses.* **NCLEX®:** Physiological Adaption **QSEN:** Patient-centered Care

18. **The nurse is assessing a client for the risk of human immunodeficiency virus infection. What assessment questions will assist in determining the client's risk? Select all that apply.**
    1. ◉ Do you ever share drug-using equipment with another person?
    2. ◉ Have you ever had a sexually transmitted infection?
    3. Do you ever use someone's toothbrush or drink from the same cup? *This is not a risk factor.*
    4. ◉ Have you ever had a blood transfusion?
    5. Do you ever use public restrooms? *- This is not a risk factor.*

Rationale: The nurse should assess risk by asking some basic questions, including if they've had a blood transfusion or used clotting factors prior to 1985; if they've shared drug-using equipment with another person (especially needles); if they've had a sexual experience without protection that included contact of the penis, vagina, rectum, or mouth; if they've had a sexually transmitted infection; or if they've had sexual contact with someone known to have HIV. Each question should be followed up by additional in-depth questioning related to the identified risk.

THIN Thinking: Nursing Process – *When the nurse knows the risks for disease they can better plan care for the client.* **NCLEX®:** Safety and Infection Control **QSEN:** Patient-centered Care

19. **A client with type 2 diabetes with neuropathy is admitted for cellulitis of the right foot after stepping on a nail. What actions should the nurse include when planning care? Select all that apply.**
    1. 💡 Educate about the importance of diabetic foot care.
    2. 💡 Assess for fall precautions.
    3. Apply hot compresses to the injured foot, twice a day. *Hot compresses could cause further skin damage.*
    4. Check blood glucose levels every 6 hours. *Clients with type 2 diabetes can check blood glucose levels less frequently.*
    5. 💡 Monitor for warmth and redness at the site of the injury.

    Rationale: This client is dealing with concerns related to diabetes, neuropathy, and cellulitis. The nurse should create a teaching plan for diabetic foot care. It is not important to check blood glucose every 6 hours; it would be better to complete them AC & HS for a client with type 2 diabetes. Fall precautions are important to assess because of the neuropathy and foot injury. Hot compresses would be contraindicated for someone with neuropathy. It is anticipated that cellulitis would cause warmth and redness, and this should be monitored for a worsening situation.

    THIN Thinking: Identify Risk to Safety - The *person with neuropathy and cellulitis is at risk for sepsis and injury. Planning for injury prevention is important.* **NCLEX®:** Safety and Infection Control **QSEN:** Safety

20. **The nurse is performing routine care for a client admitted with gout. Place the nursing actions in order of priority.**
    1. Assessment of vital signs.
    2. Assessment of pain.
    3. Apply heat to swollen joints.
    4. Medicate with NSAIDS.
    5. Evaluation of serum uric acid level.
    6. Education about low purine diet.

    Rationale: As the nurse performs daily care, vital signs should be the first assessment, followed by a pain assessment. The client with gout may have significant pain, so treatment with heat/cold and NSAIDS are the standard. The decision to apply heat before medicating would be based on least-invasive-first prioritization. Evaluation of the uric acid level will tell if the gout is improving or worsening and the education will take place once the client is feeling more comfortable.

    THIN Thinking: Nursing Process – *Techniques to prioritize care include physiological needs first and least invasive first.* **NCLEX®:** Physiological Adaption **QSEN:** Patient-centered Care

21. **A client visits his school nurse presenting with moderate right-lower-quadrant pain, abdominal distension, and nausea. The client reports the pain began one to two hours prior to this visit. The nurse palpates the abdomen and notes rebound tenderness. Which is the next appropriate nursing action?**
    1. Provide antacids and advice the client to return to class *Client needs to be seen by healthcare provider.*
    2. 💡 Call his parents and advise them to immediately seek healthcare.
    3. Monitor the student's temperature and keep the client NPO in the office *Client needs to be seen by healthcare provider.*
    4. Call for emergency transport for immediate surgical intervention *Client needs to be evaluated, but unknown at this time if surgery would be needed.*

    Rationale: The place of the pain and rebound tenderness suggest appendicitis. The parents would need to be present to consent for treatment or surgery for the client, so calling the parents would expedite the student's treatment. Prolonging the process, returning the child to class, and treating with antacids are not correct courses of action, but ambulance transportation without the parent's present will not assist unless the client is in an emergency situation.

    THIN Thinking: Top Three – *Symptoms are consistent with appendicitis which requires medical intervention.* **NCLEX®:** Reduction of Risk Potential **QSEN:** Patient-centered Care

22. **The nurse receives handoff report on each of these clients experiencing complications from untreated cystitis. Which clients should be managed first? Rank order the responses.**
    1. 54-year-old with flank pain and a temperature of 102°F (38.8°C).
    2. 28-year-old at 38 weeks gestation in preterm labor.
    3. 67-year-old with a GFR of 25%.
    4. 32-year-old with cloudy yellow urine.
    5. 81-year-old with nightly incontinence.

    Rationale: Cystitis indicates inflammation of the bladder. If left untreated it can spread to a urinary tract infection (UTI) or even to systemic infection (urosepsis) that is a life-threatening condition requiring emergency treatment. Flank pain and a high fever is a sign of pyelonephritis, a significant complication. Preterm labor can result from a UTI, but at 38 weeks, the mom is near term and will be allowed to deliver. The GFR is concerning, but not much can be done once kidney damage has occurred, cloudy urine would be anticipated with cystitis and incontinence is more of an annoyance than a medical emergency.

    THIN Thinking: Top Three – *Prioritization includes physiological needs first, ABCs, and acute versus chronic.* **NCLEX®:** Management of Care **QSEN:** Patient-centered Care

23. The nurse is caring for a client recovering from bacterial meningitis. The healthcare provider is expecting discharge the next day. The nurse reviews the collaborative note in the electronic health record. As a result of this information, what recommendation should the nurse make for discharge planning?

3/19/XX 0930 Physical Therapy	Ambulated to the door using a walker with 2-assist. States "legs feel like rubber" and knees beginning buckle. Placed in the recliner chair for two hours before returning to bed.

1. Intensive physical therapy is needed at home. *Client needs to have extended therapy.*
2. 💡 Discharge should be to an acute rehabilitation unit.
3. The client should remain hospitalized longer. *No indication client requires hospitalization.*
4. Physical therapy needs to work with the client 4-5 times each day until discharge. *Client does not require further hospitalization.*

Rationale: After the acute period has passed, the client with meningitis requires several weeks of convalescence and rehabilitation before resuming normal activities. In this period, adequate nutrition, rest, and physical therapy are important. Muscle rigidity may persist in the neck and backs of the legs. Progressive range-of-motion exercises, warm baths, and progressive ambulation are useful.

THIN Thinking: Nursing Process – *As a part of the health care team, the nurse should recommend further acute rehabilitation to prevent injuries after discharge.* **NCLEX®:** Management of Care **QSEN:** Patient-centered Care

24. The client is receiving ciprofloxacin 400 mg in 200 mL over 60 minutes IV every 12 hours for a catheter-associated urinary tract infection. The tubing drop factor is 10 gtts/mL. How many drops per minute will the nurse administer?_____ gtts/min

Answer: 33 gtts/min

Rationale:
$$\frac{200 \text{ mL} \times 10 \text{ gtts}}{60 \text{ min} \quad \text{mL}} = \frac{2000}{60} = 33 \text{ gtts/min}$$

THIN Thinking: Identify Risk to Safety – *The nurse should perform safe calculations to administer medications accurately.* **NCLEX®:** Pharmacological and Parental Therapies **QSEN:** Safety

25. While completing an admission assessment on a client with a history of systemic lupus, the client states; "My husband and I have been trying to have a baby; however, I am not sure with my lupus. What are your thoughts?" Which is the best response by the nurse?
1. 💡 How long have you been in remission with your systemic lupus?
2. Longer gestations may be seen in women with a history of lupus. *Inaccurate statement.*
3. In my opinion, it would be best if you tried to become pregnant within the first six months of being diagnosed with lupus. *Giving advice and unhelpful to client.*
4. Most women get relief of lupus symptoms when they are pregnant. *Inaccurate statement.*

Rationale: Many women become pregnant after an SLE diagnosis with a positive pregnancy and delivery. However, a good outcome is dependent upon proper treatment for SLE before pregnancy. Those whose heart and/or kidneys are not affected. The presence of SLE anti-bodies increase the chances of miscarriage.

THIN Thinking: Identify Risk to Safety – *Gathering more information can support how the nurse proceeds with the conversation.* **NCLEX®:** Health Promotion and Maintenance **QSEN:** Evidence-based Practice

26. A child is to begin a treatment regimen for human immunodeficiency virus (HIV). Prior to initiating the treatment regimen, what is a priority nursing action?
1. 💡 Test for antiretroviral drug resistance.
2. Assess for adequate urine output. *Although important, this is not the most important action.*
3. Diagnose sexually transmitted infections. *This would not be the priority concern before treatment.*
4. Obtain baseline liver function tests. *Although important, this would not be as important as determining drug resistance.*

Rationale: Prior to making a change to a treatment regimen for a child with HIV, the provider must test for antiretroviral drug resistance. Infants can acquire a drug-resistant strain of HIV from their mother. Determining the most appropriate treatment for the child leads to a more successful treatment regimen.

THIN Thinking: Nursing Process – *Gathering baseline assessment will allow the nurse to prioritize care.* **NCLEX®:** Health Promotion and Maintenance **QSEN:** Evidence-based Practice

27. **An 11 kg child diagnosed with a severe infection is to receive ceftriaxone 75 mg/ kg every 12 hrs. The concentration of ceftriaxone is 1 gram per 10 mL. What volume of medication should the nurse administer for each dose? Go to the one decimal place.**

    Answer: 8.3 mL

    Rationale: 75 mg x 11 kg = 825 mg

    $$\begin{aligned} 825 &= 1,000 \\ X &\quad\ 10 \text{ mL} \\ 8250 &= 1,000x \\ X &= 8.3 \text{ mL} \end{aligned}$$

    THIN Thinking: Identify Risk to Safety – *The nurse should perform safe calculations to administer medications accurately.* **NCLEX®:** Pharmacological and Parental Therapies **QSEN:** Safety

28. **A child is admitted to the hospital with increasing pain that localized in the right lower quadrant. Upon arriving to the unit, the child's pain was initially improved, but over the next two hours, the pain has increased and he is nauseous and has a temperature of 102.6°F. What action does the nurse take?**
    1. Administer acetaminophen *Child is nauseous and should be seen by healthcare provider.*
    2. Increase the I.V. fluids *This would not address child's pain, fever or nausea.*
    3. ⦿ Notify the primary care provider.
    4. Provide an antiemetic *While addressing nausea, it wouldn't help with other symptoms and does not address potential complications.*

    Rationale: The child is demonstrating signs of a ruptured appendix. This is a surgical emergency and the provider needs to be notified immediately. No heat should be applied to the abdomen of a client with suspected appendicitis due to the increased risk of rupture of the appendix.

    THIN Thinking: Help Quick – *The child has shown a change in condition and additional prescriptions are required.* **NCLEX®:** Physiological Adaption **QSEN:** Safety

29. **A client with pancreatitis and a nasogastric (NG) tube in place complains of nausea. Which of the following nursing interventions is most appropriate?**
    1. Administer antiemetic medicine. *Most important action would be to check tube placement.*
    2. Remove NG tube an insert a new one. *Would need to check tube placement before assuming the tube needs to be replaced.*
    3. ⦿ Aspirate the gastric contents with a syringe.
    4. Irrigate the NG tube with distilled water. *It would be dangerous to irrigate the tube without checking placement first.*

Rationale: The first step here would be to confirm placement of the NG tube. This is done by aspirating contents and checking the pH. If in the stomach, the pH should be between 0-4. You do not want to irrigate if you are not sure that the tube is in the stomach and not the lungs. The NG tube when functioning correctly, should decrease the nausea and prevent the need to administer an antiemetic and, until placement is confirmed or denied, there is no reason to pull this NG tube and insert another one.

THIN Thinking: Nursing Process – *Priority of care is further assessment to determine what is causing the nausea.* **NCLEX®:** Reduction of Risk Potential **QSEN:** Evidence-based Practice

30. **The healthcare provider placed an intracranial monitor device in a child with encephalitis and increased intracranial pressures. Which should the nurse most carefully monitor for?**
    1. Changes of breathing patterns due to the proximity to the device. *The device does not obstruct or impact the airway.*
    2. Tissue necrosis due to poor blood flow at the insertion site. *The device is more short-term and should not result in necrosis.*
    3. A rise in intracranial pressure due to insertion of the device. *The device measures intracranial pressure but does not increase it.*
    4. ⦿ Infection at the insertion site or in the brain.

    Rationale: Client's with encephalitis are hospitalized for observation including intracranial monitoring. Although intracranial monitoring does not often cause infection, the sites must be monitored for common signs of infection and inflammation.

    THIN Thinking: Identify Risk to Safety – *Nurses must assess for potential sources of infection.* **NCLEX®:** Safety and Infection Control **QSEN:** Safety

Homeostasis

Acid-base Balance / Electrolyte Imbalance / Fluid Imbalance

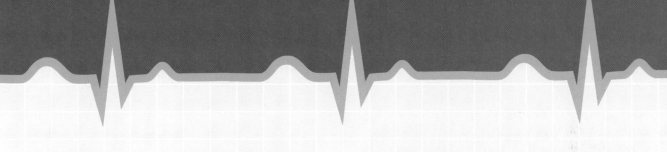

This chapter addresses how the body strives to maintain homeostasis and conditions that lead to fluid and electrolyte imbalance.

The human body exists in a delicate balance of acids/bases, fluids, and electrolytes. Nurses play a significant role in assessing and detecting changes in this balance, understanding conditions that require vigilant monitoring, and implementing strategies to promote homeostasis.

Study Hint: Turn to the inside back cover of the book and create a NurseThink® notecard for each ion listed here:

> Main extracellular electrolytes: sodium, chloride, bicarbonate

> Main intracellular electrolytes: potassium, magnesium, phosphate

Study Hint: Make sure you are comfortable assessing hydration status in clients across the lifespan!

Priority Exemplars:

> Overhydration/Fluid overload

> Dehydration/Fluid deficit/resuscitation

> Hyper/Hypocalcemia

> Hyper/Hypokalemia

> Hyper/Hypomagnesemia

> Hyper/Hyponatremia

> Hyper/hypophosphatemia

> Metabolic acidosis

> Metabolic alkalosis

> Respiratory acidosis

> Respiratory alkalosis

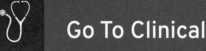
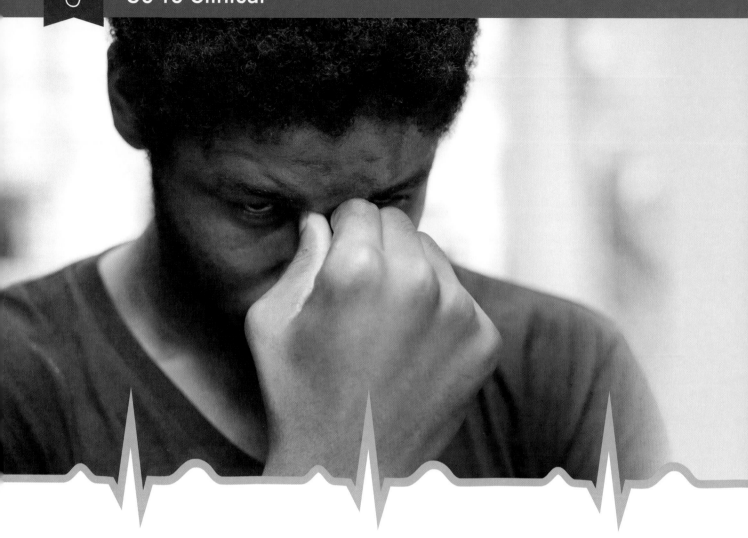

Go To Clinical Case 1

You are a registered nurse in the renal clinic. A 23-year-old man presents with swelling, fatigue, and nausea. The client reports a history of nephrotic syndrome, diagnosed at 11 years of age. He states he had a "bad cold" a few weeks ago. These infections often cause him to have a "flare up" of his disease. During these "flare ups" he reports to take prednisone and he has taken 12 days of the 14-day course, at which time he will begin the tapering dose schedule. He states he wants to "stop the prednisone right now" because of the side effects.

The client's vital signs are 99.0°F—118-22-140/92. His baseline weight is 174 pounds (79 kg.). Today he weighs 181 pounds (82.3 kg.)

Today, he reports that his "heart is pounding" in his chest, he can't get his shoes on with the swelling, and he states it is difficult to climb steps because he has "trouble breathing." You note that he has 2+ edema in both ankles. You dipstick his urine and note large amounts of protein.

Study Hint: Remember 1 kg. of weight equals 1 liter of fluid retained. In this case study, the weight gain of 7 pounds (approximately 3.3 kg) represents 3.3 liters of fluid overload.

NurseThink® Time

Using the NurseThink® system, complete the priorities. Check your answers designated by 💡 in the Overhydration/fluid overload Priority Exemplar.

Priority Assessments or Cues

1.

2.

3.

Priority Laboratory Tests/Diagnostics

1.

2.

3.

Priority Interventions or Actions

1.

2.

3.

Priority Potential & Actual Complications

1.

2.

3.

Priority Nursing Implications

1.

2.

3.

Priority Medications

1.

2.

3.

Priority Education/Discharge Issues

1.

2.

3.

Overhydration/fluid overload

Pathophysiology/Description

> Fluids and electrolytes exist in homeostasis in the body in the intravascular, intracellular, and interstitial compartments

> Diffusion, osmosis, filtration, and hydrostatic pressure maintain fluids and ensure fluids move throughout the body and meet the metabolic needs

> About 60% of adults, 55% of older adults, and 80% of infants are made up of fluids/water; decreased organ function (cardiac) may lead to overhydration

> Intake of fluids comes from water, solid foods mixed with liquids, food oxidation, and medications such as those administered via the parenteral routes

> Output of water is lost via measurable sources (urine, emesis, drainage/drains) and insensible sources (perspiration, exhale air, water in stool)

> The kidneys maintain homeostasis of fluids within the body such that increased intake, increases output; water is conserved with decreased intake and increased body needs (diaphoresis, diarrhea, vomiting)

> An elaborate system of aldosterone secretion (adrenals), antidiuretic hormone (pituitary gland), and the kidneys assist the body to maintain homeostasis

> Overload of fluids/fluid volume excess occurs when fluid intake or availability is more than needed for body functioning

> Types of overhydration
  - Isotonic overhydration/hypervolemia
    - Excessive fluid in the extracellular spaces (does not enter the cells)
    - Yields circulatory overload and interstitial edema
    - Causes include excessive intravenous fluids, kidney disease/failure, fluid retention secondary to steroid use/Cushing's syndrome
  - Hypertonic overhydration
    - Too much sodium intake, rarely occurs
    - Extracellular volume expands, intracellular volume contracts
    - Causes include increased sodium ingestion, high volume/rapid infusion of hypertonic intravenous solutions, high dose sodium bicarbonate replacement
  - Hypotonic overhydration/water intoxication
    - Fluid moves into the cells
    - Dilutional electrolyte deficiencies
    - Causes include early kidney impairment, heart failure, syndrome of inappropriate antidiuretic hormone (SIADH), excessive intravenous hypotonic or oral fluids, irrigation with hypotonic fluids, primary polydipsia, inappropriate dialysis, rapid correction of hyperglycemia with large infusions of hypotonic fluids

> May be characterized by "third-spacing" and edema (excessive fluids in interstitial spaces)

Priority Assessments or Cues

> Assess risk related to age and diagnosis (older adults, infants with immature kidney function in response to overhydration, heart failure, kidney disease)

> Assess vital signs and watch for bounding tachycardia, hypertension, dysrhythmias, tachypnea

> Assess breath sounds for crackles, shallow/rapid respirations

> Observe jugular vein distension

> Assess weight—obtain accurate weight, compare to baseline

> Assess level of consciousness including level of alertness, confusion and restlessness. The client may report muscle weakness/spasms, visual changes and a headache

> Assess skin/extremities/abdomen for edema (pitting), pale/cool skin, hepatomegaly, ascites

> Assess perfusion—edema may impair perfusion to extremities. Assess peripheral and central pulses, capillary refill, skin color and temperature, sensory and motor function

> Observe for urine output (requires adequate kidney function to excrete excess fluids)

Next Gen Clinical Judgment

1. List the steps to assessing jugular venous distension.

   _____

   _____

   _____

   _____

2. Review an online video on JVD.

3. In the video, attempt to locate the jugular veins of the client.

Priority Laboratory Tests/Diagnostics

> Decreased serum osmolality normal 275-295 mOsm/kg; decreased found in overhydration (< 275 mOsm/kg); < 265 mOsm/kg is a critical finding

> CBC—decreased hemoglobin and hematocrit

> Decreased BUN (blood urea nitrogen)

> Decreased serum sodium (may occur with other electrolyte shifts due to dilution)

> Decreased urine specific gravity <1.005

⚠ Priority Interventions or Actions

> Goal: Reduce excess body fluids, promote desired elimination
- Manage underlying cause
> Restrict dietary sodium intake
- Monitor I&O
- Administer diuretics to remove excess fluids
> Monitor client signs and electrolyte values
> Restrict oral and other fluid intake as prescribed

⚑ Priority Potential & Actual Complications

> Isotonic overhydration
  - Heart failure
  - Pulmonary edema

> Seizure
> Coma

⚕ Priority Nursing Implications

- Closely monitor intravenous fluid infusions and avoid potential fluid overload
> Provide appropriate skin care to edematous tissues
- Assessing pitting edema depression—2 mm (+1), 4 mm (+2), 6 mm (+3), 8 mm (+4)
> Nurses should be vigilant for signs of cerebral edema (secondary to overhydration, stroke, trauma, infections) and report to healthcare provider
- Monitor and maintain comfort measures for clients with edema and ascites, including easing work of breathing, skin care, and treating underlying cause

🜄 Priority Medications

- furosemide
  - loop diuretics
  - Rapid removal of excess fluid
  - Potassium-wasting—monitor serum potassium levels
  - High ceiling medication-increased doses may be given to achieve diuresis
- mannitol
  - osmotic diuretics
  - Stimulate diuresis
  - Used to decrease peripheral, intracranial, and intraocular edema, prevent renal failure
  - Potassium-wasting—monitor serum potassium levels
  - May exacerbate heart failure and pulmonary edema
  - Only given in inpatient settings as an emergency intervention

👤 Priority Education/Discharge Issues

> Counsel parents of infants that intake of high volumes of free water or incorrectly mixed formula may cause fluid overload

> Instruct parents/guardians to ensure infants do not drink water during swimming or in baths

- Ensure client/family understands the care of edematous tissues-elevation, skin care, avoid crossing legs, avoid constrictive clothing

- Reinforce that clients understand causative factors of overhydration and means of prevention

Clinical Hint

One kilogram (2.2 pounds) equals 1 liter of fluid. Loss/gain of weight is an excellent indicator dehydration/overhydration.

Go To Clinical Answers

Text designated by 💡 are the top answers for the Go To Clinical related to Overhydration/fluid overload.

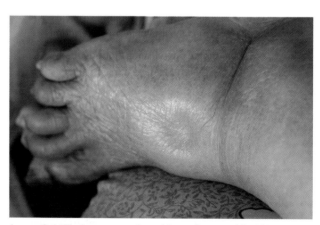

Image 8-1: What assessment would you document for this client's edema?

_____

_____

_____

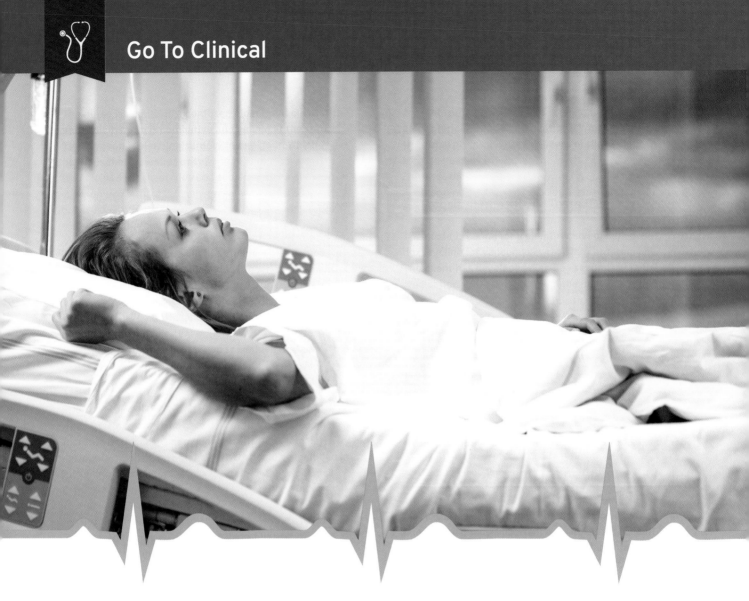

Go To Clinical Case 2

As a nurse on the adolescent unit, you have cared for many teens with type 1 diabetes mellitus. K.L. is a 14-year-old who was diagnosed at 10 years of age and she is skilled at managing her carbohydrate to insulin ratios, blood glucose monitoring, and insulin pump. K.L. became concerned about her weight and started omitting her insulin at meals. She stopped checking her blood glucose and was happy with the 5 pounds she lost in the last few weeks.

This morning she woke up vomiting and had a severe stomach ache. Her parents brought her to the emergency department where her blood glucose was 340 mg/dL and positive for ketones. Her HgbA1c was 12.5%. She is being admitted to the adolescent unit from the ED. When you transfer her from the stretcher to the bed, she reports being dizzy and feeling faint.

K.L.'s vital signs are 99.6°F— 118-26-92/62. You note that her previous vital signs at a recent clinic visit were 99.6°F—84-16-110/70. Her mucous membranes are pale and dry and you notice that her skin is also dry.

NurseThink® Time

Using the NurseThink® system, complete the priorities. Check your answers designated by 💡 in the Dehydration/fluid deficit Priority Exemplar.

Having trouble with interpreting Arterial Blood Gases? Go online and search for the Tic-Tac-Toe method of ABG interpretation! Take a break and watch a few videos—you may find them VERY helpful!

✏️ Priority Assessments or Cues

1.

2.

3.

⚗️ Priority Laboratory Tests/Diagnostics

1.

2.

3.

⚠️ Priority Interventions or Actions

1.

2.

3.

🚩 Priority Potential & Actual Complications

1.

2.

3.

⚕️ Priority Nursing Implications

1.

2.

3.

💧 Priority Medications

1.

2.

3.

👤 Priority Education/Discharge Issues

1.

2.

3.

Dehydration/fluid deficit

Pathophysiology/Description

> Fluids and electrolytes exist in homeostasis in the body in the intravascular, intracellular, and interstitial compartments

> Diffusion, osmosis, filtration, and hydrostatic pressure maintain fluids and ensure fluids move throughout the body and meet the metabolic needs

> About 60% of adults, 55% of older adults, and 80% of infants are made up of fluids/water, indicating the risk associated with fluid loss in older adults and infants

> Intake of fluids comes from water, solid foods mixed with liquids, food oxidation, and medications such as those administered via the parenteral routes

> Output is water lost via measurable sources (urine, emesis, drainage/drains) and insensible sources (perspiration, exhaled air, water in stool)

> The kidneys maintain homeostasis of fluids within the body with increased intake, increasing output; water is conserved with decreasing intake and increased body needs (examples include diaphoresis, diarrhea, vomiting)

> An elaborate system of aldosterone secretion (adrenals), antidiuretic hormone (pituitary gland), and the kidneys assist the body to maintain homeostasis

> Dehydration occurs when fluid intake is insufficient to meet the metabolic needs of the body

> Types of dehydration
  - Isotonic/hypovolemia
    - Water and electrolytes are lost, with decreased circulating blood volume and poor tissue perfusion (most common form)
    - Causes are inadequate intake of fluid/electrolytes, increased loss of fluids/electrolytes, fluid shifts
  - Hypertonic
    - More water is lost than electrolytes, excesses in electrolytes change the homeostatic balance, leading to fluid leaching into the vascular and interstitial spaces, resulting in cellular dehydration
    - Causes are increased fluid loss, as in diabetes insipidus, hyperventilation, profuse diaphoresis, ketoacidosis/osmotic diuresis, early phases of kidney failure
  - Hypotonic
    - More electrolytes are lost than water, plasma leaves the intravascular compartment into the cells, yielding low intravascular fluids and cellular swelling
    - Causes are chronic illness, hypotonic/water replacement deficient in electrolytes, kidney disease, malnutrition

Priority Assessments or Cues

> Assess for risk related to age including infants, older adults

> Assess vital signs, watch for tachycardia/weak pulse (dysrhythmias evident in late dehydration), tachypnea/dyspnea, low-grade temperature. Blood pressure may be normal or low—dramatic reductions in blood pressure are a late sign of dehydration/fluid deficit

> Assess weight—obtain accurate weight, compare to baseline

> Assess level of consciousness—alertness, reports of dizziness/syncope, orthostatic hypotension, muscle weakness, restlessness

> Assess perfusion—peripheral/central pulses, capillary refill (< 3 seconds), skin temperature, skin color, peripheral motor and sensory function, later sign: decreased urine output

> Assess hydration status—skin turgor, intake and output, moisture in mucous membranes of mouth, nose, and eyelids, decreased bowel sounds/constipation, thirst

> Assess for conditions leading to dehydration—diarrhea, poor intake, vigorous exercise, vomiting, polyuria, fluid losses (burns, trauma), clients with drains/nasogastric tube, burns/fluid shifts, overuse of diuretics

> Assess potential for injury—falls, aspiration, alterations in skin integrity

Priority Laboratory Tests/Diagnostics

> Serum electrolytes—depending upon type of dehydration, often hypernatremia

> Increased serum osmolality—Normal: 275-295 mOsm/kg; Elevated: > 295 mOsm/kg found in dehydration; >320 mOsm/kg is a critical finding

> CBC—elevated hemoglobin and hematocrit

> Elevated urine specific gravity >1.030

> Increased BUN (blood urea nitrogen)

Clinical Hint

Infants and frail older adults are prone to dehydration due to high concentration of fluids in their body, immature kidney water-conserving mechanisms, high metabolic rate, increased body surface area, and high fluid level requirements relative to size. Nurses need to assess infants carefully-capillary refill, skin turgor, fontanels, and other parameters.

⚠ Priority Interventions or Actions

> Goal of interventions—replace fluid and electrolytes to achieve homeostasis

> Closely monitor client's status and rehydration, avoid overcorrection

💡 Monitor I&O and body weight

💡 Identify and manage cause—diarrhea, vomiting, blood loss, poor intake

> Oral rehydration is priority if tolerating PO fluids

> Intravenous fluid resuscitation/replacement, general guidelines:

  • Hypertonic dehydration—hypotonic fluids-D5W (once dextrose is metabolized), 0.45% NaCl (½ normal saline)

  💡 Isotonic dehydration—isotonic fluids (normal saline solution, lactated ringers)

  • Hypotonic dehydration—hypertonic fluids (3% or 5% saline solutions)

  • Blood products in increased blood loss/trauma

> Medications to treat cause—antidiarrheals, anti-emetics, antibiotics, antipyretics

> Ingestion of food—to replace electrolytes

🚩 Priority Potential & Actual Complications

💡 Hypovolemia

💡 Hypovolemic shock

💡 Seizures/coma

> Multiorgan system failure

🩺 Priority Nursing Implications

💡 Nurses at the bedside may detect subtle changes in client's behavior that indicate dehydration and poor perfusion

💡 Nurses should consider clients at risk (children, older adults) and provide vigilant assessments to avoid dehydration

> Clients with nasogastric tubes should not drink water. This will leach out electrolytes as they are suctioned out of the stomach

> Encourage older adults to drink oral fluids. Due to decreased thirst, decreased mobility to access fluids, and reluctance to hydrate and need to urinate, older adults are often poorly hydrated

💡 Nurses should assess and provide skin care to avoid breakdown

💧 Priority Medications

> diphenoxylate with atropine
  • Opiate antidiarrheal
  • Atropine causes less dependence
  • Less sedation

> loperamide
  • Antidiarrheal
  • Less sedation and safety risk

> promethazine HCl
  • Antiemetic
  • Causes sedation and safety concerns

> acetaminophen
  • Antipyretic
  • Treat high fevers to prevent fluid loss
  • Allow low-grade fevers to increase immune function

👤 Priority Education/Discharge Issues

> Instruct clients/family to intervene early with clients with diarrhea and vomiting; encourage small, frequent fluid attempts of oral rehydration solution

> Encourage clients/families to add flavoring to oral electrolyte solutions to enhance palatability

💡 Teach clients and families to know and report early signs of dehydration

Go To Clinical Answers

Text designated by 💡 are the top answers for the Go To Clinical related to Dehydration/fluid deficit.

Next Gen Clinical Judgment

Mean Arterial Pressure (MAP) is a calculation that includes the systolic and diastolic blood pressure numbers. It is considered the most important number to determine whether there is enough blood flow, resistance, and pressure to supply blood to all major organs. A low MAP means low perfusion, a high MAP means increased perfusion pressure. Automatic blood pressure cuffs give the MAP.

1. What would be the impact for the client if the MAP is low for a period of time?

2. What would be the impact for the client if the MAP is high for a period to time?

Hyper/hypocalcemia

Pathophysiology/Description

> Calcium is an essential component of nerve/muscle/cardiac contractions, and blood clotting, along with the major element of bones and teeth

> Calcium required via daily intake, requires Vitamin D for metabolism, and requires parathormone and calcitonin to move calcium in and out of bone

> Hypercalcemia
  - High calcium levels may be associated with increased intake and mobilization from bones/metastatic processes
  - Causes include malignancies resulting in bone destruction, bone metastasis, hyperparathyroidism, decreased excretion with kidney disease, glucocorticoids, dehydration, immobilization, calcium and/or Vitamin D overdose, acidosis, milk-alkali syndrome, thiazide diuretics, and increased intake of calcium antacids

> Hypocalcemia
  - Low levels may be associated with decreased parathormone, decreased intake, and alkalosis
  - Causes include low calcium intake, lactose intolerance, parathyroidism, pancreatitis, multiple blood transfusions (citrate binds with calcium), alkalosis, laxative abuse, malabsorption syndromes, kidney disease, high phosphorus levels, Vitamin D deficiency, low magnesium levels, alcoholism, diarrhea, loop diuretics, wound drainage, and immobility

Priority Assessments or Cues

> Hypercalcemia
  - Assess clients at risk—vital signs for tachycardia, hypertension, bounding pulses
  - Assess for lethargy, weakness (may be profound), confusion, decreased reflexes, nausea/vomiting, bone pain, physiologic fractures, polyuria, and kidney stones

> Hypocalcemia
  - Assess clients at risk—vital signs for bradycardia, hypotension, weak peripheral pulses
  - Assess for tetany, Chvostek's sign, Trousseau's sign, laryngeal stridor, dysphagia, fatigue, anxiety, depression, hyperreflexia, and muscle spasms numbness/tingling of extremities and around mouth

Priority Laboratory Tests/Diagnostics

> Serum calcium levels 8.6-10.2 mg/dL and 4.5-5.5 mEq/L
> ECG changes
  - Hypercalcemia—short ST segment, wide T wave
  - Hypocalcemia—prolonged ST segment, prolonged QT segment

Priority Interventions or Actions

> Hypercalcemia
  - Determine and manage underlying cause
  - Enhance calcium excretion with diuretics
  - Hydrate with isotonic saline solutions/oral hydration of 3000-4000 mL/day
  - Low calcium diet
  - Increase weight bearing exercises

> Hypocalcemia
  - Determine and manage underlying cause
  - Enhance dietary calcium and Vitamin D intake
  - Administer IV calcium gluconate-monitor ECG and patency of IV

Priority Potential & Actual Complications

> Hypercalcemia
  - Coma
> Hypocalcemia
  - Seizures
  - Laryngospasm
  - Ventricular tachycardia

Priority Nursing Implications

> High calcium levels may be associated with renal lithiasis—strain urine and assess for kidney/flank pain
> High calcium may exacerbate digoxin toxicity
> Assess clients with neck or thyroid surgery for potential parathyroid damage
> Manage pain and anxiety of clients at risk for hypocalcemia - respiratory alkalosis may exacerbate symptoms

Priority Medications

> furosemide
  - Enhances renal excretion of calcium
> calcitonin
  - Given IM
  - Lowers serum calcium level
> pamidronate
  - Lowers calcium levels
  - Used with cancer-related hypercalcemia

Priority Education/Discharge Issues

> Teach clients safe antacid and laxative use
> Teach clients about calcium-rich foods (dairy, sardines, canned fish)
> Teach clients about the importance of mobility and weight-bearing exercises

Hyper/hypokalemia

📋 Pathophysiology/Description

> Potassium is involved in neuromuscular and cardiac function

> Potassium regulates intracellular osmolality and enhances cellular growth

> Allows glycogen to be deposited into muscle and liver cells

> Plays a role in acid-base balance

> Potassium ingested from dietary sources, excreted by the kidneys, lost also in stool and sweat

> Hyperkalemia

  • Increased K+ from impaired excretion, moving from ICF to ECF, and large intake of K+

  • Causes: Acidosis, cellular lysis (burns, injury, infection), medications maintain K+ in intravascular space, high oral intake of potassium, rapid or high dose infusion of IV potassium, renal failure, adrenal insufficiency, overuse of K+ salt substitute, tumor lysis syndrome, use of K+ sparing diuretics, and hyperuricemia

> Hypokalemia

  • Decreased K+ from loss of potassium via urine, movement of the K+ from ECF to ICF, or decreased intake

  • Causes: Diarrhea, vomiting, inadequate intake of potassium, overuse of laxatives, low magnesium levels, massive diuresis, hydration with fluids without KCl, side effect of insulin treatment with diabetic ketoacidosis, stress, delirium tremens, coronary muscle necrosis, alkalosis, wound drainage, diaphoresis, potassium-wasting diuretics, kidney disease, water intoxication, nasogastric suction

✏️ Priority Assessments or Cues

> Hyperkalemia

  • Assess vital signs for irregular pulse, bradycardia

  • Assess for clients at risk

  • Observe for irritability, anxiety, leg cramping and pain, weakness, abdominal cramps and diarrhea, cardiac dysrhythmias, and paresthesias

> Hypokalemia

  • Assess vital signs for weak, irregular pulse, shallow respirations, orthostatic hypotension

  • Assess for clients at risk

  • Observe for muscle weakness, leg weakness, paralytic ileus, hyperglycemia, paralysis, anxiety, confusion, lethargy, paresthesias, depressed deep tendon reflexes

🧪 Priority Laboratory Tests/Diagnostics

> Serum potassium levels 3.5-5.0 mEq/L

> ECG

  • Hyperkalemia—peaked T waves, prolonged PR interval, ST depression, loss of p waves, prolonged QRS

  • Hypokalemia—ST depression, flattened T wave, prolonged QRS, premature ventricular contractions

⚠️ Priority Interventions or Actions

> Hyperkalemia

  • Determine and manage underlying cause

  • Decrease oral or parenteral intake of potassium (restrict diet)

  • Increase excretion with diuretics (furosemide)

  • Potassium-binding medications

  • IV infusion of insulin with glucose to force K+ into the cells and reduce serum K+

  • IV infusion of calcium gluconate or NaHCO3 to decrease cellular cardiac excitability

  • Dialysis

> Hypokalemia

  • Oral and intravenous supplementation

🚩 Priority Potential & Actual Complications

> Hyperkalemia
  • Ventricular fibrillation
  • Complete respiratory arrest
  • Cardiac standstill/arrest

> Hypokalemia
  • Lethal cardiac dysrhythmias
  • Coma
  • Cardiac arrest

⚕️ Priority Nursing Implications

> Assess for hypotension and provide safety interventions

> All potassium chloride, oral and intravenous, must be well diluted. IV administration requires slow infusion in a well-mixed dilution via infusion pump

> Ensure renal function prior to administration of potassium

> Safety measures with hypotension

Priority Medications

> furosemide
  - Potent loop diuretic
  - Lowers potassium levels

> sodium styrene sulfonate
  - Administered orally or per rectum
  - Binds with potassium for excretion in feces

> potassium chloride (KCl)
  - Oral and IV solutions must be well diluted
  - Assess IV site for infiltration
  - Oral KCl causes nausea and vomiting, best if mixed with juice

Clinical Hint

Both hyper-and hypokalemia lead to cardiac irritability and dysrhythmias-monitor client and ECG closely, and report changes to healthcare provider.

Complete this MNEMONIC Hypokalemia Signs and Symptoms
A SIC WALT

A _____

S _____

I _____

C _____

W _____

A _____

L _____

T _____

Table 8-1: Feel free to search the Internet or create your own.

Priority Education/Discharge Issues

> Teach clients about food high in potassium: fruits (bananas, oranges), dried fruits (raisins), vegetables, fish, pork, beef, veal

> Teach clients to avoid overuse of sodium replacements that are high in potassium

> Hypokalemia potentiates digoxin toxicity-teach clients to watch for signs and symptoms, especially if on a potassium-wasting diuretic

> Instruct clients at risk about need to monitor potassium levels

> If client is changed from a potassium-wasting to a potassium sparing diet, make sure they are instructed to adjust diet accordingly

Next Gen Clinical Judgment

Potassium changes can happen quickly. What would the nurse observe if a client in diabetic ketoacidosis had a serum potassium level change? What would a nurse observe if a client with renal failure had a serum potassium level change?

Complete this MNEMONIC Hyperkalemia Signs and Symptoms
MURDER

M _____

U _____

R _____

D _____

E _____

R _____

Table 8-2: Feel free to search the Internet or create your own.

Hyper/hypomagnesemia

Pathophysiology/Description

> Essential component of cellular processes and metabolism of carbohydrates and proteins, synthesis of nucleic acids and proteins, balance phosphorus and calcium levels, assist in the function of the sodium-potassium pump

> Influences neuromuscular excitability and contractility

> Hypermagnesemia
  - High magnesium levels > 2.5 mEq/L
  - Causes include increased magnesium intake along with renal insufficiency/failure, excess intake of magnesium sulfate during pregnancy in management of eclampsia, tumor lysis syndrome, and diabetes ketoacidosis

> Hypomagnesemia
  - Low magnesium levels < 1.5 mEq/L
  - Occurs with limited intake or increased renal losses
  - Causes include diarrhea, vomiting, alcoholism, malabsorption syndrome, malnutrition, high urine output, nasogastic tube with suction drainage system, hyperaldosteronism, diabetes mellitus, prolonged parenteral nutrition, and prolonged use of diuretics

Priority Assessments or Cues

> Hypermagnesemia
  - Assess for clients at risk (renal failure/insufficiency or pregnant woman receiving magnesium sulfate for eclampsia)
  - Assess vital signs for bradycardia, hypotension
  - Assess for lethargy, nausea/vomiting, decreased deep tendon reflexes, decreased level of consciousness, flushed warm skin, muscle weakness, dysphagia

> Hypomagnesemia
  - Assess for clients at risk
  - Assess vital signs for tachycardia, hypertension
  - Assess for confusion, tremors, hyperactive deep tendon reflexes, insomnia, muscle cramps

Priority Laboratory Tests/Diagnostics

> Serum magnesium levels 1.5-2.5 mEq/L

Priority Interventions or Actions

> Hypermagnesemia
  - Determine and manage underlying cause
  - Focus is on prevention
  - Avoid magnesium containing foods (green vegetables, nuts, bananas, oranges, peanut butter, chocolate)
  - Emergency treatment for high magnesium levels-intravenous calcium gluconate or calcium chloride
  - With intact renal function promote urinary excretion with intravenous fluids, oral fluids, and intravenous furosemide
  - With impaired renal function use dialysis to draw off magnesium

> Hypomagnesemia
  - Determine and treat underlying cause
  - Dietary replacement of magnesium-supplements/magnesium containing foods
  - With significant deficits, provide intravenous magnesium

Priority Potential & Actual Complications

> Hypermagnesemia
  - Paralysis
  - Respiratory and cardiac arrest

> Hypomagnesemia
  - Seizures
  - Dysrhythmias—ventricular tachycardia, ventricular fibrillation

Priority Nursing Implications

> Magnesium, calcium, and potassium are balanced together in the body and require that nurses monitor all three in clients at risk of imbalance

> Nurses must carefully monitor intravenous infusions of magnesium—too rapid infusion may lead to cardiac or respiratory arrest

> Monitor vital signs carefully when magnesium levels are abnormal

> Magnesium enhances digoxin toxicity

Priority Medications

> furosemide
  - High ceiling, rapid acting diuretic
  - Removes excess magnesium
  - Assess hydration and serum potassium levels

Priority Education/Discharge Issues

> Counsel clients in chronic renal failure to avoid magnesium-containing drugs and limit magnesium containing foods

> Ensure that clients monitor their urine output as a reflection of renal function

> Depending upon excess or deficit, instruct clients to eat or avoid magnesium-rich foods

Clinical Hint

Although Chvostek and Trousseau signs are often the signs of hypocalcemia, they also may reflect hypomagnesemia.

Hyper/hyponatremia

Pathophysiology/Description

> Sodium maintains extracellular volume and water distribution in extracellular/ intracellular compartments and changes in sodium levels create changes in osmolality

> Functions in nerve conduction, muscle contractility, and acid-base balance

> Changes in serum sodium levels may reflect changes in amount of sodium relative to water or water relative to sodium

> Sodium is acquired from dietary sources, usually in excess of needs

> Sodium excreted in urine, feces, and sweat, regulated by the kidneys

> Hypernatremia—elevated serum sodium levels > 145 mEq/L (water loss, sodium increases)

  • Hyperosmolality

  • Fluid shift from cells to extracellular space, causing dehydration

  • Causes include diabetes insipidus, hyperosmolar tube feedings, hyperglycemia/diabetes mellitus, excessive diaphoresis, sodium intake without water (ocean water, sodium tablets), primary aldosteronism, overdose with hypertonic saline IV solution, lack of free water with tube feedings, osmotic diuretics, and diarrhea

> Hyponatremia—decreased serum sodium levels < 135 mEq/L

  • Water excess relative to sodium levels related to sodium loss or loss of sodium containing fluids

  • Fluid shifts into cells from extracellular space, causing cellular edema

  • Causes include diaphoresis, diarrhea, draining wounds, vomiting, trauma with blood loss, infusion of low sodium or no sodium fluids, IV fluids with clients in renal failure, excessive water intake, and Syndrome of Inappropriate Antidiuretic Hormone (SIADH)

Priority Assessments or Cues

> Assess clients at risk

> Hypernatremia

  • Assess vital signs for hypotension/postural hypotension

  • Assess skin for poor turgor and dry/swollen tongue

  • Assess level of consciousness for agitation, lethargy, weakness

  • Ask about thirst, sodium intake, water intake

  • Determine if client is exhibiting hypernatremia with decreased or increased extracellular volume

> Hyponatremia

  • Assess level of consciousness (changes in neurological function may be first symptoms from cerebral edema) for headache, confusion, irritability

Priority Laboratory Tests/Diagnostics

> Serum sodium levels 135-145 mEq/L

Priority Interventions or Actions

> Hypernatremia

  • Monitor serum electrolytes

  • Determine and treat underlying cause

  • Administer oral or intravenous hypotonic or isotonic fluids as prescribed

  • Limit sodium intake

  • Diuretics to pull off sodium

> Hyponatremia

  • Fluid restriction

  • Determine and treat underlying cause

  • If hyponatremia related to fluid loss, replace with sodium containing fluids

  • If seizures develop, administration of small volumes of hypertonic solutions titrated to serum osmolality and sodium levels

  • Close monitoring of serum sodium levels

Priority Potential & Actual Complications

> Hypernatremia/hyponatremia

  • Seizures

  • Coma

  • Neurological damage/coma

Priority Nursing Implications

> Hyper- and hyponatremia may occur from diarrhea—nurses need to monitor serum electrolyte levels of clients

> Carefully monitor intravenous fluid infusions

Priority Medications

> hydrochlorothiazide diuretics (HCTZ)

  • Pull off excess fluids and sodium

  • Used with diabetes insipidus

Priority Education/Discharge Issues

> Teach clients to avoid drinking seawater and prevent children from ingestion of seawater

> Discuss the decreased thirst mechanism with older clients and the need to drink when thirsty

Hyper/hypophosphatemia

📋 Pathophysiology/Description

> Most phosphorus is in bones and teeth as calcium phosphate

> Also works in function of muscle, red blood cells, and the nervous system

> Functions in the acid-base balancing system, function of ATP, cellular uptake and use of glucose, and metabolism of carbohydrates, proteins, and fats

> Excretion requires adequate kidney function. Regulation in the body is controlled by the parathyroid hormone

> Hyperphosphatemia
- Phosphorus levels > 4.5 mg/dL
- Causes include acute kidney injury or chronic kidney disease, chemotherapy, excessive ingestion of cow's milk, excessive intake of phosphorus-based laxatives/enemas, large intake of Vitamin D, hypoparathyroidism, and sickle cell anemia

> Hypophosphatemia
- Phosphorus levels < 3.0 mg/dL
- Low levels are rare
- Causes include malnutrition, malabsorption syndrome, alcohol withdrawal, use of phosphate-binding antacids, total parenteral nutrition with low phosphorus levels, recovery from diabetic ketoacidosis, respiratory alkalosis

✏️ Priority Assessments or Cues

> Hyperphosphatemia
- Assess clients at risk and monitor serum phosphorus levels
- Clients may be asymptomatic
- Assess and monitor serum calcium levels
- Symptoms of high levels of phosphorus often associated with hypocalcemia
- Assess for tetany, muscle cramps, paresthesias, numbness and tingling of extremities and around mouth, and hyperreflexia

> Hypophosphatemia
- Assess clients at risk and monitor serum phosphorus levels
- Mild hypophosphatemia is asymptomatic
- Assess and monitor serum calcium levels
- Assess for decreased level of consciousness, confusion, muscle weakness, pain, dysrhythmias, osteomalacia, rhabdomyolysis, and neuropathy

🧪 Priority Laboratory Tests/Diagnostics

> Serum phosphorus levels 3.0-4.5 mg/dL

> Serum calcium levels 9.0-10.5 mg/dL (exist in inverse proportions with phosphorus)

⚠️ Priority Interventions or Actions

> Hyperphosphatemia
- Determine and treat underlying cause
- Restrict phosphorus-containing foods
- Phosphorus-binding medications
- Dialysis
- Insulin and glucose infusion
- Ensure adequate hydration and monitor serum calcium and phosphorus levels

> Hypophosphatemia
- Oral phosphorus supplements
- Diet high in phosphorus (dairy products)
- Intravenous sodium phosphate/potassium phosphate

🚩 Priority Potential & Actual Complications

> Seizures associated with hyperphosphatemia

> Calcium/phosphorus deposits may precipitate on major organs including joints, kidneys, skin, arteries, corneas, and may lead to organ dysfunction

> Severe hypophosphatemia may result in cardiomyopathy and be fatal

⚕️ Priority Nursing Implications

> Clients receiving intravenous phosphorus infusions need to be carefully assessed for hypocalcemia

> Assess intravenous site as phosphorus may be sclerotic and cause tissue necrosis

🩸 Priority Medications

> calcium carbonate
- Bind with phosphorus in hyperphosphatemia
- Treats both hyperphosphatemia and hypocalcemia
- May cause constipation and flatulence

👤 Priority Education/Discharge Issues

> Counsel clients to not take in excessive milk products or laxatives/enemas with phosphorus

Clinical Hint

Calcium and phosphorus exist in inverse levels in the human body—high levels of phosphorus yield low calcium levels and low levels of phosphorus yield high calcium levels.

Metabolic acidosis

Pathophysiology/Description

> Deficit of base bicarbonate

> When acids accumulate in the body or bicarbonate is lost

> Compensation occurs by the release of CO_2 via rapid respirations (Kussmaul respirations) and kidney excretion of acids

> Calculate anion gap to determine cause of metabolic acidosis $Na - (Cl + HCO_3)$

> May occur with respiratory acidosis, as in cardiopulmonary arrest

> Causes include diabetic ketoacidosis, lactic acid accumulation when in shock or after a trauma, loss of HCO_3 from diarrhea, starvation, renal tubular necrosis, gastrointestinal fistulas, aspirin overdose, high-fat diets, ineffective metabolism of carbohydrates, and renal disease that impairs ability to reabsorb HCO_3

Priority Assessments or Cues

> Assess for signs and symptoms of respiratory distress

> Assess vital signs for hypotension, tachypnea, dysrhythmias

> Assess for symptoms of drowsiness, confusion, headache, warm flushed skin, nausea, vomiting, diarrhea, abdominal pain

Priority Laboratory Tests/Diagnostics

> Normal anion gap is 10-14 mEq/L (increased with acid gains related to metabolic acidosis, it is normal with bicarbonate loss)

> Arterial blood gases
  - Normal values
    - pH 7.35-7.45
    - $PaCO_2$ 35-45 mmHg
    - HCO_3 22-26 mEq/L
  - Metabolic Acidosis
    - pH decreased
    - $PaCO_2$ normal (uncompensated)
    - $PaCO_2$ decreased (compensated)
    - HCO_3 decreased

> Monitor serum potassium levels 3.5-5.0 mEq/L

Priority Interventions or Actions

> Determine and manage underlying cause

> Establish seizure precautions, as indicated

> Assess intake and output

> Provide $NaHCO_3$ via IV

> Treat DKA with insulin and hydration

> Clients with kidney disease are treated with dialysis and a low protein/high calorie diet

Priority Potential & Actual Complications

> Seizures

> Coma

> Polyuria/osmotic diuresis/diarrhea may lead to hypovolemia and shock

Priority Nursing Implications

> Read and interpret arterial blood gas findings, watching for trends and change

> Establish seizure precautions and observe/describe seizures

Priority Education/Discharge Issues

> Teach clients with diabetes about sick day care and means to avoid DKA

> Encourage clients with renal disease to report signs/ symptoms out of the ordinary to healthcare provider

Clinical Hint

To interpret blood gases, remember ROME.
RO: Respiratory opposite: pH/CO_2
ME: Metabolic equal : pH/HCO_3

Create an ABG for a client who is abusing laxatives. List lab values that indicate metabolic acidosis.	
	ABG VALUES
pH	
$PaCO_2$	
HCO_3	

Table 8-3

_____

_____

_____

_____

Metabolic alkalosis

📋 Pathophysiology/Description

> Base bicarbonate excess

> Loss of acid (vomiting or nasogastric suction) or gain in bicarbonate (eating baking soda)

> Compensation includes renal excretion of HCO_3

> May also compensate with reduction in the respiratory rate to retain carbon dioxide, this is limited by body's natural impulse to take the next breath/ventilate

> Causes include vomiting, nasogastric suctioning, diuretics, hypokalemia, increased mineral corticoids, eating baking soda/infusion of excess Na HCO_3, hyperaldosteronism, large blood transfusions wherein citrates bind with HCO_3

> May occur with respiratory acidosis (client with COPD on thiazide diuretic)

> May occur with respiratory alkalosis (hypoventilating and losing gastric acids via nasogastric drainage)

✏️ Priority Assessments or Cues

> Assess clients at risk

> Assess for increased work of breathing or respiratory distress

> Assess vital signs for tachycardia, bradypnea, dysrhythmias

> Assess for dizziness, drowsiness, confusion, headache, nausea/vomiting, anorexia, tetany, muscle cramps, tremors, hypotonicity

⚗️ Priority Laboratory Tests/Diagnostics

> **Arterial blood gases**
  - Normal values
    - pH 7.35-7.45
    - $PaCO_2$ 35-45 mmHg
    - HCO_3 22-26 mEq/L
  - Metabolic alkalosis
    - pH increased
    - $PaCO_2$ normal (uncompensated)
    - $PaCO_2$ elevated (compensated)
    - HCO_3 increased
> Monitor serum potassium levels 3.5-5.0 mEq/L

> Monitor serum calcium levels 8.6-10.2 mg/dL and 4.5-5.5 mEq/L

⚠️ Priority Interventions or Actions

> Determine and manage underlying cause

> Implement seizure precautions, as indicated

> Replace potassium

> Medications to increase excretion of bicarbonate

🚩 Priority Potential & Actual Complications

> Seizures

↻ Priority Nursing Implications

> Read and interpret arterial blood gas findings, watching for trends and change

> Maintain safety precautions with change in sensorium

> Assess clients with profuse vomiting/gastric suctioning for changes in level of consciousness

👤 Priority Education/Discharge Issues

> Instruct client on importance of hydration

> Educate client on signs and symptoms that warrant reporting to healthcare provider

Create an ABG for a client needing nasogastric suctioning for an extended period of time. List lab values that indicate metabolic alkalosis.	
	ABG VALUES
pH	
$PaCO_2$	
HCO_3	

Table 8-4

Respiratory acidosis

Pathophysiology/Description

> Occurs from carbonic acid excess (CO_2 and H_2O combine, high hydrogen ion concentration)

> Generally due to hypoventilation and CO_2 retention –lowers the pH

> Kidneys compensate with conservation of HCO_3 –renal compensation occurs within 24 hours

> May occur with metabolic alkalosis (client with COPD on thiazide diuretic)

> May occur with metabolic acidosis, as in cardiopulmonary arrest

> Causes include COPD, barbiturate/CNS depressant/opioid overdose, pneumonia, asthma, atelectasis, low respiratory rate on a mechanical ventilator/hypoventilation, conditions causing respiratory muscle weakness (Guillain-Barré, myasthenia gravis), high oxygen provision to CO_2 retainers, pulmonary edema, and pulmonary embolism

Priority Assessments or Cues

> Assess clients at risk

> Assess for respiratory depression or obstructed airway

> Assess vital signs for hypotension, bradypnea, oxygen saturation-hypoxia

> Assess for dizziness, drowsiness, confusion, headache, warm flushed skin

Priority Laboratory Tests/Diagnostics

> Arterial blood gases
  - Normal values
    - pH 7.35-7.45
    - $PaCO_2$ 35-45 mmHg
    - HCO_3 22-26 mEq/L
  - Respiratory Acidosis
    - pH decreased
    - $PaCO_2$ increased
    - HCO_3 normal (uncompensated)
    - HCO_3 increased (compensated)

> Monitor serum potassium levels 3.5-5.0 mEq/L

Priority Interventions or Actions

> Determine and treat underlying cause and manage respiratory distress

> Provide oxygen as prescribed

> Position in semi-Fowler's position

> Encourage client to turn, cough, and deep breath

> Encourage fluids to liquefy secretions, suction as needed

> Avoid medications that cause respiratory depression

> Provide respiratory treatments and antibiotics as prescribed

> Monitor for rising CO_2 and need for intubation and mechanical ventilation

> Implement seizure precautions as indicated

Priority Potential & Actual Complications

> Seizures

> Coma

> Ventricular fibrillation

> May be fatal

Priority Nursing Implications

> Monitor clients at risk for and symptoms of increasing respiratory distress

> Read and interpret arterial blood gas findings, watching for trends and change

> Respiratory distress is very frightening for clients requiring nurses to provide support and remain calm

Priority Education/Discharge Issues

> Instruct client and family to assess for deteriorating respiratory condition

> Educate client on means to prevent respiratory infections

Clinical Hint

Clients who are carbon dioxide retainers respond to the hypoxic drive to breath. If clients receive high oxygen levels, this may be extinguished causing apnea.

Create an ABG for a client found unresponsive floating in a pool. List lab values that indicate respiratory acidosis.	
	ABG VALUES
pH	
$PaCO_2$	
HCO_3	

Table 8-5

Respiratory alkalosis

Pathophysiology/Description

> Carbonic acid deficit with increased carbon dioxide excretion

> Occurs with client hyperventilation

> Related to hypoxia from respiratory distress

> Compensation usually does not occur, it may include HCO_3 being excreted or transferred into the cells

> Associated with anxiety, CNS conditions, overventilation/overstimulation of respiratory system

> Causes include hyperventilation, hypoxia, pulmonary embolism, fear, pain, fever, anxiety, overventilation during exercise, brain injury/encephalitis, septicemia, salicylate poisoning, and overventilation via mechanical ventilator

> May occur with metabolic alkalosis (hypoventilating and losing gastric acids via nasogastric drainage)

Priority Assessments or Cues

> Assess for clients at risk including those in respiratory distress

> Assess vital signs for tachycardia, tachypnea, dysrhythmias

> Assess for confusion, lethargy, headache, dizziness, nausea/vomiting, epigastric pain, tetany, numbness, tingling, and hyperreflexia

Priority Laboratory Tests/Diagnostics

> Arterial blood gases
  • Normal values
    - pH 7.35-7.45
    - $PaCO_2$ 35-45 mmHg
    - HCO_3 22-26 mEq/L
  • Metabolic alkalosis
    - pH increased
    - $PaCO_2$ decreased
    - HCO_3 normal (uncompensated)
    - HCO_3 decreased (compensated)

> Monitor serum potassium levels 3.5-5.0 mEq/L

> Monitor serum calcium levels 8.6-10.2 mg/dL and 4.5-5.5 mEq/L

Priority Interventions or Actions

> Determine and manage underlying cause
> Provide emotional support
> Encourage normal breathing patterns
> Teach client means to retain CO_2
  • Holding breath
  • Use of a rebreathing mask
  • Breathing into a paper bag

> Alleviate hypoxemia to lower respiratory rate, ensure adjustment of ventilator settings

> Implement seizure precautions, as indicated

Priority Potential & Actual Complications

> Seizures

Priority Nursing Implications

> Read and interpret arterial blood gas findings, watching for trends and change

> Assess and manage a client on mechanical ventilation

> Provide education and emotional support as indicated

Priority Medications

> calcium carbonate
  • Treats respiratory alkalosis, hyperphosphatemia, and hypocalcemia
  • May cause constipation and flatulence
  • IV infusion
  • Monitor for tetany

Priority Education/Discharge Issues

> Teaching clients breathing techniques to manage breathing pattern

> Provide referrals for emotional support as needed

Create an ABG for a patient with severe abdominal pain and hyperventilation. List lab values that indicate respiratory alkalosis.	
	ABG VALUES
pH	
$PaCO_2$	
HCO_3	

Table 8-6

1. The nurse is caring for a client in diabetic ketoacidosis. An intravenous insulin drip is infusing at a continuous rate along with normal saline infusion at 250 mL/hour. The client is becoming increasingly responsive and the glucose level has decreased each hour. Which finding would indicate that the client's metabolic acidosis is improving?
   1. Glucose 132 mg/dL.
   2. HCO_3 20 mEq/L.
   3. $PaCO_2$ 36 mmHg.
   4. pH level 7.39.

2. During assessment of the postoperative client following abdominal surgery, the nurse notes that respirations are shallow. Which priority intervention should the nurse plan for this client to avoid respiratory acidosis?
   1. Administer oxygen via nasal cannula.
   2. Auscultate lung sounds every four hours.
   3. Use of incentive spirometer every hour while awake.
   4. Administer pain medication as indicated.

3. The nurse is assessing a client who has been admitted with abdominal pain. The client reports vomiting after meals and use of oral antacids several times daily. A nasogastric tube is inserted to low intermittent suction. What assessment finding would require immediate follow-up by the nurse?
   1. Return of 200 mL dark green liquid from nasogastric tube.
   2. Complaints of dizziness and lightheadedness.
   3. Hypoventilation at rate of 10 breaths/minute.
   4. pH 7.47, $PaCO_2$ 40, HCO_3 30.

4. The nurse is caring for a client recently involved in a motor vehicle crash with prolonged extrication. The airbag was deployed, and the client has facial abrasions and bruising diagonally across the chest. The client has a dislocated fracture of the right ankle. Vital signs are blood pressure 152/100, heart rate 110, and respiratory rate 28. What medication is priority for the nurse to administer to decrease risk of respiratory alkalosis?
   1. Lorazepam 2 mg intravenous push.
   2. Morphine sulfate 4 mg intravenous push.
   3. Sodium bicarbonate one ampule intravenous push.
   4. Broad-spectrum antibiotic intravenously.

5. The nurse is caring for a client with metastatic bone cancer. Initial assessment findings include delayed skin turgor, dry mucous membranes, and cloudy urine. The client reports that she is no longer able to walk outside the home due to severe pain with ambulation. The lab results include sodium 148 mEq/L, potassium 3.2 mEq/L, calcium 13.8 mg/dL, glucose 134 mg/dL, blood urea nitrogen (BUN) 24 mg/dL. What is the nurse's priority intervention?
   1. Fully assess pain severity.
   2. Insert urinary catheter to monitor output.
   3. Initiate intravenous fluids with sodium chloride.
   4. Consult with physical therapy to increase activity tolerance.

6. The nurse is caring for a client receiving dialysis for chronic renal failure. Which assessment finding requires immediate intervention by the nurse?
   1. Potassium level 2.8 mEqL.
   2. Two diarrhea stools in past four hours.
   3. Client reports not taking daily dose of potassium.
   4. Glucose level 140 mg/dL.

7. The nurse is caring for the client with diabetes insipidus. Assessment findings include restlessness, agitation, flushed skin and dry tongue. What priority intervention should the nurse implement?
   1. Monitor daily weight measurements.
   2. Ensure the client drinks a minimum of 64 ounces of water daily.
   3. Begin intravenous fluid volume replacement.
   4. Notify dietician of sodium restriction.

8. The nurse is caring for a client experiencing new onset seizures. Which statement by the client's spouse requires further follow-up?
   1. "My spouse exercises every day by walking and stretching."
   2. "My spouse uses a small bottled enema every day because of constipation."
   3. "My spouse gets up during the night to urinate at least once or twice."
   4. "We eat a lot of whole-grain cereal, vegetables, cheese, fruits, and red meat."

9. The nurse is planning to teach high school football coaches how to recognize early signs of dehydration. Which statement by a coach requires additional education by the nurse?
   1. "I need to let the players drink water when they are thirsty."
   2. "I need to only practice in the morning or evening."
   3. "I need to limit practice time in hot weather."
   4. "Insensible water loss can occur during practice."

10. The nurse is caring for a teenage client with chronic streptococcal infections of the throat who has come to the clinic with complaints of swelling around her eyes. What is the priority nursing assessment for this client?
    1. Administer antihistamine to decrease swelling.
    2. Test urine for glucose and ketones.
    3. Assess for hypotension.
    4. Assess for generalized edema.

11. The nurse is caring for a client with acute pancreatitis and renal insufficiency who is experiencing hyperreflexia and contraction of the muscles in the hands. Which medication order requires follow-up by the nurse?
    1. Calcium gluconate 500 mg orally twice daily.
    2. Vitamin D 5000 units orally once daily.
    3. Magnesium sulfate 5 grams intravenous over 3 hours.
    4. Morphine 2 mg intravenous push every 2 hours PRN pain.

12. The nurse is providing discharge instructions for the client with chronic kidney disease. Which statement by the client indicates the need for additional teaching related to prevention of hypermagnesemia?
    1. "I should not experience changes in my urine output from hypermagnesemia."
    2. "I should not experience severe muscle weakness from too much magnesium."
    3. "I can take over-the-counter antacids for indigestion."
    4. "I should avoid eating green vegetables, chocolate, and nuts."

13. The nurse is admitting a client from a long-term care facility with new onset of confusion. The client's assessment findings include irritability, tremors in the hands, urinary incontinence and dry mucous membranes. The client has a peripheral vascular wound that has copious amounts of serosanguinous drainage. The laboratory findings include Na 128 mEq/L, K 3.5 mEq/L, Cl 88 mEq/L, and glucose 88 mg/dL. What is the priority intervention for this client?
    1. Intravenous infusion of hypotonic fluid.
    2. Insert urinary catheter.
    3. Encouraging oral fluid intake.
    4. Begin intravenous antibiotic therapy.

14. The nurse is counseling a group of teenagers about nutritional requirements and how to avoid electrolyte imbalances. Which is important to include in the teaching plan related to prevention of hypophosphatemia?
    1. Phosphate supplements do not cause adverse gastrointestinal effects.
    2. Low-fat dairy products should be included in the daily food plan.
    3. Low phosphate levels pose little risk to the teenager.
    4. Anorexia and bulimia do not impact phosphate levels.

15. The nurse is caring for a client with anorexia nervosa. Arterial blood gas results are pH 7.26, $PaCO_2$ 40 mmHg, and HCO_3 16 mEq/L. What is the nurse's priority intervention?
    1. Assist the client when moving from bed to chair.
    2. Administer medication for seizure prevention.
    3. Insert urinary catheter to monitor output.
    4. Provide meal with high potassium options.

16. The nurse is admitting a client who has overdosed on barbiturates. The nurse analyzes the initial blood gas results which show pH 7.2, $PaCO_2$ 56 mmHg, and HCO_3 24 mEq/L with a PaO_2 of 62 mmHg. What is the nurse's priority intervention?
    1. Administer bicarbonate intravenously.
    2. Apply oxygen via nonrebreather mask.
    3. Encourage the client to relax and slow breathing.
    4. Begin cardiopulmonary resuscitation.

17. The nurse is caring for a geriatric client who is severely dehydrated. Intravenous fluids are infusing at 250 mL over 30 minutes and the infusion can be repeated twice. Which assessment findings following the first infusion indicate that the nurse should repeat the infusion? Select all that apply.
    1. Crying without tears.
    2. Incontinent pad wet with urine.
    3. Normotensive blood pressure.
    4. Tachycardic heart rate.
    5. Crackles in lung bases bilaterally.
    6. Capillary refill greater than 3 seconds.

18. The nurse is administering two units of packed red blood cells into an elderly client who has experienced gastrointestinal bleeding from an ulcer. What assessment findings indicate that the client is experiencing fluid overload? Select all that apply.
    1. Oxygen saturation 97%.
    2. Auscultation of crackles in the posterior lung fields.
    3. Shortness of breath when talking to nurse.
    4. Blood urea nitrogen level 11 mg/dL.
    5. S3 heart sound.
    6. Jugular vein distention.

19. The nurse is caring for a client after abdominal surgery who has a nasogastric tube to low intermittent suction. The tube has drained 2000 mL dark green fluid over the past 12 hours. Urine output via catheter was 1000 mL over the past 12 hours. Isotonic intravenous fluids are infusing at 125 mL/hour. The client has a medical history that includes heart failure, hypertension, and diabetes. Which assessment findings cause the nurse to become concerned about risk for metabolic alkalosis? Select all that apply.
    1. $PaCO_2$ 44 mmHg.
    2. pH 7.33.
    3. HCO_3 30 mEq/L.
    4. Nasogastric tube output.
    5. Infusion of incorrect type of intravenous fluids.
    6. Bradycardia.

20. The nurse is caring for a client with liver failure. The arterial blood gas results are pH 7.61, $PaCO_2$ 34 mmHg, HCO_3 54 mEq/L, and PaO_2 76 mmHg. What interventions should the nurse implement? Select all that apply.
    1. Assess for hypothermia.
    2. Obtain emergency airway equipment.
    3. Administer oxygen at 2L/minute via nasal cannula.
    4. Implement seizure precautions.
    5. Administer acetaminophen rectally for pain relief.

21. The nurse is obtaining vital signs on a client receiving a second unit of packed red blood cells. The client's respiratory rate is 26 breaths/minutes, oxygen saturation is 95% and they are short of breath and frequently cough when responding to the nurse's questions. What is the priority order for these nurse's interventions? Rank order the responses.
    1. Stop or slow rate of blood infusion.
    2. Notify blood bank.
    3. Apply oxygen via nasal cannula.
    4. Infuse normal saline intravenously at keep vein open rate.
    5. Elevate head of bed.
    6. Notify healthcare provider.

22. The nurse is preparing to begin an intravenous infusion for a client with dehydration due to sun overexposure. In what order would the nurse perform these actions? Rank order the responses.
    1. Explain procedure to the client.
    2. Wash hands.
    3. Gather supplies and equipment.
    4. Verify order for intravenous infusion.
    5. Insert and secure IV catheter.
    6. Don gloves.

23. The nurse is caring for a client with renal failure. The client is on a special diet and strict intake and output. Which assessments are of the highest priority for this client? Select all that apply.
    1. Daily weights.
    2. Assess bowel sounds.
    3. Monitor appetite.
    4. Monitor edema in extremities.
    5. Monitor bowel movements.
    6. Monitor urine output.

24. A client is admitted with ascites from liver failure. Spironolactone 100 mg is administered. What signs or symptoms would designate a potential serious adverse reaction in this client?
    1. Blurred vision.
    2. Leg Pain.
    3. Low potassium levels.
    4. Skin Rash.

25. The nurse is monitoring a 65-year-old client's fluid volume status upon return from surgery. Upon assessing the client, fluid volume overload is suspected. Which symptoms support this condition?
    1. Hypertension, bounding pulse; weakness; as well as respiratory crackles.
    2. Oral temperature of 101°F (38.3°C), BP 90/60, thready pulse of 94.
    3. 700 mL's urine out in the OR, CVP = 6 and nystagmus.
    4. Noted lethargy with complaints of abdominal pain and headache.

26. A healthcare provider calls the charge nurse to give an order on another nurse's client who has been diagnosed with hypokalemia. The verbal order is as follows: Start 500 mL's IV Dextrose 5% in ½ Normal Saline; add 40 mEq's of KCL to the 500 mL IV bag and run over four hours. The KCl is available at 2 mEq/mL. How many milliliters of KCL should the pharmacy add to the IV solution?
    1. 25 milliliters.
    2. 10 milliliters.
    3. 20 milliliters.
    4. 15 milliliters.

27. The nurse is discussing fluids with a dialysis client. The nurse understands what aspect of care is a priority for the dialysis client?
    1. Restricting fluid intake.
    2. Eating fruits and vegetables.
    3. Daily exercise.
    4. Monitoring output.

28. The nurse is planning discharge teaching for an elderly client who has been hospitalized for dehydration. Which steps should the nurse complete when developing the education plan? Select all that apply.
    1. Write learning goals that are achievable.
    2. Choose a time to maximize client attention and minimize distraction.
    3. Ensure all materials are given to client only in writing.
    4. Evaluate client's understanding to identify knowledge gaps.
    5. Always use modern technology to provide client education.

29. The nurse is completing the intake and output record for the client recovering from bariatric surgery. The intake for 12 hours includes: Intravenous fluids infused at 125 mL/hour and oral intake of one ounce clear fluids every hour x 6, followed by 1.5 ounce/hour x 4, followed by 2 ounces per hour x 2. The client urinated two times: 450 mL and 330 mL. How many mL difference is there between intake and output?

    _____

30. The nurse is administering intravenous (IV) fluids to a pediatric client who has experienced third-degree burns. To prevent dehydration, the nurse is to administer 2 mL of lactated ringers IV solution times the body weight in kilograms times the percentage of total body surface area burned (2 mL LR x kg x %TBSA burned). One half of the IV fluids is to be delivered over the first eight hours with the remaining half delivered over the subsequent 16 hours. The client's weight is 55 pounds. Estimated burned body surfaces include 7% of each leg, 9% of the right arm and 6% of the abdomen. How many mL (in whole number) of intravenous fluid should be delivered 14 hours after the fluid resuscitation has begun?

    _____

1. The nurse is caring for a client in diabetic ketoacidosis. An intravenous insulin drip is infusing at a continuous rate along with normal saline infusion at 250 mL/hour. The client is becoming increasingly responsive and the glucose level has decreased each hour. Which finding would indicate that the client's metabolic acidosis is improving?
   1. Glucose 132 mg/dL. *Not an indicator of acidosis.*
   2. HCO_3 20 mEq/L. *Reflective of acidosis.*
   3. $PaCO_2$ 36 mmHg. *Close to normal, but on alkaline side.*
   4. ⦿ pH level 7.39.

   Rationale: pH is the indicator of acidosis or alkalosis. The pH has returned to the normal range. HCO_3 and $PaCO_2$ remain below normal; glucose level shows client is improving; however, doesn't directly indicate resolving acidosis.

   THIN Thinking: Nursing Process – *Evaluation of the client's response to treatment is an important part of the nurse's role in monitoring response to insulin.* **NCLEX®**: Safety and Infection Control **QSEN**: Patient-centered Care

2. During assessment of the postoperative client following abdominal surgery, the nurse notes that respirations are shallow. Which priority intervention should the nurse plan for this client to avoid respiratory acidosis?
   1. Administer oxygen via nasal cannula. *Not helpful if client's respirations are shallow.*
   2. Auscultate lung sounds every four hours. *Provides data but doesn't prevent acidosis.*
   3. ⦿ Use of incentive spirometer every hour while awake.
   4. Administer pain medication as indicated. *May make it easier for client to breathe but may also suppress respirations. Incentive spirometer is priority intervention.*

   Rationale: Respiratory acidosis may result from hypoventilation and atelectasis. Use of incentive spirometry decreases risk of atelectasis. There is no data in the question to support use of oxygen; administering pain medication may result in furthering shallow breathing pattern, and auscultating lung sounds is not a preventative intervention--is an assessment technique.

   THIN Thinking: Top Three – *The priority needs to be to improve gas exchange. To do this aggressive coughing and deep breathing and the use of the incentive spirometer are helpful.* **NCLEX®**: Reduction of Risk Potential **QSEN**: Patient-centered Care

3. The nurse is assessing a client who has been admitted with abdominal pain. The client reports vomiting after meals and use of oral antacids several times daily. A nasogastric tube is inserted to low intermittent suction. What assessment finding would require immediate follow-up by the nurse?
   1. Return of 200 mL dark green liquid from nasogastric

   tube. *This is expected.*
   2. ⦿ Complaints of dizziness and lightheadedness. *Dizziness may increase risk for falls and risks to safety.*
   3. Hypoventilation at rate of 10 breaths/minute. *Hypoventilation is not a priority issue since it's compensatory.*
   4. pH 7.47, $PaCO_2$ 40, HCO_3 30. *Although the client is alkalotic, the nurse would not be able to intervene on an immediate basis.*

   Rationale: The ABG results indicate metabolic alkalosis but is not so aberrant that it warrants immediate attention. Hyperventilation, dizziness, and lightheadedness are manifestations of respiratory alkalosis and may pose a safety hazard requiring immediate attention. The nasogastric tube return is expected and normal in amount and color.

   THIN Thinking: Identify Risk to Safety – *Dizziness increases the risk for falls.* **NCLEX®**: Physiological Adaptation **QSEN**: Patient-centered Care

4. The nurse is caring for a client recently involved in a motor vehicle crash with prolonged extrication. The airbag was deployed, and the client has facial abrasions and bruising diagonally across the chest. The client has a dislocated fracture of the right ankle. Vital signs are blood pressure 152/100, heart rate 110, and respiratory rate 28. What medication is priority for the nurse to administer to decrease risk of respiratory alkalosis?
   1. Lorazepam 2 mg intravenous push. *Not the priority. Need to address pain issue.*
   2. ⦿ Morphine sulfate 4 mg intravenous push.
   3. Sodium bicarbonate one ampule intravenous push. *This would worsen the alkalosis.*
   4. Broad-spectrum antibiotic intravenously. *Wouldn't affect respiratory alkalosis risk.*

   Rationale: Respiratory alkalosis is often caused by hyperventilation due to hypoxia, anxiety, pain, and fear. This client has tachypnea, pain from ankle and other injuries and fear and anxiety which would be expected following a crash of this magnitude. Pain management with morphine will decrease pain and anxiety. Lorazepam may be an option but not the first one. Sodium bicarbonate is not given unless other interventions to relieve acidosis are not effective. Broad-spectrum antibiotics will be required due to the open fracture; however, they are not priority over pain management.

   THIN Thinking: Top Three – *Pain/anxiety become the highest priority because the vital signs indicate client stability..* **NCLEX®**: Pharmacological and Parental Therapies **QSEN**: Patient-centered Care

5. The nurse is caring for a client with metastatic bone cancer. Initial assessment findings include delayed skin turgor, dry mucous membranes, and cloudy urine. The client reports that she is no longer able to walk outside the home due to severe pain with ambulation. The lab results include sodium 148 mEq/L, potassium 3.2 mEq/L, calcium 13.8 mg/dL, glucose 134 mg/dL, blood urea nitrogen (BUN) 24 mg/dL. What is the nurse's priority intervention?

1. Fully assess pain severity. *Priority is correcting fluid issue, then pain can be addressed.*
2. Insert urinary catheter to monitor output. *Priority is initiating fluids, then a catheter can be placed.*
3. ⦿ Initiate intravenous fluids with sodium chloride.
4. Consult with physical therapy to increase activity tolerance. *Not a priority. May be addressed when stable.*

Rationale: The history, physical assessment, and laboratory reports indicate hypercalcemia due to dehydration and bone cancer. The priority is high volume fluid replacement. The client will need a urinary catheter after fluids initiated to monitor output. Pain and activity assessment can take place once client is stabilized.

THIN Thinking: Top Three – *High calcium, high sodium, and physical assessment support dehydration, IV fluids are the priority with the information given.* **NCLEX®:** Pharmacology and Parenteral Therapies **QSEN:** Patient-centered Care

6. The nurse is caring for a client receiving dialysis for chronic renal failure. Which assessment finding requires immediate intervention by the nurse?

1. ⦿ Potassium level 2.8 mEqL.
2. Two diarrhea stools in past four hours. *Not as critical as potassium level.*
3. Client reports not taking daily dose of potassium. *Needs to be addressed after potassium level corrected.*
4. Glucose level 140 mg/dL. *Rationale- High, but not a critical level.*

Rationale: The potassium level is critically low and could lead to cardiac changes that are potentially life-threatening (ventricular dysrhythmias, heart block). Diarrhea and failure to take potassium supplement contributed to the hypokalemia but can be managed after initial threat resolved. Hyperglycemia can result from hypokalemia; however, this finding is not critical.

THIN Thinking: Top Three – *The K+ level is critical. Slow potassium replacement intravenously needs to be initiated quickly to prevent dysrhythmias.* **NCLEX®:** Reduction for Risk Protential **QSEN:** Safety

7. The nurse is caring for the client with diabetes insipidus. Assessment findings include restlessness, agitation, flushed skin and dry tongue. What priority intervention should the nurse implement?

1. Monitor daily weight measurements. *Important to monitor, but not most important.*
2. Ensure the client drinks a minimum of 64 ounces of water daily. *Necessary, but client needs IV fluid replacement first.*
3. ⦿ Begin intravenous fluid volume replacement.
4. Notify dietician of sodium restriction. *Important, but needs IV fluid replacement first.*

Rationale: The assessment findings indicate significant hypernatremia and dehydration. While all options are appropriate, dehydration from diabetes insipidus is most important to reverse in order to decrease dehydration of brain cells resulting in restlessness, agitation, and seizures. Failure to do so could lead to worsening mental status and coma.

THIN Thinking: Top Three – *All interventions address the dehydrated clients, but IV fluids will correct the situation the quickest and is the highest priority.* **NCLEX®:** Physiological Adaptation **QSEN:** Safety

8. The nurse is caring for a client experiencing new onset seizures. Which statement by the client's spouse requires further follow-up?

1. "My spouse exercises every day by walking and stretching." *Irrelevant to teaching.*
2. ⦿ "My spouse uses a small bottled enema every day because of constipation."
3. "My spouse gets up during the night to urinate at least once or twice." *Unrelated to issue.*
4. "We eat a lot of whole-grain cereal, vegetables, cheese, fruits, and red meat." *Unrelated to issue.*

Rationale: Seizures can be a result of hyperphosphatemia, which can be caused by phosphate enemas (Fleets enema). The other responses do not correlate with a new onset seizure.

THIN Thinking: Identify Risk to Safety – *Excessive absorption of phosphate can increase the risk for seizures, a safety concern.* **NCLEX®:** Safety and Infection Control **QSEN:** Safety

9. The nurse is planning to teach high school football coaches how to recognize early signs of dehydration. Which statement by a coach requires additional education by the nurse?
   1. 🔦 "I need to let the players drink water when they are thirsty."
   2. "I need to only practice in the morning or evening." *This would be helpful since it's often cooler during these times.*
   3. "I need to limit practice time in hot weather." *This will decrease risk of dehydration.*
   4. "Insensible water loss can occur during practice." *This is a true statement.*

   Rationale: Dehydration is manifested by thirst. To prevent dehydration, regular fluid intake should occur and not wait until symptoms appear. The remaining statements are appropriate.

   THIN Thinking: Nursing Process – *Evaluation of learning is important for the nurse to determine if the teaching was effective.* **NCLEX**®: Health Promotion and Maintenance **QSEN:** Safety

10. The nurse is caring for a teenage client with chronic streptococcal infections of the throat who has come to the clinic with complaints of swelling around her eyes. What is the priority nursing assessment for this client?
    1. Administer antihistamine to decrease swelling. *No indication that this is caused by an allergy.*
    2. Test urine for glucose and ketones. *No indication this is related to glucose levels.*
    3. Assess for hypotension. *Client would be at risk for high blood pressure.*
    4. 🔦 Assess for generalized edema.

    Rationale: The client could be experiencing acute post-streptococcal glomerulonephritis, an illness that is common following strep infections. The priority is to assess for additional evidence of fluid overload. Hypertension is common with fluid overload, while hypotension is common to fluid deficit. The periorbital edema is not allergy-related (per history given) so antihistamines are not indicated. Urine glucose and ketones are not correlated to this case.

    THIN Thinking: Nursing Process – *The connection between the infection and edema places the client at risk for glomerulonephritis. The assessment will detect this concern.* **NCLEX**®: Physiological Integrity **QSEN:** Patient-centered Care

11. The nurse is caring for a client with acute pancreatitis and renal insufficiency who is experiencing hyperreflexia and contraction of the muscles in the hands. Which medication order requires follow-up by the nurse?
    1. 🔦 Calcium gluconate 500 mg orally twice daily.
    2. Vitamin D 5000 units orally once daily. *Appropriate order, improves calcium absorption.*
    3. Magnesium sulfate 5 grams intravenous over 3 hours. *Appropriate order for electrolyte replacement.*
    4. Morphine 2 mg intravenous push every 2 hours PRN pain. *Appropriate order for pain – safe dose.*

    Rationale: The client's hypocalcemia is severe as demonstrated by Trousseau's sign (contraction of the muscles in the hand) so the calcium should be administered intravenously. The remaining medications are appropriate for this client. Dosages are all within correct ranges.

    THIN Thinking: Help Quick – *The assessment findings demonstrate severe hypocalcemia so the dose needs to be delivered IV rather than orally.* **NCLEX**®: Pharmacological and Parenteral Therapies **QSEN:** Evidence-based Practice

12. The nurse is providing discharge instructions for the client with chronic kidney disease. Which statement by the client indicates the need for additional teaching related to prevention of hypermagnesemia?
    1. "I should not experience changes in my urine output from hypermagnesemia." *Correct.*
    2. "I should not experience severe muscle weakness from too much magnesium." *Correct.*
    3. 🔦 "I can take over-the-counter antacids for indigestion."
    4. "I should avoid eating green vegetables, chocolate, and nuts." *These foods are high in magnesium and should be avoided.*

    Rationale: Hypermagnesemia typically only occurs with increased intake of magnesium in the client with renal disease. Aluminum hydroxide/magnesium hydroxide (Maalox) is a common antacid that can lead to increased magnesium levels. Urinary retention and muscle weakness are manifestations of hypermagnesemia and require follow-up. Avoiding foods containing magnesium helps avoid hypermagnesemia in a client already predisposed.

    THIN Thinking: Nursing Process – *Evaluation of understanding is important to be assured the client is retaining correct information.* **NCLEX**®: Basic Care and Comfort **QSEN:** Patient-centered Care

13. The nurse is admitting a client from a long-term care facility with new onset of confusion. The client's assessment findings include irritability, tremors in the hands, urinary incontinence and dry mucous membranes. The client has a peripheral vascular wound that has copious amounts of serosanguinous drainage. The laboratory findings include Na 128 mEq/L, K 3.5 mEq/L, Cl 88 mEq/L, and glucose 88 mg/dL. What is the priority intervention for this client?

1. Intravenous infusion of hypotonic fluid. *Would further lower sodium level.*
2. 💡 Insert urinary catheter.
3. Encouraging oral fluid intake. *Would further lower sodium level.*
4. Begin intravenous antibiotic therapy. *Not indicated.*

Rationale: Accurate intake and output is important to the treatment of this client as fluid restriction may need to be initiated and that is based on prior urine output. Oral fluids may further dilute the sodium and infusion of hypotonic fluids can cause hyponatremia. Antibiotics are not indicated for a wound draining serosanguinous fluid, nor is that the priority for this client.

THIN Thinking: Top Three – *Accurate intake and output is a high priority to measure the effectiveness of the treatment plan.* **NCLEX®:** Reduction of Risk Potential **QSEN:** Patient-centered Care

14. The nurse is counseling a group of teenagers about nutritional requirements and how to avoid electrolyte imbalances. Which is important to include in the teaching plan related to prevention of hypophosphatemia?

1. Phosphate supplements do not cause adverse gastrointestinal effects. *GI distress common with phosphate supplements.*
2. 💡 Low-fat dairy products should be included in the daily food plan.
3. Low phosphate levels pose little risk to the teenager. *Low phosphate can cause complication in all age groups.*
4. Anorexia and bulimia do not impact phosphate levels. *Clients with anorexia and bulimia may have poor nutrition and a higher risk for hypophosphatemia.*

Rationale: Dairy products are critical to maintaining normal phosphate levels. The remaining choices are false as supplements do cause GI distress, malnutrition can cause low phosphate levels and result in complications including death.

THIN Thinking: Nursing Process – *Planning teaching with this age group needs to be specific to their needs.* **NCLEX®:** Reduction for Risk Potential **QSEN:** Patient-centered Care

15. The nurse is caring for a client with anorexia nervosa. Arterial blood gas results are pH 7.26, $PaCO_2$ 40 mmHg, and HCO_3 16 mEq/L. What is the nurse's priority intervention?

1. 💡 Assist the client when moving from bed to chair.
2. Administer medication for seizure prevention. *Metabolic acidosis does not commonly cause seizures.*
3. Insert urinary catheter to monitor output. *Nothing indicates a fluid imbalance.*
4. Provide meal with high potassium options. *Metabolic acidosis often causes hyperkalemia so potassium should be avoided.*

Rationale: Hypotension, lethargy, confusion, dizziness, and muscle weakness are manifestations of metabolic acidosis; therefore, safety is priority for this response. Starvation is one cause of metabolic acidosis. Diuretic therapy and other types of fluid volume loss are a cause of metabolic alkalosis; therefore, it is unnecessary to insert urinary catheter. While nutrition is important, it is not the priority response. Seizures are a risk factor for respiratory acidosis and not metabolic acidosis.

THIN Thinking: Identify Risk to Safety – *With an altered mental status, safety and risk for falls are a concern.* **NCLEX®:** Safety and Infection Control **QSEN:** Safety, Patient-centered Care

16. The nurse is admitting a client who has overdosed on barbiturates. The nurse analyzes the initial blood gas results which show pH 7.2, $PaCO_2$ 56 mmHg, and HCO_3 24 mEq/L with a PaO_2 of 62 mmHg. What is the nurse's priority intervention?

1. Administer bicarbonate intravenously. *Bicarbonate level is normal.*
2. 💡 Apply oxygen via nonrebreather mask.
3. Encourage the client to relax and slow breathing. *Not a treatment for acidosis, would cause retention of more CO_2.*
4. Begin cardiopulmonary resuscitation. *No indication of need for this intervention, further assessment required.*

Rationale: Barbiturate overdose is a cause of respiratory acidosis from respiratory depression, which is indicated by these ABG results. The client is retaining CO_2 due to hypoventilation and oxygen should be delivered to decrease hypoxia (followed by likely intubation). The client does not need to slow their breathing as they are already breathing to slow. They are likely nonresponsive at this point and anxiety is not a factor. The bicarbonate level is normal in this uncompensated client. The client's pH indicates they are near death but do not require CPR.

THIN Thinking: Top Three – *Hypoxia indicates the need for oxygen. The nonrebreather mask prevents further elevation of CO_2.* **NCLEX®:** Health Promotion and Maintenance **QSEN:** Patient-centered Care

17. The nurse is caring for a geriatric client who is severely dehydrated. Intravenous fluids are infusing at 250 mL over 30 minutes and the infusion can be repeated twice. Which assessment findings following the first infusion indicate that the nurse should repeat the infusion? Select all that apply.
    1. ◉ Crying without tears.
    2. Incontinent pad wet with urine. *Indicates rehydration when urine output increases.*
    3. Normotensive blood pressure. *Indicates adequate hydration.*
    4. ◉ Tachycardic heart rate.
    5. Crackles in lung bases bilaterally. *Indicates too much fluid.*
    6. ◉ Capillary refill greater than 3 seconds.

    Rationale: Lack of tears, increased heart rate, and delayed capillary refill all are indicative of dehydration. Urination and blood pressure within normal range show improvement in condition, while crackles in the lungs requires further assessment prior to administration of more fluids.

    THIN Thinking: Nursing Process – Knowing the assessment for dehydration and evaluation of rehydration are important to the care of the client with fluid imbalance. **NCLEX®:** Physiological Adaptation **QSEN:** Patient-centered Care

18. The nurse is administering two units of packed red blood cells into an elderly client who has experienced gastrointestinal bleeding from an ulcer. What assessment findings indicate that the client is experiencing fluid overload? Select all that apply.
    1. Oxygen saturation 97% *Not indicative of fluid overload, normal finding.*
    2. ◉ Auscultation of crackles in the posterior lung fields.
    3. ◉ Shortness of breath when talking to nurse.
    4. Blood urea nitrogen level 11 mg/dL. *Normal level.*
    5. ◉ S3 heart sound.
    6. ◉ Jugular vein distention.

    Rationale: Crackles in the lungs anywhere, shortness of breath, S3 heart sound, and JVD are all signs of fluid excess. The oxygen saturation and BUN are within normal limits.

    THIN Thinking: Nursing Process – *Recognizing the assessment findings for fluid excess is important in the care of the client.* **NCLEX®:** Reduction of Risk Potential **QSEN:** Patient-centered Care

19. The nurse is caring for a client after abdominal surgery who has a nasogastric tube to low intermittent suction. The tube has drained 2000 mL dark green fluid over the past 12 hours. Urine output via catheter was 1000 mL over the past 12 hours. Isotonic intravenous fluids are infusing at 125 mL/hour. The client has a medical history that includes heart failure, hypertension, and diabetes. Which assessment findings cause the nurse to become concerned about risk for metabolic alkalosis? Select all that apply.
    1. ◉ $PaCO_2$ 44 mmHg.
    2. pH 7.33. *Indicates acidosis, not alkalosis.*
    3. ◉ HCO_3 30 mEq/L.
    4. ◉ Nasogastric tube output.
    5. Infusion of incorrect type of intravenous fluids. *Isotonic solution will replace volume loss in the vascular space.*
    6. Bradycardia. *Tachycardia is common in metabolic alkalosis.*

    Rationale: The pH indicates acidosis while the other two blood gas results correspond to metabolic alkalosis. Nasogastric fluid loss and increased urination from diuretics are causes of metabolic acidosis. The type of intravenous fluid replacement is correct. This client would be expected to have tachycardia rather than bradycardia.

    THIN Thinking: Nursing Process – *Assessment of acid-base status is important to the recognition of changes in the treatment plan.* **NCLEX®:** Reduction of Risk Potential **QSEN:** Patient-centered Care

20. The nurse is caring for a client with liver failure. The arterial blood gas results are pH 7.61, $PaCO_2$ 34 mmHg, HCO_3 54 mEq/L, and PaO_2 76 mmHg. What interventions should the nurse implement? Select all that apply.
    1. Assess for hypothermia. *No indication that this is needed.*
    2. ◉ Obtain emergency airway equipment.
    3. ◉ Administer oxygen at 2L/minute via nasal cannula. *Oxygen is required to ensure PaO_2 does not deteriorate.*
    4. ◉ Implement seizure precautions.
    5. Administer acetaminophen rectally for pain relief. *Contraindicated in liver failure and no indications of its need.*

    Rationale: Blood gas results indicate metabolic alkalosis and the client is in critical condition. HCO_3 levels greater than 50 mEq/L may result in seizures, hypoventilation, and coma. Hypothermia is not an immediate concern, oxygen needs to be administered via nonrebreather mask, and acetaminophen is contraindicated in liver failure.

    THIN Thinking: Help Quick – *This client requires emergency/critical care including oxygen, seizure precautions, and emergency equipment.* **NCLEX®:** Safety and Infection Control **QSEN:** Patient-centered Care

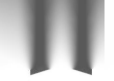

21. The nurse is obtaining vital signs on a client receiving a second unit of packed red blood cells. The client's respiratory rate is 26 breaths/minutes, oxygen saturation is 95% and they are short of breath and frequently cough when responding to the nurse's questions. What is the priority order for these nurse's interventions? Rank order the responses.
    1. Elevate head of bed.
    2. Apply oxygen via nasal cannula.
    3. Stop or slow rate of blood infusion.
    4. Infuse normal saline intravenously at keep vein open rate.
    5. Notify healthcare provider.
    6. Notify blood bank.

    Rationale: The client is experiencing circulatory overload during the transfusion. Airway and breathing are priority; elevating the head of the bed may provide immediate relief of shortness of breath. Oxygen is then applied due to low saturation level and tachypnea. Once breathing is addressed, circulatory status is the next priority and the transfusion should be stopped or slowed based on severity of clinical presentation, why blood is required, and medical history. The IV line must be kept patent and normal saline is hung with blood transfusions for this purpose. Once the immediate needs are addressed, the healthcare provider should be notified. The blood bank will need to be notified if transfusion cannot be completed or future units need to be divided into smaller amounts.

    THIN Thinking Top Three – *Priority is ABC. Airway/breathing, then circulation* **NCLEX®**: Physiological Adaptation **QSEN:** Safety

22. The nurse is preparing to begin an intravenous infusion for a client with dehydration due to sun overexposure. In what order would the nurse perform these actions? Rank order the responses.
    1. Verify order for intravenous infusion.
    2. Explain procedure to the client.
    3. Gather supplies and equipment.
    4. Wash hands.
    5. Don gloves.
    6. Insert and secure IV catheter.

    Rationale: The order should be verified before discussing with client. The procedure should be explained prior to gathering supplies in case the client refuses the treatment. Once supplies taken to room, the nurse should wash their hands before providing any care to client. Gloves must be applied prior to inserting the intravenous catheter.

    THIN Thinking: Identify Risk to Safety – *Procedures should be performed so that they are safe and protect the client for infection.* **NCLEX®**: Safety and Infection Control **QSEN:** Safety

23. The nurse is caring for a client with renal failure. The client is on a special diet and strict intake and output. Which assessments are of the highest priority for this client? Select all that apply.
    1. 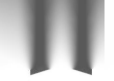 Daily weights.
    2. Assess bowel sounds. *Not a priority assessment for this client.*
    3. Monitor appetite. *Not a priority assessment for this client.*
    4. 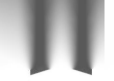 Monitor edema in extremities.
    5. Monitor bowel movements. *Not a priority assessment for this client.*
    6. 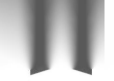 Monitor urine output.

    Rationale: Monitoring weight, edema, and urine output are all appropriate assessments of hydration. Weight gain is a sign of fluid retention, as is edema. Although bowel sounds, appetite, and bowel movements are important, they are not a priority for this client.

    THIN Thinking: Nursing Process – *Fluid status is a priority assessment for renal failure.* **NCLEX®**: Reduction of Risk Potential **QSEN:** Patient-centered Care

24. A client is admitted with ascites from liver failure. Spironolactone 100 mg is administered. What signs or symptoms would designate a potential serious adverse reaction in this client?
    1. Blurred vision. *Not an adverse reaction of this drug.*
    2. Leg Pain. *Not an adverse reaction of this drug.*
    3. Low potassium levels. *Not an adverse reaction of this drug, it is potassium sparing.*
    4. 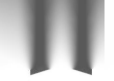 Skin Rash.

    Rationale: Blurred vision is not associated with spironolactone. Leg pain and low potassium levels are not associated with this drug as it is a potassium sparing diuretic. The skin rash may indicate an adverse reaction and may be the first sign of Stevens-Johnson Syndrome, which may be life-threatening.

    THIN Thinking: Identify Risk to Safety – *Understand potentially life-threatening side effects of medication are important to identify early.* **NCLEX®**: Pharmacology and Parenteral Therapies **QSEN:** Evidence-based Practice

25. The nurse is monitoring a 65-year-old client's fluid volume status upon return from surgery. Upon assessing the client, fluid volume overload is suspected. Which symptoms support this condition?
   1. 🔵 Hypertension, bounding pulse; weakness; as well as respiratory crackles.
   2. Oral temperature of 101°F (38.3°C), BP 90/60, thready pulse of 94. *Low BP and thready pulse indicate fluid deficit.*
   3. 700 mL's urine out in the OR, CVP = 6 and nystagmus. *Anticipated findings.*
   4. Noted lethargy with complaints of abdominal pain and headache. *Not associated with fluid overload.*

   Rationale: A bounding pulse, weakness, and respiratory crackles leads the nurse to identify fluid volume overload. Excess fluid may interfere with the exchange of oxygen and carbon dioxide. With this excess, fluid shifting may occur leading to pleural effusion.

   THIN Thinking: Nursing Process – *It is important for the nurse to assess the signs of volume overload so medical treatment can be explored.* **NCLEX®:** Reduction of Risk Potential **QSEN:** Patient-centered Care

26. A healthcare provider calls the charge nurse to give an order on another nurse's client who has been diagnosed with hypokalemia. The verbal order is as follows: Start 500 mL's IV Dextrose 5% in ½ Normal Saline; add 40 mEq's of KCL to the 500 mL IV bag and run over four hours. The KCl is available at 2 mEq/mL. How many milliliters of KCL should the pharmacy add to the IV solution?
   1. 25 milliliters.
   2. 10 milliliters.
   3. 🔵 20 milliliters.
   4. 15 milliliters.

   Rationale: 40 mEq/2 mEq/mL = 20 mL

   THIN Thinking: Safety - *Planning for safe medication administration is critical to prevent injury.* **NCLEX®:** Safety and Infection Control **QSEN:** Evidence-based Practice

27. The nurse is discussing fluids with a dialysis client. The nurse understands what aspect of care is a priority for the dialysis client?
   1. 🔵 Restricting fluid intake.
   2. Eating fruits and vegetables. *Need to be limited.*
   3. Daily exercise. *Not a priority related to fluid intake.*
   4. Monitoring output. *Not as important as measuring intake.*

   Rationale: Fruits and vegetables would not be indicated as they are high in potassium and sodium. Exercise is important but not a priority. A client on dialysis would have a very low output due to renal insufficiency. Intake of fluids is critical because dialysis is only done several times/week and too much fluid intake may overload the kidneys.

   THIN Thinking: TOP Three - *Overload of fluid may damage the kidneys and impair function.* **NCLEX®:** Management of Care **QSEN:** Teamwork and Collaboration

28. The nurse is planning discharge teaching for an elderly client who has been hospitalized for dehydration. Which steps should the nurse complete when developing the education plan? Select all that apply.
   1. 🔵 Write learning goals that are achievable.
   2. 🔵 Choose a time to maximize client attention and minimize distraction.
   3. Ensure all materials are given to client only in writing. *No indication that this is preferred. The nurse would need to assess learning needs.*
   4. 🔵 Evaluate client's understanding to identify knowledge gaps.
   5. Always use modern technology to provide client education. *This may not be appropriate for client, need to assess learning needs.*

   Rationale: It is important to evaluate knowledge gaps prior to determining where to focus teaching. Learning goals are created so that the nurse can determine if the client understands the information once taught. Comprehension will be easier if the client can focus solely on the education. While it is important to provide written materials for later review and reinforcement of knowledge, this is not the only method for providing education (internet, video, demonstration). Modern technology may not be accessible for all clients in their home environment, nor do they all know how to use it.

   THIN Thinking: Nursing Process – *When providing client education, the nurse needs to consider any learning barriers the client may have.* **NCLEX®:** Management of Care **QSEN:** Patient-centered Care

29. The nurse is completing the intake and output record for the client recovering from bariatric surgery. The intake for 12 hours includes: Intravenous fluids infused at 125 mL/hour and oral intake of one ounce clear fluids every hour x 6, followed by 1.5 ounce/hour x 4, followed by 2 ounces per hour x 2. The client urinated two times: 450 mL and 330 mL. How many mL difference is there between intake and output?

Answer: 1200 mL

Rationale: 125 mL/hour x 12 hours = 1500 mL; total oral intake is (6 x 1) + (1.5 x 4) + (2 x 2) = 16 ounces x 30 mL = 480 mL. Total intake = 1980 mL. Output total = 780 mL. Difference = 1200 mL

THIN Thinking: Safety – *Accurate evaluation of intake and output is important to monitoring fluid status.* **NCLEX®:** Basic Care and Comfort **QSEN:** Patient-centered Care

30. The nurse is administering intravenous (IV) fluids to a pediatric client who has experienced third-degree burns. To prevent dehydration, the nurse is to administer 2 mL of lactated ringers IV solution times the body weight in kilograms times the percentage of total body surface area burned (2 mL LR x kg x %TBSA burned). One half of the IV fluids is to be delivered over the first eight hours with the remaining half delivered over the subsequent 16 hours. The client's weight is 55 pounds. Estimated burned body surfaces include 7% of each leg, 9% of the right arm and 6% of the abdomen. How many mL (in whole number) of intravenous fluid should be delivered 14 hours after the fluid resuscitation has begun?

Answer: 45 mL

Rationale:
55 pounds = 25 kg; %TBSA = 7 + 7 + 9 + 6 = 29%
2 mL x 25 kg = 50 x 29% = 1450 mL
1450 mL / 2 = 725 mL over 8 hours followed by 725 mL over 16 hours
725 mL / 16 hours = 45 (45.3) mL

THIN Thinking: Safety – *Accurate calculation of fluid intake if critical to safe client outcomes.* **NCLEX®:** Pharmacological and Parenteral Therapies **QSEN:** Safety

Respiration

Oxygenation / Gas Exchange

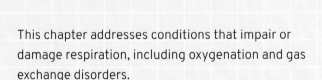

This chapter addresses conditions that impair or damage respiration, including oxygenation and gas exchange disorders.

We have learned the importance of airway patency and breathing in sustaining and living a quality life. Nurses play a significant role in assessing for changes in oxygenation and ventilation, anticipating changes in gas exchange, and providing interventions to enhance or restore respiration.

Next Gen Clinical Judgment

As you have noticed, we give you the numbers 1-3 under NurseThink® Time in all the areas. This is vital in Priority Assessments as NCLEX® really emphasizes Focused Assessment. When helping clients with gas exchange concerns, the nurse must focus. Performing unneeded or nonessential assessments can actually mean a delay in Priority Interventions.

Study Hint: Make sure you are comfortable assessing airway patency, breathing, and adequacy of respirations in clients across the lifespan!

Priority Exemplars:

> Chronic obstructive pulmonary disease
> Cystic Fibrosis
> Chest trauma/Pneumothorax
> Asthma
> Acute respiratory distress syndrome (ARDS)
> Tuberculosis
> Pneumonia
> Bronchiolitis/lower airway infections
> Upper airway infections
> Croup syndromes/epiglottitis
> Pulmonary hypertension
> Iron-deficiency anemia
> Sickle cell anemia (SSA)

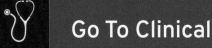
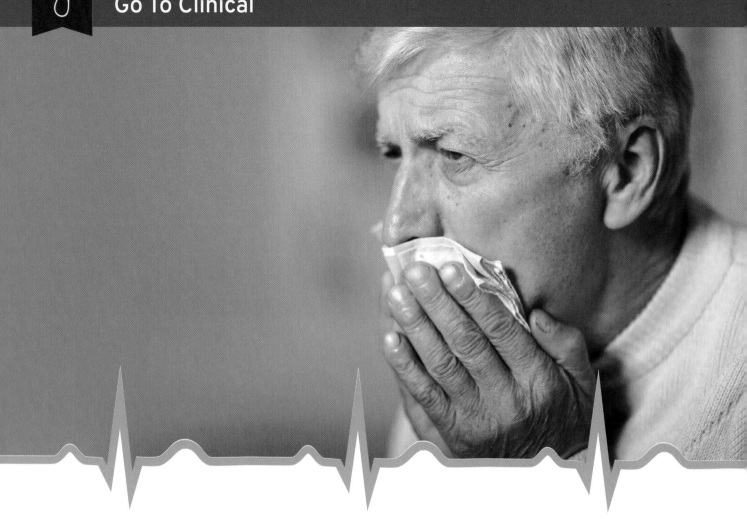

Go To Clinical Case 1

You are caring for D.B., a 64-year-old man with a history of COPD. He enters the pulmonary clinic with a 2-day history of increasing shortness of breath, and his sputum changing from his customary clear-yellow to yellow-green. He denies other symptoms except for fatigue and malaise. He has been smoking for over 30 years and continues to smoke, as does his partner.

He has been using his tiotropium and fluticasone inhalers as prescribed. He is able to speak 6-8 words before needing to take a breath and has dyspnea with exertion. D.B.'s color is pale with mild cyanosis of the lips. D.B.'s pulse oximetry is 88-89% on room air.

The nurse conducts an assessment and finds his temperature is 101°F and his breath sounds are diminished in the bases bilaterally. He reports that the last time he felt this way he was hospitalized and was treated with oral antibiotics and oral prednisone.

NurseThink® Time

Using the NurseThink® system, complete the priorities. Check your answers designated by 💡 in the COPD Priority Exemplar.

Clinical Hint

Differentiate clients with emphysema (Pink Puffers) from chronic bronchitis (Blue Bloaters). Use these descriptors to consider the characteristics of the two!

Priority Assessments or Cues

1.

2.

3.

Priority Laboratory Tests/Diagnostics

1.

2.

3.

Priority Interventions or Actions

1.

2.

3.

Priority Potential & Actual Complications

1.

2.

3.

Priority Nursing Implications

1.

2.

3.

Priority Medications

1.

2.

3.

Priority Education/Discharge Issues

1.

2.

3.

Chronic obstructive pulmonary disease (COPD)

Pathophysiology/Description

> Airway obstruction secondary to emphysema (permanent enlargement of alveoli) or chronic bronchitis (consistent, unrelieved cough) and concurrent inflammatory changes

> Symptoms related to inflammation of central airways/destruction of cilia, remodeling of peripheral airways, destruction of pulmonary parenchyma, and pulmonary vascular changes leading to ineffective gas exchange, mucus hypersecretion, hyperinflation of lungs, loss of recoil, alveolar destruction, and airflow limitation

> Generally associated with cigarette smoking/passive smoking/environmental tobacco smoke. Also related to occupational chemicals/dust, air pollution, and infections

> Genetic components associated with α1-antitrypsin deficiency

> Although symptoms present and increase with aging, it is not known if aging is a risk factor

> COPD may occur with asthma

> An increased number of women are now diagnosed with COPD (increased smoking) and may have poorer outcomes (smaller airways, decreased quality of life)

> COPD is progressive, with constant/non-fluctuating airway resistance, is not usually reversible

Priority Assessments or Cues

> Assess for risk factors including tobacco smoking, occupation, and environmental exposure

> Assess for cough, exertional dyspnea, sputum production, weight loss (monitor weight over time), later-dyspnea at rest

> Assess dyspnea through speech by counting the number of words a client can say between breaths is a measurable demonstration of dyspnea and responses to care

> Auscultate breath sounds for wheezing/crackles, prolonged expiration, decreased breath sounds

> Assess vital signs for tachypnea, cardiac dysrhythmias

> Observe for barrel chest, use of accessory muscles

> Ask about orthopnea, number of pillows used in bed

> Assess for confusion or changes in level of consciousness

> Assess and document characteristics of sputum including amount, color, thickness

> Assess client's ability to cough and expectorate sputum, provide suction as needed

Priority Laboratory Tests/Diagnostics

> Chest X-ray may show congestion and hyperinflation, flattening of diaphragm

> Arterial blood gases for hypoxemia, hypercapnia, and respiratory acidosis

> Pulmonary function tests for forced vital capacity/Forced expiratory volume (FEV_i/FVC) <70% (lower percentages = decreased capacity)

> CBC: Polycythemia

> Sputum culture and sensitivity

Priority Interventions or Actions

> Administer oxygen and titrate with pulse oximetry readings/arterial blood gases. Use caution with oxygen administration and maintain low-flow to preserve hypoxic drive to breathe—may use CPAP or BiPAP

> Place client in sitting position and/or leaning forward—use overbed table or hands to knees (tripod)

> Treatment based on symptoms and severity as in GOLD (Global Initiative for Chronic Obstructive Lung Disease) classification of airway limitation

> Administer breathing treatments and strategies to clear the airway

> Encourage small, frequent meals and hydration to liquefy secretions; encourage high calorie/high-protein diet

> Provide antibiotics in case of infection/pneumonia

> Activity as tolerated and progress as able

> Teach client to employ diaphragmatic or abdominal breathing techniques and pursed-lip breathing to maintain end-expiratory pressure and exhale carbon dioxide

Priority Potential & Actual Complications

> COPD exacerbations with increased severity and frequency

> Creation of bullae (air spaces in the tissue) and blebs (air collection in open spaces)

> Deterioration in lung capacity/pulmonary hypertension and cor pulmonale (Right heart failure)

> Acute respiratory failure

> Depression and anxiety

Priority Nursing Implications

- Be aware of many administration devices including metered dose inhalers, dry powder inhalers, nebulizers, and the use of spacers
- Nurses may work at institutions that use standardized dyspnea and COPD scales
- Assess and use oxygen delivery devices safely. Assess for skin breakdown, airway dryness, client tolerance of device, need for humidity.
- ❯ Medications for COPD are usually increased as the client's symptoms intensify
- ❯ Note that clients with COPD have lower baseline oxygen norms. Oxygen should not be increased above 2 liters/minute to avoid respiratory depression

Priority Medications

- bronchodilators
  - To decrease dyspnea and increase FEV$_1$
  - Via inhaler or nebulizer
  - Adrenergic agonist-albuterol
  - Anticholinergics-ipratropium, tiotropium
  - May be as needed (PRN) or scheduled
- ❯ mucolytics
- corticosteroids
  - Fluticasone with salmeterol
  - Oral steroids only used during exacerbations—prednisone
- antibiotics
  - Recommended if client has dyspnea, has increased sputum volume, or sputum is purulent (or if client is on mechanical ventilation)

Priority Education/Discharge Issues

- Try to avoid others with respiratory infections, crowds during high-risk periods, and ensure immunizations (influenza and pneumococcal vaccine)
- Encourage smoking cessation
- Reinforce safety aspects of oxygen therapy at home including continuous use improves prognosis, risk for combustion, carbon dioxide narcosis, oxygen toxicity, absorption atelectasis, infection, portability, maintaining oxygen supplies, battery backup, delivery mechanisms
- ❯ If dusting, use a wet cloth to avoid free-floating of dust and avoid environmental allergens/triggers such as open flames, feathers, extremes in temperatures, and dust

Go To Clinical Answers

Text designated by ♀ are the top answers for the Go To Clinical related to COPD.

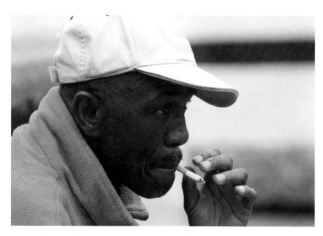

Image 9-1: Review this website https://60plus.smokefree.gov/. Based on the website, write one statement by this client that would indicate an understanding of the website. Then create a statement by the client that would indicate a need for further teaching.

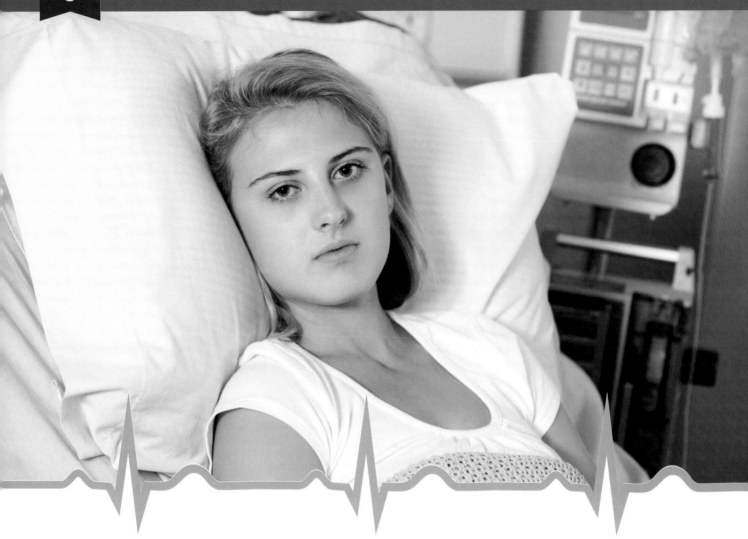

Go To Clinical Case 2

A.P. is a 16-year-old who was diagnosed with cystic fibrosis at 2 years of age. A.P. and her caregivers have successfully managed her disease and symptoms by providing chest physiotherapy (CPT) four times/day, using the percussor vest twice/day, and administering aerosolized dornase alfa and tobramycin.

A.P. takes vitamins A,D,E, & K and pancreatic enzymes.

In the last three months, A.P. has been refusing to take medications and do CPT. A.P. refused to describe her stools to her caregivers and to take pancreatic enzymes. Despite eating adequate amounts of foods, she has demonstrated some weight loss and her menstrual periods are irregular. A.P. shares with you that she is "tired of having cystic fibrosis" and "wants to be like her friends."

NurseThink® Time

Using the NurseThink® system, complete the priorities. Check your answers designated by 💡 in the Cystic fibrosis Priority Exemplar.

Clinical Hint

Cystic fibrosis is a condition where the pathophysiology, signs/symptoms, assessments, and treatments are readily related and evident as one examines client care. This case demonstrates why knowledge of all these elements is critical to provide comprehensive client care!

NurseThink® Time

✏ Priority Assessments or Cues

1.

2.

3.

⚗ Priority Laboratory Tests/Diagnostics

1.

2.

3.

⚠ Priority Interventions or Actions

1.

2.

3.

⚑ Priority Potential & Actual Complications

1.

2.

3.

℧ Priority Nursing Implications

1.

2.

3.

◐ Priority Medications

1.

2.

3.

☺ Priority Education/Discharge Issues

1.

2.

3.

Cystic fibrosis (CF)

Pathophysiology/Description

> Dysfunction of the exocrine (mucus-producing) glands, effects many systems

> Most common lethal genetic disorder of Caucasians

> Inherited as an autosomal recessive trait (if both parents carry trait, each pregnancy as a 1:4 chance of the disease)

> Cystic fibrosis transmembrane regulator (CFTR) reduces cells' transporting of chloride

> Most affected are the lungs with increased thick/tenacious mucus; yielding mucus retention/obstruction, pneumonia, hypoxia, hypercapnia, and acidosis

> Also causes increased electrolytes in the sweat, increased viscosity of the pancreatic mucus-producing glands leading to duct fibrosis and enzymes unable to reach duodenum impairing digestion

> Many males are sterile; females have copious uterine/cervical secretions. Women who conceive are at risk for preterm labor and low-birth-weight infants

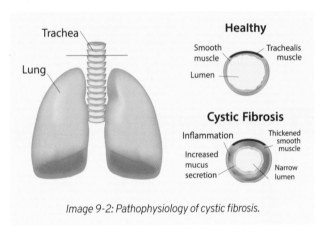

Image 9-2: Pathophysiology of cystic fibrosis.

Priority Assessments or Cues

> Assess pulmonary signs/symptoms including wheezing, dry, non-productive chronic cough, dyspnea, signs of upper and lower airway respiratory infections/involvement, decreased breath sounds over areas of atelectasis

> Assess changes in appearance including barrel chest, clubbing of fingers and toes, cyanosis, lack of weight gain despite adequate intake/growth failure, signs of anemia (pallor, fatigue, shortness of breath, tachycardia)

> Ask about history of meconium ileus, frequent respiratory infections, or dry mouth

> Assess gastrointestinal signs/symptoms such as large/bulky frothy stools containing undigested food, volume of stools increased with solid food, steatorrhea (stools float in toilet) and azotorrhea (foul smelling due to protein)

> Parents may report the child "tastes salty" from elevated sodium in the sweat

Priority Laboratory Tests/Diagnostics

> Positive sweat chloride test (pilocarpine iontophoresis)—requires 75 grams of sweat—normal <40 mEq/L (mean 18 mEq/L); Diagnosed with 2 readings of >60 mEq/L

> Negative pancreatic enzyme assessments

> Chest X-ray for pulmonary changes

> Pulmonary function testing

> Newborn screening is part of newborn panel-nonreactive trypsinogen analysis

> Genetic testing-mutations on CTR/Δ F508 gene (may be done in utero)

> Stool—72-hour samples for fats and enzymes

> Early diagnosis leads to better management

> Screening of parents may be done prenatally or prior to pregnancy

Priority Interventions or Actions

> Early treatment and prophylactic antibiotics

> Ensure airway clearance. Provide chest physiotherapy, percussion and postural drainage, high frequency chest compressions via vests, exercise, positive expiratory therapy (flutter mucus clearance device), huffing/forced expiration, handheld percussors, positive expiratory pressure mask

> Bronchodilators to break down mucus, inhaled powdered mannitol (rehydrate airway), nebulized hypertonic saline (hydrate secretions), aerosolized or intravenous antibiotics

> Long-term NSAIDs treatment (ibuprofen) to prevent inflammation

> Pancreatic enzymes that are titrated to food eaten and a high protein, high calorie, unrestricted fat diet is recommended

Priority Potential & Actual Complications

> Hyponatremia when profusely sweating or during fever

> Chronic respiratory infections (pneumonia)

> Acidosis with hypoxia and hypercapnia

> Pulmonary fibrosis or rupture of blebs causing pneumothorax

> Pulmonary hypertension and/or Cor pulmonale; may indicate need for lung transplantation

> Chronic sinusitis and bone erosion

> Pancreatic fibrosis may lead to type 1 and type 2 diabetes mellitus

> Gastroesophageal reflux

> Prolapsed rectum

> Hypoalbuminemia and generalized edema

- Bleeding related to decreased Vitamin K absorption
- Liver and biliary cirrhosis or meconium ileus equivalent/ distal intestinal obstruction syndrome
- Respiratory failure
- May be fatal

Priority Nursing Implications

- Nurses are an important part of the multidisciplinary management of CF
- The family requires considerable support and assistance; despite many breakthroughs, a diagnosis with cystic fibrosis shortens the life expectancy and presents difficulty during exacerbations
- Clients are prone to infections. Nurses need to assist clients and families in balancing isolation from infectious sources and quality of life
- Nurses should be vigilant for early signs of respiratory infections (fever, tachypnea, increased dyspnea, characteristics of sputum)
- Nurses may provide home care to provide peripherally inserted catheter (PICC) or port medications, teaching, and pulmonary care to prevent hospitalization and exposure to pathogens
- Clients are hypercapnic, therefore, oxygen must be administered carefully to prevent extinguishing the hypoxic drive to breath
- Children with CF metabolize medications differently and may need higher doses
- Pancreatic enzymes are enteric coated to be functional in the intestines. Do not crush or chew but capsule beads may be "sprinkled" over food. Enzymes may be inactivated in hot food

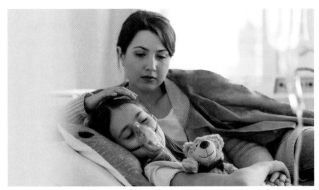

Image 9-3: The mother of a child with cystic fibrosis asks which parent gave the disease to her daughter. What is the nurse's best response?

Priority Medications

- ibuprofen
  - Antiinflammatory
  - Assess for GI erosion or bleeding
  - Monitor serum levels- maintain a blood level of 50-1000 mcg/mL

- dornase alfa
  - Antibiotic
  - Decreases viscosity of the secretions
  - Given via nebulizer
- tobramycin
  - Antibiotic
  - Given via nebulizer
  - Prevent infections
- Systemic antibiotics
  - Prevent or treat pulmonary infections
  - Nebulized or given IV via peripherally inserted central catheter (PICC) or port
- Water miscible solutions of vitamins A,D,E, & K

Priority Education/Discharge Issues

- Parents and caregivers must consider the developmental age of the child—the regimen is rigorous and children/teens may not always adhere to procedures
- Nurses are often a key component of transitioning the child with cystic fibrosis to adult services, healthcare professionals, and support groups
- Family must learn to provide pulmonary/airway clearance care at least twice/day, often 4-6 times/day
- Nurses may offer resources to the teen/young adult with cystic fibrosis to become independent with personal healthcare. The regimen for cystic fibrosis is very rigorous and clients must learn to devote a significant amount of time and energy to staying healthy
- Teach client/family how to titrate pancreatic enzymes to achieve the optimal number of stools per day and for optimal growth; reinforce the importance of a high calorie/well-balanced diet
- Teach nasal lavage to prevent/treat chronic sinusitis
- Assist client to establish an exercise program that is both fun and effective in mobilizing respiratory secretions
- Instruct parents on monitoring child for growth and achieving developmental milestones
- Reinforce the need for routine immunizations and the annual influenza vaccination
- Inform parents about community and national resources to assist in coping with this diagnosis

Go To Clinical Answers

Text designated by 💡 are the top answers for the Go To Clinical related to Cystic Fibrosis.

Chest trauma/pneumothorax

Pathophysiology/Description

> Chest trauma may be related to motor vehicle or other accidents, abuse/violence, falls, gun shot injuries, and other etiologies

> Blunt trauma (struck by an object-may include laceration of lung/cardiac tissues, compression of chest, or contralateral injuries) or penetrating trauma (open wound injuries)

> Issues include rib fracture, flail chest, pulmonary contusions, and pneumothorax; some clients may need ventilatory support related to respiratory failure

> Pneumothorax occurs when the negative pressure inside the pleural space is lost and the lung collapses

> Pneumothorax may be spontaneous (from the rupture of an emphysematous or other bleb), iatrogenic (puncture from a medical procedure or ventilator), open/traumatic (from an opening or wound in the chest wall), or tension (when there is too much positive pressure in the pleural space related to a chest injury or mechanical ventilation)

> Hemothorax is blood in pleural space. Chylothorax is lymph fluid in pleural space

Priority Assessments or Cues

> Assess for history of an injury, ventilator support, or other risk factors

> Assess respiratory status: Absent breath sounds on the affected side, cyanosis, decreased chest expansion on affected side, increased work of breathing, hypotension, tracheal deviation, tachycardia, tachypnea, sucking sound with a chest wound, subcutaneous emphysema

> Assess subjective findings: Severe chest pain, dyspnea, local pain

> Assess for bruising, abrasions, open wound

Priority Laboratory Tests/Diagnostics

> Chest X-ray to confirm pneumothorax

> Arterial blood gases to assess oxygenation/ventilation status

> Thoracentesis to confirm hemothorax

Priority Interventions or Actions

> Sit client up, apply an occlusive dressing to open wound, and apply oxygen

> Prepare client and care for client with chest tube

> Stabilize flail chest with hand and then tape

> Tension pneumothorax may require needle decompression/thoracentesis prior to or instead of chest tube drainage

> IV access and fluid resuscitation/infusion of maintenance fluids

> Medicate for pain as indicated to enhance ventilation and comfort

Priority Potential & Actual Complications

> Rib fractures are characterized by pain and impaired respirations

> Flail chest may be associated with blunt chest trauma, hemothorax, and fractured ribs-chest segment becomes paradoxical to rest of chest, leading to paradoxical respirations, dyspnea, cyanosis, severe pain, tachycardia, hypotension, and decreased breath sounds

> Acute respiratory failure and mechanical ventilation

> If open wound is covered, client may experience a tension pneumothorax

> Subcutaneous emphysema is air leaking into tissue around chest tube or wound site

> Cardiac tamponade is blood in pericardial sac compresses heart and prevents ventricular filling

Priority Nursing Implications

> Consider the fear, anxiety, and apprehension in a client suffering from chest trauma/pneumothorax and provide sensitive and caring support

> Chest tubes designed to drain and re-establish negative pressure in the pleural space

> During chest tube insertion, nurses need to teach client about the procedure as time will allow, assemble equipment, pre-medicate or sedate as able, position the client, and stay at the bedside to provide comfort and assistance as needed, along with monitoring client status

> Smaller wounds or those with less drainage may be relieved by a chest tube connected to a Heimlich/flutter valve and drainage system

> Pleural drainage systems include a drainage chamber, a water-seal chamber, and a suction chamber. The drainage chamber collects air and drainage. The water-seal fluctuates with respiration (tidaling), while the slow rolling bubbles in the suction chamber indicate suction is on. The amount of suction is regulated by the level of water-seal, not the amount of bubbling in the suction chamber

> Clamping of a chest tube is not recommended—if disconnected, place end of tube in water. Some practitioners clamp a chest tube before it is removed to assess client readiness, or clamp the tube intermittently during hospitalization, but practices differ

Priority Medications

> Comfort and sedation medications as indicated

Priority Education/Discharge Issues

> Clients may go home on flutter valve systems. Client teaching is indicated

> Teach clients about injury prevention and safety

> After a pneumothorax, educate clients about potential complications and respiratory symptoms that need to be reported to a healthcare provider

Asthma

Pathophysiology/Description

> Allergen/antigen mediated response creates a hypersensitive reaction
> Results in decreased airflow due to inflammation, bronchoconstriction, hyperresponsiveness, airway obstruction, airway edema, and mucus production and/or stasis
> Types include exercise-induced, allergic, infantile as manifested by eczema, food intolerance, allergic rhinitis
> Known as a chronic disease with acute exacerbations, classified based on severity of symptoms: Severe persistent, moderate persistent, mild persistent, and intermittent
> Increased risk factors include exposure/responses to allergens (atopy), hereditary factors; exposure to smoking or maternal smoking during pregnancy, low birth weight (LBW), and obesity, increased severity at night and early morning

Priority Assessments or Cues

> Monitor vital signs and oxygen saturation
> Respiratory effort including increased work of breathing, non- or productive cough, forced expiration, retractions, nasal flaring
> Breath sounds may include a wheeze, coarse breath sounds, prolonged expiration, decreased breath sounds (lack of air movement-ominous sign), client may speak in short/broken sentences
> Subjective data may include tightness of chest, chest pain, itching around neck, headache, fatigue, coughing at night without other respiratory symptoms
> Assess for changes in appearance such as restlessness, air hunger, tripod positioning, pursed lips, irritability, apprehension, cyanosis

Priority Laboratory Tests/Diagnostics

> Chest X-ray for infiltrates and hyperexpansion/pneumonia
> Pulmonary function tests/spirometry-presence and degree of pulmonary involvement/evaluate response to treatment
> Bronchoprovocation testing-exposure to antigens/skin testing
> Peak expiratory flow rate-peak flow meter-establish personal best and compare to peak flow at times of respiratory distress
> White blood cell count to determine infection
> Arterial blood gases for hypercapnia and respiratory acidosis

Priority Interventions or Actions

> Position client to aid in breathing-tripod or sitting with head forward, 100% oxygen therapy unless contraindicated
> Identify and alleviate triggers—environmental and lifestyle control; use of air conditioners/filters and dehumidifiers
> Medications—a combination of preventer/long-term and rescue/quick relief agents
> IV access during acute attack
> Have intubation equipment available and assess for "silent chest" or lack of air movement

Priority Potential & Actual Complications

> In children, higher incidence in boys than girls but hospitalization and death rate higher in girls
> Airway remodeling/damage to structure that is nonresponsive to anti-inflammatory and other treatments
> Hypoxemia, respiratory acidosis, respiratory failure

Priority Nursing Implications

> Teach about use of metered-dose inhalers, dry powder inhalers, spacers, nebulizers, abdominal breathing, and pursed-lip breathing
> Instruct clients about environmental and trigger control
> Teach clients benefits of breathing exercises and physical exercises as ways to enhance conditioning
> Assess for status asthmaticus-medical emergency or deterioration of status requiring oxygen and ventilatory support

Priority Medications

> Rescue/quick-relief medications
  • Short-acting beta-agonists—albuterol (caution with heart disease-tachycardia)
  • Anticholinergics-ipratropium
  • Systemic steroids-methylprednisolone
> Maintenance/long-term control medications
  • Inhaled steroids/encourage mouth care after use
  • Cromolyn and nedocromil-maintenance therapy-via nebulizer and metered-dose inhaler
  • Long-acting beta-agonists—salmeterol
  • Methylxanthines-theophylline (only when not responsive to other treatments)
  • Leukotriene modifiers
> omalizumab-monoclonal antibodies for use in clients resistant to inhaled corticosteroids

Priority Education/Discharge Issues

> Teach to avoid personal triggers such as animal dander, pollen, mold, food additives/foods, strong emotions, cold air, exercise, aspirin, upper respiratory infection (URI), exposure to cold environmental temperatures, endocrine factors, dust, cockroach antigen/feces
> Instruct clients to avoid overuse of short-acting beta-agonists to avoid rebound bronchospasm or lack of effective bronchodilation during an attack
> Encourage hydration to liquefy secretions
> Teach clients at their developmental capacity to understand treatments and care
> Ensure that clients have an asthma action plan-monitor for symptoms, assessing peak flow readings, and action steps
> Instruct clients on their personal early symptoms of asthma and to intervene or seek emergency help early

Acute respiratory distress syndrome (ARDS)

📋 Pathophysiology/Description

> Sudden and advanced progression of acute respiratory failure with large variability of impact and symptoms

> Characterized by hypoxemia, dyspnea, and decreased lung compliance despite increases in oxygen delivery

> Inflammatory response causing neutrophil collection, increased pulmonary capillary membrane permeability, vasoconstriction, decreased collagen, and microemboli

> Exists in 3 phases including injury/exudative (days 1-7, alveolar edema and atelectasis), reparative/proliferative (weeks 1-2, increased inflammation and fibrosis), and fibrotic (weeks 2-3, scarring, fibrosis, and decreased compliance)

> Related to systemic inflammatory response syndrome (SIRS), may be infectious or non-infectious and associated with multiorgan dysfunction syndrome (MODS)

✏️ Priority Assessments or Cues

> Assess for risk factors such as aspiration, viral /bacterial pneumonia, sepsis, trauma/injury, near-drowning, embolism

> Assess breath sounds which may be normal or include fine crackles to diffuse crackles and rhonchi

> Assess for symptoms of phase 1 including dyspnea, tachypnea, cyanosis, pallor, cough, retractions, and increased work of breathing

> Assess for symptoms of phase 2 including the above and increasing hypoxemia, restlessness, and tachycardia

> Assess for symptoms of phase 3 including the above, marked hypoxia, and signs of pulmonary hypertension

🧪 Priority Laboratory Tests/Diagnostics

> ABGs show hypoxia, hypoxemia, and hypercarbia (indicate fatigue and respiratory failure), respiratory alkalosis due to tachypnea and exhalation of CO_2

> CXR showing scattered infiltrates, edema of alveoli and interstitial tissues

> Pulmonary function tests showing decreased tidal volume, compliance, and functional residual capacity

> Measured via PaO_2/FIO_2 ratio (normal PaO_2 is 85-100 mmHg at 0.21 % O_2-room air = >400). Acute lung injury ratio is 200-300. ARDS ratio is <200

> Pulmonary wedge pressure < 18 mmHg

⚠️ Priority Interventions or Actions

> Identify and treat underlying cause

> Oxygen via mask, cannula, or endotracheal tube/positive pressure ventilation with positive end-expiratory pressure (PEEP)

> Check oxygen saturation frequently and keep oxygen at lowest concentration to maintain PaO_2 > 60 mmHg

> Nutrition and hydration, may include parenteral and enteral routes

> Continuous lateral rotation therapy/turning and prone positioning

> Sedation as indicated

> ECMO (extracorporeal membrane oxygenation)

🚩 Priority Potential & Actual Complications

> Sepsis/infections

> Stress ulcers

> Dysrhythmias and decreased cardiac output

> Pulmonary barotrauma

> Delirium

> Tracheomalacia or tracheal stenosis/ulceration

> MODS

> Ventilator-associated pneumonia (VAP)

> Oxygen toxicity

> May be fatal (50% mortality rate)

♻ Priority Nursing Implications

> VAP prevention to include sterile technique with suctioning, handwashing, and oral care

> Ventilator bundle to include elevate HOB 30-45 degrees, sedation holidays to assess for potential extubation, ulcer disease protocol, venous thrombosis prevention, and oral care daily with chlorhexidine

> Reduce barotrauma with lowest effective ventilator pressures

💧 Priority Medications

> dopamine/dobutamine/norepinephrine
  - Used to increase and maintain blood pressure/organ perfusion in critically ill clients
  - Carefully titrated via intravenous route and infusion pump

> furosemide
  - To decrease pulmonary hypertension and edema

👤 Priority Education/Discharge Issues

> Support client during this frightening experience, anxiety may increase oxygen hunger and physiological stress/symptoms

> Provide family education and support during this critical period by educating on disease, potential course, equipment, and treatments

> Refer to spiritual and emotional support systems

Tuberculosis

Pathophysiology/Description

> Tuberculosis (TB) caused by *Mycobacterium tuberculosis*

> Leading cause of death in world, high co-morbidity with HIV

> Previously eradicated in the US, increase in prevalence related to increased immunosuppressed populations, migration, and among those living in poverty

> Spread via airborne droplets, requires close, frequent exposure or decreased immunocompetence in recipient to be contracted

> May be primary, latent (asymptomatic/can't transmit), or reactivated; may be pulmonary or extrapulmonary

Priority Assessments or Cues

> Assess risk factors related to social and occupational history/social determinants

> Assess for dry cough, fatigue, malaise, anorexia, weight loss, low-grade fevers, and night sweats

> Later in disease, assess for dyspnea, hemoptysis, high fever, chills, flu-like symptoms, pleuritic pain, productive cough, decreased breath sounds, and afternoon temperature elevation

> In older adults, early symptoms may relate to changes in cognitive function

> With extrapulmonary forms, assess for dysuria/hematuria (renal), headache, vomiting, lymphadenopathy (tuberculin meningitis) or pain and decreased range of motion (bone and joint involvement)

Priority Laboratory Tests/Diagnostics

> Tuberculin skin test as purified protein derivative (PPD), site assessed 48 to 72 hours after injection for induration. A positive test indicates exposure to TB

> Interferon release assays

> CXR for infiltrates

> Bacteriostatic studies including sputum for acid-fast bacillus. Three consecutive morning specimens recommended for disease confirmation

Priority Interventions or Actions

> Outpatient management optimal

> Long-term antimicrobials; multidrug therapy has changed the way disease is managed and increased prognosis; several first and second line regimens available

> Follow-up CXRs and bacterial studies

> Latent TB is treated for 6-9 months with isoniazid (INH)

Priority Potential & Actual Complications

> Pulmonary scarring/pulmonary effusions/pneumonia/decreased pulmonary function

> Miliary TB with systemic spread

> Extrapulmonary may include peritonitis, meningitis, and vertebral degeneration

> May be fatal

Priority Nursing Implications

> Initiate and maintain airborne isolation including negative pressure room and high efficiency particulate air masks (HEPA)

> Considered infectious for 2 weeks after initiation of medication therapy

> Reinforce importance with long-term/complex drug therapy to ensure eradication of disease. May initiate direct observing taking medication practices (DOT)

> BCG vaccine recommended for those who are continuously exposed to TB including healthcare workers

> TB is a reportable disease and should involve local public health departments

Priority Medications

> isoniazid (INH)
> - No alcohol with medication, may increase hepatotoxicity
> - Periodic assessment of liver function

> rifampin
> - Causes orange discoloration of body fluids
> - Assess for thrombocytopenia and/or hepatitis
> - Not with liver disease or during pregnancy

> pyrazinamide
> - May enhance uric acid buildup and symptoms of gout
> - Hepatotoxic
> - May cause arthralgia

> ethambutol
> - May decrease visual acuity and require frequent monitoring
> - May inhibit green red color differentiation

Priority Education/Discharge Issues

> Teach clients the importance of adherence to medication regimen and the reasons for treatment plans to prevent drug resistance and reactivation

> Screen contacts and assess need for treatment

> While at home encourage client to sleep alone, spend time outside, encourage adequate ventilation of living spaces, and hygiene with tissues, bed linens, and strict handwashing

> Teach clients symptoms of relapse and the potential for smoking to foster relapse (encourage smoking cessation)

Pneumonia

Pathophysiology/Description

> Infection of the lung parenchyma (bacterial, viral, or mycoplasma)

> Community-acquired pneumonia (CAP) is the leading cause of death in individuals 65 years and older

> Incompetent defense mechanism (air filtration, epiglottis, cough reflex, bronchoconstriction, or the mucociliary escalator mechanism) or virulent causative factors lead to pneumonia

> Three causative mechanisms include aspiration, inhalation, or hematogenous spread from other locations in the body

> Types include community-acquired pneumonia, medical care associated pneumonia (MCAP), healthcare-associated pneumonia (HCAP), hospital-acquired pneumonia (HAP), and ventilator-associated pneumonia (VAP)

Priority Assessments or Cues

> Assess for causative factors, including exposure to air pollution, cigarette smoking, upper respiratory infections, age (> 65 years), abdominal/chest surgery, altered levels of consciousness, immobility, chronic illness, inhalation injuries, immunosuppression, smoking, malnutrition, residence in long-term care, and endotracheal intubation

> Assess for risk factors for aspiration pneumonia, including decreased level of consciousness, dysphagia, nasogastric intubation, or decreased gag or cough

> Assess for risk of opportunistic pneumonia including immunosuppression, malnutrition, or history of radiation and chemotherapy

> Assess for common symptoms including non-productive cough, chills, dyspnea, fever, tachypnea, pleuritic chest pain, green/yellow/rust sputum, fatigue, diaphoresis, anorexia, headache, and abdominal pain

> In older adults, initial and progressive symptoms may include decreased level of consciousness, confusion, and hypothermia

> Assess breath sounds for rhonchi, crackles, decreased breath sounds, and increased fremitus

Priority Laboratory Tests/Diagnostics

> Chest X-ray may show consolidation, infiltrates, and effusions

> Thoracentesis and bronchoscopy may be done if infection is refractory to other treatments

> Sputum specimen

> Blood cultures

> Arterial blood cultures demonstrate hypoxia, hypercapnia, and acidosis

> Elevated white blood cell count (> 15,000/microliter)

> C-reactive protein levels may assist with antibiotic choice/sensitivity

Priority Interventions or Actions

> Oxygen therapy

> Antibiotics

> Analgesics for chest pain

> Antipyretics

> Rest and activity as tolerated

> Adequate hydration and nutrition

Priority Potential & Actual Complications

> Pleurisy, pleural effusion, empyema, pneumothorax

> Atelectasis, lung abscess

> Bacteremia and sepsis

> Pericarditis

> Meningitis

> Acute respiratory failure

Priority Nursing Implications

> Do not delay use of antibiotics for culture results

> Implement preventative practices such as activity/ambulation, checking nasogastric tube placement, aspiration precautions, oral care, coughing and deep breathing, turning, incentive spirometry, tracheostomy care

Priority Medications

> levofloxacin
  • For clients with CAP with other health issues
  • For clients with HCAP/MCAP

> erythromycin
  • For clients with CAP in otherwise healthy individuals

Priority Education/Discharge Issues

> Avoid cigarette smoking

> Encourage the pneumococcal vaccine for at-risk individuals and older adults

> Encourage adequate nutrition, hydration, mobility, and effective coughing in immobile, postoperative, and at-risk clients

Next Gen Clinical Judgment

List 3 things a nurse can do to prevent hospital-acquired Pneumonia.

_____

_____

_____

Bronchiolitis/lower airway infections

📋 Pathophysiology/Description

> Inflammation of the bronchioles producing copious, thick mucus

> Most frequent origin is respiratory syncytial virus (RSV) which is highly virulent and communicable via contact with respiratory secretions

> Most often contracted in winter and spring

> Rare in children over 2 years of age, peak incidence at 6 months and in children at risk across childhood (risk associated with prematurity, congenital heart disease, chronic respiratory disorders, bronchopulmonary dysplasia, or immunosuppression)

> Most common cause for hospitalization of infants less than one year of age

> See also Pneumonia Priority exemplar

✏️ Priority Assessments or Cues

> Assess for early symptoms including nasal, eye, and ear drainage, copious nasal secretions, nasal crusting, pharyngitis, dry cough, sneezing, wheezing, fever, poor oral intake, and irritability

> Assess for symptoms as disease progresses including air hunger, tachypnea, retractions, crackles in the lung fields, and cyanosis

> Assess for severe disease including a respiratory rate over 70 breaths/minute, decreased breath sounds and air movement, apneic periods, significant restlessness

🧪 Priority Laboratory Tests/Diagnostics

> Culture of nasal or nasopharyngeal (NP) secretions

> Pulse oximetry to assess oxygen saturation

> Rapid immunofluorescent antibody/direct fluorescent antibody staining

⚠️ Priority Interventions or Actions

> Cool humidified oxygen

> Hydration

> Elevate head of bed

> Attempt small frequent feedings to encourage oral intake

> Suction as needed using bulb or nasopharyngeal suctioning

> Nasogastric hydration or feedings as indicated

> May require ventilatory support

🚩 Priority Potential & Actual Complications

> Pneumonia

> Respiratory failure from fatigue

> Electrolyte imbalance

> Apnea/respiratory arrest

♻ Priority Nursing Implications

> Contact (gown/gloves) and/or droplet (gown/gloves/mask) isolation practices

> Ensure a private room or cohort with other children with RSV

> Do not assign nurses to clients with RSV with other clients at risk/who are immunosuppressed

> Encourage mothers who breastfeed to pump and preserve milk if infants taking no or low oral intake

💧 Priority Medications

> palivizumab

  • Monoclonal antibody therapy

  • Prevention of RSV in high-risk groups (including preterm children born earlier than 32 weeks gestation)

  • IM injection monthly for 5 months from November to March

  • Also available IV

> ribavirin

  • Inhaled antiviral agent

  • Decreases duration and severity of viral infection

  • Potential toxic effects to exposed healthcare workers

👤 Priority Education/Discharge Issues

> Encourage breastfeeding to increase immune function

> Encourage strict handwashing

> Reinforce the need for prevention of exposure to secondhand smoke

> Teach family to instill normal saline solution nose drops before meals and at bedtime to encourage sleep and oral intake

> Encourage limiting exposure of affected clients to others who are at risk/may contract RSV

Upper airway infections

Pathophysiology/Description

> Tonsillitis is inflammation of the tonsils/lymph tissue in the pharynx

> Adenoiditis is inflammation in the glands in the posterior pharynx

> Viral nasopharyngitis (NP) is often referred to as a "URI" or the "common cold"

> Acute streptococcal pharyngitis due to Group A beta-hemolytic streptococcus (GABHS) may lead to an acute or chronic issue in clients

> Tracheobronchitis is a mild viral infection that often occurs with a "URI"

Priority Assessments or Cues

> Upper airway infections often characterized by a dry, hacking, non-productive cough which may be worse at night, rhinorrhea, chills, poor oral intake, open-mouth breathing, lethargy, nausea/vomiting, fever, and malaise

> Assess for tonsillitis including sore throat, dysphagia, fever, mouth breathing, malodorous breath, and cough

> Assess for adenoiditis including nasal speech, snoring, sleep apnea, hearing difficulties, and mouth breathing

Priority Laboratory Tests/Diagnostics

> Diagnosis based on symptoms

> GABHS throat culture/rapid antigen testing

Priority Interventions or Actions

> Mild infections treated with cool, humidified air, increasing hydration, allowing rest, and antipyretics. These infections usually resolve in 4 to 10 days

> Warm salt-water gargles may relieve symptoms

> Bacterial infections treated symptomatically and with antibiotics

> Chronic tonsillitis/adenoiditis may indicate surgical removal of tonsils and adenoids

Priority Potential & Actual Complications

> With untreated GABHS, complications include acute glomerulonephritis, scarlet fever, rheumatic fever, and cardiac valve damage/rheumatic heart disease

Priority Nursing Implications

> For clients with URI, antitussives are only recommended in select situations. They may suppress the natural cough mechanism, are to be used only with a dry cough that disrupts sleep or is annoying. Instead, expectorants are encouraged to mobilize secretions

> Nursing care for clients having tonsillectomy/adenoidectomy (T & A) may include

- Providing developmentally appropriate preoperative teaching, assessing for bleeding disorders, and assessing for infection

- Postoperative care includes analgesics, use of an ice collar as tolerated, and assessing for post-op bleeding/hemorrhage (bloody drool, frequent swallowing, pallor, or restlessness), discourage coughing/clearing throat/nose-blowing which may cause bleeding.

- Encourage client to lay on side to allow for drainage of secretions. Have suction available for emergencies

- Postoperative fluids should be clear, non-citrus, and non-carbonated. Do not use red or brown fluids which may be mistaken for blood. Avoid milk or thick fluids that may cause clearing of the throat

- Advance to a soft diet as tolerated, avoiding irritating foods

Priority Medications

> Analgesia after T & A
- morphine
  - Intravenous narcotic for severe pain
  - Watch for respiratory depression
- acetaminophen with codeine
  - For moderate postoperative pain
  - Need to eat crackers or small snack to avoid nausea/vomiting
  - May cause constipation

> Nasopharyngitis/viral/URI
- acetaminophen
  - Antipyretic
  - May be used for mild pain
- Decongestants
  - Nasal more effective than systemic
  - Not with children less than 6 years of age
  - 2 drops per nares, wait 10 minutes, repeat
  - Use for less than 3 days to prevent rebound congestion

> GABHS
- amoxicillin via oral route
- PCN G via intramuscular route
  - Used when adherence is difficult
  - May include procaine to decrease pain of injection

Priority Education/Discharge Issues

> Teach family how to make saline/salt solution for home use

> Teach family about postoperative medication and feeding of clients after a T&A including the potential for the scab to slough up to 10 days postoperatively and to observe for bleeding, to avoid sharp objects in mouth, and assess for fever

> After GABHS, get a new toothbrush 24 hours after beginning antibiotics

> Avoid spread of infections through handwashing, staying away from crowds, safe tissue handling, fluids, and rest

Croup syndromes/epiglottitis

Pathophysiology/Description

> Laryngitis is a common viral syndrome, often associated with the "common cold"

> Laryngotracheobronchitis (LTB) is the most common type of croup; most often associated with children < 5 years, may be bacterial or viral

> Epiglottitis is a bacterial form of croup, characterized by inflammation of the epiglottis and has a rapid onset
   - H. Flu immunizations (H. Influenzae type B-HIB) have decreased incidence
   - Most often in children 2-8 years but may be at any age
   - Medical emergency as may progress quickly to respiratory distress and edema of epiglottis may cause total airway obstruction

Priority Assessments or Cues

> Assess for laryngitis including headache, malaise, nasal congestion, and hoarseness

> Assess for LTB including low-grade temperature, brassy/barky cough, inspiratory stridor, retractions, cough, hoarseness, tachypnea, and restlessness. May progress to stridor, retractions, hypoxia/hypercapnia, cyanosis, and apnea

> Assess for epiglottitis including fever, drooling, pain with swallowing, dysphagia, dyspnea, restlessness, tachycardia, tachypnea, increased work of breathing, retractions, nasal flaring, and inspiratory stridor

> Assess client's position of choice/comfort. Client may tripod body position to breathe

> Assess for progression to respiratory distress

> Assess level of consciousness

Priority Laboratory Tests/Diagnostics

> Treatment often based on symptoms

> For epiglottitis, neck X-rays may be done to confirm diagnosis

> ABGs to assess for hypercapnia, hypoxia, and respiratory acidosis

> Pulse oximetry for oxygen saturation

Priority Interventions or Actions

> For laryngitis, treatment is symptomatic

> For LTB with mild croup/no stridor at rest, management may be at home using cool mist vaporizers. Counsel family to expose to cool air with respiratory distress (take child to basement, garage, open freezer door, go outside, cool shower). Encourage rest, oral hydration, elevate head of bed, analgesics, and antibiotics (if bacterial). Hospitalization indicated for increased respiratory distress or poor hydration status

> For epiglottitis
   - No oral temperatures, manipulation of mouth/visualization/no tongue depressors
   - Keep client calm/with caregivers, sitting up, in position of comfort, do not restrain
   - Cool mist oxygen therapy with least invasive method (blow-by mask held by family member)
   - Keep NPO
   - Determine ability to attain IV access, defer to airway management if child becomes upset. IV hydration and antibiotics if able
   - Analgesics and antipyretics
   - May require nasotracheal intubation/tracheostomy

Priority Potential & Actual Complications

> Airway occlusion and lack of access to airway (epiglottitis)

> Respiratory failure

> Respiratory arrest

Priority Nursing Implications

> Advocate for family participation in care to keep child calm. Allow child to sit in caregiver's lap for all care and provide age-appropriate distraction/teaching as indicated

> For epiglottitis, follow agency protocol for resuscitation equipment availability/transfer of client to the operating room for all assessments/care due to potential need for surgical intervention/tracheostomy

> Croup may require droplet isolation as a precaution in hospital until organism is specified or on antibiotics for 24 hours

> May use Heliox (helium/oxygen) to decrease edema and work of breathing

Priority Medications

> methylprednisolone
   - IV steroid
   - Decreases airway inflammation in epiglottitis

> dexamethasone
   - Oral steroids
   - Single dose for inflammation of LTB

> epinephrine
   - Nebulized, racemic
   - Reduces airway edema

Priority Education/Discharge Issues

> Teach family about emergency procedures related to epiglottitis and provide support in efforts to keep child calm and resting during respiratory distress. Teach about comfort measures and the importance of cuddling

> Teach family to avoid antitussives which depress the cough reflex

> For other croup syndromes, teach family about signs of deteriorating respiratory status

> Encourage HIB vaccine

> May provide prophylactic antibiotics for family/contacts depending upon infectious organism

Pulmonary hypertension

📋 Pathophysiology/Description

> Elevated pulmonary artery pressure resulting in resistance to blood flow in the pulmonary circulation (normally low pressure/resistance)

> An insult (hormonal, mechanical, or other) leads to pulmonary endothelial injury (smooth muscle proliferation, vascular scarring) causing pulmonary hypertension

> May be idiopathic (primary) or secondary to other disorders such as heart failure or congenital heart defects

> Secondary often due to COPD with constriction of the pulmonary vessels secondary to hypoxia and acidosis

> Cor pulmonale is enlarged right ventricle secondary to pulmonary hypertension (usually related to COPD)

✏️ Priority Assessments or Cues

> Assess for dyspnea on exertion, shortness of breath, fatigue, exertional chest pain, dizziness, or exertional syncope

> May progress to dyspnea at rest or with feeding/eating

> May occur with early heart failure symptoms including peripheral edema, dyspnea, fatigue, increased pulmonic heart sounds, fourth heart sound, hepatomegaly, distended neck veins and full, bounding pulse

> Pulse oximetry

🧪 Priority Laboratory Tests/Diagnostics

> Right-sided cardiac catheterization
> Chest X-ray
> ECG
> CT scans
> Pulmonary function tests
> CBC to assess for polycythemia secondary to chronic hypoxemia
> ABGs to assess for hypoxemia

⚠️ Priority Interventions or Actions

> In secondary pulmonary hypertension, treatment is most focused on management of the underlying disorder

> Low flow oxygen to keep saturations above 90%. O_2 may be long-term to correct hypoxemia

> Surgical intervention includes atrial septostomy, pulmonary thromboendarterectomy, or heart transplant

> Medications may include diuretics (reduce edema), anticoagulants (reduce production of thrombi), vasodilators (decrease pressure in vessels)

> Low sodium diet if Cor pulmonale or heart failure develops

> Clients with pulmonary hypertension may be candidates for lung transplantation

🚩 Priority Potential & Actual Complications

> Right ventricular hypertrophy/cor pulmonale

> Right-sided heart failure

> May be fatal

⚕️ Priority Nursing Implications

> Early intervention enhances effectiveness of treatment

> Many clients sustain significant damage prior to diagnosis

> Implement fall and safety precautions while on vasodilators and assess BP frequently

🩸 Priority Medications

> calcium channel blockers-diltiazem
  • Vasodilates to reduce pressure in the pulmonary artery and on the right ventricle
  • Should not be used with right-sided heart failure

> sildenafil
  • Smooth muscle relaxation
  • Not with nitroglycerine—may cause hypotension

> prostacyclins
  • Dilate pulmonary and systemic vessels
  • iloprost-inhaled
  • epoprostenol-intravenous
  • May cause hypotension

> bosentan
  • Endothelin receptor antagonist
  • Decreases pulmonary artery pressure
  • Monitor liver function

👤 Priority Education/Discharge Issues

> Teach client safe administration of medications and need to move/rise slowly after administration

> Instruct clients on portable oxygen devices and safety parameters around oxygen

> Ensure that clients and family understand the roles of diet, activity, and lifestyles in heart health and optimal respiratory function

_____

_____

_____

Iron-deficiency anemia

Pathophysiology/Description

> Most common hematologic disorder, affects 2-5% of adult men and post-menopausal women, may be higher among very young clients and women in the reproductive years (menstruating, pregnant)

> Causes include inadequate dietary intake, blood loss, hemolysis, malabsorption, and nutritional deficiencies associated with alcoholism

Priority Assessments or Cues

> Assess risk in pregnant and menstruating women, those with malabsorption (gastric bypass and removal), chronic blood loss (gastric bleed secondary to peptic ulcer, gastritis, hemorrhoids, and diverticulitis), chronic kidney disease (dialysis, frequent blood draws, or erythropoietin deficiencies)

> Assess for pallor, glossitis, cheilitis, headache, paresthesias, burning of tongue, fatigue, tachycardia (if severe)

Priority Laboratory Tests/Diagnostics

> Hemoglobin and hematocrit

> Red blood cells and reticulocytes

> Serum iron, ferritin, and transferrin levels

> Total iron-binding capacity (TIBC)

> Stool for occult blood (assess for blood loss)

Priority Interventions or Actions

> Identify and treat underlying cause (malnutrition, blood loss, etc.)

> Nutritional therapy with foods high in iron

> Blood transfusions with severe deficiency symptoms

> Oral and parenteral iron supplements

> Ongoing reassessment of iron and red blood cell levels

Priority Potential & Actual Complications

> Complications from unexplained blood loss

> Prolonged, untreated anemia may lead to myocardial infarction and heart failure

Priority Nursing Implications

> Counsel clients and assess clients for constipation. Encourage clients to exercise, drink adequate fluids, eat high fiber diets, and take stool softeners as needed

> Encourage clients to take iron one hour before meals and with a vitamin C source (orange juice)

> If ingestion causes gastric upset, take with meals (but decreases absorption)

> Foods high in iron include liver and muscle meats, dried fruits, eggs, legumes, dark green leafy vegetables, whole grain breads, and potatoes

> Assess clients skin color and mucous membranes with attention to baseline skin color and changes associated with iron-deficiency

Priority Medications

> ferrous sulfate
  - Oral forms of iron should be enteric coated or sustained-release to ensure absorption in the duodenum for optimal absorption
  - Liquid oral forms of iron will stain the teeth so a straw and diluting the solution is recommended

> ferrous gluconate
  - See above

> iron dextran/sodium ferrous gluconate
  - Intramuscular and intravenous forms
  - Parenteral forms of iron may stimulate allergies or anaphylaxis
  - Intramuscular forms may stain and require needle changing or z-track method

Priority Education/Discharge Issues

> Black stools are an expected side effect and are benign

> Client need to take supplements for 2-3 months after a normal hemoglobin

> Clients who are recommended to take iron supplements for life should have liver enzymes assessed routinely

Sickle cell anemia (SSA)

Pathophysiology/Description

> Inherited autosomal recessive disorders

> Sickled hemoglobin cells (Hgb S) with decreased oxygen carrying capacity cause vascular occlusion

> Sickled cells increase hemostasis which increases sickling

> Types include sickle cell anemia, Hgb C disease, sickle cell thalassemia, and sickle cell trait

> May be diagnosed later in infancy due to function of fetal hemoglobin

> Vaso-occlusive crisis (VOC) is severe and painful vessel blockage, characterized by plasma loss, tissue ischemia, necrosis, and shock

> Sequestration crisis is pooling of blood in liver

> Aplastic crisis occurs with increased destruction and decreased production of healthy red blood cells

Priority Assessments or Cues

> Assess for factors that increase cellular sickling, including fever, hypoxia, infections, emotional and physical stress, high altitude, surgery, blood loss, dehydration, acidosis, hypothermia, and surgery

> Assess for a variety of symptoms depending on number of sickled cells, during remission may only have mild anemia and mild to moderate pain

> During exacerbation, pain may be moderate to severe

> Assess for fever, swelling of joints, tenderness around liver/spleen/joints, tachypnea, hypotension, nausea/vomiting, chest pain, dyspnea, pallor/gray skin/mucous membranes, and jaundice

> Assess for priapism which is a sustained, painful, and engorged penile erection

> Assess for splenomegaly/hepatomegaly

Priority Laboratory Tests/Diagnostics

> Peripheral blood smears for Hgb S

> Skeletal X-rays

> Chest X-ray

> Serum electrolytes as indicated

> Magnetic resonance imaging for cerebral vessels/cerebrovascular accident

> Doppler studies for deep vein thromboses

> Newborn and other screening with sickle turbidity test

Priority Interventions or Actions

> Avoid crisis-precipitating factors

> Provide rest and pain management

> Provide supplemental oxygen to relieve hypoxia

> Provide IV hydration and correct electrolyte imbalances

> For leg ulcers, treat with saline soaks and assist with debridement/grafting

> For priapism, provide fluids, pain medications, nifedipine, or penile injection of epinephrine

> Provide antibiotics to treat or prevent infection

> Administer blood transfusions/red blood cell exchange transfusions to manage anemia

> Provide chelation therapy to reduce transfusion associated high iron levels

> Hematopoietic stem cell transplantation (research ongoing related to effectiveness/use)

Priority Potential & Actual Complications

> Vaso-occlusive/aplastic/sequestration crises

> Infection/pneumonia

> Leg ulcers

> Priapism

> Retinal detachment/blindness

> Osteoporosis/osteosclerosis

> Cholelithiasis/hepatomegaly

> Renal failure/hematuria

> Pulmonary failure/heart failure/cor pulmonale/pulmonary hypertension/pulmonary embolism

> Splenic scarring/functional autosplenectomy

> Acute chest syndrome including pneumonia, tissue infarction, and fat embolism

> Cerebrovascular accident (CVA)/stroke

Priority Nursing Implications

> Ensure clients with SSA receive immunizations (meningococcal/pneumococcal)

> Due to chronicity of pain, clients may become tolerant and dependent upon opiates. Nurses need to provide pain management and assist clients to deal with chronic pain

> Titrate pain medications and use client-controlled (PCA)/continuous analgesia when available (meperidine is not suggested because high/sustained doses associated with seizures)

> Support newborn screening for SSA (standard in the US)

Priority Medications

> morphine or hydromorphone
>   - IV narcotic for severe pain, may be used with PCA
>   - Assess for respiratory depression, tolerance, and dependency
> nifedipine
>   - Used to relieve priapism
> deferoxamine
>   - Parenteral chelation therapy to remove excess iron
> deferasirox
>   - Oral iron chelation therapy
> hydroxyurea
>   - Chemotherapy agent used to increase levels of fetal hemoglobin
>   - Increases red blood cell volume/decreases sickled cells
>   - Decreases sickled cell adhesion to blood vessel endothelium
>   - May prevent CVA

Priority Education/Discharge Issues

> SSA requires much teaching about assessment and prevention of many complications
> Requires ongoing monitoring and surveillance by healthcare professionals, including regular eye exams
> Encourage caregivers/clients to intervene early with infections, signs/symptoms, and potential risk factors (hydration, stress, temperature/weather changes, infections)
> Provide support and referral to resources to assist in coping with the emotional burden of SSA, including depression, anxiety, and crisis intervention
> Refer to genetic counseling for children and subsequent pregnancies

Complete this MNEMONIC

SICKLE CELL DISEASE COMPLICATIONS

S _____

I _____

C _____

K _____

L _____

E _____

Table 8-1: Feel free to search the Internet or create your own.

Next Gen Clinical Judgment

You are a nurse caring for the following three clients. What concerns you most about each of these clients?

1. An infant with a respiratory rate of 50 breaths/ minute, nasal flaring, and using his belly to breath.

2. A 12-year-old child with a history of asthma who uses his rescue inhaler 4-6 times per day.

3. A 5-year-old child who has not received immunizations presents with a high fever and is drooling.

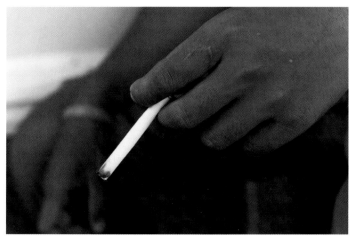

Image 9-4: List 5 things the client with sickle cell anemia can do to prevent a crisis.

1. _____

2. _____

3. _____

4. _____

5. _____

1. The nurse is caring for a client with an acute asthma exacerbation. What priority assessment would concern the nurse most?
    1. Shortness of breath and temperature above 100°F.
    2. An Oxygen saturation of 90% and pulse rate greater than 80.
    3. Inspiratory wheezing and respiratory rate greater than 30.
    4. Tachycardia and pursed-lip breathing.

2. The home care nurse is analyzing the client's understanding of caring for home oxygen equipment to treat chronic obstructive pulmonary disease. What statement by the client indicates additional teaching is needed?
    1. "I wash the nasal cannula once a month with warm water and dish soap."
    2. "I use mouthwash several times per day to deal with my dry mouth."
    3. "The company sends me new cannulas every couple of weeks."
    4. "If I have a cold, I always replace my cannula as soon as I feel better."

3. The nurse is planning care for a client with a diagnosis of cystic fibrosis living in the community. What is the priority goal to be included?
    1. Increase activity level to 20 minutes per day.
    2. Recognize risk factors for respiratory infections.
    3. Family members will support client's care.
    4. Genetic testing will be considered in the future.

4. The nurse is caring for a client with pulmonary hypertension who asks "Am I going to die?" What is the best response by the nurse?
    1. "Of course you aren't going to die, we are taking good care of you."
    2. "Pulmonary hypertension is a scary diagnosis but it won't kill you."
    3. "You sound frightened, can you tell me more about that?"
    4. "We can give you medications to control your symptoms."

5. The nurse caring for a client with adult respiratory distress syndrome (ARDS) is evaluating the plan of care. What is the priority safety goal that needs to be evaluated?
    1. Deep breathing and coughing on a regular basis to remove secretion.
    2. Identify and address potential causes of agitation.
    3. Encourage adequate nutritional intake especially protein intake.
    4. Assess client's understanding of the diagnosis.

6. The nurse is assessing a client with a diagnosis of asthma who reports having a dry cough and episodic hoarseness. What information is the highest priority for the nurse to collect?
    1. Potential seasonal allergies that may compound the asthma symptoms.
    2. Whether a spacer is being used with inhalation corticosteroids.
    3. Any recent prescriptions for bronchodilators for cold symptoms.
    4. Compliance with prescribed medications to control asthma symptoms.

7. The nurse is instructing an unlicensed assistive personnel (UAP) regarding the care of a male client with a diagnosis of chronic obstructive pulmonary disease (COPD). What is the highest priority nursing action to share with the UAP?
    1. Encourage the client to ambulate as much as possible.
    2. Keep the head of the bed elevated to 45 degrees.
    3. Never leave the client alone when he is out of bed.
    4. Offer to help the client with activities of daily living.

8. The home health nurse is assessing the learning needs of a client with a diagnosis of cystic fibrosis recently discharged following a brief hospitalization. What statement by the client would alert the nurse that additional teaching is needed?
    1. "I am able to take a shower and get dressed without becoming overly fatigued."
    2. "My coughing seems to stay under control as long as I continue to use my medications."
    3. "My neighbor likes to visit with his dog and my coughing gets worse."
    4. "I have talked with my social worker about the costs of my medications."

9. The clinic nurse is evaluating the over-the-counter medications that a client with a diagnosis of asthma reports taking on a regular basis. Which medications should be of concern?
    1. Multivitamin.
    2. Low dose aspirin.
    3. Probiotic.
    4. Ginseng.

10. The nurse is planning care for a client with a diagnosis of chronic obstructive pulmonary disease (COPD) with a high anxiety level that causes shortness of breath. Which action should the nurse take given the client's reaction to anxiety?
    1. Administer prescribed anti-anxiety medications as needed.
    2. Teach pursed-lip breathing to use when feeling anxious.
    3. Discourage visitors who may cause anxiety to increase.
    4. Teach proper use of inhalers to control anxiety.

11. The nurse is implementing the plan of care for a client with cystic fibrosis. What is the priority nursing goal for the client's care?
    1. Administering medication as prescribed.
    2. Encouraging adequate nutrition.
    3. Maintaining adequate airway clearance.
    4. Assessing for clear breath sounds.

12. The nurse is assessing a client with a diagnosis of adult respiratory distress syndrome. What findings will the nurse anticipate?
    1. Lethargy, muscle cramping, and shortness of breath.
    2. Restlessness, confusion, and agitation.
    3. Hypotension, diaphoresis, and anxiety.
    4. Bradycardia, hyperventilation, and nausea.

13. The nurse has completed the assessment for a client in the clinic with a diagnosis of chronic asthma. What would be the priority goal the nurse should discuss with the client?
    1. Maintaining a regular exercise routine.
    2. Complying with medication instructions.
    3. Recognizing triggers that cause asthma attacks.
    4. Understanding physical limitations caused by this disease.

14. The nurse is preparing a client with a diagnosis of cystic fibrosis for discharge from the hospital. What category of medications will the nurse anticipate in the discharge prescriptions?
    1. Beta-blockers.
    2. Antihypertensives.
    3. Prophylactic antibiotics.
    4. Anticholinergics.

15. The nurse is assessing a client with secondary pulmonary hypertension. What statement by the client requires further assessment by the nurse?
    1. "There is no cure for this so I might as well just give up now."
    2. "I need to pay close attention to what causes me to be short of breath."
    3. "Regardless of how I feel, I need to make sure I drink plenty of fluids."
    4. "My wife will be a big help at home so I don't have to exert myself."

16. The nurse is reviewing the plan of care for a client with a diagnosis of adult respiratory distress syndrome. What goals should the nurse expect to be included in the plan of care? Select all that apply.
    1. PaO_2 of 60 mmHg or greater.
    2. SaO_2 of 45 mmHg or less.
    3. Lungs clear on auscultation.
    4. SaO_2 greater than 90%.
    5. Normal ph.
    6. Respiratory rate greater than 20 breaths/minute.

17. The nurse is assessing a client brought into the emergency room with respiratory distress and a provisional diagnosis of asthma. What findings should the nurse anticipate with the asthma diagnosis? Select all that apply.
    1. Wheezes on auscultation.
    2. Friction rub on auscultation.
    3. Restlessness.
    4. Bradycardia.
    5. Intercostal retractions.
    6. Cyanosis.

18. The nurse is teaching the client pursed-lip breathing techniques. What guidelines should the nurse include? Select all that apply.
    1. Inhale slowly and deeply through the mouth.
    2. Exhalation should be 3 times as long as inhalation.
    3. Purse lips like whistling to exhale.
    4. Puff cheeks while doing pursed-lip breathing.
    5. Use pursed-lip breathing before and after activities.

19. The home care nurse is evaluating the environment prior to starting a client with chronic obstructive pulmonary disease on home oxygen therapy. What factors should be of most concern? Select all that apply.
    1. Another client in the home receiving oxygen.
    2. A family member who smokes lives in the home.
    3. Presence of blankets that cause static.
    4. Remodeling in process with cans of paint around.
    5. Bathroom is too small to accommodate additional large equipment.

20. The nurse is teaching the client to do huff coughing. In what order will the nurse instruct the client to perform the steps? Place the steps in the correct order.
    1. Breathe out through the mouth in a slow but forceful manner, making a "who" sound.
    2. Breathe in slowly and deeply through the nose, holding breath for a few seconds.
    3. Assume sitting position on a chair or at edge of the bed, with feet on floor.
    4. Relax, then repeat the steps, ending with a strong cough to get rid of mucus from lungs.
    5. Position head so there is a slight upward tilt of the chin.

21. The clinic nurse is assessing a client with cystic fibrosis about the technique for using a metered dose inhaler. When asked to demonstrate the technique, in what order should the client demonstrate the procedure? Place the steps in the correct order.
    1. Wait about 1 minute before repeating.
    2. Breath in slowly through mouth while pressing down on inhaler once.
    3. Continue to breathe in slowly.
    4. Exhale completely to clear lungs as much as possible.
    5. Hold breath for 10 seconds if possible.
    6. Shake the inhaler vigorously.

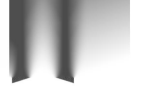

22. The interdisciplinary team is meeting to discuss discharge planning for a client with cystic fibrosis. What priorities will the team want to include in the plan? Select all that apply.
   1. Medication teaching related to new prescriptions.
   2. Assessment of need for support in the community.
   3. Discussion of financial means to manage costs of treatment.
   4. Genetic counseling for client and spouse.
   5. Need for parenteral nutritional therapy.

23. A nurse is making a home visit with a client with iron-deficiency anemia. The client's hemoglobin (Hgb) one week ago was 11.2 g/dL. What assessment data alerts the nurse to the need for follow-up?
   1. Heart rate 88 beats per minute.
   2. Capillary refill of 1 – 2 seconds.
   3. Client states, "I'm a little tired today."
   4. Dyspnea at rest.

24. The nurse is preparing to teach a client newly diagnosed with sickle cell disease. What information does the nurse need to include to help the client prevent a sickle cell crisis?
   1. The need to drink about 64 ounces or 2 liters of water every day.
   2. Refrain from getting a flu shot due to high-risk of infection.
   3. The importance of including high impact aerobics for 30-40 minutes every day.
   4. High stress environments help improve coping skills.

25. The nurse is caring for a client with acute chest syndrome resulting from sickle cell anemia. What are the priority nursing actions? Select all that apply.
   1. Monitor the client's lung sounds.
   2. Administer antibiotics and oxygen as prescribed.
   3. Encourage the client to use incentive spirometer every 2 hours.
   4. Teach the client to eat beef, oysters and clams.
   5. Administer hydroxyurea as prescribed.

26. The nurse is reviewing an immunization record for a 4-year-old child to determine the risk for epiglottitis. Which will indicate the lowest risk for the child to contract the illness?
   1. Hepatitis B—all doses before two years of age.
   2. Rotavirus—all doses before six months of age.
   3. Haemophilus influenzae type b (Hib)—all doses before 15 months of age.
   4. Pneumococcal—all doses before 18 months of age.

27. The nurse is caring for a 4-month-old infant brought in by his 17-year-old sister who was babysitting while the infant's parents are out of town. The child has bronchiolitis and requires urgent intubation for severe respiratory distress. How should the nurse obtain consent for the procedure?
   1. Allow the sister to sign the consent, since the parent's implied consent when leaving the infant to the care of the sibling.
   2. Have the sister contact the parents and obtain verbal consent over the phone.
   3. Have the health care provider provide written consent.
   4. Complete consent once the parents are at the facility.

28. A non-English speaking client comes into the emergency department with a 4-week onset of a productive cough, fever, night sweats, and weight loss. Through an interpreter, you learn that he has been living in Mexico and recently came to the United States. What should the nurse do next?
   1. Collect a sputum specimen.
   2. Determine when he last ate a balanced meal.
   3. Place him on airborne precautions.
   4. Determine his support systems.

29. The nurse is presenting a workshop in a senior community center about the prevention of pneumonia. Which observations should the nurse address with the group? Select all that apply.
   1. A man is coughing into his hand.
   2. A group of participants smoking outside the community center.
   3. A woman is eating an apple without cutting it up first.
   4. Two participants are washing their hands without soap.
   5. A person is saying that they could not sleep last night.

30. The nurse receives the following discharge instructions for a client recently admitted with active tuberculosis (TB). How will the nurse best explain how to take these medications?

DISCHARGE MEDICATIONS
8/29/XX   First Take: isoniazid (INH) 300 mg PO daily, rifampin (RIF) 600 mg PO daily, ethambutol (EMB) 1000 mg PO daily, & pyrazinamide (PZA) 1000 mg PO daily - 7 days/week for 56 doses.
Then Take INH & RIF PO daily - 7 days/week for 126 doses.

   1. You will complete these TB medications in eight weeks.
   2. There are several medications, and they should be taken exactly as prescribed.
   3. You will take the ethambutol for the entire period.
   4. Your medications will be done in 48 weeks.

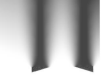

1. **The nurse is caring for a client with an acute asthma exacerbation. What priority assessment would concern the nurse most?**
   1. Shortness of breath and temperature above 100°F. *No temperature with asthma attack.*
   2. An Oxygen saturation of 90% and pulse rate greater than 80. *The oxygen saturation is not as concerning as inspiratory wheezing.*
   3. Inspiratory wheezing and respiratory rate greater than 30.
   4. Tachycardia and pursed-lip breathing. *Signs not as indicative of an asthma attack as wheezing and increased respiratory rate.*

   Rationale: An acute asthma attack is characterized by wheezing, poor movement of the diaphragm, increased respiratory rate, usually higher than 30 breaths/minute and heart rate higher than 120 beats/minute. With these findings, the client is forced to sit forward to allow for more effective breathing. Additionally, an acute attack causes the client to use accessory muscles located in the neck to lift the diaphragm and when percussed, hyperresonance can be heard in the lung fields. It is also common for the client to display agitation, secondary to hypoxemia. Auscultation of the lungs indicates inspiratory or expiratory wheezing.

   THIN Thinking: Nursing Process – *Assessment findings are the priority and include wheezing and tachypnea.* **NCLEX®:** Management of Care **QSEN:** Patient-centered Care

2. **The home care nurse is analyzing the client's understanding of caring for home oxygen equipment to treat chronic obstructive pulmonary disease. What statement by the client indicates additional teaching is needed?**
   1. "I wash the nasal cannula once a month with warm water and dish soap."
   2. "I use mouthwash several times per day to deal with my dry mouth." *Valid response.*
   3. "The company sends me new cannulas every couple of weeks" *Valid response.*
   4. "If I have a cold, I always replace my cannula as soon as I feel better." *Accurate response.*

   Rationale: The highest risk for infection is the cannula because there is the potential for bacterial growth due to the humidity. Washing the cannula with mild liquid soap and rinsing thoroughly at least once per week is recommended.

   THIN Thinking: Identify Risk to Safety – *Infection is a risk for the client with a compromised pulmonary system. Proper care and cleaning can prevent pneumonia.* **NCLEX®:** Safety and Infection Control **QSEN:** Safety

3. **The nurse is planning care for a client with a diagnosis of cystic fibrosis living in the community. What is the priority goal to be included?**
   1. Increase activity level to 20 minutes per day. *Although helpful, this is not the priority.*
   2. Recognize risk factors for respiratory infections.
   3. Family members will support client's care. *Important, but not the priority.*
   4. Genetic testing will be considered in the future. *Helpful, but not a priority.*

   Rationale: Cystic fibrosis is a chronic disease and reduction of potential risk of an infection is a priority. The client needs to be able to recognize risk factors that could lead to respiratory infections which would exacerbate the cystic fibrosis.

   THIN Thinking: Top Three – *The compromised client with cystic fibrosis is at risk for infection and early identification and intervention is needed.* **NCLEX®:** Health Promotion and Maintenance **QSEN:** Evidence-based Practice

4. **The nurse is caring for a client with pulmonary hypertension who asks "Am I going to die?" What is the best response by the nurse?**
   1. "Of course you aren't going to die, we are taking good care of you." *False reassurance.*
   2. "Pulmonary hypertension is a scary diagnosis but it won't kill you." *Untrue.*
   3. "You sound frightened, can you tell me more about that?"
   4. "We can give you medications to control your symptoms." *True, but unhelpful as it doesn't address the client's concerns.*

   Rationale: The treatment of pulmonary hypertension can be challenging and early diagnosis can prevent permanent heart damage. Encouraging the client to talk about fears and anxiety can be helpful but never provide false reassurances that are not warranted.

   THIN Thinking: Nursing Process – *Therapeutic communication is empathetic and asks open-ended questions.* **NCLEX®:** Psychosocial Integrity **QSEN:** Patient-centered Care

5. The nurse caring for a client with adult respiratory distress syndrome (ARDS) is evaluating the plan of care. What is the priority safety goal that needs to be evaluated?
   1. Deep breathing and coughing on a regular basis to remove secretion. *Not a safety goal.*
   2. 🔘 Identify and address potential causes of agitation.
   3. Encourage adequate nutritional intake especially protein intake. *Not a safety goal.*
   4. Assess client's understanding of the diagnosis. *Not a priority.*

   Rationale: The priority safety consideration focuses on reducing client agitation. The nurse needs to help identify potential causes of agitation. Using sedatives to control agitation can impact the client's already compromised respiratory system.

   THIN Thinking: Top Three – *The goal of treatment is to reduce the oxygen demands for the client. Agitation will increase the client's need for O_2.* **NCLEX®**: Physiological Adaptation **QSEN**: Evidence-based Practice

6. The nurse is assessing a client with a diagnosis of asthma who reports having a dry cough and episodic hoarseness. What information is the highest priority for the nurse to collect?
   1. Potential seasonal allergies that may compound the asthma symptoms. *Not the priority information for this client.*
   2. 🔘 Whether a spacer is being used with inhalation corticosteroids.
   3. Any recent prescriptions for bronchodilators for cold symptoms. *Not a priority for this client.*
   4. Compliance with prescribed medications to control asthma symptoms. *Important, but learning how corticosteroids are administered is more important.*

   Rationale: Chronic inflammation is a primary component of asthma which is treated with corticosteroid inhalers. Hoarseness and a dry cough are frequent side effects of inhaled corticosteroids. Use of a spacer can reduce or prevent these symptoms.

   THIN Thinking: Help Quick – *The use of the spacer with inhaled corticosteroids can reduce hoarseness.* **NCLEX®**: Pharmacological and Parental Therapies **QSEN**: Evidence-based Practice

7. The nurse is instructing an unlicensed assistive personnel (UAP) regarding the care of a male client with a diagnosis of chronic obstructive pulmonary disease (COPD). What is the highest priority nursing action to share with the UAP?
   1. Encourage the client to ambulate as much as possible. *Not the priority.*
   2. 🔘 Keep the head of the bed elevated to 45 degrees.
   3. Never leave the client alone when he is out of bed. *May not be necessary.*
   4. Offer to help the client with activities of daily living. *Not the priority.*

   Rationale: Clients with COPD experience dyspnea even at rest. Keeping the head of the bed elevated to 45 degrees can help the client breathe easier.

   THIN Thinking: Help Quick – *The head of the bed elevation will ease respiration and may be done by the UAP* **NCLEX®**: Basic Care and Comfort **QSEN**: Patient-centered Care

8. The home health nurse is assessing the learning needs of a client with a diagnosis of cystic fibrosis recently discharged following a brief hospitalization. What statement by the client would alert the nurse that additional teaching is needed?
   1. "I am able to take a shower and get dressed without becoming overly fatigued." *Positive comment.*
   2. "My coughing seems to stay under control as long as I continue to use my medications" *Positive comment.*
   3. 🔘 "My neighbor likes to visit with his dog and my coughing gets worse."
   4. "I have talked with my social worker about the costs of my medications" *Positive comment.*

   Rationale: The overall goals for the client with cystic fibrosis is maintaining airway clearance and avoiding any triggers that may result in complications. Bringing a dog into the home may be impacting the client's airway resulting in an exacerbation of coughing.

   THIN Thinking: Help Quick – *The introduction of allergens and irritants will worsen the client's situation and risk for injection.* **NCLEX®**: Reduction of Risk Potential **QSEN**: Safety

9. The clinic nurse is evaluating the over-the-counter medications that a client with a diagnosis of asthma reports taking on a regular basis. Which medications should be of concern?
   1. Multivitamin. *Not a concern.*
   2. 🔘 Low dose aspirin.
   3. Probiotic. *Not a concern.*
   4. Ginseng. *Not a concern.*

   Rationale: Clients with asthma should avoid taking any medications that contain aspirin. Aspirin is known to be a trigger for asthma attacks for many people.

   THIN Thinking: Nursing Process – *The nurse needs to recognize all over-the-counter medications that can interact with the client's illness or other medications.* **NCLEX®**: Health Promotion and Maintenance **QSEN:** Evidence-based Practice

10. The nurse is planning care for a client with a diagnosis of chronic obstructive pulmonary disease (COPD) with a high anxiety level that causes shortness of breath. Which action should the nurse take given the client's reaction to anxiety?
    1. Administer prescribed anti-anxiety medications as needed. *Non-pharmacological methods should be tried first.*
    2. 🔘 Teach pursed-lip breathing to use when feeling anxious.
    3. Discourage visitors who may cause anxiety to increase. *This would likely increase anxiety.*
    4. Teach proper use of inhalers to control anxiety. *Important, but not as effective as teaching client pursed-lip breathing technique.*

    Rationale: Pursed-lip breathing can be effective when the client is experiencing shortness of breath. Anti-anxiety medications may be effective, but they also have potential respiratory side effects.

    THIN Thinking: Top Three – *Pursed-lip breathing can reduce anxiety quickly and low tachypnea.* **NCLEX®**: Psychosocial Integrity **QSEN:** Evidence-based Practice

11. The nurse is implementing the plan of care for a client with cystic fibrosis. What is the priority nursing goal for the client's care?
    1. Administering medication as prescribed. *Important, but not as important as maintaining airway.*
    2. Encouraging adequate nutrition. *Not as important as maintaining airway.*
    3. 🔘 Maintaining adequate airway clearance.
    4. Assessing for clear breath sounds. *Not as important as maintaining airway.*

    Rationale: The plan of care for the client with cystic fibrosis should focus on management of pulmonary issues and maintaining an adequate airway. Measures to clear an airway may be evaluated by assessing breath sounds. Nutrition and medications prescribed are important, but breathing is always the priority.

    THIN Thinking: Identify Risk to Safety – *Impaired airway from excess secretions can place the client in jeopardy of airway obstruction.* **NCLEX®**: Physiological Adaptation **QSEN:** Evidence-based Practice

12. The nurse is assessing a client with a diagnosis of adult respiratory distress syndrome. What findings will the nurse anticipate?
    1. Lethargy, muscle cramping, and shortness of breath. *Incorrect.*
    2. 🔘 Restlessness, confusion, and agitation.
    3. Hypotension, diaphoresis, and anxiety. *Incorrect.*
    4. Bradycardia, hyperventilation, and nausea. *Incorrect.*

    Rationale: With acute respiratory distress restlessness, confusion, agitation, and combative behavior could suggest inadequate O_2 delivery to the brain. These symptoms require immediate action.

    THIN Thinking: Help Quick – *Restlessness, confusion, and agitation are early signs of hypoxia.* **NCLEX®**: Safety and Infection Control **QSEN:** Safety

13. The nurse has completed the assessment for a client in the clinic with a diagnosis of chronic asthma. What would be the priority goal the nurse should discuss with the client?
    1. Maintaining a regular exercise routine. *Helpful, but not the priority.*
    2. Complying with medication instructions. *Important, but not the priority.*
    3. Recognizing triggers that cause asthma attacks.
    4. Understanding physical limitations caused by this disease. *Important, but not the priority.*

    Rationale: The priority goal is asthma control as evidenced by minimal symptoms both during the day and at night. While medication compliance is important, recognizing triggers that cause symptoms is the priority to control symptoms.

    THIN Thinking: Nursing Process – *Identification of asthma triggers can prevent asthma attacks.* **NCLEX®:** Reduction of Risk Potential **QSEN:** Patient-centered Care

14. The nurse is preparing a client with a diagnosis of cystic fibrosis for discharge from the hospital. What category of medications will the nurse anticipate in the discharge prescriptions?
    1. Beta-blockers. *These would cause bronchoconstriction.*
    2. Antihypertensives. *No need to lower blood pressure.*
    3. Prophylactic antibiotics.
    4. Anticholinergics. *No need for this medication.*

    Rationale: Acute care for a cystic fibrosis client includes interventions such as antibiotics, oxygen therapy and aggressive CPT. Clients are also encouraged to maintain an adequate food and fluid intake.

    THIN Thinking: Top Three – *Because of the risk for infection, antibiotics are anticipated.* **NCLEX®:** Health Promotion and Maintenance **QSEN:** Evidence-based Practice

15. The nurse is assessing a client with secondary pulmonary hypertension. What statement by the client requires further assessment by the nurse?
    1. "There is no cure for this so I might as well just give up now."
    2. "I need to pay close attention to what causes me to be short of breath." *Accurate statement.*
    3. "Regardless of how I feel, I need to make sure I drink plenty of fluids." *Accurate statement.*
    4. "My wife will be a big help at home so I don't have to exert myself." *Positive statement.*

    Rationale: Although there is no cure for pulmonary hypertension, there are strategies to control the symptoms. Secondary pulmonary hypertension may improve when primary illness is treated. Clients with chronic diseases may think their life is over because of the lack of a cure. The nurse always needs to be alert to any statement that could potentially suggest the client is considering suicide.

    THIN Thinking: Help Quick – *The client with pulmonary hypertension will need to learn how to best manage their chronic illness even though it is not curable.* **NCLEX®:** Psychological Integrity **QSEN:** Safety

16. The nurse is reviewing the plan of care for a client with a diagnosis of adult respiratory distress syndrome. What goals should the nurse expect to be included in the plan of care? Select all that apply.
    1. PaO_2 of 60 mmHg or greater.
    2. SaO_2 of 45 mmHg or less. *This is too low.*
    3. Lungs clear on auscultation.
    4. SaO_2 greater than 90%.
    5. Normal ph.
    6. Respiratory rate greater than 20 breaths/minute *Not a positive outcome.*

    Rationale: With appropriate therapy, overall goals include a PaO_2 of 60 mmHg or higher and adequate lung ventilation to maintain normal pH. Specific goals for a client with ARDS include (1) PaO_2 within normal limits for age or at baseline on room air, (2) SaO_2 greater than 90%, (3) resolution of the precipitating factor(s) for ARDS, and (4) clear lungs on auscultation.

    THIN Thinking: Top Three – *Maintaining oxygenation is the priority concern for a client with ARDS. Maintaining PO_2, SaO_2, and normal acid-base balance is the key.* **NCLEX®:** Physiological Adaptation **QSEN:** Evidence-based Practice

17. The nurse is assessing a client brought into the emergency room with respiratory distress and a provisional diagnosis of asthma. What findings should the nurse anticipate with the asthma diagnosis? Select all that apply.
    1. 💡 Wheezes on auscultation.
    2. Friction rub on auscultation. *This is not a sign seen in asthma.*
    3. 💡 Restlessness.
    4. Bradycardia. *Heart rate will likely be increased.*
    5. 💡 Intercostal retractions.
    6. 💡 Cyanosis.

    Rationale: Assessment findings commonly seen with an acute asthmatic attack include: restlessness, absent or diminished lung sounds along with crackles, confusion, upright or forward leaning body position, diaphoresis, wheezing, hyperresonance on percussion, sputum (thick, white, tenacious), increased work of breathing with use of accessory muscles, intercostal and supraclavicular retractions, cyanosis of the nailbed and around the mouth, tachypnea with hyperventilation, nasal polyps, prolonged expiration, eczema, tachycardia, pulsus paradoxus, discharge from the nares, jugular venous distention, hypertension or hypotension, and premature ventricular contractions.

    THIN Thinking: Nursing Process – *The nurse should understand the assessment findings that are consistent with this diagnosis.* **NCLEX®:** Safety and Infection Control **QSEN:** Safety

18. The nurse is teaching the client pursed-lip breathing techniques. What guidelines should the nurse include? Select all that apply.
    1. Inhale slowly and deeply through the mouth. *Inhale through nose.*
    2. 💡 Exhalation should be 3 times as long as inhalation.
    3. 💡 Purse lips like whistling to exhale.
    4. Puff cheeks while doing pursed-lip breathing. *Facial muscles should stay relaxed.*
    5. 💡 Use pursed-lip breathing before and after activities.

    Rationale: Pursed-lip breathing should be used before and after any activities that may cause shortness of breath. Inhale slowly through the nose and exhale slowly through purse lips (like whistling). Keep facial muscles relaxed and do not puff checks. Exhalation should be 3 times as long as inhalation.

    THIN Thinking: Top Three – *To perform pursed-lip breathing the client should breathe slowly through pursed lips with slow exhalation.* **NCLEX®:** Basic Care and Comfort **QSEN:** Evidence-based Practice

19. The home care nurse is evaluating the environment prior to starting a client with chronic obstructive pulmonary disease on home oxygen therapy. What factors should be of most concern? Select all that apply.
    1. Another client in the home receiving oxygen. *Not a concern.*
    2. 💡 A family member who smokes lives in the home.
    3. 💡 Presence of blankets that cause static.
    4. 💡 Remodeling in process with cans of paint around.
    5. Bathroom is too small to accommodate additional large equipment. *Home oxygen therapy equipment may be compact sized.*

    Rationale: Safety factors to consider with home oxygen include family members or visitors who smoke in the house, the presence of any fabrics that may cause static, and also the presence of any flammable liquids such as paint, paint thinners, etc.

    THIN Thinking: Identify Risk to Safety – *The priority when starting a client on O_2 at home is to assess for safety concerns.* **NCLEX®:** Safety and Infection Control **QSEN:** Safety

20. The nurse is teaching the client to do huff coughing. In what order will the nurse instruct the client to perform the actions? Rank order the responses.
    1. Assume sitting position on a chair or at edge of the bed, with feet on floor.
    2. Position head so there is a slight upward tilt of the chin.
    3. Breathe in slowly and deeply through the nose, holding breath for a few seconds.
    4. Breathe out through the mouth in a slow but forceful manner, making a "who" sound.
    5. Relax, then repeat the steps, ending with a strong cough to get rid of mucus from lungs.

    Rationale: The huff technique is a simple, yet effective way to force the separation of mucous from the wall of the lungs, thus making it easier to cough up and expel from the airway. For clients with conditions that cause tenacious mucous, like cystic fibrosis, this technique is particularly helpful.

    THIN Thinking: Nursing Process – *Performing interventions in the proper order will be most beneficial for the client.* **NCLEX®:** Physiological Adaptation **QSEN:** Evidence-based Practice

21. The clinic nurse is assessing a client with cystic fibrosis about the technique for using a metered dose inhaler. When asked to demonstrate the technique, in what order should the client demonstrate the procedure? Place the steps in the correct order.
1. Shake the inhaler vigorously.
2. Exhale completely to clear lungs as much as possible.
3. Breath in slowly through mouth while pressing down on inhaler once.
4. Continue to breathe in slowly.
5. Hold breath for 10 seconds if possible.
6. Wait about 1 minute before repeating.

Rationale: Steps for proper use of a metered dose inhaler: Take the top off and shake the inhaler. Breathe all the way out. Breath in slowly through the mouth and press down inhaler once (dose will be administered). Continue to breathe in slowly to move medication to lungs. Hold breath for 10 seconds if possible to hold the medication in the lungs. Wait at least one minute before repeating procedure if more than one puff is prescribed.

THIN Thinking: Nursing Process – *Performing interventions in the proper order will be most beneficial for the client.* **NCLEX®:** Pharmacology and Parenteral Therapies **QSEN:** Evidence-based Practice

22. The interdisciplinary team is meeting to discuss discharge planning for a client with cystic fibrosis. What priorities will the team want to include in the plan? Select all that apply.
1. 🔵 Medication teaching related to new prescriptions.
2. 🔵 Assessment of need for support in the community.
3. 🔵 Discussion of financial means to manage costs of treatment.
4. Genetic counseling for client and spouse. *Not a priority.*
5. Need for parenteral nutritional therapy. *No indication this is needed.*

Rationale: Client teaching regarding new prescriptions is always a priority when planning for discharge. Clients with a diagnosis of cystic fibrosis may need considerable support and resources especially following an acute episode. Compliance with medications and treatment is a priority to avoid further exacerbations. Many times, the costs of care are a significant concern that clients are not comfortable talking about unless asked by the interprofessional team. Genetic counseling is not a priority but may be something to be considered in the future if the client wants to have children. There is no indication the client needs parenteral nutrition therapy.

THIN Thinking: Top Three – *Detailed discharge instructions are important for the client with cystic fibrosis to avoid complications.* **NCLEX®:** Management of Care **QSEN:** Evidence-based Practice

23. A nurse is making a home visit with a client with iron-deficiency anemia. The client's hemoglobin (Hgb) one week ago was 11.2 g/dL. What assessment data alerts the nurse to the need for follow-up?
1. Heart rate 88 beats per minute. *Normal range.*
2. Capillary refill of 1 – 2 seconds. *Normal range.*
3. Client states, "I'm a little tired today." *Not unusual.*
4. 🔵 Dyspnea at rest.

Rationale: The client's hemoglobin one week ago indicated the client was experiencing mild anemia. Clients with mild anemia may experience palpitations, dyspnea on exertion and fatigue. Dyspnea at rest is a symptom of severe anemia. This symptom indicates that the client's anemia may be worsening and requires follow-up by the nurse.

THIN Thinking: Top Three – *Since hemoglobin carries oxygen, difficulty with breathing and oxygenation are the priority concerns.* **NCLEX®:** Management of Care **QSEN:** Safety

24. The nurse is preparing to teach a client newly diagnosed with sickle cell disease. What information does the nurse need to include to help the client prevent a sickle cell crisis?
1. 🔵 The need to drink about 64 ounces or 2 liters of water every day.
2. Refrain from getting a flu shot due to high-risk of infection. *Client should obtain flu shot to avoid infection.*
3. The importance of including high impact aerobics for 30-40 minutes every day. *Low impact exercise as tolerated is recommended.*
4. High stress environments help improve coping skills. *Stress can trigger attack.*

Rationale: Clients with sickle cell disease need to stay hydrated to prevent sickle cell crisis. Because sickle cell disease predisposes a client to infection, getting preventative immunizations is important. Emotional and physical stress contribute to oxygen loss. Therefore, clients with sickle cell disease should avoid strenuous activity and stressful environments.

THIN Thinking: Identify Risk to Safety – *Hydration helps to prevent crisis.* **NCLEX®:** Health Promotion and Maintenance **QSEN:** Patient-centered Care

25. The nurse is caring for a client with acute chest syndrome resulting from sickle cell anemia. What are the priority nursing actions? Select all that apply.
    1. ⦿ Monitor the client's lung sounds.
    2. ⦿ Administer antibiotics and oxygen as prescribed.
    3. ⦿ Encourage the client to use incentive spirometer every 2 hours.
    4. Teach the client to eat beef, oysters and clams. *Not indicated.*
    5. ⦿ Administer hydroxyurea as prescribed.

Rationale: Acute chest syndrome includes acute pulmonary complications, such as pneumonia and tissue infarction, that is commonly seen in clients with sickle cell disease. It can be fatal. If a client has acute chest syndrome, it is essential to monitor for and treat this serious condition. Appropriate nursing actions include assessing lung sounds, administering antibiotics and oxygen, and encouraging the client to use an incentive spirometer to manage respiratory complications. Hydroxyurea is the only medication that has been shown to be beneficial in decreasing the number of sickled cells. Clients with sickle cell disease need to consume diets high in folic acid. Beef, oysters and clams are high in iron, not folic acid.

THIN Thinking: Top Three – *Greatest concerns are with oxygenation and complications.* **NCLEX®:** Physiological Adaptation **QSEN:** Patient-centered Care

26. The nurse is reviewing an immunization record for a 4-year-old child to determine the risk for epiglottitis. Which will indicate the lowest risk for the child to contract the illness?
    1. Hepatitis B—all doses before two years of age. *Does not offer protection for this illness.*
    2. Rotavirus—all doses before six months of age. *Does not offer protection for this illness.*
    3. ⦿ Haemophilus influenzae type b (Hib)—all doses before 15 months of age.
    4. Pneumococcal—all doses before 18 months of age. *Does not offer protection for this illness.*

Rationale: Haemophilus influenzae type b (Hib) conjugate vaccines protect against a number of serious infections caused by Hib, especially bacterial meningitis, epiglottitis, bacterial pneumonia, septic arthritis, and sepsis (Hib is not associated with the viruses that cause influenza, or "flu").

THIN Thinking: Top Three – *The nurse needs to understand the illness that various immunizations prevent.* **NCLEX®:** Health Promotion and Maintenance **QSEN:** Safety

27. The nurse is caring for a 4-month-old infant brought in by his 17-year-old sister who was babysitting while the infant's parents are out of town. The child has bronchiolitis and requires urgent intubation for severe respiratory distress. How should the nurse obtain consent for the procedure?
    1. Allow the sister to sign the consent, since the parent's implied consent when leaving the infant to the care of the sibling. *Sister is not legal guardian.*
    2. ⦿ Have the sister contact the parents and obtain verbal consent over the phone.
    3. Have the health care provider provide written consent. *If possible, need to obtain parents' consent.*
    4. Complete consent once the parents are at the facility. *In urgent situation, this might not be soon enough to prevent injury.*

Rationale: There are certain times when requiring parental consent to treat children who are minors can be bypassed. These exceptions include times when immediate surgical or medical intervention is needed, and the child's parent(s) cannot be reached or if the parents can be reached, they do not consent. When legal guardians of the child or parents are not present, persons in charge of the child may be permitted by the parents to give informed consent by proxy if established ahead of time in written form. In this case, obtaining verbal consent over the phone would be appropriate. In emergencies, including danger to life or the possibility of permanent injury, appropriate care should not be withheld or delayed because of problems obtaining consent. All efforts that are made to receive consent must be carefully documented by the nurse.

THIN Thinking: Identify Risk to Safety – *Urgent and legal consent is needed.* **NCLEX®:** Management of Care **QSEN:** Patient-centered Care

28. **A non-English speaking client comes into the emergency department with a 4-week onset of a productive cough, fever, night sweats, and weight loss. Through an interpreter, you learn that he has been living in Mexico and recently came to the United States. What should the nurse do next?**
    1. Collect a sputum specimen. *Priority is to prevent spread of infection.*
    2. Determine when he last ate a balanced meal. *Priority is to prevent spread of infection.*
    3. 💡 Place him on airborne precautions.
    4. Determine his support systems. *Priority is to prevent spread of infection.*

Rationale: This client is experiencing the classic signs of tuberculosis, productive cough, fever, night sweats, and weight loss. Airborne precautions are used if the organism can cause infection over long distances when suspended in the air (e.g., TB, rubeola). It is anticipated that a specimen will be collected, but the priority is to place the client in isolation to prevent further exposure of others.

THIN Thinking: Identify Risk to Safety – *When a client presents with symptoms of tuberculosis and has risk factors, immediate isolation is required to prevent the spread of illness.* **NCLEX®:** Safety and Infection Control **QSEN:** Safety

29. **The nurse is presenting a workshop in a senior community center about the prevention of pneumonia. Which observations should the nurse address with the group? Select all that apply.**
    1. 💡 A man is coughing into his hand.
    2. 💡 A group of participants smoking outside the community center.
    3. A woman is eating an apple without cutting it up first. *Not a concern.*
    4. 💡 Two participants are washing their hands without soap.
    5. 💡 A person is saying that they could not sleep last night.

Rationale: Pneumonia can result in significant respiratory problems and so it is important that measures are taken to reduce the risk of getting the condition. Nurses should educate individuals on the importance of preventative measures which include proper hand washing, smoking cessation, limiting close contact with persons with pneumonia, and covering a cough. Eating a healthy diet, staying hydrated, and getting enough sleep at nights are also good habits to help prevent pneumonia.

THIN Thinking: Identify Risk to Safety – *Recognition of health concerns is the role of the community-based nurse.* **NCLEX®:** Reduction of Risk Potential **QSEN:** Patient-centered Care

30. **The nurse receives the following discharge instructions for a client recently admitted with active tuberculosis (TB). How will the nurse best explain how to take these medications?**

DISCHARGE MEDICATIONS	
8/29/XX	<u>First Take:</u> isoniazid (INH) 300 mg PO daily, rifampin (RIF) 600 mg PO daily, ethambutol (EMB) 1000 mg PO daily, & pyrazinamide (PZA) 1000 mg PO daily - 7 days/week for 56 doses. <u>Then Take</u> INH & RIF PO daily - 7 days/week for 126 doses.

1. You will complete these TB medications in eight weeks. *Incorrect.*
2. 💡 There are several medications, and they should be taken exactly as prescribed.
3. You will take the ethambutol for the entire period. *Incorrect.*
4. Your medications will be done in 48 weeks. *Incorrect, it is for 26 weeks.*

Rationale: Because of the growing prevalence of multi-drug resistant-TB, the client who has active tuberculosis must be, managed aggressively. There are two phases to drug therapy for TB; these are the initial and continuation phases. Usually, treatment for clients with previously untreated TB consists of a 2-month initial phase with four drugs (isoniazid, rifampin, pyrazinamide, and ethambutol). Ethambutol is usually removed from the regimen if it is determined that all four drugs are effective against the bacteria. There are conditions, such as pregnancy or liver disease, that prevent the prescription of pyrazinamide from being a part of initial drug therapy. In those cases, isoniazid, rifampin and ethambutol are used. The regimen indicates a course of 26 weeks.

THIN Thinking: Identify Risk to Safety – *It is important for nurses to instruct clients to take all medications as prescribed.* **NCLEX®:** Pharmacological and Parental Therapies **QSEN:** Safety

Regulation

Cellular / Intracranial / Thermoregulation

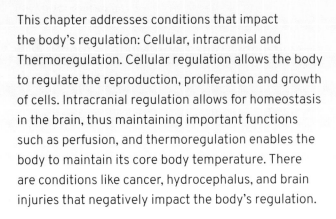

This chapter addresses conditions that impact the body's regulation: Cellular, intracranial and Thermoregulation. Cellular regulation allows the body to regulate the reproduction, proliferation and growth of cells. Intracranial regulation allows for homeostasis in the brain, thus maintaining important functions such as perfusion, and thermoregulation enables the body to maintain its core body temperature. There are conditions like cancer, hydrocephalus, and brain injuries that negatively impact the body's regulation.

Nurses are integral to the care of clients with conditions related to impaired regulation. They play a significant role in assessing for status changes pertaining to the specific regulation disorder, planning appropriate care, providing effective interventions, evaluating effectiveness of care to ensure the best possible outcomes, and providing client education to foster good follow-up care.

Priority Exemplars:

> Hydrocephalus
> Blood-borne cancers
> Lymph cancers
> Skin cancers
> Other cancers
> Acute traumatic brain injury
> Polycythemia
> Thrombocytopenia
> Hyperthermia
> Hypothermia

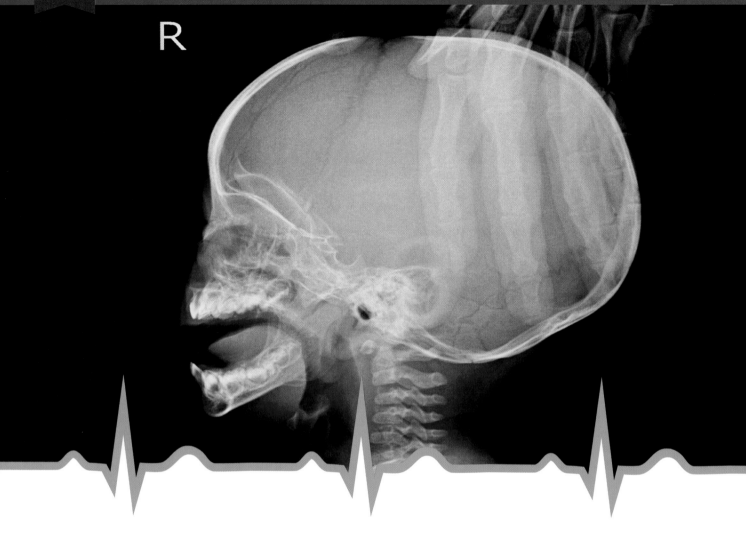

R

Go To Clinical Case 1

A 12-week-old male infant is brought to the emergency department by his mother. The mother states that the baby has not been eating well for the past 3 days and seems to be "shunning" the breast. He vomited several times in the past week. She states that the baby is not happy anymore and has become very irritable and fussy. Further, the mother is worried that something is wrong with her baby's head because it seems much larger than when she brought him home and when she touches the soft area on the baby's head, it appears swollen.

Health history reveals that the infant was born premature and spent 2 weeks in the neonatal intensive care unit but was doing well at home until recently. Vital signs are: Temperature 36.2°C, Pulse 145, Respirations 40, Blood pressure 90/60 mmHg, Weight 4.0 kg, length 50 cm.

Neurological assessment and imaging in the ED shows that the baby has hydrocephalus and he is being admitted to your unit for a ventriculoperitoneal shunt placement.

NurseThink® Time

Using the NurseThink® system, complete the priorities. Check your answers designated by 💡 in the Hydrocephalus Priority Exemplar.

✏️ Priority Assessments or Cues

1.

2.

3.

🧪 Priority Laboratory Tests/Diagnostics

1.

2.

3.

⚠️ Priority Interventions or Actions

1.

2.

3.

🚩 Priority Potential & Actual Complications

1.

2.

3.

⚕️ Priority Nursing Implications

1.

2.

3.

💧 Priority Medications

1.

2.

3.

👤 Priority Education/Discharge Issues

1.

2.

3.

Hydrocephalus

Pathophysiology/Description

> In normal functioning, cerebrospinal fluid (CSF) flows freely between the four ventricles of the brain then is reabsorbed into the bloodstream

> Cerebrospinal fluid brings nutrients to and removes waste from the brain, provides a cushioning effect for the brain and acts as a compensatory mechanism for changes in the amount of blood within the brain

> Conditions that impede the flow or absorption of CSF will result in excess accumulation and increased intracranial pressure against the brain, causing hydrocephalus

> Hydrocephalus can be defined as:
> - Congenital, meaning present at birth and the cause might be genetic or an event that occurred in fetal development
> - Acquired, meaning caused by conditions that develop after birth

> Treatment goal is to decrease pressure in the brain with a shunt or by performing a ventriculostomy (hole in the ventricle)

Priority Assessments or Cues

Complete neurological assessment to determine deficits

Watch for change in infant's positioning. A change from flexion to extension is a sign of worsening neurological status

A change from flexion to extension is a sign of worsening neurological status

Measure head, looking for an increased circumference

> Assess infant's fontanel. A bulging and non-pulsating fontanel is indicative of hydrocephalus

> Assess for McEwen's sign which is a cracked-pot sound from the thinly separated bones of the infant's head, when the head is percussed

> Observe eyes. With hydrocephalus, eyes can be bulging with downward deviation (called sunsetting)

> Ask caregivers(s) about poor feeding, irritability, vomiting, sleepiness, seizures, high-pitched cry, all signs and symptoms of hydrocephalus

> Monitor vital signs

Priority Laboratory Tests/Diagnostics

Ultrasound to determine the size of the ventricles in the brain

Magnetic resonance imaging (MRI) to view cross-sectional images of the brain

Computed tomography (CT) scan to view cross-sectional images of the brain (CT provides less detailed imaging than an MRI and is used mostly in an emergency)

Priority Interventions or Actions

> Prepare infant for surgery
> Post shunt Interventions
> - Position flat on the unaffected side to decrease pressure on the shunt and the likelihood of rapid reduction of ICF. Elevate head of bed 15-30 degrees if ICP increases. This creates gravity and fosters flow of ICP through the shunt
> - Monitor intracranial pressure to ensure functioning of the shunt
> - Measure head circumference at ordered frequency
> - Check level of consciousness, pupillary reaction, and observe for seizures every 2- 4 hours, or more frequently if needed
> - Inspect dressing immediately postoperative, hourly for first 3-4 hours and then at least every 4 hours thereafter
> - Administer medications as ordered and observe for adverse effects
> - Observe for signs of infection

Priority Potential & Actual Complications

If left untreated at birth, high likelihood it will result in brain damage, physical disabilities, stunted growth, seizures and may be fatal

> Complications post-surgery
> - Blockage, disconnection and infection of shunt
> - Seizures
> - Drowsiness
> - Irritability
> - Headache
> - Pain in abdomen if location of shunt valve is abdomen
> - Tenderness to the skin along path the shunt tube follows

Priority Nursing Implications

Crucial assessments after surgery must focus on proper functioning of the shunt, decreasing intracranial pressure and preventing infection

There must be a baseline head circumference measurement and periodic measurements after surgery to determine effectiveness of the surgery

> Keep environment calm for the infant and caregivers(s) to decrease anxiety

Educate caregivers on surgery site care, signs of shunt failure and infection, and answer their questions in simple to understand responses

> Medications (acetazolamide and furosemide) are used with low birth weight infants who have low success rate with shunts but there is no evidence they increase the infant's survival rate

> Understand the need for social interaction with the infant, incorporating talk and play as appropriate

⬤ Priority Medications

> Use of medication is controversial. Usually used to treat post hemorrhagic hydrocephalus in infants

💡 acetazolamide (Carbonic anhydrase inhibitor)

- Decreases production of CSF

- Administered via oral and intravenous routes

- Watch for early adverse effects of tinnitus, paresthesia, nausea and vomiting

💡 furosemide (Loop diuretic)

- Works better when used in combination with acetazolamide

- Administered orally (parenteral in infants given only if unable to take oral)

- Watch for common side effects of low blood pressure, hearing loss and dehydration

👤 Priority Education/Discharge Issues

> Shunt replacement as infant grows

💡 Wash incision daily with mild soap, rinse and dry by patting gently

💡 Monitor for complications and malfunctioning of shunt

💡 List of symptoms that require an immediate call to the health care provider

_____

_____

_____

_____

_____

_____

_____

_____

Go To Clinical Answers

Text designated by 💡 are the top answers for the Go To Clinical related to Hydrocephalus.

Hydrocephalus

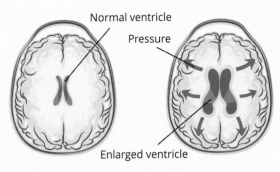

Normal ventricle

Pressure

Enlarged ventricle

Image 10-1: The increased pressure in the brain disrupts regulation globally in the client.

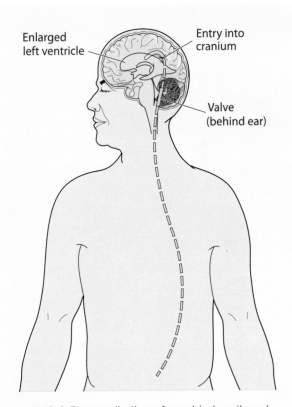

Enlarged left ventricle

Entry into cranium

Valve (behind ear)

Image 10-2: The complications of a ventriculoperitoneal shunt can arise at anytime. Review the Hydrocephalus Association's website (www.hydroassoc.org) for discussions about these problems. This will help you on NCLEX® with questions that address the Reduction of Risk Potential client needs.

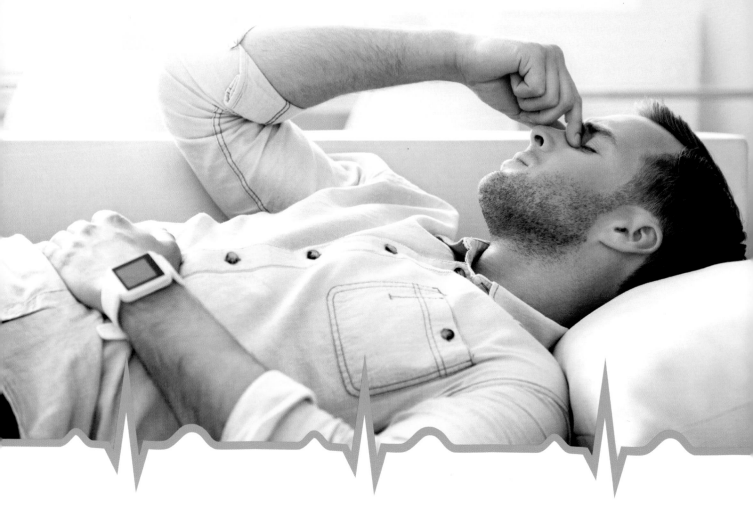

Go To Clinical Case 2

H. L. is a 22-year-old Caucasian male who presents to the emergency department (ED), reporting "weakness and just not feeling well" over the past two weeks. He looks emaciated and pale and says that he hasn't been eating well as he seems to have lost his appetite. He further states that his joints feel weak and all that he has been wanting to do is just stay in bed. He notices that his gums bleed when he brushes his teeth. His mother is accompanying him and is very worried about her son. She adds that last week when he took his shirt off, she noticed bruising on his body and thought he may have been in a fight. He denied being in a fight and was not aware of how he got the bruises. His mother is distraught and wants to know what is wrong with her son.

Vital signs in the ED: Temperature 38.2°C, Pulse 102, Respirations 18, Blood pressure 122/70 mmHg.

Preliminary assessment and labs are done in the ED and acute lymphocytic leukemia is suspected. H.L. is admitted to the oncology unit for further work up and possible treatment.

You are the nurse who admits H. L. and since you work a consistent day shift, you also care for him over the next few weeks as he is tested, diagnosed and undergoes a bone marrow transplant with cells donated by his older brother.

NurseThink® Time

Using the NurseThink® system, complete the priorities. Check your answers designated by 💡 in the Blood-borne cancers Priority Exemplar.

✏ Priority Assessments or Cues

1.

2.

3.

🧪 Priority Laboratory Tests/Diagnostics

1.

2.

3.

⚠ Priority Interventions or Actions

1.

2.

3.

🚩 Priority Potential & Actual Complications

1.

2.

3.

⚕ Priority Nursing Implications

1.

2.

3.

💧 Priority Medications

1.

2.

3.

👤 Priority Education/Discharge Issues

1.

2.

3.

Blood-borne cancers

Pathophysiology/Description

> Acute lymphocytic leukemia (ALL) is an aggressive cancer of the blood and bone marrow caused by out of control growth of abnormal white blood cells (WBC). It invades the blood system quickly

> The exact cause of ALL is unknown but possible risk factors are exposure to chemicals and radiation, being Caucasian versus African American, male versus female, and having had viral infections

> A bone marrow transplant for ALL replaces the bad WBCs with healthy matched donor cells. The process is done in several phases

Priority Assessments or Cues

- Ask about influenza-like symptoms, which are fatigue, fever, anorexia, shortness of breath and pain/tenderness to bones or joints. This is because some leukemia symptoms resemble those seen with influenza

- Assess for bleeding, bruising, bone soreness, swollen lymph nodes, enlargement of spleen, and infection. Infection results from neutropenia

- Assess results of blood counts

> Conduct thorough assessment of all body systems (respiratory, renal and cardiac are crucial)

> Monitor vital signs

> Determine social support as client is likely to need ongoing physical support when discharged

> Assess client's understanding of treatment protocol

> Assess for graft-versus-host-disease (GVHD). This indicates a rejection of the host tissue by the implanted donor tissue

Priority Laboratory Tests/Diagnostics

- Complete blood count with differential. Likely to see low platelets causing bruising and bleeding, low red blood cells (RBC) causing tiredness and shortness of breath, and low-normal white blood cells, increasing risk of infection

- Blood chemistries and coagulation to determine kidney and liver problems caused by the cancer spreading or by side effects of chemotherapy

- Bone marrow aspiration and biopsy. Result will identify leukemic blasts, which are immature cells

> Lumbar puncture to determine metastasis to brain and spinal cord

> Computed tomography (CT), magnetic resonance imaging (MRI), ultrasound. These determine any organ enlargement and/or metastasis of the cancer

Priority Interventions or Actions

> Prepare client for bone marrow biopsy and assess for bleeding, pain and client's level of consciousness post procedure

- Maintain thorough hand washing, keeping environment clean and using strict aseptic technique for all procedures. These actions protect client from infection

> Ensure client is educated about the process of bone marrow transplant and side effects, and is prepared to start the conditioning phase

> Conditioning Phase is aimed at destroying damaged cells

- Administer several regimens of high dose chemotherapy and monitor for side effects

- Administer RBCs, platelets and antibiotics as ordered

- Support through radiation if combined with chemotherapy

- Monitor for hemorrhagic cystitis

- Watch for low neutrophil count and place client in positive pressure isolation if required. An absolute neutrophil count of less than 500 cells/uL is considered severe neutropenia

> Infusion and engraftment phase

- Administer and monitor infusion

- Assess for signs of bleeding and sepsis

- Administer drugs to prevent GVHD

- Administer immunosuppressants, antiemetics and antibiotics as ordered

> Post-transplant

- Assist with scheduling of follow-up visits

- Determine psychosocial status

- Assess for late effects of BMT

Priority Potential & Actual Complications

- Graft-versus-host-disease (GVHD)

- Stem cell failure

> Viral and fungal infections

- Bleeding

> Sterility, cataracts, gastrointestinal and liver complications

Priority Nursing Implications

- Understand effects of chemotherapy drugs and radiation; conduct frequent assessment for adverse effects of therapy

- Most chemotherapy drugs are vesicants that can cause significant damage if leaked from veins; be watchful for swelling, redness or pain at the client's intravenous site

> Provide supportive care and assess client for means of

social support upon discharge

💡 Create an environment that decreases the risk of infection

> Ensure thorough client education and health maintenance on disease process

> Epoetin alfa can cause life-threatening heart or circulatory problems

> Prednisone can cause corticosteroid withdrawal if stopped abruptly

> Be careful with vincristine administration. Several deaths have been reported from administration of the drug intrathecally. It must only be administered intravenously

> Methotrexate at high doses causes severe bone marrow suppression so must be given with a rescue antidote called leucovorin

💧 Priority Medications

💡 vincristine, daunorubicin, asparaginase, methotrexate
- Chemotherapy
- Administered intravenously, intramuscularly in large muscle, or orally
- Common side effects of chemotherapy drugs are myelosuppression, hair loss, nausea and vomiting, fatigue and infection

💡 prednisone
- Corticosteroid used to treat possible allergic reactions caused by chemotherapy drugs
- Administered in liquid or tablet form. Given with food or milk to decrease stomach upset
- Usual dose is 5-60 mg daily. Dosage is tapered to prevent prednisone withdrawal

> epoetin alfa
- Hemopoietic growth factor that promotes red blood cell growth
- Administered via intravenous or subcutaneous routes and dosage is weight based
- Usual range of dose is 2,000–40,000 units 1-3 times weekly

💡 filgrastim (commonly known as G-CSF)
- Colony-stimulating factor that treats neutropenia
- Administered daily subcutaneous or intravenous. Stopped when absolute neutrophil is above 10,000 cells/mm^3
- Common range of dose is 5-10 mcg/kg/day

👤 Priority Education/Discharge Issues

> Educate on the following:

   💡 Signs and symptoms of GVHD, cell graft failure, infection and bleeding prevention

   💡 Being around people, animals, flowers and the risk each contributes to the individual's health

   - Physical and sexual activity
   - Exposure to sun

- Not stopping prednisone abruptly to avoid prednisone withdrawal
- Cleanliness of environment
- Social support
- Nutritional intake

💡 Using toothbrush with soft bristles to brush teeth

- Female not becoming pregnant while getting chemotherapy drugs (toxic to fetus)
- Driving and return to normal activities (Work, school, etc.)

Go To Clinical Answers

Text designated by 💡 are the top answers in the Go to Clinical related to Blood-borne cancers.

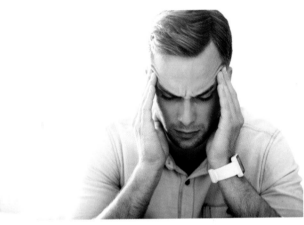

Image 10-3: Because the symptoms of blood-borne cancers can be so vague and mimic another disease, the nurse must consider various presentations.

_____

_____

_____

_____

_____

_____

_____

_____

Skin cancers

📋 Pathophysiology/Description

> Skin cancer is uncontrolled growth of abnormal skin cells

> Most common cancer in United States

> Three types of skin cancer
> - Basal cell carcinoma
> - Squamous cell carcinoma
> - Melanoma

> Melanoma is the least common, but the most lethal of the three
> - Occurs when melanocytes (cells that produce pigment) mutate and become cancerous
> - Peaks between ages 20 and 45
> - Risk factors are ethnicity (Caucasian most common), ultraviolet rays, fair-skinned in complexion and skin with large moles
> - Uses TNM staging system and is staged based on the thickness of the tumor

✏️ Priority Assessments or Cues

> Perform thorough skin assessment in good lighting. Palpate lymph nodes in area of lesions

> Use the ABCDEs to assess moles on the body:
> - **A**symmetry, which is an unbalanced lesion with irregular surface
> - **B**order is irregular and indistinct
> - **C**olor is variegated and not uniformly colored. A blue shade is bad (ominous)
> - **D**iameter, with moles larger than 6 mm being more suspicious
> - **E**levation or evolution (change over time)

> Conduct complete and thorough client history by asking about pain, pruritus, and tenderness of mole (These do not exist in a nevus that is benign). Ask about family history (melanoma occurs in families)

🧪 Priority Laboratory Tests/Diagnostics

> Biopsy gives information on the thickness of the cancerous lesion as well as the type and level of invasion. A biopsy confirms the disease

> After diagnosis is made stage the extent of the disease by performing
> - Complete blood count
> - Liver function test
> - Computed tomography (CT) scan

⚠️ Priority Interventions or Actions

> Prepare client for excision of lesion

> Administer and monitor chemotherapy and immunotherapy

> Assess client for pain related to surgical excision

> Monitor excision site for bleeding, healing and signs of infection

> Monitor graft site (if grafting of skin is done)

> Provide emotional and holistic support (surgery may cause disfiguring)

> Provide client education about course of treatment (To defray anxiety and doubt)

> Monitor symptoms to determine metastasis

🚩 Priority Potential & Actual Complications

> Surgical site infection

> Metastasis (Deeper and thicker melanoma tissue has higher risks of metastasis)

> Recurrence of melanoma

🩺 Priority Nursing Implications

> Know that client will need emotional support because surgery may cause disfigurement

> Awareness that melanoma is familial so provide client teaching about the importance of follow-up with other close family members

> Understand complications of melanoma and provide client education

> Client must be taught how to detect the early signs of melanoma

> If temozolomide capsule is opened accidentally, do not inhale or touch the contents. Flush with water if contact

> Interleukin causes the serious reaction of capillary leak syndrome, especially in high doses. This results in low blood pressure and poor blood flow to the internal organs. Shaking the medication container or syringe may render the medication ineffective

🩸 Priority Medications

> Radiotherapy
> - Uses a series of radiation over several days to kill cancer cells
> - Used alone or in combination with chemotherapy, immunotherapy or surgery
> - Blistering, redness, peeling, itching and weeping of the skin are side effects of radiation

> dacarbazine, temozolomide, paclitaxel
  - Chemotherapy agents
  - Administered intravenously or orally
  - Assess for bleeding, fatigue and infection. Monitor red and white blood cell counts and platelets

> interferon-alpha, interleukin-2
  - Cytokines for immunotherapy
  - Administered intramuscularly, intravenously, subcutaneously or directly in the lesion
  - Injection site reaction, flu-like symptoms, dizziness, GI upset, and headaches are common side effects

> pembrolizumab
  - PD-1 inhibitor (newer form of treatment) for immunotherapy
  - Administered as intravenous infusion every 2-3 weeks
  - Common side effects are constipation, nausea, fatigue, hyponatremia and joint pain

👤 Priority Education/Discharge Issues

> Teach client how to do skin self-examination monthly (Will need a hand-held as well as full-length mirror, and good lighting)

> Ensure client understands the signs of melanoma and what findings to report to the physician

> Teach about side effects of treatment and complications of the condition

> Ensure client understands the importance of getting an annual health assessment

> Teach client how to avoid sun exposure
  - Wear sunscreen (Must block ultraviolet A and B radiation)
  - Apply sunscreen about 15 minutes before exposure and every 2 hours while exposed
  - Avoid the sun on the hottest days
  - Avoid getting sunburned
  - Avoid tanning beds
  - Avoid sunbeds and sunlamps

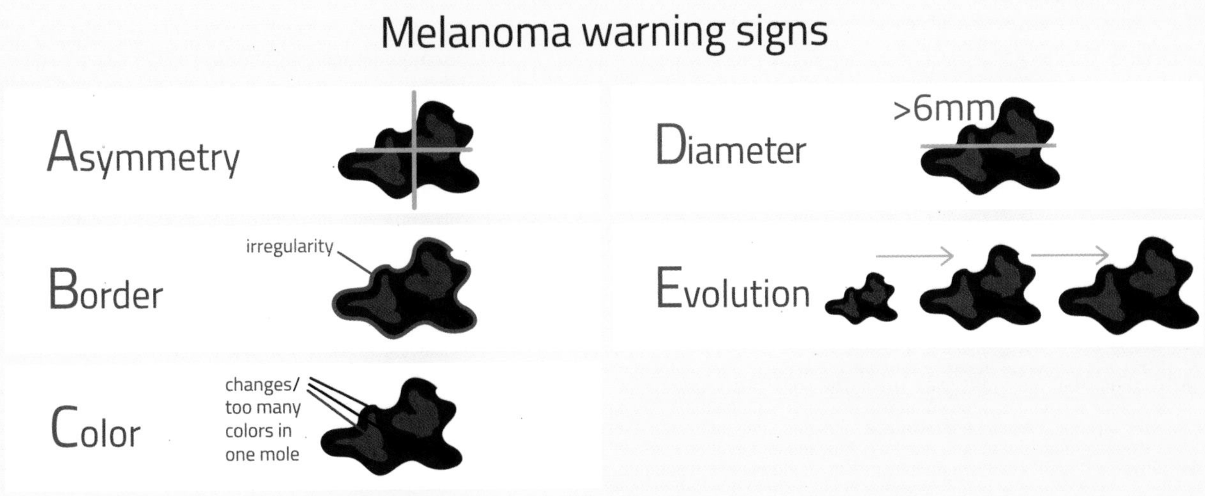

_____

_____

_____

_____

_____

_____

_____

_____

_____

Melanoma warning signs

Asymmetry

Border — irregularity

Color — changes/ too many colors in one mole

Diameter — >6mm

Evolution

Image 10-4: Conduct an internet search for pictures of skin cancer and compare to this chart. Can you identify the ABCDEs in this chart on the pictures you are reviewing?

Lymph cancers

Pathophysiology/Description

> Lymphoma is a type of cancer that has its origin in lymphocytes. There are two types, Hodgkin's and Non-Hodgkin's

> Hodgkin's Lymphoma (HL)
>   • Starts anywhere in the body where there is lymph tissue but is often found in a lymph node. The HL cells are called Reed-Sternberg cells
>   • Peaks in early 20s and after age 50. Has familial tendency
>   • Seen in military men who had Agent Orange exposure. Commonly seen in those receiving chronic immunosuppressive therapy
>   • Linked to the Epstein-Barr virus. There are four stages to HL and Lugano classification is used to stage the disease

Priority Assessments or Cues

> Assess body for enlarged painless lumps in the neck, under the arm, or in the groin

> Determine alcohol intake (Lumps may cause pain when alcohol is consumed)

> Assess for invasion of HL to other organs, indicated by abdominal pain, cough, bone pain, and jaundice

> Ask client about B symptoms to help staging
>   • B symptoms may predict how the cancer is likely to behave and which treatments might be best to start with. These symptoms are drenching night sweats, fever and weight loss
>   • B symptoms are most common in more rapidly growing lymphomas

> Assess for understanding of the disease and treatment options

Priority Laboratory Tests/Diagnostics

> Lymph node biopsy shows Reed-Sternberg cells

> X-ray and computed tomography (CT) scan of chest, abdomen and pelvis will help to define the clinical stage

> Positron emission tomography (PET) scan help to stage the disease as well as determine response to therapy

> Complete blood count (CBC), erythrocyte sedimentation rate (ESR) and platelet count do not diagnose the disease but help to determine involvement of other organs

Priority Interventions or Actions

> Prepare client for biopsy procedure

> Administer chemotherapy and monitor for adverse effects

> Administer prednisone and filgrastim and monitor for adverse effects

> Support through radiation

> Minimize risk of infections

> Manage system problems that may arise because of the cancer

Priority Potential & Actual Complications

> Complications are treatment related, including weakened immune system, herpes infections, cardiomyopathy, pericarditis, pneumococcal sepsis, development of second malignancies, and infertility

Priority Nursing Implications

> Understand that risk for infection is major for this client

> Raynaud's phenomenon, which is discoloration of fingers and toes, is a consideration with ABVD therapy

> vinblastine causes constipation

> Withhold etoposide for platelet count below 50,000 mm^3 or absolute neutrophil count below 500 mm^3

> Administer injection carefully to prevent leakage of drug into tissue; severe damage can occur with drug leakage

> dexamethasone and prednisone can cause corticosteroid withdrawal if stopped abruptly

Priority Medications

> adriamycin, bleomycin, vinblastine, dacarbazine (ABVD therapy)
>   • Chemotherapy agents
>   • Administered via intravenous infusion or injection, intramuscular or subcutaneous
>   • Assess for bleeding, fatigue and infection. Monitor red and white blood cell counts and platelets

> mechlorethamine, doxorubicin, vinblastine, vincristine, bleomycin, etoposide, prednisone (Stanford V therapy)
>   • Chemotherapy agents
>   • Administered via tablet and intravenous routes
>   • Causes increased risk of infection, anemia and bleeding due to decreased platelets, red and white blood cells

> prednisone
>   • Corticosteroid used to treat possible allergic reactions caused by chemotherapy drugs
>   • Administered in liquid or tablet form. Given with food or milk to decrease stomach upset
>   • Usual dose is 5-60 mg daily. Dosage is tapered to prevent prednisone withdrawal

> filgrastim (commonly known as G-CSF)
>   • Colony-stimulating factor that treats neutropenia
>   • Administered daily subcutaneous or intravenous. Stopped when absolute neutrophil is above 10,000 cells/mm^3
>   • Common range of dose is 5-10 mcg/kg/day

Priority Education/Discharge Issues

> Educate client on
>   • Prevention of infection, long-term complications of the disease, not stopping prednisone abruptly, hair loss, and verbalization of feelings. Also discuss infertility and the fact that men may need to consider sperm banking if they desire to have children

> Eliminating factors that increase the risk of other cancers

Other cancers

Pathophysiology/Description

> Breast cancer
  - Out of control malignant cells in the breast
  - Can invade surrounding tissue or metastasize to distant areas of the body
  - Can start anywhere in the breast but point of origin is quite often the ducts that carry milk to the nipple
  - Symptoms are hard, painless lump with irregular edges (but some lumps might also be soft and round), breast swelling, dimpling, irritation, pain, discharge, redness and retraction of nipple
  - No sure way to prevent breast cancer but risk factors are obesity, inactivity, birth control, having had no children, first child after age 30, post-menopause hormone therapy and alcohol intake
  - Staging is with the TNM staging system is used (stages 0 -IV). Higher stage means greater spread of the cancer

> Brain cancer
  - Defined as primary (develop from cells in the brain) or secondary (travel from somewhere else in the body to the brain, called metastasis)
  - Metastatic brain cancer is much more common than primary cancer
  - Signs and symptoms are confusion, memory loss, seizures, headaches, vision problems, gait disturbances, paralysis, aphasia
  - Treatment of metastatic brain cancer is palliative. If no treatment then median survival is one month. With treatment, survival is 3-6 months
  - Treated with surgery, radiation and chemotherapy
  - Brain cancer is not staged but graded as I-IV, with higher grade indicating more rapid growth

> Bone cancer
  - Defined as with brain cancer (primary vs secondary)
  - Abnormal bone is formed, or bone is destroyed
  - Secondary (metastatic) bone cancer is the most common
  - Several types of bone cancer. The name is based on the cells that form the tumor or the part of the bone and tissue that is affected. Some types are multiple myeloma, osteosarcoma, chondrosarcoma, fibrosarcoma and Ewing's sarcoma
  - Metastatic bone cancer primarily affects the femur, humerus, spine and skull
  - Treatment of metastatic bone cancer is palliative
  - Grading is as with brain cancer above (I- IV)

> Lung cancer
  - Defined as with bone cancer above (primary vs secondary)
  - Metastatic (secondary) lung cancer is the most common
  - Most lung cancer cases are related to inhalation of carcinogens, like cigarette smoke and asbestos. Carcinogen binds to the cell's DNA and causes damage. This causes abnormal growth of the cells and cell changes, leading to malignancy
  - Lung cancer is classified as small-cell and non-small-cell. There is further classification for the non-small cell type
  - Non-small cell type is the most common lung cancer, 75-80% of all cases
  - Staged as I-IV, with stage I being the first stage of the condition and having the highest cure rate

Priority Assessments or Cues

> Assessment common to breast, brain, bone and lung cancers
  - Perform a complete physical assessment
  - Complete a detailed health history
  - Provide client education and preparation on what to expect pre, during and post-surgery
  - Review vital signs and labs
  - Assess for evidence of surgical or other infections
  - Assess impact of the client's illness on the family and work with others on the healthcare team to address these impacts
  - Assess baseline pain level and use it to inform changes in pain intervention

> Breast cancer
  - Assess client's feelings about diagnosis, treatment and possible breast reconstruction
  - Ongoing assessment of client's feelings about body image disturbance post-surgery

> Brain cancer
  - Conduct a thorough initial and ongoing focused neurological assessment
  - Emaciation and muscle wasting are common in clients with brain cancer so assess nutrition
  - Assess client's readiness to verbalize feelings about fear of dying, altered lifestyle or changed appearance

> Bone cancer
  - Assess for degree of disability, as bone cancer often ends in amputation of limbs
  - Assess for signs and symptoms of hypercalcemia (muscle weakness, vomiting, nausea, seizures). Hypercalcemia is a common, and serious occurrence in bone cancer
  - Ask about fractures or related symptoms
  - Assess for numbness and tingling as cancer in the spine can elicit these symptoms
  - Ongoing focused assessment on musculoskeletal system

> Lung cancer
  - Assess for persistent cough, shortness of breath, wheezing that has new onset, respiratory infections, hoarseness, chest pain worsened by laughing, breathing or coughing, blood in sputum
  - Ask about exposure to risk factors
  - Ongoing focused assessment on respiratory and cardiac systems

Other cancers

⚗ Priority Laboratory Tests/Diagnostics

> Breast cancer
  - Clinical breast exam
  - Screening mammograms, ultrasound, magnetic resonance imaging, breast tomosynthesis or 3D mammography (this is a newer test) are used to diagnose the disease
  - Breast biopsy is used to diagnose the disease

> Brain Cancer
  - Computed tomography (CT) scan and magnetic resonance imaging (MRI). An MRI can find small tumors that a CT scan might miss

> Bone cancer
  - Computed tomography (CT) scan, magnetic resonance imaging (MRI), X-rays, bone scans and bone biopsy. These are used to diagnose the tumor

> Lung cancer
  - Chest X-ray, computed tomography (CT) scan, sputum cytology or fiberoptic bronchoscopy and lung biopsy. These are used to diagnose the tumor

⚠ Priority Interventions or Actions

> Interventions common to breast, brain, bone and lung cancers
  - Provide information related to before and after surgery
  - Assess surgical site for bleeding and signs of infection
  - Assess client's readiness to view surgical site for first time
  - Discuss after surgery treatment, including chemotherapy
  - Administer and monitor chemotherapy treatment
  - Provide medications to manage side effects of chemotherapy
  - Monitor for side effects of radiation therapy
  - Assess oral cavity daily (at risk for stomatitis)
  - Discuss hair loss and regrowth with client and family
  - Remove unpleasant odors and sights from environment during mealtime. They can stimulate anorexia and client already experiences increase in nausea and vomiting
  - Encourage frequent rest periods to conserve energy (treatment depletes energy)
  - Manage pain

> Breast cancer
  - Initiate client's arm and shoulder exercise, as restoration of arm function is priority
  - Manage surgical drains
  - Administer hematopoietic growth factor to help in reduction of chemotherapy-induced neutropenia

> Brain cancer
  - Frequent neurological assessment and monitoring to detect subtle new changes that may impact outcome

> Bone cancer
  - Provide prompt treatment of hypercalcemia that can occur from bone breakdown
  - Prepare client for bone graft, if bone grafting is being performed
  - Assess client's readiness to talk about loss of limb; discuss phantom pain
  - Discuss use of prosthesis

> Lung cancer
  - Prepare client for invasive testing procedures, like bronchoscopy and biopsy
  - Maintain proper airway clearance by performing suction, teaching client deep-breathing exercises and coughing
  - Administer oxygen
  - Monitor client's activity and ensure that energy conservation measures are used
  - Help client and family cope with the usual rapid progression of this disease
  - Assess readiness to discuss end-of-life treatment options

⚑ Priority Potential & Actual Complications

> Complications common to breast, brain, bone and lung cancers include, bleeding, infection, pain

> Breast cancer complications include hematoma or seroma, lymphedema, depression, loss of interest in sex, metastasis to brain, bone or lungs, and death

> Brain cancer complications include cerebral herniation, hydrocephalus, hemorrhage and stroke, coma and persistent vegetative state, and death

> Bone cancer complications include weakening of bones with susceptibility to fractures, hypercalcemia (dangerously high levels can occur), osteomyelitis, metastasis

> Lung cancer complications include respiratory failure with mechanical ventilation, pneumonitis, diminished cardiopulmonary function

℧ Priority Nursing Implications

> Breast cancer
  - Many do not consider the fact that men also get breast cancer and so many healthcare providers do not take the time to speak with men about breast cancer
  - Many persons believe that all breast cancer lumps are painless, with irregular edges. However, some lumps have round edges and are painful so teach clients to see a healthcare professional for any new lumps observed in the breast
  - Lower doses of epirubicin should be considered in clients with severe renal or liver impairment
  - With docetaxel, corticosteroid tablet is used to decrease the severity of allergic reaction and fluid retention caused by the drug
  - Dexamethasone and prednisone can cause corticosteroid withdrawal if stopped abruptly

> Brain cancer
  - Consider that this client is at high-risk for a deep vein thrombosis and pulmonary embolism, but anticoagulant is usually not prescribed because of the high-risk of brain hemorrhage. Nursing measures should be taken to minimize the above complications
  - Consider the significant physical, psychosocial and financial burden that the complications of brain cancer have on the client and caregivers. It is important to provide holistic care to the client and family
  - Do not use bevacizumab within 28 days before or after a planned surgery as it interferes with wound healing
> Bone cancer
  - Bones can be weakened by cancer and fracture can occur
  - Disfigurement can occur, especially with amputations. Be sensitive to body image disturbances with client
  - Bones may become weakened and need structural support and stabilization to prevent pathological fractures. Bone cement, internal fixation or arthroplasty may be used to achieve stabilization
> Lung cancer
  - Lung cancer is a very subtle disease in that its growth is insidious

Priority Medications

> doxorubicin, epirubicin, daunorubicin, paclitaxel, docetaxel, temozolomide, bevacizumab, vincristine, procarbazine, mitotane, cisplatin, etoposide
  - Chemotherapy drugs used in a variety of combinations and vary in duration
  - Administered via intravenous, injection or infusion
  - Assess for bleeding fatigue, and infection. Monitor red and white blood cell counts and platelets
> filgrastim (commonly known as G-CSF)
  - Colony-stimulating factor that treats neutropenia
  - Administered daily subcutaneous or intravenous. Stopped when absolute neutrophil is above 10,000 cells/mm^3
  - Common range of dose is 5-10 mcg/kg/day
> dexamethasone, prednisone
  - Corticosteroids used to suppress immune response and reduce inflammation
  - Administered intravenous or oral, with food or milk to decrease stomach upset
  - Drugs must be tapered
> epoetin alfa
  - Hemopoietic growth factor that promotes red blood cell growth
  - Administered via intravenous or subcutaneous routes and dosage is weight based
  - Usual range of dose is 2,000 – 40,000 units 1-3 times weekly
> mannitol
  - Diuretic used to decrease fluid in brain
  - Administered via intravenous solution
  - Test dose is to be done in clients with renal impairment

> phenytoin
  - Antiepileptic drug to prevent seizures in clients with brain cancer
  - Administered intravenous and oral but mostly give via the oral route
  - Gingival hyperplasia is a common adverse effect
> calcitonin
  - Administered via subcutaneous or intramuscular routes
  - Used to decrease bone destruction
  - May cause increased bone pain in first few months of treatment

Priority Education/Discharge Issues

> Education common to breast, brain, bone and lung cancers
  - Provide education and expectations of after surgery treatment, like chemotherapy
  - Ensure that client knows the side effects of chemotherapy, which are nausea, vomiting, hair loss, bad taste in mouth, mucositis and fatigue
  - Teach management of complications such as antiemetics for nausea and bicarbonate solution for mucositis
  - Determine readiness to assume self-care and fill in any gaps in knowledge that may exist
  - Instruct on when to engage in pre-surgery activities
  - Educate on care of incision site
  - Teach the importance of timely follow-up care
> Breast Cancer
  - Provide instructions about drain care and how to measure drainage to determine when it is less than 30 mL
  - Teach care of incision site and when to apply lotions and creams (when completely healed)
  - Teach range of motion exercises to affected arm
  - Teach about phantom sensations, feeling like the breast is still present. Make client aware that this feeling usually stays for a few months but will slowly go away
  - Client and partner may benefit from many community resources so assist with locating resources
> Brain cancer
  - Teach that there may be potential reoccurrence or worsening of brain cancer symptoms
  - Teach that the client may require 24-hour long-term care
  - Identify community resources
  - Teach proper dental care due to gingival hyperplasia effect from phenytoin
> Bone cancer
  - Discuss use of prosthesis and have client demonstrate donning and doffing
  - Ensure client knows how to secure assistive devices
> Lung cancer
  - Teach client about ways to keep airway clear
  - Teach about the importance of conserving energy
  - Assist client and family with pulmonary rehabilitation consultation if ordered

Acute traumatic brain injury

Pathophysiology/Description

> Defined as a disruption in the brain's normal function due to some type of trauma
  - Penetrating force to the head
  - Blow received to the head
  - Bumping the head
  - Jolt to the head

> A seemingly minor head injury can result in disrupted blood flow, poor tissue perfusion and major brain damage

> Signs and symptoms of traumatic brain injury (TBI) can occur immediately, or can be delayed

> Traumatic brain injury is considered mild or moderate-severe
  - Mild: neurological function loss is temporary and there is no visible structural damage (as in a concussion)
  - Moderate-severe: From minimal brain damage (bruising) to more widespread damage (damage to brain hemispheres, intracranial bleeding)

> Far-reaching physical and psychological effects can result from TBI

Priority Assessments or Cues

> Initial assessment only
  - Ask about the time, cause and source of the injury. If client unconscious, elicit information from family members or others who may have witnessed the injury
  - Physical assessment to determine if other injuries exist on any other part of body
  - Measure vital signs

> Initial and ongoing assessment
  - Glasgow Coma Scale
  - Neurological assessment (must be very thorough). Head injury may impact several neurological functions

> Respiratory assessment
  - Injury to brain can alter respiratory function
  - Can experience hypoxemia due to systemic changes from head injuries

> Cardiovascular assessment
  - At risk for deep vein thrombosis because of immobility (if unconscious)
  - May develop cardiac dysrhythmias, hypo or hypertension

> Integumentary assessment
  - Immobility due to unconsciousness causes risk of skin breakdown

> Assess other systems as symptoms present

Priority Laboratory Tests/Diagnostics

> Detailed neurological exam

> Magnetic resonance imaging (MRI) shows extent of brain injury

> Computed tomography (CT) scans are done ongoing to monitor the injury

> Intracranial pressure monitoring determines pressure in the brain

Priority Interventions or Actions

> Anticipate client's needs as injury may prevent ability to make needs known

> Assess client initially and as frequently as the client's needs dictate
  - Monitor level of consciousness and motor function, looking for changes in neurological status
  - Level of consciousness is the best indicator of change in neurological function
  - Manage the airway. An obstructed airway fosters CO_2 retention which can cause the vessels in the brain to dilate, creating an increase in intracranial pressure (ICP)
  - Assess for signs of possible hematoma or brain hemorrhage

> If client is unconscious
  - Maintain head of bed at 30 degrees to decrease venous ICP
  - Suction effectively as secretions elicit coughing, which increases ICP
  - Monitor blood gasses as they need to be in normal range to support flow of blood to brain

Priority Potential & Actual Complications

> Complications are many and can go from mild to severe. Here are a few of the more serious ones
  - Cerebral edema and herniation
  - Hematomas and hemorrhage
  - Decreased cerebral perfusion
  - Impaired ventilation and oxygenation
  - Seizures
  - Headaches

> Long-term complications
  - Disability
  - Death

Priority Nursing Implications

> Baseline and ongoing neurologic assessments are crucial, so that subtle changes can be identified quickly

> Understand the association between vital signs and the client's ICP

- Increasing systolic blood pressure, slowed heart rate and widening pulse pressure are indicative of increasing ICP

> All body systems are potentially impacted by a brain injury, so the nurse must ensure measures that support all body systems

> Client and family will need long-term community involvement to help with long-term needs of client

> Monitor potassium when on furosemide as the drug is potassium-wasting

💧 Priority Medications

> mannitol, furosemide
- Diuretics used to decrease fluid and reduce pressure in brain
- Administered via intravenous solution
- Test dose of mannitol is to be done in clients with renal impairment

> nimodipine
- Calcium channel blocker
- Widens blood vessels and fosters improved blood flow to brain
- Administered orally and can be given via gastric tube

> phenytoin
- Antiepileptic drug to prevent seizures
- Administered intravenous and oral
- A loading dose is usually given, followed by a maintenance dose

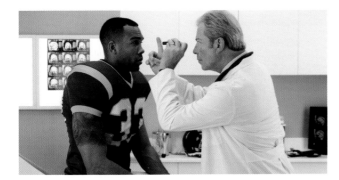

Image 10-5: Write out 3 statements by this football player that could indicate there is a brain injury.

_____

_____

_____

👤 Priority Education/Discharge Issues

> If client is being discharged to home
- Teach and reinforce client's prognosis with client and family
- Ensure client's limitations are understood by client and family
- Teach self-care management strategies
- Reinforce safety for the client, such as fall prevention techniques
- Teach about complications that require a call to the neurologist
- If being discharged with seizure medications, provide teaching about the medication
- Teach family about home care environment modifications that are to be made to accommodate the client

> If client is being discharged to rehabilitation or long-term care
- Assist family with locating rehabilitation or long-term care placement
- Educate on what to expect at these two levels of care

BEHAVIOR	RESPONSE
Eye Opening	4. Spontaneously 3. To speech 2. To pain 1. No response
Verbal	5. Oriented to time, person and place 4. Confused 3. Inappropriate words 2. Incomprehensible sounds 1. No response
Motor	6. Obeys command 5. Moves to localized pain 4. Flex to withdraw from pain 3. Abnormal flexion 2. Abnormal extension 1. No response

Image 10-6: Be sure to practice using the Glasgow Coma Scale.

Polycythemia

Pathophysiology/Description

> Polycythemia: Bone marrow makes excess red blood cells. Platelets and white blood cells are usually in excess as well

> Blood becomes thickened, increasing potential for blood clots and subsequent stroke or heart attack

> More common in older adults

> With treatment, survival is over 10 years. Survival decreases to 6-18 months without treatment

> Two classifications of polycythemia

  • Primary (Polycythemia Vera): the result of genes that have mutated. Platelet, erythrocyte and leukocyte counts are elevated but the highest count is erythrocyte. Hematocrit may exceed 60%

  • Secondary: excessive erythropoietin production in response to situations where oxygen is reduced (i.e. high altitude). No treatment is necessary as it resolves when the cause is removed

Priority Assessments or Cues

> Conduct a complete health history

  • Ask about symptoms experienced

  • Ask about any previous associated illnesses like a stroke, blood clot or heart attack

  • Assess for any abnormal bleeding and ask about risk factors

  • Determine social history, especially alcohol intake

> Ask about over-the-counter (OTC) supplements. Iron is in many vitamins and it can further stimulate the production of red blood cells

> Perform physical assessment

  • Important to check spleen for splenomegaly

  • Assess for gastric fullness or bloating, symptoms caused by enlarged spleen

  • Assess for itching, a common problem with the condition

> Measure vital signs

Priority Laboratory Tests/Diagnostics

> Complete blood count (CBC)

  • Erythrocytes, platelets, leukocytes, hemoglobin and hematocrit levels are elevated

> Blood smear will indicate shape, size and condition of blood cells

> Erythropoietin test (EPO). Erythropoietin directs the production of red blood cells. The level in polycythemia is low because it is not directing RBC production. A mutated gene is doing the direction

Priority Interventions or Actions

> Phlebotomy is important therapy

  • Remove 500 mL blood weekly to decrease viscosity of blood and deplete iron store so client will be iron deficient. This prevents the continuous excessive production of erythrocytes

> Administer and monitor for adverse effects of medications and phlebotomy treatment

> Manage side effects of medications

Priority Potential & Actual Complications

> Tiredness from repeated phlebotomy

> Damaged veins from repeated phlebotomy

> Thrombosis, which can cause blood clots, stroke, heart attack and pulmonary embolism

> Enlarged spleen

> Long-term complications

  • Myelofibrosis where bone marrow no longer produces healthy functioning cells and scar tissue forms

  • Leukemia occurring over time. The longer the condition exists, the higher the risk of leukemia

Priority Nursing Implications

> Consider the impact of treatment on the client and understand that tiredness will be evident. The client's status must be factored in when planning daily nursing care

> Ensure that client is educated on the significant risk of blood clots

> This condition causes potentially fatal or life-threatening neuropsychiatric, autoimmune, and infectious disorders. Occasional clinical evaluations are recommended

Priority Medications

> hydroxyurea
> - An antimetabolite, chemotherapy agent
> - Administered orally as pill form. May be dissolved in water
> - Myelosuppression, edema, headache and drowsiness are the most common side effect

> busulfan
> - Chemotherapy agent
> - Administered oral or intravenous; tablet form only available as brand name, Myleran
> - Infection, bleeding and anemia are common side effects

> interferon-alpha
> - Cytokines for immunotherapy
> - Administered intramuscularly, intravenously, subcutaneously or directly in the lesion
> - Injection site reaction, flu-like symptoms, dizziness, GI upset, and headaches are common side effects

> anagrelide
> - Platelet reducing agent
> - Decrease platelet count and reduce the risk of thrombotic events
> - Administered orally as capsules

Priority Education/Discharge Issues

> Teach client about side effects of medications
> Teach about long-term complications of the condition, like myelofibrosis
> Discuss conditions that can exacerbate the condition, like smoking or high altitude
> Educate on how to reduce risk of getting a blood clot
> - Refrain from crossing the legs as it impedes blood flow. Do not wear clothing that is tight or restrictive
> - Refrain from sedentary lifestyle, walk frequently
> Decrease intake of alcohol to help reduce the risk of bleeding
> Do not take iron as it causes red blood cell production
> To help the itching
> - Use sodium bicarbonate in bath water
> - Apply cocoa butter to body
> - Use lotion and bath products that have oatmeal
> - Use cool or tepid bath water
> - Pat skin dry after bath; do not dry skin vigorously
> Teach importance of follow-up care

Thrombocytopenia

📋 Pathophysiology/Description

> Thrombocytopenia is low platelet count. The normal range of platelets in the blood is 150,000 to 450,000 per microliter. With thrombocytopenia, the count is less than 150,000 per microliter

> There are a few causes for thrombocytopenia and a myriad of reasons for these causes, such as medications and other disease processes

> Thrombocytopenia is evidenced by increased destruction of platelets, decreased production of platelets or increased consumption of platelets

✏️ Priority Assessments or Cues

> Review the result of the most recent complete blood count. The platelet count determines the severity of the client's symptoms
>   - When count is less than 20,000, petechiae (tiny red spots on skin) and bleeding can occur
>   - When count is less than 5,000, gastrointestinal and potentially lethal central nervous system hemorrhage can occur

> Assess skin for petechiae and bruising

> Assess for bleeding primarily from the nose and gastrointestinal system

> Ask about prolonged bleeding after a cut, surgery or dental procedure; blood in bowel movement or urine; medication history as some, like heparin, can induce thrombocytopenia

> Ask female about menstrual bleeding. Menstruation is excessive with thrombocytopenia

> If client is being administered heparin, assess for heparin-induced thrombocytopenia (HIT)

🧪 Priority Laboratory Tests/Diagnostics

> Complete blood count: Less than 150,000 platelets per microliter of blood indicates thrombocytopenia

⚠️ Priority Interventions or Actions

> Address intervention for underlying cause. If it is heparin-induced, stop the heparin

> Administer, and monitor platelet transfusion

> Administer corticosteroid and monitor for side effects as well as effectiveness of the drug. A corticosteroid is first drug of choice if condition is related to an issue with the immune system

> Ensure daily labs (CBC) are drawn on time and platelet count is reviewed

> Assess client's skin for petechiae and bruising

> Assess client for bleeding

🚩 Priority Potential & Actual Complications

> Hemorrhage and significant blood loss

> Spontaneous bleeding when platelet count is less than 10,000

> If client is on the blood thinner heparin, this drug can induce thrombocytopenia, called heparin-induced thrombocytopenia (HIT). With HIT, the client is at significant risk for developing a deep vein thrombosis or pulmonary embolism

☺ Priority Nursing Implications

> Understand the impact of various platelet levels on the symptoms experienced by the client

> It is important to know the specific cause of the client's thrombocytopenia so that inducing elements can be avoided

> Be mindful that false thrombocytopenia, called pseudo thrombocytopenia is common and occurs when platelets clump together on a complete blood count, causing a false low result. The blood must be redrawn if this is suspected

> Understand that bleeding is a major risk in a client with thrombocytopenia so ensure daily assessment for bleeding

> Dexamethasone and prednisone can cause corticosteroid withdrawal if stopped abruptly

🩸 Priority Medications

> dexamethasone, prednisone
>   - Corticosteroids used to suppress immune response and the antibodies for platelets
>   - Administered orally with food or milk to decrease stomach upset
>   - Must not be stopped abruptly

> argatroban, bivalirudin and angiomax
>   - Used for heparin-induced thrombocytopenia only
>   - Administered via intravenous injection
>   - Significant risk of hemorrhage

👤 Priority Education/Discharge Issues

> Teach client that delayed treatment might cause potentially fatal problems such as a heart attack or a pulmonary embolism

> Teach client to avoid any known agent that induced the condition, like heparin or alcohol

> Teach client the signs of disease exacerbation and how to contact the provider

> Educate client on assessing skin for petechiae and bruising

> Reinforce the importance of preventing actions that can result in bleeding including straining to have stools, constipation, using straight razors for shaving, using toothbrush with hard bristles

> Teach that if the platelet count is below 10,000 sexual intercourse should not be vigorous/rough due to risk of bleeding

> Teach side effects of steroids. The most important is infections

> Teach client to be cautious when using over-the-counter medications that can impair platelet function, such as aspirin and ibuprofen. Tell client to speak with pharmacist before taking a new drug

Hyperthermia

Pathophysiology/Description

> Hyperthermia is abnormally high body temperature where the body's system that regulates heat fails to manage the heat from the environment. Body temperature then rises too high to the point where it threatens health

> Sustained body temperature that is usually greater than 102.2°F (39°C)

> Forms of hyperthermia
> • Heat stroke, heat cramps, heat exhaustion, heat fatigue and heat syncope

> There are many risk factors. The list below is not exhaustive
> • Lifestyle such as inadequate intake of fluids, lack of air conditioning, overcrowding, poor or lack of access to transportation, immobility issues and homelessness
> • Health-related factors such as cardiac or renal diseases, salt-restricted diets, reduced sweating, dehydration, over/under weight and intake of alcohol

Priority Assessments or Cues

> Assess vital signs (pulse might be weak and thready with increased rate)

> Ask about what may have triggered the condition

> Assess for presenting symptoms to determine the form of hyperthermia

> Assess neuro status as there can be confusion, especially with heat exhaustion

> Assess urine status as dehydration occurs with hyperthermia

> Ask about living and health conditions

> Perform physical assessment

> If client is unconscious, measure pulmonary artery or central venous pressure to determine fluid status

Priority Laboratory Tests/Diagnostics

> Electrolytes, primarily sodium. Sodium will be low because of profuse sweating

Priority Interventions or Actions

> Monitor temperature. Tympanic or rectal gives more accurate core body temperature

> Monitor heart rate and blood pressure. As hyperthermia worsens, these vital signs increase

> Anticipate the need for oxygen therapy and have it ready. Metabolic demand for oxygen is increased with hyperthermia

> Remove excess clothing and covers from client

> Monitor environmental temperature and adjust as indicated

> Encourage and provide fluids by mouth if no contraindication

> Provide cooling mattress and cool packs

> Bathe client in tepid water

> Adjust cooling process based on the client's response

> Anticipate administration of normal saline (NS) so ensure a patent intravenous line. Normal saline restores fluid loss

> Administer and monitor internal cooling measures in severe cases with use of rectal and gastric ice water lavage

Priority Potential & Actual Complications

> Complications of hyperthermia occur when the condition is not treated
> • Sustained mental confusion
> • Coma
> • Death, occurring more commonly in elderly persons and the very young

Priority Nursing Implications

> In educating individuals on hyperthermia, consider that the risk for hyperthermia increases with a combination of the individual's health status, lifestyle choices and the outside environment

> In a severe and prolonged heat wave, older adults who live alone without air conditioning may need assistance to move to safer dwelling temporarily. As the nurse, you may have to initiate the steps to securing that safer dwelling

Priority Medications

> No specific medications to treat hyperthermia but if body systems are affected, then medications may be used to support the system issue

> Normal saline to replace fluid loss

Priority Education/Discharge Issues

> Educate client and family members about the signs and symptoms of hyperthermia

> Teach the importance of adequate fluid intake, especially in hot weather

> Instruct older adults to remain inside in hot weather. If outside, wear a hat and stay hydrated

> Instruct on adherence to air pollution alerts

> If no air conditioning in the home, instruct to go to places that have air conditioning like shopping malls, libraries, or senior centers

> Educate on seeking out cooling stations/centers that religious groups or health agencies set up in the community

> Educate on alcohol intake as it may impair thermoregulation

> Encourage intake of 8 glasses of water daily, if not contraindicated

> Teach immediate treatment of suspected hyperthermia
> • Drink adequate fluids, water or fruit/vegetable juices
> • Take a shower or sponge bath with cool water
> • Place cold wet cloth to areas where blood passes close to the surface of the skin, like armpits, neck, groin and wrists. This helps to cool the blood

Hypothermia

📋 Pathophysiology/Description

> Hypothermia occurs when the core body temperature decreases to below 95°F (35°C). Heat that the body produces cannot compensate for heat that it looses to the environment

> Stages of hypothermia are based on severity
> - Mild (mental confusion, shivering, increased heart and respiratory rates). With these responses, the body is trying to maintain heat. Body temperature ranges from 93.2 to 96.8°F (34-36°C)
> - Moderate (Shivering is more pronounced, movements slowed, fingers/toes/lips/ears turn blue, paleness occurs, heart and respiratory rates slow, metabolic rate decreases). Body temperature ranges from 89.6 to 93.2°F (32-34°C)
> - Severe (gross confusion, heart/respiratory/blood pressure rates decrease, metabolism shuts down, behavior is irrational, skin appears blue, reflexes absent, pupils fixed). Body temperature is below 89.6°F (32°C)

> Causes are
> - Exposure to cold temperature
> - Any condition that increases the loss of heat or decreases the production of heat

> Paradoxical undressing
> - Seen with moderate to severe hypothermia where the individual undresses. There is a sudden surge of blood causing the individual to feel overheated

> Risk factors
> - Homelessness, substance abuse, poor clothing, living in extremely cold environments and some chronic health conditions, like hypothyroidism

✏️ Priority Assessments or Cues

> Assess airway, breathing and circulation

> Assess vital signs (Temperature must be taken with a special low-temperature thermometer and esophageal measurement is the most accurate)

> Assess for presenting symptoms. These symptoms indicate the extent and dictate appropriate treatment

> Assess result of electrocardiogram as it will be classic for what's termed Osborn J wave which closely resembles the ST elevation that is evident in a myocardial infarction

> Ask about
> - Living conditions (homelessness is a risk factor)
> - Social history (substance abuse is a risk factor)
> - Existing health conditions (some conditions, like hypothyroidism, are risk factors)

> Perform physical assessment to determine damage to body, such as discoloration of body parts

> Assess neurological status as confusion can be evidenced in all stages of hypothermia

> Assess for hypoglycemia, which is often associated with hypothermia

🧪 Priority Laboratory Tests/Diagnostics

> Measurement of core body temperature and client's presenting symptoms

> Other tests may be done depending on impact on body systems

⚠️ Priority Interventions or Actions

> Mild hypothermia
> - Provide warm beverages
> - Put warn clothing on client
> - Encourage physical activity
> - Ongoing measurement of temperature

> Moderate hypothermia
> - Place heating blankets on client
> - Administer intravenous fluid that is warmed. Rewarming is ongoing with a goal of an increase in the body temperature to 90°F (32°C)
> - Ongoing measurement of temperature

> Moderate and severe hypothermia
> - May need to manage extracorporeal membrane oxygenation (ECMO)
> - Manage cardiopulmonary bypass
> - Ongoing measurement of temperature
> - If client has no pulse, then intervene with cardiopulmonary resuscitation (CPR)

> Treat any other systemic effects of hypothermia, like hypoglycemia

> For all types of hypothermia assess sensation to distal parts of the body

🚩 Priority Potential & Actual Complications

> Frostbite (freezing and crystallization of body tissue), coma and death

℧ Priority Nursing Implications

> Understand that because most regular thermometers do not measure below temperatures of 93.9°F (34.4°C), with hypothermia, a low-temperature thermometer must be used. Temperature is measured in the esophagus, bladder or rectum

> Understand the implications for the client with hypothermia after discharge. Community resources may be needed to return the client to safe living conditions and/or safe modified lifestyle

> Frostbite may cause loss of body parts; psychological and physical support may be needed

● Priority Medications

> No specific medications to treat hypothermia but if body systems are affected, then medications may be used to support the system issue

● Priority Education/Discharge Issues

> Teach about proper dress when planning outside trips

> Educate on the possible impact of alcohol intake on hypothermia, especially in outdoor activities, and discuss importance of having one sober individual present

> If homebound, recommend someone checks on client regularly and ensure the home temperature is at least 64°F (18°C)

> Assist homeless individuals with resources such as location of shelters to go in cold weather

> Assist poor and elderly individuals to secure resources of clothing, shelter and financial assistance

> Educate on the importance of taking medications for existing health conditions that may impact body temperature, like hypothyroidism

> Educate on the complications of hypothermia

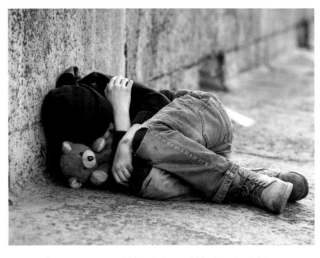

Image 10-7: An 11-year-old boy is brought in by a taxi driver to the emergency department and there are concerns of hypothermia. For each of the following 3 areas (mild / moderate / severe hypothermia) create a set of vitals and at least 2 other assessment findings that would be congruent for this child if he were suffering from that state of hypothermia.

Mild Hypothermia:

_____

_____

_____

_____

Moderate Hypothermia:

_____

_____

_____

Severe Hypothermia:

_____

_____

_____

1. What statement made by a client who just received discharge teaching on polycythemia indicates the need for further education?
   1. "I know that I must drink a lot of water when I go home."
   2. "I must be careful how much activity I do so I do not get fatigued."
   3. "I must call my doctor if my chest starts to hurt."
   4. "I do not think my children will get polycythemia."

2. The spouse of a client with thrombocytopenia who experienced cerebral hemorrhage and is now on a mechanical ventilator states, "I was very upset with my husband for being confused but then he fell. He was having a stroke and I didn't even know it. I just don't know what to do now that he cannot speak to me." What is an appropriate response by the nurse?
   1. "It is quite normal for you to feel guilty at a time such as this."
   2. "He should rest. Please sit quietly with him and I'll be outside if you need me."
   3. "Your husband may still hear you. I can leave the room, so you can speak with him."
   4. "The hospital chaplain is available to meet with you as you appear to be upset."

3. What assessment findings for a client with a calcium level of 14.0 mg/dL and who is being administered intravenous fluid of 2.5 liters daily, indicate effectiveness of the therapy?
   1. Clear lung sounds.
   2. Better use of muscles.
   3. Blood pressure of 110/68.
   4. Breakfast intake of 75%.

4. What is a nursing assessment priority for a client who is being administered temozolomide for a brain tumor?
   1. Labs for platelet and absolute neutrophil count.
   2. Mucous membranes for mouth excoriation.
   3. Level of consciousness for changed status.
   4. CT scan results for change in tumor status.

5. The nurse assesses a client who had a left mastectomy earlier today and finds the client's left arm is slightly edematous. The client reports a pain level of 4 out of 10. What is the priority nursing action?
   1. Discuss body image disturbance with the client.
   2. Provide pain medication and teach exercises for the arm and shoulder.
   3. Present information on further treatment for the cancer.
   4. Perform assessments to determine the client's risk factor for breast cancer.

6. A nurse is caring for a client who has Hodgkin's lymphoma and is receiving chemotherapy. What can the nurse delegate to the unlicensed assistive personnel (UAP)?
   1. Explain the need for the client to avoid large crowds and people with infections.
   2. Ensure the client's room is clean and odor-free when meals are delivered.
   3. Evaluate temperature trends every 4 hours.
   4. Encourage the client to talk about the impact of hair loss on self-image.

7. A nurse is caring for a client newly diagnosed with acute myelogenous leukemia (AML). Which assessment finding needs to be reported to the client's health care provider immediately?
   1. Absolute neutrophil count 1500 cells/mm^3.
   2. Oral temperature 99.0°F [37.2°C].
   3. New onset of headache.
   4. Hgb 10.5 g/dL.

8. A nurse completed health promotion teaching for a client at risk for developing lung cancer. Which statement made by the client requires follow-up by the nurse?
   1. "I need to let my health care provider know if I have a cough that won't go away."
   2. "I should have my house tested for radon."
   3. "My 60-year-old mother who has been smoking 2 packs a day for the past 40 years should have a CT scan every year."
   4. "I will not get lung cancer since I have never smoked cigarettes."

9. The nurse is planning care for a 23-year-old married male client recently diagnosed with Hodgkin's lymphoma who will be receiving chemotherapy and radiation. What information is essential for the nurse to provide?
   1. Contact information for local support groups for cancer survivors.
   2. The need to discuss different options for sperm banking with his wife.
   3. Different options for end-of-life care including palliative care.
   4. The signs and symptoms of anemia and thrombocytopenia.

10. The nurse is caring for a client who has just been admitted from an outpatient clinic with a diagnosis of multiple myeloma. The client has the following laboratory values: Na 138 mEq/L; K 4.0 mEq/L; glucose 110 mg/dL; total Ca 13.2 mEq/L; creatinine 1.2 mg/dL. What is the priority nursing action?
    1. Initiate intravenous fluids as prescribed.
    2. Administer allopurinol as prescribed.
    3. Provide a high-fiber diet to prevent constipation.
    4. Assess for splenomegaly.

11. A nurse is providing care to a client who experienced heat exhaustion while running a marathon. The client is in a cool environment and is receiving 100 mL 0.9% normal saline IV. What finding by the nurse requires immediate follow-up?
    1. Radial pulses +1 bilaterally.
    2. Heart rate 102 beats per minute.
    3. Temperature 104°F [40°C].
    4. Decreased level of consciousness.

12. A nurse completed health promotion teaching about skin cancer prevention. What statement made by the client indicates the teaching was effective?
    1. "Since I have dark-colored skin, I do not need to worry about developing skin cancer."
    2. "As long as I wear sunscreen, I will not develop skin cancer."
    3. "Indoor tanning booths are safer than being in the sun."
    4. "I need to let my doctor know if I develop a spot on my skin that has different colors."

13. The nurse is planning care for a client who has hydrocephalus from a glioblastoma. What statement from the client indicates the need for further assessment?
    1. "I have started hearing things every now and then that no one else can hear."
    2. "I need to have someone help me brush my hair and teeth sometimes."
    3. "Sometimes I have problems saying what I want to say."
    4. "I have been talking with my family about my treatment options. It's been really difficult, but we have gotten much closer."

14. The nurse is caring for a client who has multiple dysplastic nevi. Based on this assessment finding, what does the nurse identify as a priority need for client education?
    1. Prevention of cellulitis.
    2. The importance of getting immunized for herpes zoster.
    3. Candidiasis prevention and treatment.
    4. Self-examination of skin lesions.

15. The nurse is teaching a group of adolescents about means to prevent brain injury. What is a priority to include in the lesson plan?
    1. Airbags.
    2. Car door locks.
    3. 4-wheel drive.
    4. Seatbelts.

16. A client with chemotherapy-induced anemia has a prescription for 75 mg of iron-dextran to be given intramuscularly (IM). The pharmacy sent 2 mL single-dose vials that are labeled 50 mg/mL. How much medication does the nurse need to prepare in the syringe?

_____

17. The nurse is assessing a client who is near the end-of-life because of end-stage breast cancer. Which subjective data indicates the client may not be coping with her illness?
    1. Loss of 2 pounds in the past 2 weeks.
    2. Inability to concentrate while answering questions.
    3. Her husband reports she is having difficulty sleeping.
    4. Denying that she is at the end-of-life.

18. The nurse is caring for a client who is identified to have signs and symptoms of hypothermia. Which nursing actions does the nurse need to implement? Select all that apply.
    1. Wrap the client in warm blankets.
    2. Provide warm caffeinated beverages.
    3. Cover the top of the client's head.
    4. Administer antipyretics as prescribed.
    5. Monitor the client's vital signs.
    6. Assess for sensation in distal tissues.

19. A nurse is assessing a client who is in the emergency department with a concussion after falling down the stairs at home. What assessment findings require immediate follow-up by the nurse? Select all that apply.
    1. Glasgow Coma Scale score goes from 15 to 13 over an hour.
    2. The client has a headache of 2 on a pain scale of 0–10.
    3. The client has nystagmus when gazing to the far left-hand side of the room.
    4. The client cannot remember falling down the stairs.
    5. The client is sleepy but easily aroused.

20. A nurse is caring for a client diagnosed with acute lymphocytic leukemia who had a bone marrow biopsy with IV sedation. What does the nurse include in the assessment following the procedure? Select all that apply.
    1. The client's pain.
    2. Determine if there is bleeding at the biopsy site.
    3. Inspect the dressing and ensure it remains clean and nonocclusive.
    4. Ask the client to explain the results of the biopsy.
    5. The client's level of consciousness.

21. The nurse is assessing a client who has hydrocephalus. Which assessment techniques indicate the client's functions of Cranial Nerves III, IV and VI are intact? Select all that apply.
    1. The client reads a Snellen chart accurately.
    2. The client can follow the movement of the nurse's finger with the eyes in each of the 6 directions of gaze.
    3. The ability to distinguish sharp and dull sensations on the face.
    4. The client's smile is symmetrical.
    5. Pupils are equal in size, round, and reactive to light and accommodation.
    6. The eyelid remains open.

22. A nurse is caring for a client with end-stage lung cancer. The client's health care provider prescribed morphine to be administered by intravenous bolus. The client has an IV of normal saline infusing at 100 mL/hour. In what order would the nurse perform these actions to administer the medication? Rank order the responses.
    1. Select and clean injection port closest to the client with antiseptic swab.
    2. Occlude IV line by pinching the tubing just above the injection port, pull back to aspirate blood return.
    3. Perform hand hygiene and apply clean gloves.
    4. Connect syringe with medication to IV port.
    5. Release tubing and inject medication over amount of time recommended by agency policy, pharmacist, or medication reference manual.
    6. Dispose uncapped syringe in puncture-proof, leak-proof container.

23. The nurse is planning care for a client with lung cancer. Which activities can the nurse delegate to the nursing assistant? Select all that apply.
    1. Checking the pulse oximeter reading.
    2. Verifying the client's oxygen is being delivered per nasal prongs as prescribed.
    3. Assessing the client's breath sounds.
    4. Reporting if the client states pain is becoming worse.
    5. Walking the client in the hallway as prescribed.
    6. Teaching the client the importance of smoking cessation.

24. The nurse is caring for a client admitted for observation for possible head injury following a motor vehicle accident in which the client has no memory of what happened. Which assessment data would be a priority for the nurse?
    1. "Can you tell me what happened?"
    2. "Do you have a history of black-outs, frequent falls, or seizures?"
    3. "Was anyone else with you?"
    4. "What medications do you take?"

25. A client began receiving prednisone for treatment of immune thrombocytopenic purpura (ITP) on 10/17. Based on the information in the client's chart below, what laboratory information indicates the prednisone is being effective?
    1. Hemoglobin and hematocrit.
    2. Glucose.
    3. White blood cell count.
    4. Platelet count.

Diagnosis: Immune Thrombocytopenic Purpura Allergies: None		
Order date	Lab	Result
10/17	Hgb Hct WBC PLT Glucose	12.2 g/dL 33% 4950/mm³ 8,000/mm³ 150 mg/dL
10/25	Hgb Hct WBC PLT Glucose	14 g/dL 38% 5600/mm³ 10,500/mm³ 145 mg/dL

26. A 6-year-old with acute lymphocytic leukemia received induction chemotherapy. The client's absolute neutrophil count is zero, the client has fatigue, and experiences mild nausea. Which nursing actions are highest priority?
    1. Administer antiemetics and assess nutrition and hydration status.
    2. Limit contacts with infected visitors and place in positive pressure isolation.
    3. Assess for sources of bleeding and provide pressure on wounds.
    4. Monitor energy levels and begin energy conserving techniques.

27. The nurse explains the effects of chemotherapy to an adolescent diagnosed with leukemia. The nurse notes that there is increased risk for injury due to neutropenia. Which comment by the client indicates teaching was effective?
    1. "I will brush my teeth using a soft-bristle toothbrush."
    2. "Using an alcohol-based mouthwash twice a day is best."
    3. "A humidifier will help when I sleep at night."
    4. "I will eat only fresh uncooked fruits and vegetables."

28. The nurse is caring for a child with increased intracranial pressure. Which change in assessment would require immediate notification of the health care provider?
    1. Change in level of consciousness from lethargic to alert.
    2. An increase in the child's body temperature of 0.1°F.
    3. A Glasgow Coma Scale modified for children score of 15.
    4. A change from flexion posturing to extension posturing.

29. The parent of a preschooler who received chemotherapy last week, calls the clinic to report that the child has a temperature of 101.9°F. What is the most appropriate response by the nurse?
    1. "Please bring your child to the lab right away so a CBC level can be determined."
    2. "Do any of your family members or close friends have a fever at this time?"
    3. "Please bring your child to the clinic now so we might do further assessment."
    4. "You must give the child the antibiotic that was prescribed by the oncologist."

30. A nurse is providing teaching to a client with thrombocytopenia. Which statement by the nurse should be included in teaching?
    1. "You should monitor for weakness and fatigue."
    2. "You should monitor for dizziness and vomiting."
    3. "You should monitor for bruising and petechiae."
    4. "You should monitor for confusion and light-headedness."

1. **What statement made by a client who just received discharge teaching on polycythemia indicates the need for further education?**
   1. "I know that I must drink a lot of water when I go home." *Accurate statement.*
   2. 💡 "I must be careful how much activity I do so I do not get fatigued."
   3. "I must call my doctor if my chest starts to hurt." *Accurate statement due to the risk of clots.*
   4. "I do not think my children will get polycythemia." *Accurate statement.*

   Rationale: Clients with polycythemia are at high-risk for developing clots. Therefore, they need to stay hydrated and walk frequently to prevent blood clots. Angina is a sign that the client may be developing clots. Although polycythemia has a genetic link, it is not typically inherited.

   THIN Thinking: Identify Risk to Safety – *The potential complication of clot formation is the greatest concern with polycythemia. Understanding that will improve safety.* **NCLEX®**: Safety and Infection Control **QSEN:** Safety

2. **The spouse of a client with thrombocytopenia who experienced cerebral hemorrhage and is now on a mechanical ventilator states, "I was very upset with my husband for being confused but then he fell. He was having a stroke and I didn't even know it. I just don't know what to do now that he cannot speak to me." What is an appropriate response by the nurse?**
   1. "It is quite normal for you to feel guilty at a time such as this." *This statement does not address wife's concerns.*
   2. "He should rest. Please sit quietly with him and I'll be outside if you need me." *This doesn't address wife's concerns.*
   3. 💡 "Your husband may still hear you. I can leave the room, so you can speak with him."
   4. "The hospital chaplain is available to meet with you as you appear to be upset." *The nurse should be able to offer the wife support.*

   Rationale: Clients who are critically ill and their family members are experiencing crisis. It is important for nurses to establish a therapeutic relationship, ensure a therapeutic environment, provide education to the client and family, and include family members in the client's care if they desire. None of the other nurse's responses demonstrate use of therapeutic communication.

   THIN Thinking: Top Three – *The statement by the spouse demonstrates remorse. It is important to establish communication at this time.* **NCLEX®**: Psychosocial Integrity **QSEN:** Patient-centered Care

3. **What assessment findings for a client with a calcium level of 14.0 mg/dL and who is being administered intravenous fluid of 2.5 liters daily, indicate effectiveness of the therapy?**
   1. Clear lung sounds. *This is not an indication of calcium levels.*
   2. 💡 Better use of muscles.
   3. Blood pressure of 110/68. *This is not an indication of calcium levels.*
   4. Breakfast intake of 75%. *This is not an indication of calcium levels.*

   Rationale: This client is experiencing hypercalcemia. Treatment includes IV hydration and bisphosphonate therapy. Treatment is effective when the signs and symptoms of hypercalcemia, such as fatigue and muscle weakness, resolve and calcium levels return to normal. Clear lung sounds and the client's blood pressure indicate the client is tolerating the IV fluids. It is important for clients with cancer to maintain healthy nutritional levels. None of these findings indicate the effectiveness of the treatment for hypercalcemia.

   THIN Thinking: Nursing Process – *Evaluation of a prescribed therapy is important to determining its effectiveness and determining if additional treatments are necessary.* **NCLEX®**: Physiological Adaptation **QSEN:** Safety

4. **What is a nursing assessment priority for a client who is being administered temozolomide for a brain tumor?**
   1. 💡 Labs for platelet and absolute neutrophil count.
   2. Mucous membranes for mouth excoriation. *Not the priority.*
   3. Level of consciousness for changed status. *Not the priority.*
   4. CT scan results for change in tumor status. *Not the priority.*

   Rationale: Temozolomide is an oral chemotherapeutic agent. It causes myelosuppression. Therefore, it is important to assess the client's absolute neutrophil and platelet count before administering the medication to ensure it is safe to administer. The other assessment findings in this question are important but are not needed to determine if it is safe to administer temozolomide.

   THIN Thinking: Nursing Process – *The nurse needs to understand safety prior to the administration of all medications. A part of that is knowing the critical assessments that need to take place first.* **NCLEX®**: Pharmacological and Parenteral Therapies **QSEN:** Safety

5. The nurse assesses a client who had a left mastectomy earlier today and finds the client's left arm is slightly edematous. The client reports a pain level of 4 out of 10. What is the priority nursing action?
   1. Discuss body image disturbance with the client. *Need to address physical concerns first.*
   2. 📍 Provide pain medication and teach exercises for the arm and shoulder.
   3. Present information on further treatment for the cancer. *Client has already been treated for cancer.*
   4. Perform assessments to determine the client's risk factor for breast cancer. *Client has already been treated for cancer.*

   Rationale: Pain control and restoring arm function are the priorities immediately following a mastectomy. Thus, it is most important at this time for the nurse to manage the client's pain and gradually start arm and shoulder exercises. Talking with the client about altered body image is important but it is not the priority at this time. Health care providers should discuss treatment options with clients. The client already has a diagnosis of breast cancer, so assessing for risk factors for breast cancer is not a priority currently.

   THIN Thinking: Nursing Process – *Understanding proper interventions for the care of the client post-mastectomy will allow the nurse to determine an appropriate plan of care.* **NCLEX®:** Basic Care and Comfort **QSEN:** Patient-centered Care

6. A nurse is caring for a client who has Hodgkin's lymphoma and is receiving chemotherapy. What can the nurse delegate to the unlicensed assistive personnel (UAP)?
   1. Explain the need for the client to avoid large crowds and people with infections. *Nursing assistants cannot perform teaching.*
   2. 📍 Ensure the client's room is clean and odor-free when meals are delivered.
   3. Evaluate temperature trends every 4 hours. *UAPs cannot monitor a client's condition.*
   4. Encourage the client to talk about the impact of hair loss on self-image. *Nursing assistants should not be counseling clients.*

   Rationale: Clients diagnosed with Hodgkin's lymphoma are usually treated with a combination of chemotherapeutic agents. Chemotherapy causes a variety of symptoms including leukopenia, alopecia, and anorexia, nausea and vomiting. All the actions listed in this question are important nursing interventions. The only task that can be delegated to a nursing assistant is to ensure the client's environment is pleasant during mealtimes. The other interventions must be completed by a nurse.

   THIN Thinking: Identify Risk to Safety – *The nurse must know the role and scope of practice for all practitioners in order to delegate safely.* **NCLEX®:** Management of Care **QSEN:** Safety

7. A nurse is caring for a client newly diagnosed with acute myelogenous leukemia (AML). Which assessment finding needs to be reported to the client's health care provider immediately?
   1. Absolute neutrophil count 1500 cells/mm³. *Although low, this is common for clients with AML.*
   2. Oral temperature 99.0°F [37.2°C]. *This is not significant.*
   3. 📍 New onset of headache.
   4. Hgb 10.5 g/dL. *Although low, this is not uncommon for a client with AML.*

   Rationale: The onset of AML is acute and abrupt. Clients can have serious infections and abnormal bleeding at the onset of the disease because of the proliferation of myeloblasts. Fatigue, weakness, low WBC count and anemia are common. The new onset of a headache needs to be reported immediately as it could indicate the client is experiencing a cerebral hemorrhage related to low levels of platelets.

   THIN Thinking: Top Three – *Priorities include bleeding and infection – need to prioritize based on symptoms. Headache could indicate an actual bleed, whereas low ANC indicates the risk for an infection.* **NCLEX®:** Safety and Infection Control **QSEN:** Safety

8. A nurse completed health promotion teaching for a client at risk for developing lung cancer. Which statement made by the client requires follow-up by the nurse?
   1. "I need to let my health care provider know if I have a cough that won't go away." *Accurate statement.*
   2. "I should have my house tested for radon." *Accurate statement.*
   3. "My 60-year-old mother who has been smoking 2 packs a day for the past 40 years should have a CT scan every year." *Accurate statement.*
   4. 📍 "I will not get lung cancer since I have never smoked cigarettes."

   Rationale: Although the risk for lung cancer is increased in people who smoke, people who do not smoke also develop lung cancer. Therefore, this response requires the nurse to provide further education. Having a cough that does not go away is a warning sign of lung cancer and should be reported. Exposure to radiation, such as radon, is a risk factor for lung cancer. Annual low dose CT scans are recommended for adults from 55-80 years old with a 30-pack year smoking history or who currently smoke.

   THIN Thinking: Nursing Process – *Evaluation of client understanding is an important part of the nursing process.* **NCLEX®:** Health Promotion and Maintenance **QSEN:** Patient-centered Care

9. The nurse is planning care for a 23-year-old married male client recently diagnosed with Hodgkin's lymphoma who will be receiving chemotherapy and radiation. What information is essential for the nurse to provide?
   1. Contact information for local support groups for cancer survivors. *This would be helpful, but is not as essential as exploring sperm bank options.*
   2. ⦿ The need to discuss different options for sperm banking with his wife.
   3. Different options for end-of-life care including palliative care. *There is no indication that the client is near death.*
   4. The signs and symptoms of anemia and thrombocytopenia. *This would be helpful, but is not the most important action.*

   Rationale: Chemotherapy and radiation treatment may cause reduced or loss of fertility. Thus, discussing fertility options with the client before treatment begins is the priority. Include the family in these discussions when appropriate. Hodgkin's lymphoma frequently affects young adults and has a long-term survival rate of over 80% for all stages. Because this client is recently diagnosed and has not started treatment yet, referring the client to a support group for cancer survivors, discussing end-of-life care and the signs and symptoms of anemia are currently not priority needs.

   THIN Thinking: Top Three – *Chemotherapy and radiation can cause a decrease in sperm counts and infertility. The nurse should discuss options with clients about future family planning prior to treatment.* **NCLEX®**: Psychosocial Integrity **QSEN:** Patient-centered Care

10. The nurse is caring for a client who has just been admitted from an outpatient clinic with a diagnosis of multiple myeloma. The client has the following laboratory values: Na 138 mEq/L; K 4.0 mEq/L; glucose 110 mg/dL; total Ca 13.2 mEq/L; creatinine 1.2 mg/dL. What is the priority nursing action?
    1. ⦿ Initiate intravenous fluids as prescribed.
    2. Administer allopurinol as prescribed. *Allopurinol may be given to prevent renal damage but is not the priority action.*
    3. Provide a high-fiber diet to prevent constipation. *This is true, but not the priority action.*
    4. Assess for splenomegaly. *This is a common finding with multiple myeloma, but is not the priority action.*

Rationale: This client has significant hypercalcemia caused by the breakdown of bones related to multiple myeloma. Identifying and treating hypercalcemia is the priority. Priority nursing interventions for clients with hypercalcemia include providing adequate hydration to attain a urine output of 1.5 – 2 L/day. None of the other options will influence the client's calcium level. Multiple myeloma may cause splenomegaly. Allopurinol may be given with chemotherapy to prevent renal damage from uric acid accumulation from the breakdown of cancer cells. A high fiber diet helps to prevent constipation related to pain management and immobility.

THIN Thinking: Help Quick – *Hypercalcemia can cause significant side effects. Delivery of IV fluids can improve calcium levels.* **NCLEX®**: Physiological Adaptation **QSEN:** Safety

11. A nurse is providing care to a client who experienced heat exhaustion while running a marathon. The client is in a cool environment and is receiving 100 mL 0.9% normal saline IV. What finding by the nurse requires immediate follow-up?
    1. Radial pulses +1 bilaterally. *Indicates a decrease of perfusion from hypovolemia, but not as concerning as a decreased level of consciousness.*
    2. Heart rate 102 beats per minute. *Mild tachycardia, not concerning.*
    3. Temperature 104°F [40°C]. *Hyperthermia but not a sign of physiological compromise.*
    4. ⦿ Decreased level of consciousness.

Rationale: Clients with heat exhaustion typically experience a weak, thready pulse, tachycardia, temperature from 99.6° to 105.8°F [37.5° to 41°C], and mild confusion. Worsening mental status, such as decreased level of consciousness and hallucinations, indicates the client may not be responding to treatment and is progressing to heatstroke, which is a medical emergency.

THIN Thinking: Help Quick – *A decrease in level of consciousness indicates decreased perfusion to the brain and is a priority concern.* **NCLEX®**: Pharmacological and Parental Therapies **QSEN:** Safety

12. **A nurse completed health promotion teaching about skin cancer prevention. What statement made by the client indicates the teaching was effective?**
    1. "Since I have dark-colored skin, I do not need to worry about developing skin cancer." *Skin cancer is still a risk for people with dark skin.*
    2. "As long as I wear sunscreen, I will not develop skin cancer." *Sunscreen decreases risk but does not eliminate the risk.*
    3. "Indoor tanning booths are safer than being in the sun." *Tanning beds are more of a risk than sun exposure.*
    4. ⊕ "I need to let my doctor know if I develop a spot on my skin that has different colors."

    Rationale: When teaching about skin cancer prevention, it is helpful to use the mnemonic ABCDE to help clients remember the signs of skin cancer. The mnemonic stands for Asymmetry, Border irregularity, Color, Diameter, and Evolving in appearance. Having a non-uniform color is a reportable symptom for a skin lesion. People with dark-colored skin and people who use sunscreen or indoor tanning booths can develop skin cancer.

    THIN Thinking: Identify Risk to Safety – *Changes in skin requires further assessment to detect early signs of skin cancer.* **NCLEX®:** Reduction of Risk Potential **QSEN:** Patient-centered Care

13. **The nurse is planning care for a client who has hydrocephalus from a glioblastoma. What statement from the client indicates the need for further assessment?**
    1. ⊕ "I have started hearing things every now and then that no one else can hear."
    2. "I need to have someone help me brush my hair and teeth sometimes." *This is not concerning.*
    3. "Sometimes I have problems saying what I want to say." *This is not as concerning as hearing things.*
    4. "I have been talking with my family about my treatment options. It's been really difficult, but we have gotten much closer." *This is a positive event.*

Rationale: This client is describing symptoms that may indicate the onset of simple focal seizures. Clients with hydrocephalus and brain tumors are at risk for developing seizures. The nurse needs to assess the client further to determine if the client is experiencing other symptoms consistent with seizures, notify the client's health care provider and possibly implement seizure precautions. Glioblastomas do not have a good prognosis. Thus, talking about treatment options with the family is a healthy behavior. Impaired mobility and aphasia are common symptoms associated with brain tumors. However, this client's need for safety related to possible seizure activity is the highest priority.

THIN Thinking: Top Three – *Seizures create a risk for safety and early identification can reduce the risk of injury.* **NCLEX®:** Reduction of Risk Potential **QSEN:** Safety

14. **The nurse is caring for a client who has multiple dysplastic nevi. Based on this assessment finding, what does the nurse identify as a priority need for client education?**
    1. Prevention of cellulitis. *Not a concern.*
    2. The importance of getting immunized for herpes zoster. *Not a concern.*
    3. Candidiasis prevention and treatment. *Not a concern.*
    4. ⊕ Self-examination of skin lesions.

Rationale: Dysplastic nevi (DN), or atypical moles, are nevi that have irregular borders, are various shades of color, and are larger than usual (greater than 5 mm across). They may have the same characteristics of melanoma but they are not as noticeable. The risk of developing melanoma increases when the client has more than one DN; thus, this client needs to know how to assess the skin for signs of melanoma using the ABCDE rule (Asymmetry, Border irregularity, Color change and variation, Diameter of 6 mm or more, Evolving in appearance). The other options in this question are different types of skin infections and are not correlated with DN.

THIN Thinking: Nursing Process – *Assessment and planning for self-examination teaching is the highest priority. This allows the client autonomy for identifying a change in the lesion's appearance.* **NCLEX®:** Health Promotion and Maintenance **QSEN:** Patient-centered Care

15. **The nurse is teaching a group of adolescents about means to prevent brain injury. What is a priority to include in the lesson plan?**
    1. 🌐 Airbags.
    2. Car door locks. *This would not impact risk for brain injuries.*
    3. 4-wheel drive. *This would not impact risk for brain injuries.*
    4. Seatbelts. *This might help decrease risk for brain injuries, but not as effectively as the use of airbags.*

    Rationale: Adolescents are at high-risk for experiencing acute brain injuries. Health promotion teaching includes making choices that protect the head in case of an injury, such as wearing a seatbelt when driving and a helmet when riding a bicycle. Airbags help prevent chest and other injuries in car accidents, but they can cause concussions and are more effective if the person in the car is wearing a seatbelt. They are not something an adolescent can choose to use. Car door locks and 4-wheel drive are other car safety features but do not prevent head injuries.

    THIN Thinking: Identify Risk to Safety – *The use of airbags can prevent the head from hitting the dashboard or windshield.* **NCLEX**®: Health Promotion and Maintenance **QSEN:** Safety

16. **A client with chemotherapy-induced anemia has a prescription for 75 mg of iron-dextran to be given intramuscularly (IM). The pharmacy sent 2 mL single-dose vials that are labeled 50 mg/mL. How much medication does the nurse need to prepare in the syringe?**

    Answer: 1.5 mL

    Rationale: To determine the appropriate amount of medication to give, first the nurse needs to recognize that the answer will be expressed in mLs. To calculate the dosage using dimensional analysis, the nurse goes through these steps:

    $$X\ mL = \frac{1\ mL}{50\ \cancel{mg}} \times 75\ \cancel{mg}$$

    $$X\ mL = \frac{1\ mL \times 75}{50} = 1.5\ mL$$

    THIN Thinking: Identify Risk to Safety – *Medication calculation requires safe practice.* **NCLEX**®: Pharmacological and Parenteral Therapies **QSEN:** Safety

17. **The nurse is assessing a client who is near the end-of-life because of end-stage breast cancer. Which subjective data indicates the client may not be coping with her illness?**
    1. Loss of 2 pounds in the past 2 weeks. *Not subjective data.*
    2. Inability to concentrate while answering questions. *Not subjective data.*
    3. Her husband reports she is having difficulty sleeping. *Not subjective data.*
    4. 🌐 Denying that she is at the end-of-life.

    Rationale: All these assessment findings indicate the client may not be coping with her illness. Subjective findings are reported by client and are verbal descriptions of health problems. Denial is a common subjective finding at the end-of-life. The other assessment findings listed here are objective findings.

    THIN Thinking: Top Three – *Subjective data is what is said by the client and may be the best indicator of client coping.* **NCLEX**®: Psychosocial Integrity **QSEN:** Patient-centered Care

18. **The nurse is caring for a client who is identified to have signs and symptoms of hypothermia. Which nursing actions does the nurse need to implement? Select all that apply.**
    1. 🌐 Wrap the client in warm blankets.
    2. Provide warm caffeinated beverages. *Caffeine would not be recommended.*
    3. 🌐 Cover the top of the client's head.
    4. Administer antipyretics as prescribed. *Client does not have a fever.*
    5. 🌐 Monitor the client's vital signs.
    6. 🌐 Assess for sensation in distal tissues.

    Rationale: Priority nursing actions for a client experiencing hypothermia include keeping the client warm by covering the client in warm blankets and covering the top of the client's head with a blanket or a cap. It is also important to assess the client's vital signs, especially the temperature, to determine the client's response to treatment. Decreased sensation in the extremities, such as the tip of the nose, earlobes, fingers and toes, indicates the client has possibly developed frostbite. Provide hot liquids such as soup and do not give clients with hypothermia caffeinated beverages. Antipyretics decrease body temperature and should not be given to a client with hypothermia.

    THIN Thinking: Nursing Process – *The nurse should understand the interventions that can raise body temperature to prevent complications.* **NCLEX**®: Physiological Adaptation **QSEN:** Safety

19. **A nurse is assessing a client who is in the emergency department with a concussion after falling down the stairs at home. What assessment findings require immediate follow-up by the nurse? Select all that apply.**
    1. ⓥ Glasgow Coma Scale score goes from 15 to 13 over an hour.
    2. The client has a headache of 2 on a pain scale of 0–10. *This would be expected.*
    3. ⓥ The client has nystagmus when gazing to the far left-hand side of the room.
    4. The client cannot remember falling down the stairs. *Short-term amnesia is common.*
    5. The client is sleepy but easily aroused. *This is a normal response.*

    Rationale: Glasgow Coma Scale (GCS) Scores range from 15 – 3 with 15 indicating full alertness. A decrease in the GCS indicates declining neurological function and needs to be reported immediately. Nystagmus is an involuntary rhythmical oscillation of the eyes and indicates potential disorder of the cranial nerves that innervate the eye muscles, which also needs to be reported. The other assessment findings indicate expected signs and symptoms of a concussion and do not need to be reported at this time.

    THIN Thinking: Identify Risk to Safety – *Identification of complications of a concussion include signs of cerebral edema. Frequent re-assessment is required for safety.* **NCLEX®:** Safety and Infection Control **QSEN:** Safety

20. **A nurse is caring for a client diagnosed with acute lymphocytic leukemia who had a bone marrow biopsy with IV sedation. What does the nurse include in the assessment following the procedure? Select all that apply.**
    1. ⓥ The client's pain.
    2. ⓥ Determine if there is bleeding at the biopsy site.
    3. Inspect the dressing and ensure it remains clean and nonocclusive. *Dressing is sterile.*
    4. Ask the client to explain the results of the biopsy. *Results would not be available.*
    5. ⓥ The client's level of consciousness.

Rationale: Complications following bone marrow biopsy include pain and bleeding. Thus, it is important to assess the client's pain and monitor for bleeding at the biopsy site. Nurses also need to assess the client's level of consciousness following IV sedation. A sterile pressure dressing is applied after the procedure. The biopsy must be sent to a laboratory for analysis. Thus, the results of the biopsy will not be known immediately after the procedure. The client's health care provider will provide the results to the client.

THIN Thinking: Top Three – *The nurse should provide assessment and interventions to improve pain and identify if bleeding is occurring.* **NCLEX®:** Reduction of Risk Potential **QSEN:** Patient-centered Care

21. **The nurse is assessing a client who has hydrocephalus. Which assessment techniques indicate the client's functions of Cranial Nerves III, IV and VI are intact? Select all that apply.**
    1. The client reads a Snellen chart accurately. *This is testing cranial nerve II.*
    2. ⓥ The client can follow the movement of the nurse's finger with the eyes in each of the 6 directions of gaze.
    3. The ability to distinguish sharp and dull sensations on the face. *This is testing cranial nerve V.*
    4. The client's smile is symmetrical. *This is testing cranial nerve VII.*
    5. ⓥ Pupils are equal in size, round, and reactive to light and accommodation.
    6. ⓥ The eyelid remains open.

Rationale: These 3 nerves help move the eye, so they are tested together by having the client move the eyes through 6 directions of gaze. Cranial nerve III also is tested by examining the client's pupils and the ability of the eyelid to remain open. The Snellen chart is used to test cranial nerve II, the facial nerve (CN VII) is responsible for symmetry in the client's smile, and cranial nerve V is tested by having the client distinguish between sharp and dull sensations on the face.

THIN Thinking: Nursing Process – *The nurse should identify the assessment findings for cranial nerves.* **NCLEX®:** Basic Care and Comfort **QSEN:** Patient-centered Care

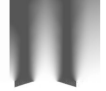

22. **A nurse is caring for a client with end-stage lung cancer. The client's health care provider prescribed morphine to be administered by intravenous bolus. The client has an IV of normal saline infusing at 100 mL/hour. In what order would the nurse perform these actions to administer the medication? Rank order the responses.**
    1. Perform hand hygiene and apply clean gloves.
    2. Select and clean injection port closest to the client with antiseptic swab.
    3. Connect syringe with medication to IV port.
    4. Occlude IV line by pinching the tubing just above the injection port, pull back to aspirate blood return.
    5. Release tubing and inject medication over amount of time recommended by agency policy, pharmacist, or medication reference manual.
    6. Dispose uncapped syringe in puncture-proof, leak-proof container.

    Rationale: This is the order in which to administer a medication by IV bolus. It is important to identify the client, ensure the 6 rights of medication administration and provide client education before beginning the procedure. Wear gloves to avoid contact with body substances. Cleaning the port prevents introduction of microorganisms during medication administration. In some cases, especially with a smaller gauge IV needle, blood return may not be aspirated. If the IV is infusing without difficulty and has no signs of infiltration, proceed with IV push medication administration. Give IV medications slowly according to agency policy. Administering IV medications too quickly can be fatal.

    THIN Thinking: Identify Risk to Safety – *The delivery of IV medication is a safety concern and safety protocol must be in place at all times.* **NCLEX®:** Safety and Infection Control **QSEN:** Safety

23. **The nurse is planning care for a client with lung cancer. Which activities can the nurse delegate to the nursing assistant? Select all that apply.**
    1. Checking the pulse oximeter reading.
    2. Verifying the client's oxygen is being delivered per nasal prongs as prescribed. *Assessing should be completed by the nurse.*
    3. Assessing the client's breath sounds. *Assessing is a nursing function.*
    4. Reporting if the client states pain is becoming worse.
    5. Walking the client in the hallway as prescribed.
    6. Teach the client the importance of smoking cessation. *Teaching is to be performed by the nurse.*

Rationale: When planning care, it is important for the nurse to determine which activities can be delegated to a nursing assistant. Nurses cannot delegate the steps of the nursing process, medication administration, or client education because these steps require nursing knowledge and judgment. Nurses can delegate tasks, such as checking the client's pulse oximeter. The nursing assistant can walk the client in the hallway and should report to the nurse if the client is in pain. Verifying oxygen is being delivered as prescribed, assessing breath sounds and teaching about smoking cessation are responsibilities of the nurse and cannot be delegated.

THIN Thinking: Identify Risk to Safety – *The process of delegation needs to include safe and appropriate delegation based on the scope of practice and stability of the client.* **NCLEX®:** Management of Care **QSEN:** Safety

24. **The nurse is caring for a client admitted for observation for possible head injury following a motor vehicle accident in which the client has no memory of what happened. Which assessment data would be a priority for the nurse?**
    1. "Can you tell me what happened?" *Client has no memory of what happened.*
    2. "Do you have a history of black-outs, frequent falls, or seizures?"
    3. "Was anyone else with you?" *This would not be the priority question.*
    4. "What medications do you take?" *This would not be the priority question.*

Rationale: Generalized seizures are characterized by tonic- clonic movements, loss of consciousness, falling to the ground or slumping in a chair, cyanosis, incontinence, and a post-ictal stage (soreness, fatigue, sleepy). Focal seizures involve symptoms of one side of the brain, can have loss of awareness or a dreamlike state, and demonstrate symptoms from the side of the brain affected. Atypical absence seizures (usually in children) can occur, where the client briefly "blanks out", stares off, and may have chewing, blinking, or other movements. Clients with a seizure disorder should not sustain injuries when a seizure occurs. They should experience physical functioning that is of a high-level while being administered anti- seizure medications and their level of psychosocial and psychological functioning should be optimal as well. These factors are pertinent goals for clients who have seizure disorder. Adults with seizures may not drive usually until they are on medication and have been on that medication for a specific length of time (3 months to one year) and are seizure-free. The policy varies from state to state.

THIN Thinking: Identify Risk to Safety – *By asking about previous history of black-outs, the nurse can identify if something led up to the accident that could have caused it.* **NCLEX®**: Basic Care and Comfort **QSEN:** Safety

25. **A client began receiving prednisone for treatment of immune thrombocytopenic purpura (ITP) on 10/17. Based on the information in the client's chart below, what laboratory information indicates the prednisone is being effective?**
    1. Hemoglobin and hematocrit. *These levels are not affected by prednisone.*
    2. Glucose. *Prednisone would increase blood glucose levels.*
    3. White blood cell count. *These levels would not be affected by prednisone.*
    4. 💡 Platelet count.

Diagnosis: Immune Thrombocytopenic Purpura **Allergies:** None		
Order date	**Lab**	**Result**
10/17	Hgb Hct WBC PLT Glucose	12.2 g/dL 33% 4950/mm³ 8,000/mm³ 150 mg/dL
10/25	Hgb Hct WBC PLT Glucose	14 g/dL 38% 5600/mm³ 10,500/mm³ 145 mg/dL

Rationale: Treatment of ITP typically begins with administration of glucocorticosteroids, such as prednisone, to suppress the phagocytic response of splenic macrophages and depress antibody formation. This alters the spleen's recognition of the platelets and increases the platelets' lifespan. In this client, the increase in the platelet count indicates the client is responding appropriately to the prednisone. A side effect of prednisone is elevated blood glucose levels. The hemoglobin, hematocrit, and white blood cell count changes are not related to administration of prednisone.

THIN Thinking: Nursing Process – *Labs are an important part of the nursing assessment and should be a regular part of the data collection to determine a medication's effectiveness.* **NCLEX®**: Pharmacological and Parenteral Therapies **QSEN:** Safety

26. **A 6-year-old with acute lymphocytic leukemia received induction chemotherapy. The client's absolute neutrophil count is zero, the client has fatigue, and experiences mild nausea. Which nursing actions are highest priority?**
    1. Administer antiemetics and assess nutrition and hydration status *Necessary, but not as essential as preventing infection.*
    2. 💡 Limit contacts with infected visitors and place in positive pressure isolation.
    3. Assess for sources of bleeding and provide pressure on wounds *No indication that bleeding is a risk factor.*
    4. Monitor energy levels and begin energy conserving techniques *Not as essential as preventing infection.*

Rationale: An absolute neutrophil count of zero indicates no immune response to infection, therefore, strategies to prevent infection are paramount. Avoiding vomiting, fatigue, and bleeding is important, but not more critical than prevention of infection in this client.

THIN Thinking: Identify Risk to Safety – *With an ANC of zero, the child has no ability to fight infection and is at extremely high-risk of dying from an infection.* **NCLEX®**: Safety and Infection Control **QSEN:** Safety

27. **The nurse explains the effects of chemotherapy to an adolescent diagnosed with leukemia. The nurse notes that there is increased risk for injury due to neutropenia. Which comment by the client indicates teaching was effective?**
    1. 💡 "I will brush my teeth using a soft-bristle toothbrush."
    2. "Using an alcohol-based mouthwash twice a day is best." *This would not be recommended.*
    3. "A humidifier will help when I sleep at night." *This would have no effect.*
    4. "I will eat only fresh uncooked fruits and vegetables." *This would not be recommended.*

Rationale: Using a soft-bristle toothbrush or toothette avoids damaging the fragile oral mucosa. Mouthwashes containing alcohol are very drying and can cause damage to the oral mucosa. Humidifiers harbor bacteria so their use should be avoided. Fruit and vegetables should be cooked or peeled due to the risk of ingesting bacteria on the skin of fruit and vegetables.

THIN Thinking: Identify Risk to Safety – *A client that is neutropenic has a high-risk of infection. The nurse needs to understand how to evaluate a client's understanding.* **NCLEX®**: Safety and Infection Control **QSEN:** Safety

28. **The nurse is caring for a child with increased intracranial pressure. Which change in assessment would require immediate notification of the health care provider?**
    1. Change in level of consciousness from lethargic to alert. *This is a positive change in client status.*
    2. An increase in the child's body temperature of 0.1°F. *This is not significant.*
    3. A Glasgow Coma Scale modified for children score of 15. *This is not significant.*
    4. 🔘 A change from flexion posturing to extension posturing.

    Rationale: A change from flexion to extension posturing is an ominous sign that indicates a worsening of neurological functioning. Therefore, the health care provider should be notified immediately when this occurs. A slight increase in temperature is expected with increased intracranial pressure. A Glasgow Coma Scale modified for children score of 15 indicated there is no impairment of neurological functioning.

    THIN Thinking: Top Three – *Increased intracranial pressure can lead to permanent neurological damage and tissue death. The nurse needs to be in tune with minor condition changes.* **NCLEX®**: Management of Care **QSEN:** Safety

29. **The parent of a preschooler who received chemotherapy last week, calls the clinic to report that the child has a temperature of 101.9°F. What is the most appropriate response by the nurse?**
    1. "Please bring your child to the lab right away so a CBC level can be determined." *This requires an order from the health care provider.*
    2. "Do any of your family members or close friends have a fever at this time?" *The source of a possible infection is not as important as treatment.*
    3. 🔘 "Please bring your child to the clinic now so we might do further assessment."
    4. "You must give the child the antibiotic that was prescribed by the oncologist." *Child needs to be assessed first.*

Rationale: The most appropriate action by the nurse is to have the child evaluated in the oncology clinic. The child may have a serious infection and needs to be evaluated prior to treatment. Though it is important to know if the child was exposed to any illnesses, it is not the most appropriate action.

THIN Thinking: Help Quick – *A rapid assessment needs to be made so that treatments can be started quickly.* **NCLEX®**: Physiological Adaptation **QSEN:** Safety

30. **A nurse is providing teaching to a client with thrombocytopenia. Which statement by the nurse should be included in teaching?**
    1. "You should monitor for weakness and fatigue." *This is not a usual issue with this disorder.*
    2. "You should monitor for dizziness and vomiting." *This is not a usual issue with this disorder.*
    3. 🔘 "You should monitor for bruising and petechiae."
    4. "You should monitor for confusion and light-headedness." *This is not a usual issue with this disorder.*

Rationale: Clients with thrombocytopenia have an issue with their clotting factors, therefore you are looking for a clotting type of answer. Weakness, fatigue, confusion and light-headedness occur with decreased number of red blood cells and the resulting hypoxia. Dizziness and vomiting is not an appropriate answer.

THIN Thinking: Top Three – *The priority concern with thrombocytopenia is bleeding. Assessments need to be focused on this concern.* **NCLEX®**: Physiological Adaptation **QSEN:** Patient-centered Care

Nutrition

Digestion / Elimination

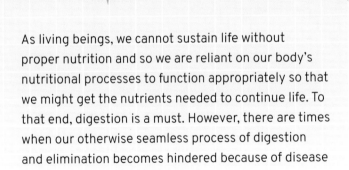

As living beings, we cannot sustain life without proper nutrition and so we are reliant on our body's nutritional processes to function appropriately so that we might get the nutrients needed to continue life. To that end, digestion is a must. However, there are times when our otherwise seamless process of digestion and elimination becomes hindered because of disease conditions that afflict our bodies.

Illnesses impacting the gastrointestinal system are prevalent and as nurses, you will spend a significant part of your role managing these illnesses. It is therefore paramount that you have a firm understanding of the diseases that can impact digestion and elimination so that you might positively impact the care of clients with these health conditions.

Priority Exemplars:

> Inflammatory bowel disease: Crohn's disease/ ulcerative colitis
> Cleft lip and palate
> Gastroesophageal reflux
> Gastritis
> Peptic ulcer disease
> Celiac disease
> Gallbladder conditions
> Constipation
> Intestinal obstruction
> Diverticular disease
> Colorectal cancer
> Cirrhosis
> Hepatitis
> Pyloric stenosis
> Obesity
> Benign prostatic hypertrophy/prostate cancer
> Chronic kidney disease/end-stage renal disease
> Acute kidney disease/injury

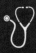
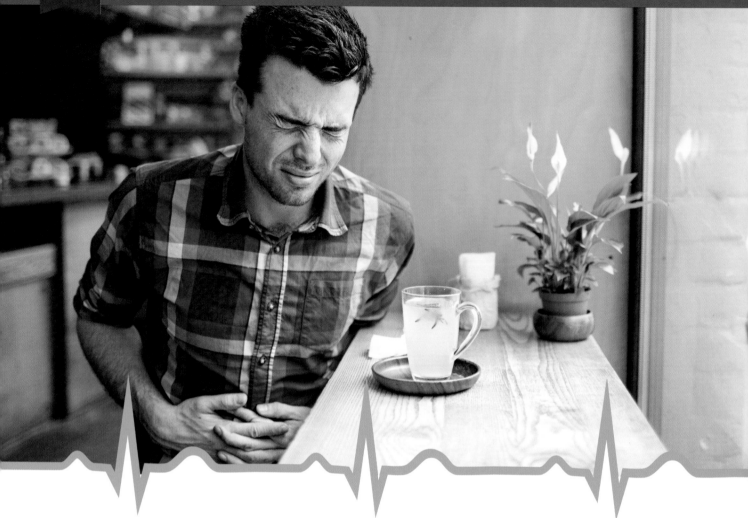

Go To Clinical Case 1

J.B. is a 25-year-old man who presents to the emergency department with abdominal pain that he describes as "cramping." He states that the pain started two days ago and has been accompanied by diarrhea. J.B. admits that he had this same thing happen previous times, but he just passed it off as something he ate or the stomach flu. He has never noticed blood in his stools. He has had 3 bowel movements today and feels very weak right now.

Health history reveals no significant medical conditions. Family history reveals an older brother who has Crohn's disease and a mother who has lupus erythematosus. Vital signs are: Temperature 100.2°F, Pulse 88, Respirations 18, Blood pressure 122/84.

An inflammatory bowel disease is suspected and J.B. is admitted to your unit for further testing. Results of further testing confirms that J.B. has Crohn's disease. You are the nurse caring for J.B.

NurseThink® Time

Using the NurseThink® system, complete the priorities. Check your answers designated by 💡 in the Inflammatory bowel disease: Crohn's disease/ulcerative colitis Priority Exemplar.

✏ Priority Assessments or Cues

1.

2.

3.

🧪 Priority Laboratory Tests/Diagnostics

1.

2.

3.

⚠ Priority Interventions or Actions

1.

2.

3.

🚩 Priority Potential & Actual Complications

1.

2.

3.

⚕ Priority Nursing Implications

1.

2.

3.

💧 Priority Medications

1.

2.

3.

👤 Priority Education/Discharge Issues

1.

2.

3.

Inflammatory bowel disease: Crohn's disease/ulcerative colitis

Pathophysiology/Description

> Inflammatory bowel disease (IBD) describes an incurable, chronic condition that is marked by inflammation of the gastrointestinal tract. The condition is not continuous but presents with periods of exacerbations and remissions. Crohn's disease and ulcerative colitis are the 2 conditions that are classified as IBD

> Factors associated with IBD
> • Genetics: it is seen that there are frequent occurrences of IBD in family members of individuals with IBD
> • Environmental: smoking, stress, air pollutants, among others, cause increase susceptibility to IBD
> • Dietary: intake of foods high in polyunsaturated fats, and meat increase the risk of getting IBD

> Crohn's disease usually affects any part of the GI system, from the mouth to the anus, but it quite commonly occurs in the proximal colon and the terminal ileum

> Ulcerative colitis is more localized and involves the rectum, spreading up toward the cecum

> It is common for both conditions to affect teenagers, adults in their third decade of life and those after 60-years-old

> The GI inflammation seen with ulcerative colitis is continuous while with Crohn's, inflammation is seen in a skipped pattern (commonly termed skipped lesions), meaning that there can be areas of normal bowel between portions that are diseased. All layers of the bowel are involved with Crohn's causing deep ulcerations and the classic "cobblestone" look. However, with ulcerative colitis, only the mucosal layer is involved

> Abscess and peritonitis are likely in Crohn's because of bowel perforation, causing bowel contents to leak into the peritoneal cavity. Narrowed lumen, ulcerations, scarring and fistulas are common in Crohn's disease

> With ulcerative colitis, inflamed mucosa prevents the absorption of electrolytes and water and the lack of absorption causes the client to have diarrhea with electrolyte loss. Finger-like projections (called pseudopolyps) may be formed because of the inflamed mucosa. These are not common to Crohn's disease

> Certain dietary measures can be taken to decrease the risk of both diseases. Eating a high intake of vegetables is known to decrease the risk of ulcerative colitis, while the risk of Crohn's can be decreased with high fruit and fiber consumption

Priority Assessments or Cues

💡 Assess for fever, cramping abdominal pain, diarrhea with pus, rectal bleeding and weight loss with Crohn's disease. Weight loss occurs as a result of malabsorption from inflammation

💡 Assess for mild to severe constant abdominal pain, bloody diarrheal stools and tenesmus (painful and constant need to empty bowel), indicative of ulcerative colitis. Assess number of bowel movements daily, expect 4-20 with ulcerative colitis

> Assess stools for infection.

> Complete client's health history

> Assess for anemia, as blood loss in stools can cause anemia. Bleeding occurs more in ulcerative colitis than Crohn's

💡 Assess for nutritional deficiency due to malabsorption. Assess for dehydration and electrolyte imbalance due to fluid and electrolytes loss in liquid stools

> Assess vital signs, hypotension, tachycardia and fever, likely due to fluid issues and inflammation

> Assess for malnutrition, expect that it may be more pronounced in Crohn's disease due to malabsorption issues

> Assess for signs and symptoms of peritonitis, occurring from bowel perforation, more likely with Crohn's disease

> Assess client's understanding of surgery, if indicated

> Assess client's readiness to look at surgical site and learn self-care, if surgery was indicated

Healthy

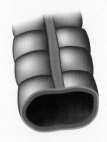

Crohn's disease

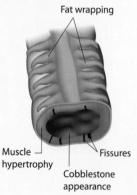

Fat wrapping

Muscle hypertrophy

Fissures

Cobblestone appearance

Ulcerative colitis

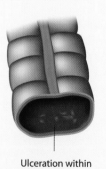

Ulceration within the mucosa

Image 11-1: Pathophysiology found in Crohn's disease and Ulcerative colitis.

🧪 Priority Laboratory Tests/Diagnostics

- 💡 C-reactive protein and white blood cell count elevated due to inflammation. Stool test shows mucus, blood and pus. Stool culture shows infection

- 💡 Metabolic profile shows decreased potassium, sodium, bicarbonate, chloride due to diarrhea and vomiting and low albumin because of inadequate nutrition

- 💡 Imaging such as computed tomography, magnetic resonance imaging (MRI), barium enema, small bowel follow through, help in the diagnosis. Colonoscopy and endoscopy are used to look for diseased areas in various parts of the gastrointestinal tract

- ❯ Complete blood count shows anemia because of blood loss in stools

⚠ Priority Interventions or Actions

- ❯ Prepare client for imaging tests
- ❯ Collect stool samples and send to lab
- 💡 Weight client daily, numerous diarrhea and fluid loss causes weight loss. Monitor intake and output
- 💡 Maintain client nothing by mouth (NPO) in acute phase. Administer intravenous fluids and electrolytes to replace loss from diarrhea. Restrict activity to decrease intestinal motility. Provide diet high in proteins, vitamins and caloric value to compensate for malabsorption and malnutrition

- ❯ Dietary consults for client's nutritional needs
- ❯ Monitor stools noting consistency and amount. Note presence of blood
- ❯ Monitor for bowel perforation, which may include tachycardia, restlessness, abdominal distention, increased temperature
- ❯ Monitor bowel sounds, abdominal tenderness and pain
- ❯ Clean client's peri area with plain water and apply barrier cream to prevent skin breaks from frequent diarrhea
- ❯ If surgery is indicated
  - Perform preoperative care
  - Insert nasogastric tube if prescribed
  - Perform post-surgical care as prescribed
  - Manage post-surgical devices such as ileal pouch
  - Manage care of surgical site. Assess for bleeding, infection and viability of stoma
  - Allow client to participate in self-care of surgical site, in preparation for home care
  - Monitor for initial ileostomy output, which may be up to 1800 mL/24 hours
- 💡 Administer medications as ordered

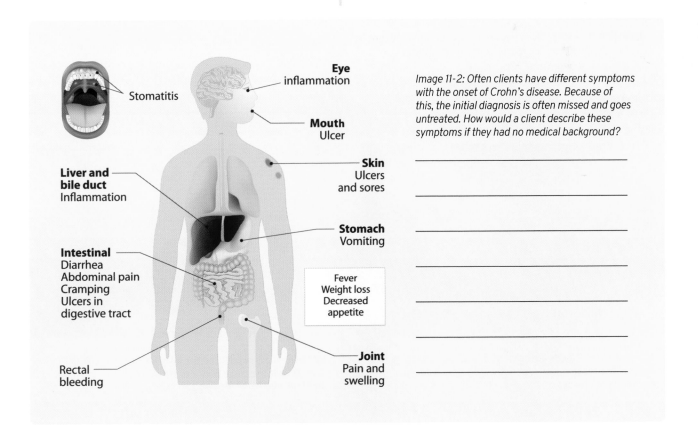

Image 11-2: Often clients have different symptoms with the onset of Crohn's disease. Because of this, the initial diagnosis is often missed and goes untreated. How would a client describe these symptoms if they had no medical background?

_____

_____

_____

_____

_____

_____

_____

⚑ Priority Potential & Actual Complications

- 💡 Fistulas and abscess of the perineal area, strictures, perforation causing peritonitis with hemorrhage

- 💡 Toxic megacolon requiring colectomy, colorectal cancer (primarily with ulcerative), small intestinal cancer (primarily with Crohn's)

- 💡 May be fatal

⚕ Priority Nursing Implications

- 💡 If client has surgery and will need to wear an ileal pouch, body image disturbances may occur so, be sensitive and allow client to deal with this emotional issue

- ❯ Teach men taking sulfasalazine that long-term therapy may result in abnormal production of sperm, which can cause infertility

- 💡 Clients with ulcerative colitis can be significantly fatigued from the numerous bowel movements they have in a day. Rest periods must be considered when performing care to the client with this condition in the acute setting

- ❯ A yellow-orange discoloration of the skin may be caused by taking sulfasalazine, so client must be made aware

- ❯ 6-mercaptopurine and azathioprine can cause suppression of bone marrow so complete blood count must be monitored when these drugs are being taken

- ❯ methotrexate has serious side effect of hepatoxicity and bone marrow suppression, so CBC must be monitored frequently. Teach female clients taking the drug not to become pregnant because the drug can cause fetal defects and death

- ❯ natalizumab, one of the biologic and targeted therapies, has a risk of progressive multifocal leukoencephalopathy. Therefore, its use is restricted, and it can only be had through a restricted program

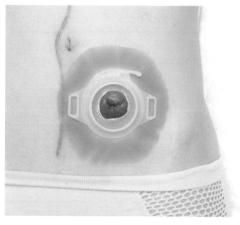

Image 11-4: Find online videos of people with colostomies talking about problems or concerns. List 3 important strategies to prevent complications when helping clients care for their ileostomy or colostomy.

1. _____

   _____

   _____

2. _____

   _____

   _____

3. _____

   _____

   _____

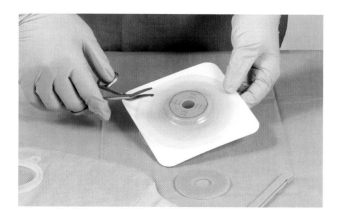

Image 11-3: Often, clients are great resources when it comes to managing the ileostomy or colostomy well. Be sure to inquire about their preferences.

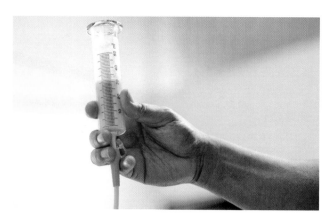

Image 11-5: Some clients have such severe inflammatory bowel disease that they do not absorb enough nutrition with regular food and they need tube feeding.

Priority Medications

sulfasalazine

- Main drug to maintain remission and prevent exacerbations (flare-ups)
- Dose for active disease is 3 to 4 grams orally in evenly divided doses, taken daily
- Maintenance dose is 2 grams orally in evenly divided doses, taken daily

olsalazine

- Main drug to maintain remission and prevent exacerbations (flare-ups)
- Dose for active disease is 500 mg to 1 gram orally each day, administered in 2 equally divided doses. For severe cases 500 mg up to 4 times a day can be administered
- Maintenance dose is 500 mg orally twice daily

mesalamine

- Main drug to maintain remission and prevent exacerbations (flare-ups)
- Dose for active disease is administered using several variations of dosages, both oral and rectal
- Dose for maintenance therapy is administered using several variations of oral dosing

> Corticosteroids
- Different ones in the class are used and dosages depend on the drug and severity of the condition. Two commonly used ones are below
- prednisone administered orally 5-6 mg daily and hydrocortisone administered 100 mg rectally via enema nightly for 21 days. It can be administered for longer if symptoms require
- Intravenous corticosteroids may be used for short duration with severe inflammation

> 6-mercaptopurine
- Immunosuppressant
- Has delayed onset of action so must not be used for active disease
- Maintenance dose is 1.0 to 1.5 mg/kg of body weight daily

> azathioprine
- Immunosuppressant
- Dose for both acute and maintenance Crohn's disease therapy is 1.5 to 4 mg/kg daily for 10 days, up to 52 weeks.
- Dose for ulcerative colitis is administered intravenously using various variations of dosages

> methotrexate
- Used for clients with Crohn's disease who are dependent on corticosteroids
- Dosage is dependent on prescriber's choice, Usual is 25 mg weekly via intramuscular injection.
- Methotrexate causes birth defects and fetal demise

> Biological and targeted therapy

- Several medications in this class of drugs used to treat Crohn's disease
- Used mostly to induce and maintain remission in clients who have had no success with other treatments
- They are either given intravenous or subcutaneous

Priority Education/Discharge Issues

Teach client to perform frequent and proper perineal care due to multiple bowel movements. Educate on not using harsh soaps that might be irritating to fragile skin. A skin barrier cream may be used to preserve skin integrity

Teach client to eat a diet high in protein, calories and vitamins to maintain nutritional status.

> Teach the importance of stress reduction as stress can worsen the symptoms of the conditions

> Teach client to get adequate rest as anemia and malnutrition can cause fatigue

> Teach coping strategies or assist client to schedule psychotherapy to deal with the emotional toll of a chronic condition and/or issues surrounding body image disturbances from ostomy device

> Teach the symptoms of the disease and when to contact the healthcare provider

> Explain the importance of smoking cessation for clients who smoke, as smoking can worsen both Crohn's disease and ulcerative colitis

> If surgery was done
- Teach client how to empty and change ostomy device
- Teach client how to care for, and assess stoma
- Have client do return demonstration of ostomy care
- Teach client signs of infection and to assess stoma site for infection
- Teach client that a second surgery may be needed to complete the process, especially if the first surgery was a proctocolectomy with ileal pouch/anal anastomosis
- Educate client on Kegel exercises that serve to strengthen the sphincter muscles and pelvic floor

> Teach that once discharged from acute care, it may take several weeks before client feels well enough to resume normal activities

Teach how to administer medications and about adverse effects for which the healthcare provider must be notified

> Teach importance of keeping follow-up appointments

Go To Clinical Answers

Text designated by 💡 are the top answers for the Go To Clinical related to Inflammatory bowel disease: Crohn's disease/ulcerative colitis.

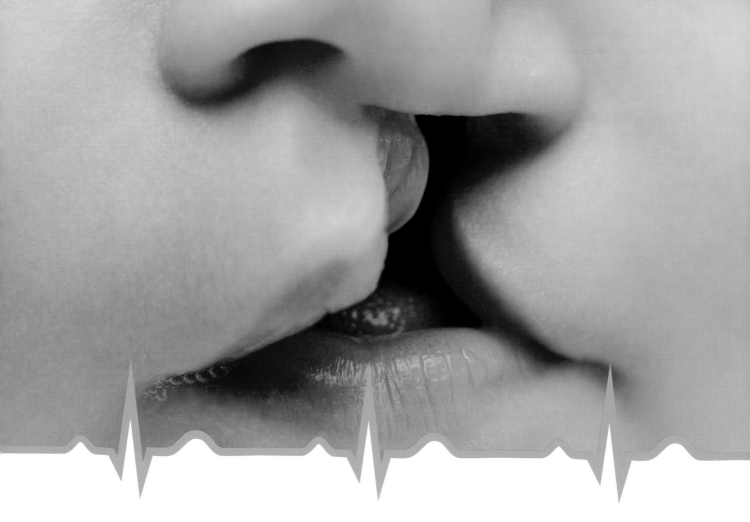

Go To Clinical Case 2

D. K. is a 7-month-old baby girl who is being admitted for repair of a cleft lip and palate. D.K. is with her mother who answers all your questions as you admit D. K. to the unit. The mother reports that D.K. has been having a "difficult time" eating and that the feeding just runs out her nose at times. She states that D. K. has been treated for 2 ear infections since birth.

Observation and physical assessment of D.K. reveal what appears to be a cleft of the hard and soft palate with a cleft lip on one side. Several of D. K.'s teeth are misaligned.

Vital signs are: Temperature 97.8°F, Pulse 142, Respirations 50, Blood pressure 88/50.

NurseThink® Time

Using the NurseThink® system, complete the priorities. Check your answers designated by 💡 in the Cleft lip and palate Priority Exemplar.

✏ Priority Assessments or Cues

1.

2.

3.

⚗ Priority Laboratory Tests/Diagnostics

1.

2.

3.

⚠ Priority Interventions or Actions

1.

2.

3.

⚑ Priority Potential & Actual Complications

1.

2.

3.

⚕ Priority Nursing Implications

1.

2.

3.

💧 Priority Medications

1.

2.

3.

👤 Priority Education/Discharge Issues

1.

2.

3.

Cleft lip and palate

Pathophysiology/Description

> Cleft lip and palate are congenital anomalies that cause abnormalities in closure of the lip and palate. Tissue that makes up the palate and lip normally fuse together in the second and third months in pregnancy. However, the fusion never occurred, or only partially occurred for babies born with cleft lip and palate.

> Cleft lip and palate can occur bilaterally or unilaterally

> Causes

- Genetics, with high incidence in children with family history of cleft lip/palate defects

- Chromosomal abnormality syndrome

- Exposure to teratogens while pregnant

- Mother having diabetes before pregnancy. Obesity during pregnancy

> Surgery is the only means of fixing a cleft lip and palate. A cleft lip is usually repaired first at around the third month of life.

> Cleft palate is repaired in several surgeries over the child's first 18 years, because of bone growth. The first surgery occurs between 6 to 12 months. Focus of the first surgery is on the creation of a palate that is functional and that minimizes the likelihood of fluid accumulating in the middle ear. This first surgery also helps the child develop facial bones and teeth

Priority Assessments or Cues

- Assess baby for difficulty feeding. Examine baby's lip and palate, will observe abnormal openings in lip and palate. Ask caregiver about regurgitation of fluids through the baby's mouth and nose

- Ask caregiver about ear infections as chronic ear infections are common with cleft lip and palate

> Examine baby's teeth (if there are teeth yet), expect misalignment of teeth

- Assess baby's ability to breathe without having difficulty

> Assess baby's voice, usually sounds nasal with cleft lip and palate

> Assess nutritional and fluid intake, may be poorly nourished because of difficulty eating

> Complete health history on the baby with the caregiver as historian

> Complete physical exam of the baby

Priority Laboratory Tests/Diagnostics

- Cleft lip and palate can be diagnosed 16 weeks into a woman's pregnancy. However, the physical appearance of the newborn after birth confirms the diagnosis of cleft lip and cleft palate

Priority Interventions or Actions

- Feed baby using a special nipple. Hold baby in a semi-upright seated position and stabilize the baby's head with one hand while feeding with the next. Keep a bulb suction to suction feeding from the nasal passage if needed.

- Feed using the ESSR method of feeding: Enlarge the nipple, Stimulate the reflex for sucking, allow baby to Swallow and Rest to give the baby time to swallow what is in its mouth. Feed baby small amounts and burp baby often. Monitor daily weights

> Allow caregiver (s) to verbalize feelings about the baby's appearance

> Prepare baby for surgery

- Postoperative interventions

- Assess surgery site for bleeding and signs of infection. A metal bar may be used on the face to protect the cleft lip surgery incision. Adhesive strips (Steri Strips) may also be used

- Keep restraint on baby's hands and arms, unless in room with baby

- Place baby to sleep on side and back and not stomach, to prevent pressure on incision

- Change dressings using sterile technique to minimize risk of infection

- Clean baby's mouth after feeding to prevent feeding from staying on the incision, causing an infection

- Apply antibiotic ointment as prescribed

- Administer pain medication to manage baby's pain

- Monitor surgical packing that is secured to the child's palate, if used. Assess for bleeding

- Since the child with palate repair surgery can be older, instruct child and caregiver not to brush child's teeth

- Do not place objects in child's mouth while assessing palate incision as objects may damage the incision

- Initiate appropriate consults such as to dietician, dentist and speech therapist

🚩 Priority Potential & Actual Complications

- 💡 Speech difficulties
- 💡 Impaired sucking ability and decreased nutrition, ear infections and hearing loss
- 💡 Dental problems
- › Parental psychological distress at disfigurement and impairment. Child having challenges coping with appearance as child grows

☘ Priority Nursing Implications

- 💡 The child born with a cleft lip and palate can be very distressing for the parents as they may see their child as being disfigured. Be sensitive about this fact and allow parents to verbalize their feelings. Provide them with referral to counseling if needed

💧 Priority Medications

- 💡 Analgesics: Used for managing child's pain after surgery. The choice and dose of medication is at the discretion of the physician

👤 Priority Education/Discharge Issues

- 💡 Teach caregiver how to use the ESSR method to feed baby, as it promotes safe feeding
- › Provide caregiver with information on cleft lip and palate support groups, if they need it
- › Inform caregiver of whom to contact with questions and concerns
- › Teach caregiver that as the baby grows, more surgery will be needed to repair the baby's palate
- 💡 Do not place anything hard, like a spoon, in baby's mouth after surgery. Give baby a small amount of water after feeding to cleanse the mouth of food that might cause buildup of bacteria in mouth, causing infection
- 💡 Place baby to sleep on back or side and not prone, to keep pressure off the surgery site. Cradle baby when holding to prevent from hurting the surgery site on your shoulder or chest
- › Baby will wear a restraint for a few weeks to prevent from rubbing or touching the incision. Remove the restraint when with the baby
- › Teach caregiver not to use aspirin for baby's pain as it may cause Reye syndrome in children, Acetaminophen may be prescribed
- › Teach caregiver to soothe baby by cradling, rocking, singing to, cooing at or any other therapeutic action

Go To Clinical Answers

Text designated by 💡 are the top answers for the Go To Clinical related to Cleft lip and palate.

Complete this MNEMONIC
CLEFT LIP Post-op Care
C _____
L _____
E _____
F _____
T _____
L _____
I _____
P _____

Table 11-1: Feel free to search the Internet or create your own.

_____

_____

_____

_____

_____

_____

_____

_____

_____

_____

Gastroesophageal reflux

Pathophysiology/Description

> Gastroesophageal reflux (GER) is a common upper gastrointestinal (GI) problem that results from the backflow (reflux) of gastric contents into the esophagus. Pepsin and hydrochloric acid irritates the esophagus and produce inflammation.

> Inflammation can be mild or severe depending on the contents that are refluxed

> Factors that predispose an individual to GER
> - A lower esophageal sphincter (LES) that does not function properly. This is the most common cause
> - Gastric emptying that is delayed
> - Motility from the esophagus that is impaired
> - Delayed stomach emptying
> - Hiatal hernia
> - Obesity
> - Cigarette smoking

> Normal function of the lower esophageal sphincter is to prevent food in the stomach from coming back up into the esophagus but with a non-functioning LES, food is allowed to backflow, especially when the individual is in a lying position.

> It has been observed that the intake of certain foods, such as caffeinated beverages, fatty foods, peppermint, and alcohol cause the pressure of the LES to be decreased, while certain medications, such as metoclopramide causes increased pressure to the LES

> In extreme cases of where individual has not responded to medical management, surgery may be indicated. The most common surgery for GER involves a fundoplication, where a portion of the gastric fundus around the esophageal sphincter is wrapped

Priority Assessments or Cues

> Assess for heartburn (pyrosis) and pain in the epigastric areas

> Assess for pain in upper, center part of the abdomen, called dyspepsia

> Ask client about onset of heartburn, usually starts after eating foods that decrease LES pressure

> Ask client about meal intake, to determine intake of foods that cause GER

> Ask about smoking habits, as smoking is a trigger for GER

> Ask about regurgitation of insipid tasting (described as sour or bitter) fluid in the mouth or throat.

> Ask about difficulty swallowing, may occur from irritation and inflammation to the throat

> Assess for wheezing and/or coughing, as regurgitation may cause aspiration into the lungs resulting in airway irritation and swelling

> Assess for hoarseness

> Assess for a feeling of fullness in the throat due to presence of inflammation and soreness

Priority Laboratory Tests/Diagnostics

> Upper GI endoscopy will show status of LES. Expect to see scarring and inflammation with GER

> Esophageal biopsy to differentiate between esophageal cancer and Barrett's esophagus (change in esophageal cell type that is reversible but a precursor to esophageal cancer)

> Radionuclide test shows gastric content reflux and how fast the esophagus is clearing the reflux

> Manometric studies shows LES pressure and movement of the esophagus

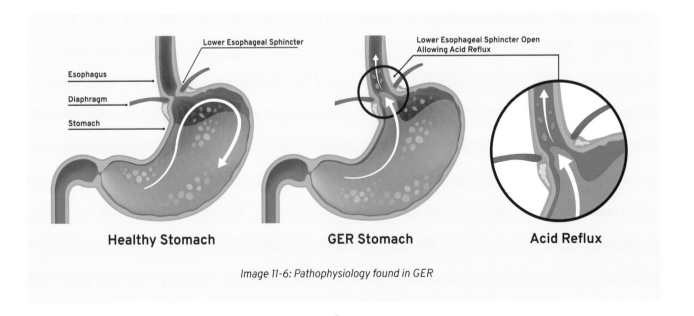

Lower Esophageal Sphincter

Esophagus

Diaphragm

Stomach

Lower Esophageal Sphincter Open Allowing Acid Reflux

Healthy Stomach　　　**GER Stomach**　　　**Acid Reflux**

Image 11-6: Pathophysiology found in GER

⚠ Priority Interventions or Actions

> Elevate client's head by using 4 to 6-inch blocks, bricks or a long wedge pillow, to decrease likelihood of reflux

> Manage diet to ensure client's meal does not contain foods that induce reflux (aforementioned)

> Ensure client is not served anything to eat or drink 2 hours before bedtime so as not to cause reflux of food eaten into the esophagus

> Administer prescribed medications

> If client is having fundoplication surgery (in extreme cases), prepare client for surgery. Surgery is usually done laparoscopically

> Monitor vital signs

🚩 Priority Potential & Actual Complications

> Esophagitis

> Barrett's esophagus

> Several respiratory complications such as laryngospasms, bronchospasms, asthma, pneumonia

> Dental carries for prolonged exposure to stomach acid

℧ Priority Nursing Implications

> Older adults with GER may have symptoms that are like angina pain. They may experience the pain as a squeezing in the chest area that radiates to the jaw and back. However, the pain will be relieved by using antacids

> The risk of fractures is increased when client takes a proton pump inhibitor (PPI) on a long-term basis

🜄 Priority Medications

> Proton pump inhibitors
  - Several drugs in this class are used. They decrease hydrochloric acid secretion and decrease gastric and esophageal mucosa irritation
  - This class of drug is among the most effective and common in treating GER
  - Available over-the-counter or by prescription

> Histamine receptor blockers
  - Several drugs in this class are used. They decrease hydrochloric acid secretion and decrease gastric and esophageal mucosa irritation
  - Like the proton pump inhibitors, this class of drugs is effective and commonly used
  - Available both as over-the-counter and prescription

> Cholinergic drug
  - Urecholine is the only drug used in this class
  - Used to increase the pressure of LES and improve esophageal emptying
  - Usual dose ranges from 10 to 50 mg three or four times daily

> Antacids
  - Several types of antacids in this class
  - Taken 1-3 hours after a meal and at bedtime, it neutralizes hydrochloric acid
  - Dosage is dependent on the drug used

👤 Priority Education/Discharge Issues

> Instruct client on administration of prescribed medications

> Provide client with list of factors that cause decreased LES pressure and teach avoidance

> Instruct client not to eat 2 hours before bedtime, as this increases gastric acid secretion and likelihood of reflux

> Teach client that eating small meals at frequent intervals and drinking fluids in between meals help to decrease reflux activity

> Teach client to seek assistance of pharmacist before taking over-the-counter medications as some medications can increase likelihood of gastric acid reflux

> Encourage smoking cessation for clients who smoke

> Encourage client who is obese to start a weight loss program

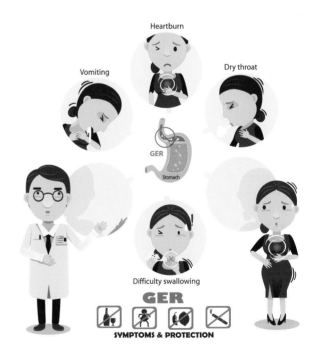

Image 11-7: Create 3 realistic statements by the client that would indicate the possibility of them having GER.

Gastritis

Pathophysiology/Description

> Gastritis is inflammation of the gastric mucosa. It is classified as acute or chronic

> Acute gastritis occurs acutely and usually has a duration of hours to a few days. The mucosa is usually completely healed after the episode

> Chronic gastritis occurs over extended periods. Atrophy of stomach mucosa occurs causing loss of parietal cells. This results in loss of intrinsic factor needed for absorption of vitamin B_{12}, which is essential in red blood cell maturation

> The etiology of gastritis relates to a breakdown in the normal mucosal barrier. This mucosal barrier breakdown allows hydrochloric acid to damage the mucosa causing irritation, erosion, edema and inflammation

> There are several risk factors for gastritis
> - Dietary, such as eating spicy foods, large amounts of food or intaking alcohol
> - Pathogens, such as Helicobacter pylori (H. pylori), which is a very common causative agent for gastritis
> - Drugs, such as non-steroidal anti-inflammatory drugs (NSAIDs)
> - Environmental, such as smoking
> - Disease processes, such as Burns
> - Autoimmune atrophic gastritis, where immune response damages stomach cells. This is an inherited condition seen in women of northern European descent

Priority Assessments or Cues

> Assess for nausea, vomiting, feeling of fullness, anorexia and epigastric tenderness

> Assess client for gastric hemorrhage, which indicates alcohol associated gastritis

> Assess client for excessive belching that can be caused from inflammation and presence of bacteria in stomach

> Assess for anemia, caused by lack of vitamin B12 with chronic gastritis

> Ask client about intake of foods that cause gastritis

> Perform ongoing assessment of vital signs, hypotension and tachycardia may indicate bleeding

> Ask client about exposure to environmental factors that cause gastritis

> Complete health history to determine other health conditions that cause gastritis

> Assess for sour taste in mouth, occurring more with chronic gastritis

> Assess for vitamin B 12 deficiency, occurring with chronic gastritis

> Complete tests to detect presence of H. pylori infection

Priority Laboratory Tests/Diagnostics

> Test for H. Pylori via breath, blood and stool, will be positive

> Stool tested for occult blood, may be positive

> Endoscopy stomach examination and biopsy will show H. Pylori and biopsy can rule out gastric cancer

> Complete blood count may indicate anemia because of lack of B12

Priority Interventions or Actions

> Acute gastritis
> - Maintain nothing by mouth (NPO) to minimize nausea and vomiting
> - Administer intravenous fluids to prevent dehydration. Monitor intake and output
> - Insert nasogastric (NG) tube in severe gastritis and monitor for bleeding
> - If no NG tube inserted, check vomitus for signs of gastric bleeding
> - Administer antiemetics as prescribed
> - Re-introduce a clear liquid diet when symptoms have subsided
> - Administer medications to manage gastritis symptoms
> - Administer antibiotics to treat Pylori, in chronic gastritis
> - Administer cobalamin for pernicious anemia, in chronic gastritis

Priority Potential & Actual Complications

> Peptic ulcer
> Pernicious anemia
> Cancer called gastric mucosa-associated lymphoid tissue (MALT) lymphoma because of chronic H. pylori gastritis

Priority Nursing Implications

> Clients with pernicious anemia from chronic gastritis must be educated on the fact that they will need to take B12 injections for life

Priority Medications

> Proton pump inhibitors
> - Several drugs in this class are used. They decrease hydrochloric acid secretion and decrease gastric mucosa irritation
> - This class of drug is among the most effective and common in treating GER
> - Available over-the-counter or by prescription
> Histamine receptor blockers
> - Several drugs in this class are used. They decrease hydrochloric acid secretion and decrease gastric and esophageal mucosa irritation
> - Like the proton pump inhibitors, this class of drugs is effective and commonly used
> - Available both as over-the-counter and prescription

Priority Education/Discharge Issues

> Instruct client on administration of prescribed medications

> Teach client to avoid spicy and well-seasoned foods, as they are irritating to the gastric mucosa

> Instruct client on prevention of alcohol intake. Assist with locating alcoholics anonymous for client, if requested

> Instruct client to stop smoking. Assist client with smoking cessation plans, if requested

> Instruct client to take all of the prescribed antibiotics for H. pylori, even if symptoms have subsided

> Teach client to increase diet back to normal, as tolerated, after an acute episode

> Encourage the intake of 6 small meals instead of large meals

> Teach client to monitor for signs and symptoms of gastric bleeding and contact healthcare provider immediately

> Teach client administration of B12 injections and have client do a return demonstration if client will be self-administering the drug

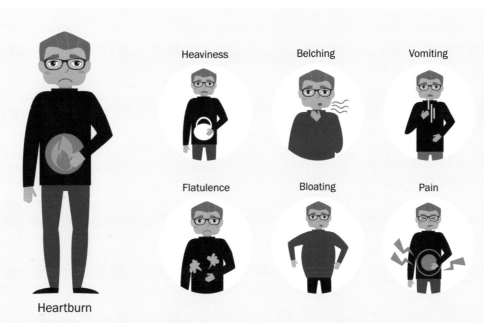

Image 11-8: Create 3 realistic statements by the client that would indicate the possibility of them having gastritis.

_____

_____

_____

Peptic ulcer disease

Pathophysiology/Description

> A peptic ulcer is an ulceration in the gastric mucosa. It can occur in several locations in the gastrointestinal (GI) system, esophagus, stomach, pylorus and duodenum. Peptic ulcers thrive in an acid environment and so any situation that causes excess acid production in the GI system contributes to peptic ulcer formation

> Classification of peptic ulcers
  - Acute vs chronic
  - Esophageal, gastric or duodenal. Gastric and duodenal are the most common types of ulcers

> Acute ulcers
  - Short duration
  - Healed quickly with treatment
  - Erosion is superficial
  - Minimal inflammation

> Chronic ulcer
  - Continues for long duration, months to sometimes years
  - Erosion is deep, going through the muscle wall
  - Occur more commonly than acute ulcers

> Gastric ulcers
  - Less common than duodenal ulcers
  - Adults over 50 years and women have the highest incidence of gastric ulcers
  - Higher risk of causing obstruction than duodenal ulcers and mortality rate higher due to age of persons with gastric ulcers

> Duodenal ulcers
  - Most peptic ulcers are duodenal ulcers
  - Unlike gastric ulcer the age of highest incidence is 35-45 years
  - H. pylori is the most common cause of duodenal ulcers

> Factors that predispose to peptic ulcers
  - Dietary, such as eating spicy foods, large amounts of food or intaking alcohol
  - Helicobacter pylori (H. pylori) can live for a long time in the gastric cells, causing production of certain chemicals that aid in activation of inflammatory agents that foster cell damage
  - Certain drugs, such as non-steroidal anti-inflammatory drugs (NSAIDs) and corticosteroids can cause erosion of gastric mucosa and decrease the protective capability of the mucosa
  - Caffeine and alcohol stimulate gastric acid secretion and smoking which delay gastric ulcer healing
  - Certain diseases predispose an individual to peptic ulcers, especially duodenal ulcers. These include liver cirrhosis, chronic pancreatitis, chronic kidney disease, among others
  - Stress is also known to negative impact peptic ulcer disease and ulcer healing

Priority Assessments or Cues

> Complete history, important to determine conditions that are risk factors for peptic ulcer disease

> Assess for pain occurring in the mid-epigastric region or toward the back. Clients usually describe it as a burning pain that occurs about 1 ½ to 3 hours after a meal, indicating a duodenal ulcer

> Ask about sleep pattern. With a duodenal ulcer, the pain usually awakens client at nights

> Assess for pain occurring in the high epigastric region. Clients usually describe it as a gnawing pain that worsens 30 to 60 minutes after a meal, indicating a gastric ulcer

> Ask client about pain relieving strategies used. Eating a meal aggravates a gastric ulcer while eating relieves pain caused by a duodenal ulcer

> Assess duration of symptoms. Duodenal ulcers may occur for a long duration, like a few months, disappear for a long while and then recur

> Assess for nausea, vomiting and bloating, experienced by some clients

> If vomiting occurs, assess for hematemesis, which indicates a gastric ulcer

> Ongoing assessment of vital signs, looking for signs of bleeding, such as hypotension

> Assess for active bleeding

> If client had surgery, ongoing assessment of all body systems to detect postoperative complications

Priority Laboratory Tests/Diagnostics

> Test for H. Pylori via breath, blood and stool, will be positive

> Stool tested for occult blood, may be positive

> Endoscopy stomach examination and biopsy will show H. Pylori and biopsy can rule out gastric cancer.

> Rapid urease testing is done for H. pylori using a biopsy sample. H. pylori secretes the urease enzyme and test will be positive for the bacteria

> Barium contrast study to detect gastric ulcers if a client cannot do an endoscopy. It also diagnoses gastric outlet obstruction

> Complete blood count may indicate anemia due to bleeding

Priority Interventions or Actions

> Acute Care
  - Maintain nothing by mouth (NPO) to minimize nausea and vomiting
  - Administer intravenous fluids to prevent dehydration
  - Monitor intake and output
  - Insert nasogastric (NG) tube and connect to suction

- If no NG tube inserted, check vomitus and stools for active bleeding
- Administer medications to heal ulcer, as prescribed
- If actively bleeding, monitor closely for hypovolemic shock and treat accordingly
- Maintain patency of NG tube to prevent blockage of the tube and risk of client getting an abdominal distention
- Assess for perforation, which may be manifested as a sudden, severe upper abdominal pain coupled with a rigid, hard abdomen
- Administer analgesics as prescribed
- Provide client with a quiet, calm and restful environment
- Administer blood transfusion, if prescribed, and monitor for transfusion reaction
- Monitor intake and output
- Central venous monitoring if perforation and severe bleeding
- Re-introduce a clear liquid diet when symptoms have subsided

> Additional interventions if surgical procedure (partial gastrectomy, vagotomy, pyloroplasty or closure of perforation)
  - Ongoing monitoring of vital signs to ensure hemodynamic stability
  - Maintain NPO until peristalsis returns and oral intake is tolerated
  - Monitor for postoperative complications (see priority complications for list)
  - Ongoing bowel assessment, looking for signs of bowel obstruction

Priority Potential & Actual Complications

> Hemorrhage
> Perforation
> Gastric outlet obstruction
> Postoperative complications:
  - Hemorrhage at surgery site, dumping syndrome, bile reflux, hypoglycemia (postprandial) vitamin B12 deficiency

Priority Nursing Implications

> The client who has a gastrectomy must be taught the symptoms of dumping syndrome and how to control it
  - Cause of dumping syndrome: Stomach no longer has control over the amount of chyme that enters the small intestines so large amounts of hypertonic fluid enter the intestine pulling fluid with it into the bowel. This causes distention of the lumen and rapid movement so that within a few minutes after eating the client gets the strong urge to have a bowel movement, associated with sweating, palpations and dizziness
  - Managing dumping syndrome: Eat six small meals instead of a few large meals and chew food properly. Do not eat concentrated sweets as they can cause diarrhea. Increase protein and complex carbohydrate intake instead of fatty foods. Do not drink fluids with, or within 30 minutes after a meal, and refrain from eating dairy products

> The risk of fractures is increased when client takes a proton pump inhibitor on a long-term basis
> It is important to note that some over-the-counter drugs contain aspirin. Clients must understand that they must seek advice from healthcare providers and pharmacists before taking OTC drugs and herbal remedies to ensure they are not increasing their risk of bleeding
> Clients with renal failure should not take antacids containing magnesium due to a potential risk of magnesium toxicity. Use antacids that contain sodium cautiously in older adults with conditions such as heart failure and hypertension as it may cause fluid retention

Priority Medications

> Proton pump inhibitors (PPI)
  - Several drugs in this class are used. They decrease hydrochloric acid secretion and decrease gastric mucosa irritation
  - This class of drug is among the most effective and common in treating peptic ulcers. Often used in combination with antibiotics to treat ulcers when the cause is H. pylori
  - Available over-the-counter or by prescription
> Histamine receptor blockers
  - Several drugs in this class are used. They decrease hydrochloric acid secretion and promote healing of ulcer
  - Like the proton pump inhibitors, this class of drugs is effective and commonly used
  - Available both as over-the-counter and prescription, and administered either oral or intravenous
> Antacids
  - Work by neutralizing hydrochloric acid
  - Several drugs in this class, available over-the-counter or with prescription
  - Best taken after meals for a longer effect
> Antiulcer protectant
  - Only one used is sucralfate
  - Taken on an empty stomach for maximum effect
  - Dose is 1 gram orally 4 times daily. Therapy lasts 4 to 8 weeks
> amoxicillin
  - Antibiotic
  - Used in triple-drug therapy with a PPI, and clarithromycin to treat H. pylori infection
  - Dose is 1 gram orally every 12 hours for 14 days
> clarithromycin
  - Antibiotic
  - Used in triple-drug therapy with a PPI, and amoxicillin to treat H. pylori infection
  - Dose is 500 mg orally every 12 hours for 10 to 14 days
> tetracycline
  - Antibiotic
  - Used in quadruple drug therapy with a PPI, bismuth, and metronidazole to treat H. pylori infection
  - Dose is 500 mg orally every 6 hours for 14 days

> metronidazole
  - Antibiotic
  - Used in quadruple drug therapy with a PPI, bismuth, and tetracycline to treat H. pylori infection
  - Dose is 250 mg orally 4 times daily for 10 to 14 days
> bismuth
  - Antacid and antidiarrheal
  - Used in quadruple drug therapy with a PPI, metronidazole and tetracycline to treat H. pylori infection
  - Dose is 524 mg orally 4 times daily

Priority Education/Discharge Issues

> Instruct client on strict administration of prescribed medications to ensure full healing of ulcer
> Instruct client to take all of the prescribed antibiotics for H. pylori, even if symptoms have subsided
> Instruct client the healthcare provider may discontinue the PPIs and histamine receptor blockers once the ulcer is healed
> Educate client that an endoscopic follow-up examination will be done about 3-6 months after treatment to evaluate the ulcer
> Instruct client to avoid foods that are irritating to the ulcer, such as pepper, hot and spicy foods, caffeinated and carbonated beverages
> Teach client that aspirin and NSAID's must not be taken for 4-6 weeks

> Teach client not to interchange brands of medications without first speaking with the healthcare provider
> If client had surgery, teach signs and symptoms of postoperative complications and when to contact the healthcare provider, Teach surgical site care
> Instruct client on prevention of alcohol intake. Assist with locating alcoholics anonymous for client, if requested
> Instruct client to stop smoking. Assist client with smoking cessation plans, if requested
> Teach client to advance diet back to normal, as tolerated, after an acute episode
> Encourage the intake of 6 small meals instead of large meals
> Teach client to monitor for signs and symptoms of gastric bleeding or perforation and to contact healthcare provider immediately
> Teach client administration of B12 injections and have client do a return demonstration, if client will be self-administering the drug
> Instruct client to modify routine to ensure adequate rest that is needed to foster healing of the ulcer
> Educate client on the importance of managing stress and other emotional issues as stress negatively impacts wound healing

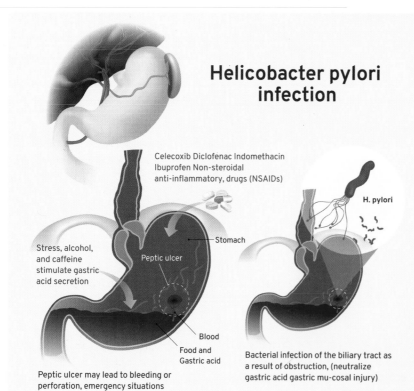

Helicobacter pylori infection

Celecoxib Diclofenac Indomethacin Ibuprofen Non-steroidal anti-inflammatory, drugs (NSAIDs)

H. pylori

Stomach

Stress, alcohol, and caffeine stimulate gastric acid secretion

Peptic ulcer

Blood

Food and Gastric acid

Peptic ulcer may lead to bleeding or perforation, emergency situations

Bacterial infection of the biliary tract as a result of obstruction, (neutralize gastric acid gastric mu-cosal injury)

Image 11-9: Create 3 notecards. Each notecard will be the GENERIC name of a medication used to treat a Helicobacter pylori infection and related peptic ulcer disease. On the back of each card, list 3 priority nursing concerns for that medication.

Celiac disease

Pathophysiology/Description

> Celiac disease is an autoimmune disease where there is damage to the small intestines from intake of rye, wheat and barley. The disease is also commonly known as gluten sensitive enteropathy or celiac sprue

> There are specific peptides in gluten that bind to the celiac disease human leukocyte antigen and initiate an inflammatory response. The inflammation causes destruction of the microvilli and brush border of the small intestine. This results in a decrease in surface area that is needed for nutrient absorption to occur

> Risk factors
> - European ancestry (common in this ethnic group)
> - First and second-degree relatives to someone with celiac disease
> - Ninety percent of persons with Celiac disease have the antigen for the disease

> Symptoms of celiac disease are most often seen in childhood, between the ages of 1 to 5 years

Priority Assessments or Cues

> Assess client for flatulence and fatty stool (steatorrhea) from poor fat absorption

> Assess for diarrhea and foul-smelling diarrhea, from malabsorption

> Assess for abdominal distention from gas accumulation due to poor nutrient absorption

> Assess for muscle wasting and weight loss due to poor absorption of protein and fats

> Assess for nausea and vomiting

> Assess for folate and iron-deficiency. Assess vitamin B12 levels

> Examine mouth, poor dentition is likely

> Ask client or caregiver about lactose intolerance, which is likely with celiac disease

> Examine skin for vesicular lesions on various parts of the body that are pruritic (itchy)

> Complete health history, other autoimmune diseases are likely

> Assess for osteoporosis due to bone weakening from inadequate vitamin D absorption and poor calcium intake

> Assess for celiac crisis: profuse watery diarrhea, nausea, vomiting

> Assess for dehydration and electrolyte imbalances, can occur with celiac crisis

> Assess vital signs, may be tachycardic and hypotensive

> Perform meticulous skin care and apply skin barrier to prevent skin breakdown from profuse diarrhea

Priority Laboratory Tests/Diagnostics

> Tissue Transglutaminase Antibodies (tTG-IgA) test, will be positive in about 98% of patients with celiac disease who are on a gluten-containing diet.

> Biopsy of small intestines will show loss of villi and flattened mucosa, damage that is consistent with celiac disease

> Genetic testing for the HLA-DQ2 and/or HLA-DQ8 antigens, will show an increased risk for celiac disease

Priority Interventions or Actions

> Refer client to have a dietary consult

> Ensure that client is served meals that are gluten-free

> Administer all necessary vitamins such as A, D, E, K, folic acid and iron. Malabsorption causes client to be deficient in these

> If client is in a celiac crisis, do not give oral food. Keep NPO until crisis is resolved and client can tolerate foods by mouth

> Provide intravenous fluids to prevent dehydration

> Administer electrolytes to compensate for electrolyte imbalance

Priority Potential & Actual Complications

> Increased risk of Hodgkin's lymphoma and gastrointestinal cancers

Priority Nursing Implications

> Ensure that the client and/or caregiver is provided with adequate discharge teaching and resources on how to live a gluten-free life. Provide information for community, local and national resources, such as the Celiac Disease Foundation and the Celiac Sprue Association

Priority Medications

> Corticosteroids (several in the class)
> - Several drugs in this category can be used. Choice of drug depends on severity
> - Used to manage refractory celiac disease (when a gluten-free diet doesn't work)
> - Dosages vary based on which corticosteroid is prescribed

Priority Education/Discharge Issues

> Encourage screening of close relatives with the disease

> Educate client and/or caregiver on eating a diet free from gluten, avoiding barley, oats, wheat and rye

> Assist with locating community resources from which to purchase gluten-free products

> Teach client and/or caregiver how to read food labels, as many food additives contain gluten

> Explain to client and/or caregiver that a gluten-free diet will need to be maintained for life

> Provide the celiac disease website to client as an excellent source for resources, www.celiac.org

Gallbladder conditions

Pathophysiology/Description

> Diseases of the gallbladder are very common in the United States. These include gallstones (cholelithiasis) and gallbladder inflammation (cholecystitis)

> Cholelithiasis occurs more in women than men and is more commonly seen in women over 40 years. Because cholesterol production is impacted by oral contraceptives and causes saturation of cholesterol in the gallbladder, younger women who take contraceptives have a high-risk of getting gallbladder disease. The same is true for women who are postmenopausal and take hormone replacement

> Obesity is also known to increase the likelihood of getting gallbladder disease because obesity causes an increased secretion of cholesterol in bile

> There is also a noted tendency for gallbladder disease to be in families

> Cholelithiasis
> • Supersaturation of bile with cholesterol occurs causing cholesterol to precipitate into stones
> • Protein, bile salts and calcium also precipitate into stones in the gallbladder
> • Conditions such as pregnancy, obstructive lesions or inflammation of the biliary system and immobility, decrease flow and/or stasis of bile and increase the risk of gallstones formation
> • Gallstones frequently stay in the gallbladder but may move to the ducts, causing obstruction and pain. If bile is unable to flow out from the ducts, this can precipitate an inflammation (cholecystitis)

> Cholecystitis
> • Can occur as acute or chronic. Acute gallbladder inflammation occurs as a result of obstruction that is caused by biliary sludge or gallstones
> • Chronic disease is caused when the wall of the gallbladder becomes scarred and tissue becomes fibrotic, causing a shrunken gallbladder and decreased function
> • In acute cholecystitis, the gallbladder becomes swollen, and usually contains pus
> • Cholecystitis can occur in the absence of gallstones, called acalculous cholecystitis. This predisposes the client to infections

Priority Assessments or Cues

> Assess for pain that client may describe as severe, steady and colicky. Pain that usually goes away after an hour, leaving a feeling of tenderness in the right upper quadrant, usually indicate cholelithiasis

> Assess for pain in the epigastric region that client might describe as radiating to the right scapula shoulder area, indicating cholecystitis

> Ask client what factors precipitate the pain. Pain with cholelithiasis/cholecystitis is usually precipitated by intake of a meal high in fat

> Assess for nausea and vomiting

> Assess for belching, flatulence and indigestion, primarily with cholecystitis

> Additional assessments if bile flow is obstructed
> • Assess client for signs of infection, such as fever
> • Assess for jaundice, indicating obstruction. Bile is not flowing into the duodenum and bilirubin is accumulating in the blood
> • Examine urine, will be dark brown in color and foamy, indicting bilirubin is being excreted by the kidneys and not going to the small intestines for conversion as is the norm
> • Assess stools, will show fat (steatorrhea) and clay color due to lack of fat digestion in the absence of bile
> • Ask client about itching skin (pruritus), due to bile salts being deposited on skin
> • Assess for bleeding. Vitamin K is not being absorbed which causes a decrease in the production of clotting factor, prothrombin
> • Assess vital signs, temperature may be elevated due to obstruction causing reflux of bacteria into systemic circulation from biliary tract
> • Assess for bleeding due to decreased production of prothrombin by the liver

Priority Laboratory Tests/Diagnostics

> Abdominal ultrasound shows gallstones

> Endoscopic retrograde cholangiopancreatography (ERCP) to examine the biliary structures and remove bile for culture, if infection suspected

> Percutaneous transhepatic cholangiography, done as a follow-up test if a blockage of the bile duct is shown on ultrasound. May show poor filling of biliary and hepatic ducts

> Liver enzymes may be elevated. Bilirubin level may be elevated

> Complete blood cell (CBC), may show increased white blood cell count due to inflammation

Priority Interventions or Actions

> Administer pain medications as prescribed. Administer antiemetics for nausea and vomiting

> Maintain nothing by mouth (NPO) status, to prevent stimulation of the gallbladder

> Insert nasogastric (NG) tube if client has severe nausea and vomiting. Maintain gastric decompression

> Administer intravenous fluids

> Initiate low-fat diet when intake by mouth is started

> Administer fat-soluble vitamins

> Monitor intake and output

> Provide client with frequent mouth care when vomiting

> Explain to client the process of removal of stones via papillotomy or lithotripsy

> Administer anti-pruritic medication as prescribed, if client is experiencing itching

- Postoperative interventions (cholecystectomy)
  - Monitor punctures to abdomen for signs of infection and bleeding
  - Manage T-tube if an open cholecystectomy was performed. Monitor and measure drainage
  - Administer pain medications as needed
  - Prevent respiratory problems. Ensure adequate ventilation
  - Encourage coughing and deep breathing to prevent respiratory compromise
  - Position client on left side with right knee flexed to minimize the common complaint of pain to the shoulder caused by the CO_2 used in surgery
  - Assist client to ambulate to prevent complications of immobility

🚩 Priority Potential & Actual Complications

- Acalculous cholecystitis with perforation and infection
- Bleeding from decreased production of prothrombin
- Injury to common bile duct during laparoscopic cholecystectomy

℧ Priority Nursing Implications

- Acalculous cholecystitis occurs more commonly in clients who are critically ill due to increased viscosity of bile from various pathological processes related to the critical illness, such as dehydration and fever.

💧 Priority Medications

- Non-steroidal anti-inflammatory drugs (NSAIDs)
  - Used to treat mild pain
  - There are several NSAIDs that can be used
  - Most significant adverse effect of NSAIDs is gastrointestinal bleeding
- morphine
  - Used initially in acute phase to manage pain and NSAIDs used after
  - Can be administered via several routes. Usual morphine oral dose is 15 to 30 mg orally every 4 hours as needed
  - Causes depressed respirations so monitor client's respiratory rate
- Anticholinergic and antispasmodic drugs
  - Used to decrease biliary ductal tone and relax the smooth muscles
  - Several drugs in the two classes
  - A common anticholinergic used is atropine. Dose is 0.4 mg to 0.6 mg, intravenous, intramuscular or subcutaneous
- ursodeoxycholic acid
  - Dissolve gallbladder stones
  - Not widely used because of the risk of gallstones returning
  - Dose is 8 to 10 mg/kg/day orally in 2 or 3 divided doses

- cholestyramine
  - Used to treat pruritus (itching)
  - Initial dose is 4 grams (1 packet or level scoop) orally once or twice a day
  - Maintenance dose is 8 to 16 grams (2 to 4 packets or level scoops) orally in 2 divided doses

👤 Priority Education/Discharge Issues

- Teach client proper medication administration such as vitamin replacement and medications for pain and spasms
- Inform client that discharge after a laparoscopic cholecystectomy is usually the day of or the day after surgery
- Teach client how to care for surgical puncture or open incisional site after a cholecystectomy
- Teach client signs and symptoms of infection
- If client has a transhepatic biliary catheter placement to drain bile, educate on cleaning skin at the insertion site with antiseptic daily to maintain cleanliness. Teach client to observe for and report any signs of catheter obstruction manifested as fever, nausea and sudden pain in abdomen. Teach client to drink beverages that contain electrolytes to replace fluid lost in the biliary drainage
- Teach client the importance of avoiding foods that are high in saturated fats
- Teach client to eat small meals and ensure intake of high fiber
- Teach client who had cholecystectomy to increase diet gradually, from liquid to regular as tolerated
- Instruct client who had cholecystectomy not to lift anything heavy for 4-6 weeks
- Instruct client on a weight reduction plan, if obese
- Remind client to keep follow-up medical appointments

Constipation

Pathophysiology/Description

> Constipation is the difficult and infrequent passage of stools that are hard and dry

> Causes
> - Not defecating when there is an urge
> - Inadequate fluid intake
> - Sedentary, decreased physical activity
> - Decreased intake of fiber
> - Disease conditions such as Parkinson's disease, hypothyroidism and stroke, among others
> - Drugs, such as opioids are commonly known to cause constipation

> When the urge to defecate is ignored, it causes water absorption and drying of stools. The mucosa and muscles of the rectum can also become insensitive to the presence of stool when the urge to defecate is ignored repeatedly. Both factors increase the risk of constipation

> Some individuals take laxatives regularly if they do not have a daily bowel movement. This results in a dependence on laxatives to have bowel movements. They are not able to defecate without taking a laxative. Their colon becomes dilated and lacks tone

Priority Assessments or Cues

> Assess for abdominal distention and bloating

> Assess for abdominal pain

> Assess for presence of rectal hemorrhoids, as these are common with chronic constipation

> Ask about quality of bowel movements. Stools are usually dry and hard

> Ask about difficulty passing stools. Straining is common because hard feces is difficult to pass

> Assess for bowel perforation, which may be indicated by nausea, vomiting, abdominal pain, and fever in the presence of constipation

> Assess for fissures and ulcers to the rectal mucosa, caused by repeated straining and irritation from dry stools

> Complete a health history

> Ask client about bowel movement habits and patterns

Priority Laboratory Tests/Diagnostics

> Abdominal X-rays will likely show constipation

> Colonoscopy shows entire colon and can detect complications of constipation, such as polyps, and cancer

> Sigmoidoscopy, shows hemorrhoids, polyps and fissures

> Barium enema can see impacted fecal matter or can detect complications such as polyps

> Anorectal manometry and rectal balloon expulsion tests are used to measure muscle tone of the anal sphincter and coordination between the rectal and anal muscles. An anal sphincter that is too tight during a bowel movement can cause constipation

> Colonic transit test, used to determine how long it takes food to travel through the colon, will likely show a delay with constipation

Priority Interventions or Actions

> Prepare client for diagnostic tests, such as barium enema

> Provide diet high in fiber

> Provide adequate liquids

> Administer laxative and/or enema in acute constipation

> Check client's rectal vault for impaction, if indicated

> Understand the uses and contraindications for the various types of enemas and provide the client with the one that is best suited for the client's situation

> Provide adequate privacy for client to defecate

> Use a safe odor eliminator to minimize odor from bowel movement

> Keep client nothing by mouth (NPO) if nausea and vomiting

> Provide diet as tolerated when client has had a fecal evacuation and nausea and vomiting has subsided

Priority Potential & Actual Complications

> Perforation of colon

> Diverticulosis

> Rectal ulcers

> Surgery with use of fecal diversions (such as colostomy)

Priority Nursing Implications

> Important for client to know the risk of repeated straining to have a bowel movement, called Valsalva maneuvers. Can cause decreased heart rate, less return of blood to the heart, and less blood flow from the heart when straining. When the straining is stopped, several physiological changes occur that can cause a fatal outcome. Clients with heart conditions and/or swelling in the brain are particularly at risk

> Surgery because of constipation is not common. However, if constipation does not resolve with all possible treatments, a continent fecal diversion, colostomy or ileostomy may be done

Priority Medications

> Laxatives and enemas are used in an acute situation and used very cautiously and sparingly because of the risk of dependence. Several types from which to choose. Below is an example of one drug in a few of the most commonly used classes

> Stool softeners
  - Soften feces by lubricating intestinal tract
  - Usually cause bowel movement in 72 hours
  - docusate, usual dose is 50 to 400 mg orally administered in 1 to 4 equally divided doses daily or 200 to 283 mg rectally administered as an enema once or twice.

> Bulk-forming laxatives
  - Absorb water and cause increase bulk, thus stimulating peristalsis
  - Usually cause bowel movement within 24 hours
  - psyllium: 1-2 teaspoons/wafers/packets/capsules PO 1-3 times/day. Take each dose with a full glass of water, doses may vary

> Stimulants
  - Work by irritating colon wall and increasing peristalsis
  - Usually cause bowel movement in 10 to 12 hours
  - bisacodyl: usual dose is 5 to 15 mg (1 to 3 tablets) orally once daily as needed, 10 mg (1 suppository) rectally once daily as needed or 10 mg rectal liquid once daily as needed

> Saline and osmotic solutions
  - Work by retaining fluid in the intestines
  - Usually cause bowel movement in 20 minutes to 3 hours
  - Magnesium citrate: usual dose is 240 mL orally one time

Priority Education/Discharge Issues

> Teach client to eat foods high in fiber. Provide a list of foods that contain high fiber such as raw vegetables, prunes, legumes and whole grain breads among others

> Educate client on drinking 8 glasses of water daily, if not contraindicated

> Educate on daily exercise

> Instruct client on defecating when the urge is felt and not suppressing the urge

> Teach client to create a schedule for bowel movements (like every morning before breakfast) and keep to that schedule as best as possible

> Teach client to tighten abdominal muscles daily to increase muscle tone

> Teach client that placing feet on a small footstool while defecating allows the thighs to be flexed, which improves passage of stool

> Discuss client's beliefs about defecation and teach that daily laxative usage removes the natural urge to defecate and replaces it with dependence on laxatives to have a bowel movement

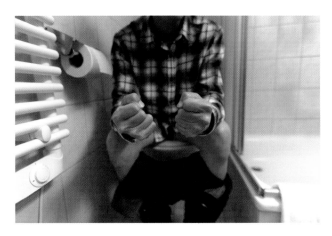

Image 11-10: Without looking at the Priority Exemplar, list 3 non-pharmacological interventions that can be used to treat constipation.

1. _____

_____

2. _____

_____

3. _____

_____

_____

_____

_____

_____

_____

_____

Intestinal obstruction

📋 Pathophysiology/Description

> Intestinal obstruction results when passage of intestinal content through the gastrointestinal (GI) tract is impaired

> When obstructions occur, contents accumulate proximal to the obstruction. The bowel evacuates distal to the obstruction but then it collapses. Distention in the proximal bowel causes pressure in the bowel to increase. This triggers a series of actions resulting finally in the intestinal muscles being fatigued, causing peristalsis to stop

> Bowel obstruction, in the presence of poor blood flow can cause major problems. Tissues can become edematous and cyanotic leading to gangrene and intestinal infarction. This is a medical emergency requiring quick attention to prevent the possibility of septic shock and death

> Obstruction can be complete or partial
> - Complete obstruction blocks the entire intestinal lumen so that gas and fluid cannot pass through the lumen
> - Partial obstruction occludes only a part of the lumen allowing some fluid and gas to pass through

> Obstruction can be described as strangulated or simple
> - With a strangulated obstruction there is no blood supply
> - A simple obstruction still has blood supply

> Mechanical bowel obstruction (physical obstruction of intestinal lumen): Causes
> - Adhesions from surgery

> One part of intestines folds into another (Intussusception)
> - Bowel twisting on itself (volvulus)
> - Colorectal cancer
> - Crohn's disease
> - Diverticular disease
> - Pseudo obstruction (obstruction with no obvious cause)

> Nonmechanical bowel obstruction (obstruction due to altered neuromuscular transmission or bowel innervation): Causes
> - Paralytic ileus (most common cause)
> - Inflammatory responses
> - Electrolyte imbalances
> - Interruption to blood supply to the intestines

> Types of surgery, if required
> - Resecting of the obstructed part of the bowel
> - Ileostomy
> - Colectomy
> - Colostomy

✏️ Priority Assessments or Cues

> Assess for abdominal distention

> Examine abdomen for scars indicating recent surgeries that may have increased client's risk of a paralytic ileus

> Assess bowel sounds. Bowel sounds may be auscultated initially but they usually decrease over time with an obstruction

> Assess for abdominal pain that client may describe as colicky

> Ask about onset and severity of pain. This can indicate the location of the obstruction. For example, with obstructions in the small bowel, pain usually occurs suddenly

> Assess for nausea and vomiting

> Ask about quality of vomiting as it can indicate the area of obstruction. For example, with distal obstruction vomiting is gradual and has a foul, fecal smell

> Ask about last bowel movement, client is usually constipated

> Assess vital signs. If strangulation, expect elevated temperature, indicating inflammation and infection

> Assess abdomen for visible masses

> If client had surgery, perform ongoing assessment of surgical site to ensure no infection and bleeding

> Assess urine and drainage from surgical drains (if used) for proper functioning

🧪 Priority Laboratory Tests/Diagnostics

> Abdominal X-rays and computed tomography (CT) scans will likely show obstruction

> Colonoscopy and sigmoidoscopy show entire colon obstruction of colon will be visualized

> Sigmoidoscopy, shows hemorrhoids, polyps and fissures

> Complete blood count will show elevated white blood cell count if perforation or strangulating has occurred. Decreased hematocrit and hemoglobin may indicate bleeding

> Metabolic profile may show electrolyte imbalances due to dehydration

⚠️ Priority Interventions or Actions

> Administer pain medications as prescribed

> Maintain client nothing by mouth (NPO) until obstruction is resolved

> Insert nasogastric (NG) tube for decompression and check every 4 hours to ensure patency

> Administer intravenous fluids using lactated ringers or normal saline to prevent dehydration

> Monitor intake and output. Empty drains and urinary catheter

> Start client on clear liquid diet when able to eat, increase diet as tolerated

> Perform good mouth care as bowel obstruction leaves a bad taste in the client's mouth

> Additional interventions if surgery is indicated
> - Perform preoperative care
> - Insert urinary catheter, if prescribed
> - Perform post-surgical care as prescribed
> - Manage post-surgical devices such as ileal pouch
> - Manage care of surgical site. Assess for bleeding, infection and viability of stoma
> - Allow client to participate in self-care of surgical site, in preparation for home care

Priority Potential & Actual Complications

> Perforation of bowel
> Strangulated and necrotic bowel
> Septic shock
> Surgery with permanent use of fecal diversions (such as colostomy)
> May be fatal

Priority Nursing Implications

> If client has surgery and will need to wear an ileal pouch, body image disturbances may occur so be sensitive and allow client to deal with this emotional issue

Priority Medications

> There are a myriad of different classes of pain medications that can be used to treat the client's abdominal pain, if medication is needed. The healthcare provider decides the best choice

Priority Education/Discharge Issues

> Instruct client on defecating when the urge is felt and not suppressing the urge
> Teach client to create a schedule for bowel movements (like every morning before breakfast) and to keep to that schedule as best as possible
> Teach client symptoms of bowel obstruction and when to contact healthcare provider
> Educate client on the risk factors for bowel obstruction
> Teach client how to minimize the risk of a paralytic ileus, especially after a surgery
> If surgery was done
>   • Teach client how to empty and change ostomy device
>   • Teach client how to care for, and assess stoma
>   • Have client do return demonstration of ostomy care
>   • Teach client signs of infection and how to assess stoma site for infection
>   • Provide client with information on resources for ostomy supplies
> Teach that once discharged from acute care, it may take several weeks before client feels well enough to resume normal activities
> Teach importance of keeping follow-up appointments

Write in the top 5 characteristics of:

SMALL BOWEL OBSTRUCTION

1. _____

2. _____

3. _____

4. _____

5. _____

LARGE BOWEL OBSTRUCTION

1. _____

2. _____

3. _____

4. _____

5. _____

Table 11-2: Bowel obstructions.

Diverticular disease

Pathophysiology/Description

> Diverticular disease encompasses two conditions, diverticulosis and diverticulitis. Diverticula are herniation or saccular dilations of the intestinal mucosa. When there are many of these diverticula present, it is called diverticulosis. When one or more diverticula become inflamed, diverticulitis occurs

> Diverticula occur mostly at points in the intestines where the wall is weak, and they can be formed anywhere in the gastrointestinal tract. However, they are most commonly located in the descending, sigmoid colon

> Causes
> • Low intake of fiber
> • Constipation
> • Obesity
> • Excessive alcohol intake
> • Western populations
> • Smoking

> Diverticular disease is often asymptomatic, diagnosed only when an individual has a screening colonoscopy

Priority Assessments or Cues

> Assess for nausea and vomiting

> Assess for abdominal pain in the left lower quadrant that usually worsens when client lifts, strains or coughs

> Assess for a palpable abdominal mass

> Ask client about flatulence, which is common with diverticulitis

> Assess for blood in the stool, can occur if the diverticula bleed or if diverticulitis develops

> Assess for bowel perforation and signs of peritonitis, which may be manifested as hard distended abdomen from bleeding, and fever and chills indicating infection

> Complete client's health history

> Assess client's understanding of surgery, if surgery indicated

> Assess client's readiness to look at surgical site after surgery and learn self-care, if surgery was indicated

Priority Laboratory Tests/Diagnostics

> Colonoscopy and sigmoidoscopy show entire colon and diverticular disease will be visualized

> Chest and abdominal X-rays determine if there are other associated diseases for the abdominal pain

> Computed tomography (CT) scan with contrast shows inflamed diverticula

> Complete blood cells show elevated white blood cell count

> Blood cultures may show infection in blood

Priority Interventions or Actions

> Keep client nothing by mouth in acute phase, to let the colon rest and heal

> Initiate intravenous fluids to prevent dehydration

> Provide clear liquids after the acute phase and progress diet as tolerated

> Administer antibiotics

> Administer analgesics and antiemetics if needed

> Administer stool softeners as prescribed

> Monitor intake and output

> Monitor for bowel perforation which may include tachycardia, restlessness, abdominal distention, increased temperature

> If surgery is indicated (resection of diseased part of colon, temporary colostomy)
> • Perform preoperative preparation and care
> • Insert nasogastric tube if prescribed
> • Perform post-surgical care as prescribed
> • Manage post-surgical devices such as ostomy pouch

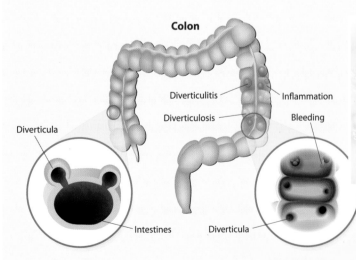

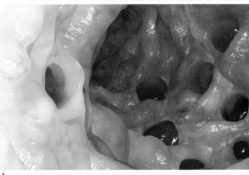

Image 11-11: Pathophysiology found in diverticular disease.

- Nasogastric (NG) tube to suction
- Manage care of surgical site. Assess for bleeding, infection and viability of stoma
- Allow client to participate in self-care of surgical site, in preparation for home care
- Allow early mobility to prevent post-surgery complications, such as pneumonia and blood clots

Priority Potential & Actual Complications

> Bowel perforation
> Peritonitis
> Permanent bowel diversion device (like colostomy)
> Sepsis
> May be fatal

Priority Nursing Implications

> Most clients with acute diverticulitis have no symptoms and in an acute attack, can be managed outside of the acute care setting. However, with severe cases, where clients are very ill and have systemic symptoms, hospitalization is necessary

Priority Medications

> Laxatives of various classes and types may be used for clients with diverticular disease. Below is an example of one drug in a few of the most commonly used classes
> Stool softeners
  - Soften feces by lubricating intestinal tract
  - Usually cause bowel movement in 72 hours
  - docusate: usual dose is 50 to 400 mg orally administered in 1 to 4 equally divided doses daily or 200 to 283 mg rectally administered as an enema once or twice
> Bulk-forming laxatives
  - Absorb water and cause increase bulk, thus stimulating peristalsis
  - Usually cause bowel movement within 24 hours
  - psyllium: 1-2 teaspoons/wafers/packets/capsules PO 1-3 times/day. Take each dose with a full glass of water, doses may vary
> Stimulants
  - Work by irritating colon wall and increasing peristalsis
  - Usually cause bowel movement in 10 to 12 hours
  - bisacodyl: usual dose is 5 to 15 mg (1 to 3 tablets) orally once daily as needed, 10 mg (1 suppository) rectally once daily as needed or 10 mg rectal liquid once daily as needed
> Saline and osmotic solutions
  - Work by retaining fluid in the intestines
  - Usually cause bowel movement in 20 minutes to 3 hours
  - Magnesium citrate: usual dose is 240 mL orally one time

> Several different types of antibiotics used to treat acute diverticulitis. Below is one example with dosage
> Metronidazole
  - Antibiotic
  - Loading dose: 15 mg/kg intravenous once and administered over 1 hour
  - Maintenance dose: 7.5 mg/kg intravenous administered over 1 hour every 6 hours for 7 to 10 days

Priority Education/Discharge Issues

> Teach client to consume a high fiber diet. These include legumes and whole grain, among others
> Stress the importance of avoiding excessive fat and meat intake
> Encourage adequate fluid intake to prevent constipation, at least 2000 mL daily
> Teach client to defecate when the urge occurs. Not doing so will cause constipation, which increases the risk of diverticulitis
> Teach client not to engage in activities that increase intraabdominal pressure, such as heavy lifting, straining or bending as they can cause an attack of diverticulitis
> Teach symptoms of the disease and when to contact the healthcare provider
> Explain the importance of smoking cessation for clients who smoke, as smoking is a risk factor for diverticular disease
> Encourage weight reduction if client is obese as obesity is a risk factor for diverticulitis

Next Gen Clinical Judgment

List 3 statements by a client that indicates a need for further teaching on dietary management of diverticulosis.

1. _____

_____

_____

2. _____

_____

_____

3. _____

_____

_____

Colorectal cancer

Pathophysiology/Description

- Colorectal cancer is a malignant growth that occurs in the rectum and/or colon. It is the third most common cancer in the United Sates and ranks as the second leading cause of death from all cancers
- Risk factor
  - First-degree family or personal history of colorectal polyps
  - Family history of colorectal cancer
  - Personal history of inflammatory bowel disease
  - Personal history of diabetes mellitus
  - Age, usually seen in older than 50 years
  - Smoking
  - Obesity
  - Excessive alcohol intake, usually more than 4 to 5 drinks weekly
  - Consumption of large amounts of red meat, usually greater than 6-7 servings weekly
- Metastasis is a major concern with colorectal cancer because as it spreads to the liver (a common site of metastasis), it can then move from the liver to several other parts of the body
- Colorectal cancer is staged using the commonly used Tumor Node Metastasis (TNM) staging system. Stages are from 0 to IV and as the stages increase, prognosis worsens
- There are several types of surgical ostomies that can be done with colorectal cancer. The choice of ostomy is dependent on the location of the tumor and the severity of the cancer

Priority Assessments or Cues

- Assess for appearance of blood in stool, both melena and hematochezia, which are very common manifestations
- Ask client about change in bowel habits, diarrhea or constipation. This can indicate the location of the tumor. For example, with tumors in the ascending colon, stools may be diarrhea
- Ask about size of stools, as in a decrease from large stools to pencil-sized. This change can indicate partial obstruction
- Assess for nausea, vomiting, anorexia and weight loss
- Assess for presence of an abdominal mass, which indicates late-stage cancer
- Assess appearance of abdomen, will appear distended, especially in late-stage cancer
- Assess for ascites, which indicates liver involvement
- Assess for muscle wasting (cachexia), which is usually a late-stage sign
- Assess for bowel perforation and signs of peritonitis, which may be manifested as hard distended abdomen from bleeding, fever and chills indicating infection

- Complete client's health history
- Assess client's understanding of surgery
- Assess client's psychological status and intervene accordingly
- Assess client's readiness to look at surgical site after surgery and learn self-care
- Assess client's acceptance of diagnosis, especially if tumor is inoperable and prognosis is poor.

Priority Laboratory Tests/Diagnostics

- Colonoscopy shows entire colon, polyps visualized can be removed and tissue biopsy done
- Fecal occult and fecal immunochemical tests show blood in stool. Since bleeding from tumor does not occur continuously, these tests must be done frequently
- Stool DNA test (New test called Cologuard) can show DNA markers that can indicate colorectal cancer
- Computed tomography (CT) scan, magnetic resonance imaging (MRI) and abdominal ultrasound to look for metastasis of the cancer
- Barium enema to look for structural abnormalities
- Complete blood cells may show elevated white blood cell count and anemia
- Liver function tests, to determine involvement of the liver, may show elevated liver enzymes
- Blood culture may show infection in blood
- Carcinoembryonic antigen (CEA) level may be elevated

Priority Interventions or Actions

- Keep client nothing by mouth in acute phase
- Initiate intravenous fluids to prevent dehydration
- Administer analgesics and antiemetics if needed. Administer antibiotics
- Monitor intake and output
- Monitor for bowel perforation which may include tachycardia, restlessness, abdominal distention, increased temperature
- Prepare client for radiation to decrease tumor size, if indicated
- Administer chemotherapy drugs and monitor for adverse effects
- Allow client time to verbalize feelings, especially if prognosis is poor
- Surgical interventions (polypectomy during colonoscopy, abdominal-perineal resection, colectomy with ostomy)
  - Perform preoperative preparation and care
  - Insert nasogastric tube to suction
  - Manage post-surgical devices such as ostomy pouch
  - Perform colostomy irrigations
  - Manage surgical drains, empty and document drainage
  - Assess for surgical site infection

- Assess viability of stoma and report any negative findings, such as a brown-black stoma color, which indicates necrosis. Healthy stoma is pink in color
- Initiate consult with the hospital's wound, ostomy and continence nurse (WOCN)
- Initiate consult with dietician to discuss, modifications in diet
- Give close attention to surgical site in the immediate postoperative period. Reinforce dressings as needed and monitor for excessive bleeding. Perform ongoing sterile dressing changes
- Provide clear liquids after the acute phase and progress diet as tolerated
- Allow client to participate in self-care of surgical site, in preparation for home care
- Allow early mobility to prevent post-surgery complications, such as pneumonia and blood clots

⚑ Priority Potential & Actual Complications

- Bowel obstruction and perforation
- Hemorrhage and peritonitis
- Fistula
- Permanent bowel diversion device (like colostomy)
- Sepsis
- May be fatal

℧ Priority Nursing Implications

- Colorectal cancer usually does not manifest until the disease has progressed to an advanced stage. Therefore, clients must be provided with information on the importance of getting a screening colonoscopy at scheduled intervals
- Having a bowel diversion device on the body and dealing with everything that comes with that device and the diagnosis of cancer, can be challenging and distressing for clients. It is important that clients get presurgical psychological preparation as this will increase the likelihood of better coping after the surgery

◊ Priority Medications

- 5-fluorouracil, oxaliplatin, irinotecan, bevacizumab, panitumumab, trifluridine/tipiracil, aflibercept, regorafenib,
  - Chemotherapy drugs used in a variety of combinations and dosages to treat colorectal cancer in its various stages. Used before surgery to decrease size of tumor, after surgery to decrease likelihood of cancer returning (adjuvant therapy) and as palliative therapy (when surgery is not an option)
  - Administered via oral and intravenous routes
  - Assess for bleeding fatigue, and infection. Monitor red and white blood cell counts and platelets

👤 Priority Education/Discharge Issues

- Teach client how to properly care for surgical site at home, such as empty device, change device, assess stoma, irrigate colostomy, assess for signs of infection, protect skin, reduce odor
- Have WOCN provide detailed client teaching on care of ostomy. Reinforce education provided by WOCN
- Teach client how to contact the WOCN with concerns or questions
- Educate client on where to get ostomy supplies
- Teach client about phantom rectal pain and the need to have a bowel movement. Let client know that this is normal and will subside over time
- Explain to client that excessive gas for the first two weeks after surgery is normal
- Educate client on eating a balanced meal and taking vitamins to prevent deficits in nutrition
- Teach client to drink adequate fluids, at least 2000 to 3000 mL daily to prevent dehydration
- Teach client to avoid foods that produce excessive gas and odor, such as broccoli, eggs and cheese, among others
- Teach client with an ileostomy to expect that stools will be liquid and to provide meticulous skin care around the stoma to prevent skin breaks
- Educate client on chemotherapy regimen and answer client's questions and concerns
- Ensure client has psychological support to cope with diagnosis and change in lifestyle due to new bowel diversion device
- Encourage client to verbalize future care needs on topics such as palliative and end-of-life care
- Assist client and family with securing hospice or palliative care if needed
- Teach client importance of keeping all follow-up medical appointments
- Teach client importance of educating family members on timely colorectal screens, since there is a genetic predisposition to the condition. Provide client with list of when screenings must be done based on risk factors

_____

_____

_____

_____

_____

Cirrhosis

Pathophysiology/Description

> Cirrhosis is chronic end-stage liver disease that is characterized by irreversible destruction and degeneration of liver cells

> Scar tissue forms in the liver due to repeated injury to the cells. The cells try to regenerate but the process is abnormal, resulting in poor blood flow. The new growth of cells and connective tissue causes the lobes of the liver to have irregular size and shape, which prevents normal blood flow to the liver. The eventual result of this process is poor liver function

> Causes of cirrhosis
>   • Chronic hepatitis, excessive alcohol intake, nonalcoholic steatohepatitis (liver damage caused by accumulation of fat in liver), extreme dieting, biliary conditions and hepatic encephalopathy

Priority Assessments or Cues

> Assess for anorexia, nausea and vomiting. Assess for ascites, measure abdominal girth

> Assess for muscle wasting from poor nutritional status

> Assess color of urine, color is dark brown in presence of jaundice

> Assess stools, color is tan or gray in presence of jaundice

> Assess respiratory status, dyspnea and hyperventilation are common issues because of ascites

> Complete physical assessment

> Assess for presence of jaundice, manifested as yellowing of skin around the eyes and mouth

> Ask client about itching, common in liver failure due to accumulation of bile salts under the skin

> Assess for melena or hematemesis, can occur from bleeding varices

> Assess client for bleeding esophageal and gastric varices (a medical emergency)

> Assess client for symptoms of hepatorenal syndrome a complication of cirrhosis. Symptoms include a sudden decrease in urine output with decreased excretion of urine sodium and increased levels of blood urea nitrogen (BUN) and creatinine

> Assess client for symptoms of hepatic encephalopathy manifested by impaired consciousness, sleep disturbances, paresthesia of feet, apraxia and asterixis (rapid flexion and extension of hands when the arm/hands are stretched out)

> Assess for a sweet, musty odor on client's breath (called fetor hepaticus), because of accumulated liver byproducts

Priority Laboratory Tests/Diagnostics

> Esophagogastroduodenoscopy (EGD), will show esophageal and stomach varices

> Liver biopsy used to make definitive diagnosis of cirrhosis

> Liver function test, enzymes will be elevated at first because they are released from inflamed cells but may be normal in end-stage cirrhosis due to damage of hepatocytes

> Increased bilirubin and decreased serum protein and albumin are expected

> Ultrasound elastography, shows liver fibrosis. Liver with cirrhosis will be stiffer than healthy one

> Complete blood cell (CBC), may show increased white blood cell count due to inflammation

Priority Interventions or Actions

> Provide good oral hygiene before meals to help client eat better

> Administer antipruritic and diuretic medications as prescribed

> Administer medication to correct hyponatremia

> Administer beta blockers as prescribed, used to decrease high portal pressure and decrease likelihood of bleeding from varices

> Administer lactulose to foster removal of ammonia from the body in hepatic encephalopathy

> Monitor intake and output

> Weigh client daily. If client can eat, provide diet high in calories to manage nutritional deficits

> Monitor for orthostatic hypotension with bleeding varices

> Administer intravenous fluids if blood loss from varices

> Assist with insertion of balloon tamponade to mechanically compress bleeding varices

> Administer supplemental vitamins

> Elevate head of bed to help client breathe better

> Measure abdominal girth throughout treatment to determine effectiveness of treatment for ascites

> Allow client to remain on bedrest until ascites starts to resolve

> Assist client with deep breathing and coughing exercises to prevent pneumonia

> Provide range of motion exercises to minimize risk of blood clots

> Monitor and document fluid and electrolyte imbalances. Administer electrolyte replacement

> If client is not able to eat or is severely malnourished, administer enteral or parenteral feedings

> Provide good skin care. Edematous skin is susceptible to breakdown. Ensure client is turned every two hours or more frequent if needed. Elevate extremities that are edematous

- Administer albumin infusion to help with maintenance of intravascular volume, if prescribed
- Prepare client for procedure to remove fluid from the abdominal cavity (paracentesis)
- Allow client time to verbalize feelings regarding disease and physical appearance
- Assist with placement of transjugular intrahepatic portosystemic shunt (TIPS), if prescribed
- Stabilize and transfer client with severe bleeding varices to the intensive care unit

Priority Potential & Actual Complications

- Portal hypertension, ascites, jaundice, hepatorenal syndrome
- Bleeding esophageal varices, defects in coagulation, encephalopathy, and may be fatal

Priority Nursing Implications

- When a balloon tamponade is used for bleeding varices, it is important that each tube is labeled so they are easily identified. The tube must be secured to prevent accidental occlusion of airway and balloons deflated per the hospital's policy

Priority Medications

- albumin
  - Used to help maintain intravascular volume and adequate urine output in ascites
  - Initial dose of albumin 5% is 250 or 500 mL intravenous administered at a rate of 1 to 2 mL per minute
  - Administer additional albumin within 15 to 30 minutes if response to initial dose was inadequate
- spironolactone
  - Several diuretics use to treat ascites, spironolactone is a commonly used drug in the class
  - Used to treat ascites and does not cause potassium to be depleted
  - Usual dose is 25 to 200 mg oral daily in single or divided doses
- tolvaptan
  - Used to treat hyponatremia that is common in cirrhosis
  - Initial dose is 15 mg orally once daily
  - Maintenance dose: 60 mg once daily for a maximum of 30 days
- nadolol
  - Used to treat clients with esophageal or gastric varices. Reduce portal pressure and decrease risk of varices rupturing and hemorrhage
  - Initial dose is 40 mg orally once daily

- Usual maintenance dose range is 40 to 80 mg orally once daily
- octreotide acetate
  - Used to stop the bleeding in varices so additional intervention can be started
  - Causes vasoconstriction and decreases portal blood flow, thus decreasing portal hypertension
  - Usual dose is 25 to 100 mcg intravenous bolus, followed by continuous intravenous infusion of 25 to 50 mcg/hour for 2 to 5 days
- lactulose
  - Used to treat hepatic encephalopathy
  - Initial dose is 30 mL orally 3 times daily or 300 mL in 700 mL normal saline or water as an enema every 4 to 6 hours. Enema must be retained for 30 to 60 minutes
  - Maintenance dose is 30 to 45 mL orally 3 times daily
- rifaximin
  - Used to reduce risk of hepatic encephalopathy
  - May cause dizziness
  - Dose is 550 mg orally twice daily
- cholestyramine
  - Used to treat pruritus (itching)
  - Initial dose is 4 grams (1 packet or level scoop) orally once or twice a day
  - Maintenance dose is 8 to 16 grams (2 to 4 packets or level scoops) orally in 2 divided doses

Priority Education/Discharge Issues

- Teach client experiencing pruritus to use knuckles to rub itchy area, instead of using nails
- Teach client the importance of not drinking alcohol
- Teach client that straining to have a bowel movement, sneezing or vomiting can increase the risk of bleeding, if client has varices or portal hypertension
- Assist client with information on help with quitting alcohol intake, like Alcoholics Anonymous
- Instruct client to follow the sodium restricted diet carefully. Usually have no more than 2 grams of sodium daily, to manage ascites. Less is prescribed if ascites is severe
- Educate on how to read food labels for sodium content
- Instruct client on intake of high calorie diet and oral nutritional supplement
- Instruct client on symptoms and when to contact healthcare provider
- Teach client with esophageal or gastric varices to not take medications that can induce bleeding, such as NSAIDs
- Remind client to keep follow-up medical appointments as cirrhosis requires ongoing medical care
- Teach client to speak with pharmacist before taking any over-the-counter medications

Hepatitis

Pathophysiology/Description

> Hepatitis is inflammation of the liver caused by viruses, or other toxic substances such as alcohol or medications. When hepatitis occurs, the virus causes many liver cells to be killed, which triggers a myriad of impaired functions in the body

> There are five different types of viral hepatitis
> - Hepatitis A virus (HAV)
> - Hepatitis B virus (HBV)
> - Hepatitis C virus (HCV)
> - Hepatitis D virus (HDV)
> - Hepatitis E virus (HEV)

> Even though there are commonalities among all types of viral hepatitis in terms of clinical manifestations, each has its own specific mode of transmission

> Hepatitis A virus
> - Transmission: primarily via fecal-oral route
> - At risk: crowded conditions, poor hygiene of food handlers, poor sanitation
> - Incubation: 15 to 50 days
> - Prevention: Good handwashing, HAV vaccine (need 2 doses at least 6 months apart)

> Hepatitis B virus
> - Transmission: via blood or body fluids
> - At risk: Health care workers, intravenous drug abusers, individuals who reside with persons who have HBV, Individuals who undergo dialysis
> - Incubation: 45 to 160 days
> - Prevention: Good handwashing, HBV vaccine, needle precautions, avoiding unprotected contact with body fluids of infected persons, blood donor screening, testing of women who are pregnant

> Hepatitis C virus
> - Transmission: via blood or body fluids
> - At risk: Health care workers, intravenous drug users, high-risk sexual practices, blood transfusions administered prior to 1992
> - Incubation: 14 to 180 days
> - Prevention: Good handwashing, blood donor screening, needle precautions, avoid unprotected sex with infected persons. No vaccine available

> Hepatitis D
> - Transmission: Same as B. HDV must have HBV in order to replicate and causes infection only when there is active HBV infection
> - At risk: same as B, except that this is predominant in Middle Eastern Countries but uncommon in the United States
> - Incubation: 2 to 26 weeks
> - Prevention: Same as HBV. No vaccine available

> Hepatitis E
> - Transmission: Same as HAV but not very common in the United States
> - At risk: Same as HAV
> - Incubation: 15 -64 days
> - Prevention: same as HAV. A vaccine was registered in China but is not yet registered and used worldwide

Priority Assessments or Cues

> Acute hepatitis
> - Assess for nausea and vomiting that usually appears in the acute stage of hepatitis
> - Ask about bowel habits, constipation or diarrhea usually occurs
> - Ask client about meal intake, as anorexia and weight loss are usually complaints in acute viral hepatitis
> - Assess for flu-like symptoms, fatigue, and a feeling of malaise
> - Ask about aches and pains, myalgias and arthralgias usually occur with acute hepatitis
> - Ask client about living conditions, crowded living condition is a risk factor for HAV
> - Assess for risky sexual behaviors and intravenous drug abuse as these are risk factors for HBV, HCV and HDV
> - Ask about meal preparation and food and water sources as HAV and HEV are transmitted via fecal-oral route
> - Ask about recent travels, as HEV and HDV are not prevalent in the United States but are common to other countries
> - Ask about the client's work as healthcare works are at increased risk of contracting hepatitis
> - Assess liver and spleen, both are likely to be enlarged
> - Assess client in acute phase for fulminant hepatitis (see symptoms in priority complications below)
> - Assess client's sense of taste and smell. Both are decreased in acute hepatitis
> - Assess color of urine, color is dark brown in presence of jaundice
> - Assess stools, expect clay-colored stools
> - Complete physical assessment
> - Assess client's tolerance for eating. Tolerance is usually low in acute phase
> - Assess for presence of jaundice, manifested as yellowing on skin, in eyes and mouth
> - Ask client about itching to skin
> - Assess vital signs, likely to find elevated temperature

> Additional assessment for chronic hepatitis
  - Determine type of hepatitis infection as HCV is more likely to be chronic
  - Assess integumentary system, likely to find red palms (palmar erythema) and small branching arteries showing on the surface of the skin (spider angiomas)
  - Assess for edema, likely to see edema to lower extremities and ascites, as the plasma oncotic pressure reduces
  - Assess for swollen lymph nodes (lymphadenopathy)
  - Assess neurologic system. Confusion may be seen due to encephalopathy
  - Assess for bruising and bleeding. Impaired coagulation is a complication of chronic hepatitis and liver disease as the liver can no longer produce clotting factors
  - Assess client for asterixis (rapid flexion and extension of hands when the arm/hands are stretched out), which is common in liver encephalopathy

🧪 Priority Laboratory Tests/Diagnostics

> There is a myriad of tests to distinguish between the various viral hepatitis to determine the specific one the client has. For example, there is Anti-HAV immune globulin M (IgM) for hepatitis A and Anti-HCV (antibody to HCV) for hepatitis C, among many others
> Aspartate aminotransferase (AST) alanine aminotransferase (ALT) will be elevated at first because they are released from inflamed cells but will decrease as hepatitis is resolved and jaundice disappears
> Serum and urine bilirubin increased due to liver damage
> Alkaline phosphatase and y-Glutamyl transpeptidase increased due to liver damage
> Prothrombin time is prolonged due to decreased production in the liver
> Liver biopsy for chronic hepatitis, will show the degree of chronic injury to the liver
> Ultrasound elastography, shows liver fibrosis. Liver with cirrhosis will be stiffer than healthy one
> FibroSure is a biomarker serum test that determines the extent of liver fibrosis

⚠️ Priority Interventions or Actions

> Allow client to rest in acute hepatitis as it helps with regeneration of liver cells
> Administer antipruritic medications as needed
> Administer antiemetics for nausea

> Administer medications for HBV to suppress replication of the virus
> Administer direct-acting antivirals as prescribed
> Provide client with a balanced nutritional diet as tolerated
> Encourage small, frequent meals instead of large meals, to help with nausea and vomiting
> Administer intravenous nutrition if unable to tolerate foods by mouth due to vomiting
> Provide adequate fluids. Encourage intake of 2500 to 3000 mL daily
> Monitor intake and output. Maintain fluid and electrolyte balance
> Place patient in a private room for HAV if client exhibits poor hygiene or has bowel incontinence
> Provide range of motion exercises to minimize risk of blood clots while client is on bedrest

🚩 Priority Potential & Actual Complications

> Chronic liver disease
> Fulminant hepatitis
> Cirrhosis
> Encephalitis
> Liver cancer
> Liver failure
> May be fatal

⚕️ Priority Nursing Implications

> Clients with hepatitis must be made aware of fulminant hepatitis, a serious complication of acute hepatitis. It causes liver failure which then triggers a myriad of other serious malfunctions in the body, including the possibility of death. Fulminant hepatitis is manifested as gastrointestinal bleeding, encephalopathy, renal failure, respiratory failure, disseminated intravascular coagulopathy and hypoglycemia, among a myriad of other severe imbalances. Prognosis is poor, and a liver transplant is the cure
> Understand that there are risk factors for acute viral hepatitis to progress to a chronic stage. These include fatty liver disease, metabolic syndrome, co-infection with HIV, alcohol intake and being male
> When a food handler contracts HAV, all food handlers at the client's place of work should be vaccinated with hepatitis A immune globulin (IG)

🔴 Priority Medications

> Direct-acting antivirals: There are several in the class. Example of one drug in the class below
>   - Drug: simeprevir, administered with another drug called sofosbuvir
>   - Works by preventing HCV replication
>   - Usual dose is 150 mg orally once daily with food for 12 weeks
> sofosbuvir
>   - Works by preventing HCV replication
>   - Administered with simeprevir
>   - Usual dose is 400 mg orally once daily for 12 weeks
> Antiemetics: There are several in the class. Example of one drug in class is below
>   - promethazine
>   - Used to treat nausea and administered via several routes
>   - Usual dose is 12.5 to 25 mg intravenous, rectal or oral every 4 to 6 hours as needed
> Nucleoside and nucleotide analogs: There are several in the class. Example of one drug in class is below
>   - lamivudine
>   - Works by inhibiting viral replication in chronic HBV and liver inflammation
>   - Usual dose is 100 mg orally once daily

👤 Priority Education/Discharge Issues

> Provide client information on vaccines for hepatitis
> Explain the importance of rest to client who is in the acute phase, if treated at home
> Teach client the method of proper hand washing
> Teach preventative measure to clients in high-risk categories
> Teach client how to prevent infecting others
> Teach the importance of maintaining good personal hygiene
> Teach clients living or working in crowded areas to maintain good environmental hygiene
> Teach client with known travel to hepatitis prevalent countries, especially for HEV and HDV, to take precautions to prevent infection
> Instruct client to avoid drinking alcohol as it can increase the rate of progression of HBV and HCV
> Teach about complications of hepatitis and how to recognize symptoms of complications
> Teach client that HBV and HCV can relapse. Teach symptoms of relapse and when to contact health care provider for symptoms
> Teach client who has HBV and HCV that they should not donate blood
> Instruct client on keeping follow-up medical appointments

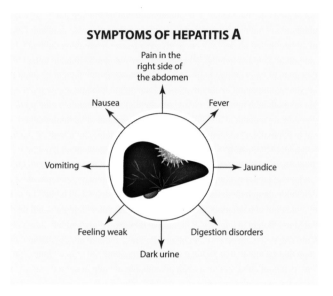

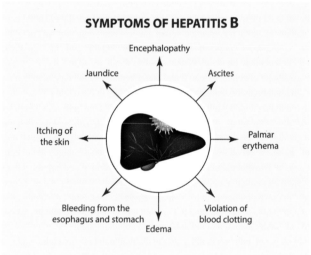

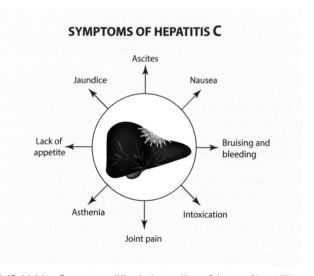

11-12: List top 3 commonalities between these 3 types of hepatitis. Next circle one unique characteristic of each that is not a part of the other two types of hepatitis.

Pyloric stenosis

Pathophysiology/Description

> Narrowing of the pyloric canal between the stomach and duodenum as a result of hypertrophy of the muscles of the pylorus. The result of this is a blockage of food from entering the small intestines causing forceful vomiting and constant hunger. Pyloric stenosis is not present at birth but develops after

> A definitive cause of a baby having pyloric stenosis is not known but possible risk factors have been identified

> Risk factors
> * More common in Caucasians who are of Northern European ancestry
> * Familial tendency. Higher rates of the condition found in babies born to mothers who had the condition
> * Mothers who were treated with antibiotics in late pregnancy
> * Babies who were treated with antibiotics in the first weeks after birth
> * Occurs more in male babies than females
> * Bottle feeding
> * Babies born prematurely
> * Smoking in pregnancy

> Treatment for pyloric stenosis is always surgical. Surgery is a Laparoscopic pyloromyotomy which opens a wider channel in the pylorus to allow food to pass through. The surgery is almost always done laparoscopically unless there are complications in surgery that cause a change to the open surgical procedure

Priority Assessments or Cues

> Assess for vomiting after feeding. Vomiting may be projectile. Assess baby for belching

> Assess for vomitus that usually contains feeding and some blood

> Ask caregiver about the baby's bowel movements. With food not getting to the intestines, baby may be constipated

> Examine skin for an olive-shaped lump by the baby's umbilicus, in the epigastric area

> Inspect baby's abdomen, wave-like contractions may be seen across baby's stomach caused by the muscles if the stomach trying to push food through the pylorus that is narrowed

> Weigh the baby. Compare baby's weight now to birthweight. Expect weight loss from lack of nutrients getting to the baby's small intestines

> Ask about baby's urination and how many diapers are changed daily. Baby may be dehydrated

> Assess baby's feeding habits. Babies with pyloric stenosis are always hungry and desire feeding after vomiting

> Assess for irritability

> Assess baby's activity, usually less active with pyloric stenosis

Priority Laboratory Tests/Diagnostics

> Ultrasound to look at the pylorus, confirms the diagnosis

> Blood tests to look for electrolyte imbalance or dehydration

Priority Interventions or Actions

> Monitor intake and output
> Obtain daily weights
> Prepare baby for surgery (laparoscopic pyloromyotomy)
> Place nasogastric tube preoperatively to decompress stomach
> Postoperative interventions
> * Maintain the baby nothing by mouth (NPO) until able to tolerate oral feeding
> * Monitor nasogastric tube
> * Monitor intake and output
> * Monitor for abdominal distention
> * Monitor surgical wound for bleeding, and infection
> * Change dressing using aseptic technique
> * Initiate small feedings
> * Administer pain medication as prescribed

Priority Potential & Actual Complications

> Failure to thrive
> Jaundice
> Dehydration
> Electrolyte imbalances
> Erosion and bleeding of the stomach/aspiration

Priority Nursing Implications

> A child with pyloric stenosis will likely show signs of poor hydration and will be hungry all the time because of excessive vomiting and food not getting to the small intestines

Priority Medications

> Analgesics: Used for managing child's pain after surgery. The choice and dose of medication is at the discretion of the physician

Priority Education/Discharge Issues

> Teach caregiver to report the following to the healthcare provider
> * The baby has increased pain and pain medication is not helping
> * The baby is not able to have a bowel movement
> * Fever greater than 101.3°F by oral or rectal thermometer
> * The baby is vomiting even after drinking only clear liquids
> * Redness, bleeding or pus at the surgical incision site
> * The baby has a fever, with a temperature greater than 101.3

> Teach the importance of keeping follow-up medical appointments

Obesity

Pathophysiology/Description

- Obesity, a major disease globally, is characterized by excessive amounts of body fat that is beyond the individual's physical body requirements. Obesity can be characterized as primary or secondary and can be classified in several ways. Primary obesity is the most common form
- Cause of primary obesity
  - Occurs with excessive calorie intake and not enough expenditure of energy
- Causes of secondary obesity
  - Lesions in the central nervous system
  - Metabolic imbalances
  - Congenital anomalies
  - Drugs
- Classifications of obesity
  - Body mass index: obese is 30 kg/m^2 and greater
  - Waist-to-hip ratio: greater than 0.8 increases the risk of health problems
  - Waist circumference: increased health risk if greater than 30 inches in men and greater than 35 inches in women
  - Body shape: apple and pear-shaped bodies have greater risks of health conditions
- Genetics, environmental and psychological contributory factors
  - Genes recently identified as having linkage to obesity
  - Greater access to fast and unhealthy foods
  - Increased tendency to eat outside the home
  - Reliance on use of technology and less physical activity
  - Increased portion sizes of meals. Use of food for comfort and reward
  - Lack of areas for recreational activities in poorer neighborhoods. Lower socioeconomic status
  - Use of food for comfort and reward
- Obesity can be managed with diet and exercise but there are times when an individual chooses to have a bariatric surgery to help with weight loss. This is surgery on the stomach and/or intestines that reduces capacity of the stomach and allows the individual to consume less food.
- Bariatric surgery procedures
  - Sleeve gastrectomy: portion of stomach removed, and remainder has a sleeved shape
  - Adjustable gastric banding: inflatable band placed around the stomach to decrease the size. Stomach size can be manipulated by injecting fluid in an inflatable/deflectable port
  - Intragastric balloons: balloon placed in stomach and is filled with saline, gives sense of fullness in the stomach so client eats less
  - Roux-en-Y gastric bypass: this is the gold standard for bariatric surgeries. A small gastric pouch is created and attached directly to the small intestines. Dumping syndrome is an issue with this procedure because of contents emptying too rapidly in the small intestines
  - Implantable gastric stimulation: Device planted in abdomen that allows client to send signal of stomach fullness to the brain

Priority Assessments or Cues

- Assess for cause of obesity
- Complete health history and be sure to discuss health conditions that predispose to obesity
- Head-to-toe physical assessment to determine existence of complications from obesity
- Assess weight and height. Assess motivation to lose weight and barriers to weight loss
- Ask about current diet
- Pre and postoperative assessment for bariatric surgery
  - Assess for use of assistive devices such as continuous positive air pressure machine (CPAP)
  - Preoperatively, teach client how to cough and deep breathe, use incentive spirometry and reposition in bed postoperatively and assess client's knowledge of the teaching
  - Assess all body systems pre and postoperatively
  - Assess vital signs pre and postoperatively
  - Assess client's knowledge of the surgical procedure
  - Assess skin to ensure no skin breaks from immobility after surgery
  - Assess surgical dressing for bleeding
  - Assess surgical site for wound dehiscence, evisceration or infection
  - Assess respiratory status to ensure no compromise, such as pneumonia

Priority Laboratory Tests/Diagnostics

- There are no specific labs for obesity. Labs and diagnostics are done based on symptoms from complications of obesity

Priority Interventions or Actions

- Restrict dietary meal intake to below energy requirement
- Initiate dietary consult
- Discuss weight loss goals with client and assist client with initiating weight loss plans
- Offer praise when weight goals are met
- Preoperative interventions for bariatric surgery
  - Coordinate care across specialties if client has other comorbidities
  - Gather all appropriately sized equipment that will be used pre and postoperative
  - Initiate intravenous access
  - Perform preoperative care
- Postoperative interventions
  - Administer pain medications as prescribed
  - Keep the client's head positioned at 35 to 40 degree angle to foster lung expansion and reduce pressure on the abdomen
  - Assist client to ambulate the evening after surgery

- Empty urinary catheter and measure output
- Assist client to use incentive spirometry
- Monitor intravenous fluid and insertion site. Document intake and output
- Provide water and sugar-free clear liquids in the immediate postoperative period

Priority Potential & Actual Complications

> Cancer, obesity is a risk factor for several cancers
> Musculoskeletal problems due to stress on joints
> Cardiovascular problems such as hypertension
> Gastrointestinal problems such as gallstones
> Endocrine problems such as diabetes
> Respiratory problems such as sleep apnea
> Psychological problems mainly from having to manage the stigma of obesity

Priority Nursing Implications

> In caring for clients with obesity, it is important to keep in mind that the Hispanic and African American ethnic groups have higher rates of obesity than Caucasians so education on complications of obesity and weight management must be considered when caring for these populations

Priority Medications

> bupropion/naltrexone (a combination drug)
  - Antidepressant/opioid antagonist
  - Initial dose is one 8 mg/90 mg tablet taken orally in the morning and 1 in the evening for the first 3 weeks
  - Maintenance dose starting in week 4 is two 8 mg/90 mg tablets twice daily naltrexone

> orlistat
  - Blocks the breakdown of fat and its absorption in the intestines
  - Has unpleasant side effect of flatulence and leakage of stool
  - Usual dose is 120 mg orally three times daily with each main meal containing fat

> lorcaserin
  - Suppress appetite causes sense of fullness
  - Selective serotine agonist
  - Usual dose is 10 mg orally twice daily

> liraglutide
  - Glucagon-like peptide that induces fullness
  - Week one dose is 0.6 mg subcutaneously once daily. Dose is increased every week until maintenance dose is reached in week five
  - Maintenance dose: 3 mg subcutaneously once daily

> Phentermine/topiramate

- Sympathomimetic anorectic/antiseizure drug that works to increase satiety
- Initial dose is one capsule of phentermine 3.75 mg/topiramate 23 mg extended-release orally once daily in the morning for the first 14 days
- Maintenance dose is one capsule of phentermine 7.5 mg/topiramate 46 mg extended-release orally once daily in the morning.

Priority Education/Discharge Issues

> Teach client to eat a balanced meal
> Familiarize client with the MyPlate guidelines
> Encourage client to drink adequate water
> Explain the risk of fad diets
> If client taking weight loss drugs, teach proper administration and side effects
> Teach client that drugs must be combined with diet and exercise to be effective in losing weight
> Teach client that weight loss requires a lifestyle change
> Teach client to set realistic weight loss goals
> Assist client with locating community social support for weight loss
> Explain the importance of starting an exercise program
> Teaching specific to post bariatric surgery
  - Explain to client that vomiting usually occurs in the early postoperative phase. Teach client to eat small meals
  - Instruct client to eat slowly and do not eat past fullness
  - Instruct client to not eat and drink at the same time
  - Teach the importance of eating a diet high in protein and low in carbohydrates and fats, as carbohydrates can trigger dumping syndrome
  - Teach not to drink large amounts of fluids as fluids promote dumping syndrome. Some clients are restricted to fluids of 1000 mL daily
  - Teach signs and symptoms of wound infection
  - Teach signs of wound dehiscence and evisceration and who to contact if either occurs
  - Explain the importance of walking daily to prevent blood clots, skin breaks and respiratory problems, such as pneumonia
  - Alert client to the fact that weight loss will be significant in first few months and to not be alarmed with loose skin
  - Let client know that complications can occur late in recovery, so it is important to keep follow-up medical appointments

_____

_____

_____

_____

Benign prostatic hypertrophy/prostate cancer

📋 Pathophysiology/Description

> Benign prostatic hypertrophy (BPH) is the increase of the prostate gland causing disruption in the outflow of urine. Conversely, prostate cancer is a slow-growing, malignant growth of the prostate gland that can spread to various parts of the body

> Decrease in testosterone as men age, coupled with an excess dihydrotestosterone, and higher proportion of estrogen may account for increase cell growth, causing BPH

> The urethra is compressed as the prostate grows causing partial obstruction and urinary difficulty

> Risk factors for BPH
> - Genetic predisposition with family history of first-degree relative having BPH
> - Erectile dysfunction, diabetes
> - Alcohol intake, smoking, obesity, physical inactivity

> Risk factors for prostate cancer
> - Age 50 and older
> - Ethnicity, as higher incidence seen in African American men
> - Diet low in vegetables and fruits but high in fats, red and processed meats
> - Interactions with chemicals such as pesticides in farming

> Both prostate cancer and BPH are slow growing and the client may not see manifestations until prostate is large and/or cancer has progressed beyond the early stage

> Prostate cancer is staged using the commonly used Tumor, Node Metastasis (TNM) staging system. Stages are from I to V, with V being the most poorly differentiated cells

✏️ Priority Assessments or Cues

> Ask about nocturia, as this is usually one of the first symptoms the client has to indicate BPH and/or prostate cancer

> Ask about urinary frequency and urgency, dysuria and bladder pain as these may indicate the added problems of infection or inflammation

> Ask client to describe the urine stream, decreased force is associated with BPH and prostate cancer

> Ask about the time it takes to start a urine stream, usually delayed with both conditions

> Ask about dribbling at the end of the stream, as the bladder struggles to try and empty in the presence of a decreased urethra diameter

> Assess for pelvic lymphadenopathy, which usually appears as a late sign of prostate cancer

> Use the American Urological Association symptom index for BPH tool to guide assessment of symptoms of voiding related to BPH

> Palpate bladder, may find that it is distended. Assess for painless, gross hematuria, indicating prostate cancer

> Assess for pathological fractures, indicating metastasis of prostate cancer to the bone

> Assess for bone pain, especially in legs and back. Bone is a common site for prostate cancer metastasis

> Assess client's understanding of surgery

> Postoperative assessment for BPH and prostate cancer surgery
> - Assess for symptoms of transurethral resection syndrome (TUR), manifested by nausea, vomiting, hypertension, bradycardia, increased intracranial pressure, disorientation
> - Assess for bladder spasms. Assess for infection and bleeding
> - Examine color of irrigation drainage to determine effectiveness of irrigation. It should be light pink in color and with no clots
> - Ongoing assessment of vital signs, primarily to determine signs of infection

BENIGN PROSTATIC HYPERPLASIA

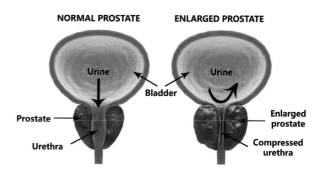

PROSTATE CANCER

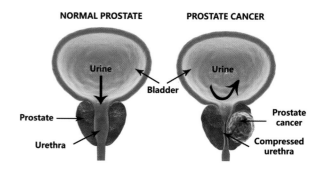

Images 11-13a and 11-13b: Pathophysiology of BPH compared to Prostate Cancer.

🧪 Priority Laboratory Tests/Diagnostics

> Digital rectal examination tells the size and consistency of the prostate

> Urinalysis shows elevated white blood cell count or hematuria, indicating inflammation or infection

> Prostate-specific antigen (PSA) will be elevated in BPH and prostate cancer

> Transrectal ultrasound to differentiate between BPH and prostate cancer and to do a biopsy of the tumor

> Magnetic resonance imaging (MRI) ultrasound fusion biopsy, a new biopsy technique that examines cancer tumor

> Serum creatinine to rule out insufficiency of renal system

> Uroflowmetry determines volume of urine that is coming from the bladder, which can then determine degree of urethral blockage

> Cystoscopy to look at inside of urethra and bladder and view the prostate enlargement

> Postvoid residual urine shows the extent of the urine flow obstruction

> Serum alkaline phosphatase will be increased if prostate cancer has metastasized to the bone

⚠ Priority Interventions or Actions

> Administer antibiotics preoperatively as prescribed. Administer antiemetics for nausea

> Insert urinary drainage preoperatively, may need to use a catheter with a special tip and insert lidocaine gel to facilitate a painless entry into the bladder

> Provide opportunity for client and partner to discuss the effect of surgery on sexual function

> Initiate chemotherapy for the client with prostate cancer, as palliative treatment

> Initiate administration of drugs for androgen deprivation therapy, if used

> Assist with procedure to remove testes(orchiectomy) to augment androgen deprivation therapy

> Prepare client for radiation, used with or without surgery

> Postoperative specific interventions for BPH and prostate cancer
  - Irrigate bladder either manually or continuously after TURP, as prescribed to prevent clots
  - Administer analgesics for pain. Administer antispasmodics for bladder spasms as prescribed
  - Have client practice Kegel exercises to strengthen pelvic floor several times while awake
  - Clean perineal area well after each bowel movement, especially if client had a radical prostatectomy, to prevent infection
  - Change dressings using sterile technique. Empty and document drainage from surgical drains
  - Dressing from a suprapubic prostatectomy procedure will drain urine at the surgical site, change dressing often and perform good site care
  - Remove suprapubic catheter when residual urine volume is less than 75 mL and client is consistently emptying the bladder
  - Monitor hematocrit and hemoglobin levels
  - Administer stool softeners to prevent client from straining at stools postoperatively
  - Assist client to ambulate early postoperatively to minimize complications of post-surgical immobility, such a blood clot

🚩 Priority Potential & Actual Complications

> TUR, hemorrhage, urinary retention, deep vein thrombosis, wound dehiscence, sexual dysfunction, sterility

☡ Priority Nursing Implications

> It is important to recognize a potentially serious complication of the TURP procedure, called transurethral resection syndrome (TUR), manifested by nausea, vomiting, hypertension, bradycardia, disorientation. The syndrome occurs as a result of bladder irrigation that is prolonged in surgery, and hyponatremia

> When the client has a perineal prostatectomy, rectal probes, tubes, thermometers must not be used as they increase the risk of trauma, which can cause infection and/or bleeding

> It is important to consider health and cultural beliefs of the client. Prostate cancer and BPH affect a man's sensitive part of his body and in some cultures, surgery on that part of the body is viewed as a significant onslaught on his manhood and how he is perceived as a "man." At some point pre or post treatment, this issue should be broached and discussed

🩸 Priority Medications

> finasteride
  - 5a-Reductase Inhibitor, a common drug used to reduce the size of the prostate
  - Must not be handled by pregnant women as it may cause anomalies with a male fetus
  - Usual dose is 5 mg orally once daily

> dutasteride/tamsulosin
  - 5a-Reductase Inhibitor, a common drug used to reduce the size of the prostate
  - This is a combination therapy so both drugs are taken together
  - Usual dose is dutasteride 0.5 mg/tamsulosin 0.4 mg orally once daily approximately 30 minutes after the same meal each day

> dutasteride
  - 5a-Reductase Inhibitor, a common drug used to reduce the size of the prostate
  - May also lower the risk of prostate cancer
  - Usual dose is 0.5 mg orally once daily

> alfuzosin
  - a-Adrenergic receptor blocker relaxes smooth muscles making urination better in BPH
  - Causes hypostatic hypotension, and is worsened if taking antihypertensive drugs
  - Dose is 10 mg extended-release tablet orally once daily, immediately after the same meal each day

> silodosin
  - a-Adrenergic receptor blocker relaxes smooth muscles making urination better in BPH
  - Dose is 8 mg orally once daily taken with a meal
  - If difficulty swallowing, open capsule and sprinkle on applesauce

> prazosin
  - a-Adrenergic receptor blocker relaxes smooth muscles making urination better in BPH
  - Initial dose is 1 mg orally 2 or 3 times daily
  - Maintenance dose is 1 to 20 mg orally, daily in divided dose

> tadalafil
  - Erectogenic drug that decreases the symptoms of BPH
  - Has added benefit of helping erectile dysfunction that is sometimes associated with BPH
  - Dose is 5 mg orally once daily at approximately the same time

> oxybutynin
  - Antimuscarinic, used to treat bladder spasms in BPH and prostate cancer
  - Can be administered via other routes as well
  - Dose is 5 mg orally 2 to 3 times daily.

> Several drugs from various classes are used for androgen deprivation therapy in prostate cancer. Below are a few common ones
  - leuprolide: can be dosed in many ways one way is 1 mg by subcutaneous injection once daily
  - triptorelin: can be dosed in many ways, one way is 3.75 mg by intramuscular injection every 4 weeks
  - degarelix: Initial dose is 240 mg administered as two injections of 120 mg each at a concentration of 40 mg/mL, administered subcutaneously. Maintenance dose is 80 mg administered subcutaneously at a concentration of 20 mg/mL, every 28 days.

- bicalutamide: dose is 50 mg orally once daily, administered at the same time each day

> The use of chemotherapy in prostate cancer is palliative and not curative. Several drugs are used Below are just a few
  - cabazitaxel: dose is 25 mg/m^2 intravenous over 1 hour every three weeks
  - docetaxel and prednisone: dose is 75 mg/m^2 intravenous over 1 hour every 3 weeks; prednisone 5 mg orally 2 times daily is administered continuously
  - estramustine: dose is 14 mg/kg/day orally in 3 or 4 divided doses

Priority Education/Discharge Issues

> Teaching for active surveillance (for BPH) or androgen suppression therapy (for prostate cancer)
  - Decrease intake of caffeine, spicy foods and artificial sweeteners, as they can act as irritants to the urinary tract by increasing bladder distention
  - Fluid intake of up to 2000 to 3000 mL daily. Restrict fluids at night before bed
  - Take medications as prescribed to decrease size of prostate gland
  - Monitor symptoms carefully to determine if they are worsening
  - Contact healthcare provider for worsening symptoms
  - Have annual PSA and digital rectal examination
  - Avoid alcohol intake
  - Speak with pharmacist before taking over-the-counter medications and herbal remedies as some can exacerbate BPH symptoms
  - Do not suppress the urge to urinate as it causes stasis of urine
  - Teach about proper administration and side effects of drugs used for androgen suppression
  - Teach that if orchiectomy is done along with androgen deprivation therapy, weight gain may occur

> Teaching for client after surgery for BPH and prostate cancer
  - Proper handling of surgical site, to prevent infection.
  - Assessing site for bleeding and infection
  - Instruct regarding the possibility of retrograde ejaculation and erectile dysfunction
  - Return of sexual function may be 1 to 2 years, depending on if surgery was for a BPH or prostate cancer
  - Take medications prescribed to help sexual function
  - Be aware of incontinence and that it should resolve over time
  - Drink water and urinate 2 to 3 times daily to clear the urinary tract
  - Signs and symptoms to report immediately and who to call

Chronic kidney disease/end-stage renal disease

Pathophysiology/Description

> Chronic kidney disease (CKD) is progressive, irreversible loss of kidney function impacting millions of Americans. End-stage renal disease with the need for dialysis or kidney transplantation is the result of CKD

> Unlike acute kidney injury that is sudden, CKD has a slow onset, often progressing over several years and is characterized by significantly decreased glomerular filtration rate (less than 60 mL/min for more than 3 months) and kidney damage (for more than 3 months)

> There are 5 stages of CKD. Stage 1 manifests kidney damage with glomerular filtration rate (GFR) of 90 mL/min or greater. As the stages progress and CKD worsens, GFR decreases until the 5th stage, kidney failure, is reached with a GFR of less than 15 mL/min. At this stage the client requires dialysis or kidney transplantation to sustain life

> Because all body systems are reliant of effective functioning of the kidneys to function effectively, when CKD occurs, all body systems are negatively impacted

> Diabetes and hypertension are the predominant causes of CKD. Urologic and cystic conditions are also contributing factors. African Americans, Hispanics and Native Americans have much higher rates of CKD than do Caucasian Americans

> With end-stage renal disease, the client will need dialysis or kidney transplantation. There are several types of dialysis

> Peritoneal dialysis
> • The peritoneum is used as a semipermeable membrane to perform dialysis treatment via a catheter that is inserted through the client's abdomen. Dialysate is instilled in client's abdomen and dwells there for a few hours, pulling toxins via the peritoneum's semipermeable membrane. It is then drained from the abdomen

> Hemodialysis
> • Removal of waste from a client's body by use of a hemodialyzer (artificial kidney). A fistula or graft is created in a client's body, usually in the lower or upper arm and these are accessed and connected to the dialyzer. One lumen takes blood from the client to the dialyzer and the other brings blood back from the dialyzer to the client

> Continuous renal replacement therapy
> • Double lumen catheter placed in the client's femoral or jugular vein and connected to a hemofilter where solutes are removed, and the client's blood is filtered of toxins

> Kidney transplantation
> • Receipt of a donor kidney to replace a client's non-functional kidney

Priority Assessments or Cues

> Assess for anorexia, nausea and vomiting, lethargy and fatigue, indicative of very high BUN level

> Assess for metallic taste to mouth and uremic fetor (urine like smell) from ammonia buildup

> Assess for signs of neurological impairment, which may manifest as confusion, headache, drowsiness and encephalopathy due to accumulation of ammonia from nitrogenous waste

> Assess for peripheral neuropathy. Clients may indicate a feeling of burning in the feet

> Assess for asterixis (rapid flexion and extension of hands when the arm/hands are stretched out)

> Assess for fractures of small bones, caused by associated mineral and bone disorder, from imbalances of calcium, vitamin D and parathyroid hormone

> Assess skin for itching caused by uremic frost, crystallization of uremia on skin due to elevated BUN

> Ask client about use of prescription and over-the-counter medications as many drugs are toxic to the kidneys

> Assess client's emotional status as the myriad of system complications associated with CKD can cause dysfunctional coping

> Assess for signs of fluid overload as CKD progresses, which includes edema and hypertension, pulmonary edema, heart failure, among other signs. When on dialysis, client may have anuria, but some clients still produce some urine

> Assess blood glucose, may find hyperglycemia due to impaired glucose metabolism

> Ongoing assessment of potassium level, expect hyperkalemia from kidney's decreased excretion of potassium

> Examine electrocardiogram strips, widening of QRS complex and ST segment depression may indicate hyperkalemia

> Assess for symptoms of metabolic acidosis due to kidney's inability to excrete excess acid

> Assess cardiovascular system, may find heart failure, coronary artery disease, among other conditions. Ongoing assessment of cardiovascular system

> Assess respiratory system, may find pneumonia, pulmonary edema, among other conditions

> Assess respirations, may find Kussmaul respirations because of metabolic acidosis, caused by depletion of sodium bicarbonate

> Assess for bleeding due to decreased coagulopathy

> Assess for infections as CKD places client at risk for several system infections

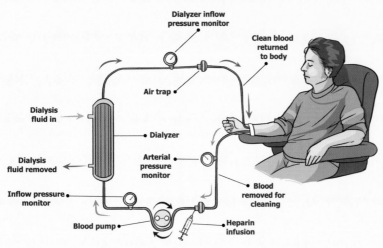

Hemodialysis

Dialyzer inflow pressure monitor

Clean blood returned to body

Air trap

Dialysis fluid in

Dialyzer

Dialysis fluid removed

Arterial pressure monitor

Inflow pressure monitor

Blood removed for cleaning

Blood pump

Heparin infusion

Image 11-14a: Hemodialysis priority nursing concerns.

Priority nursing concerns:

HEMODIALYSIS

Before:

1. _____
2. _____
3. _____

During:

1. _____
2. _____
3. _____

After:

1. _____
2. _____
3. _____

Table 11-3a

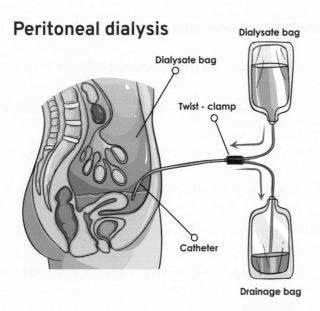

Peritoneal dialysis

Dialysate bag

Dialysate bag

Twist - clamp

Catheter

Drainage bag

Image 11-14b: Peritoneal dialysis priority nursing concerns.

Priority nursing concerns:

PERITONEAL DIALYSIS

Before:

1. _____
2. _____
3. _____

During:

1. _____
2. _____
3. _____

After:

1. _____
2. _____
3. _____

Table 11-3b

- Examine electrocardiogram strips, widening of QRS complex and ST segment depression may indicate hyperkalemia
- Assess client's long-term support system, since CKD and end-stage renal disease are life-altering conditions
- Assessment for client on hemodialysis
  - Assess client for hypotension due to rapid removal of blood volume
  - Assess for nausea vomiting chest pain and visual changes due to rapid fluid removal
  - Assess for muscle cramps associated with low sodium dialysis solution
  - Assess post dialysis bleeding from factors such as poor rinsing of blood for the dialyzer
  - Assess the fistula by feeling the thrill (purring at the fistula site) and listening to the bruit (sound of rushing water, like a washing machine) with a stethoscope, sounds created by the high flow of blood through the vein
  - Assess client for steal syndrome (shunting of blood from distal extremity in dialysis), manifested by pain distal to the access site, poor capillary refill and numbness that worsens with dialysis.
  - Assess insertion site for bleeding, hematoma or infection
- Additional assessment for client on peritoneal dialysis (PD)
  - Assess the catheter insertion site for infection, which may manifest as redness, and drainage at the site
  - Assess for peritonitis, evidenced by rebound tenderness, cloudy dialysis effluent with elevated white blood cell count, abdominal pain
  - Assess for hernias and back pain, due to weight of the dialysate causing increased pressure in the abdomen
  - Assess respiratory status for complications such as pneumonia, and atelectasis due to pressure on diaphragm from dwelling of the dialysis fluid

⚗ Priority Laboratory Tests/Diagnostics

- Urine dipstick protein will show proteinuria
- Urine will show elevated albumin, white blood cell count, protein, casts and glucose
- Glomerular filtration rate (GFR) shows degree of kidney damage
- Electrolytes show elevated potassium, blood urea nitrogen (BUN) and creatinine levels
- Kidney ultrasound to look for obstructions and/or other abnormalities of the urinary system
- Computed tomography (CT) scan to look for complications of the condition, such as renal masses and vascular abnormalities
- Renal scan to look at renal tubular function and kidney blood flow
- Renal biopsy is used to determine cause of the kidney disease and is considered the most definitive

⚠ Priority Interventions or Actions

- Administer diuretics as ordered, to treat fluid overload
- Weigh client daily using the same scale and at the same time. Note that weight increase 0.5 to 1-pound daily is indicative of fluid retention
- Administer antihypertensive drugs as prescribed and measure orthostatic blood pressures
- Administer phosphate binders and vitamin D to help in management of bone disease from CKD. Restrict phosphate once client starts dialysis
- Administer exogenous erythropoietin to replace the kidney's decreased production
- Administer iron due to depletion of iron stores from the need for iron to support erythropoiesis
- Administer stool softeners to manage constipation for iron administration
- Administer medications for dyslipidemia
- Refer client to dietitian for nutritional counseling
- Monitor client taking nephrotoxic drugs
- Allow client adequate rest as buildup of nitrogenous waste causes fatigue
- Maintain fluid restriction, as prescribed for client on dialysis
- Maintain client on sodium restricted diet to include no more than 4 grams daily
- Maintain client's phosphate intake at no more than 1 gram daily
- Assist client to initiate a conversation about kidney transplantation with the correct personnel
- Provide information to client on all types of dialysis procedures
- Provide prescribed diet, may be a low protein diet to decrease the work on the kidneys and high carbohydrates and fats to prevent ketosis. Sodium is restricted due to edema in oliguric phase
- Provide measures to prevent blood clots from immobility, such as compression devices
- Provide measures to prevent skin breaks, since the client may be in bed for prolonged periods
- Provide measures to manage itching
- Monitor for restless leg syndrome, common during dialysis treatment
- Assess for burning and tearing of eyes, caused by calcium deposits
- Administer enteral feeding if client cannot tolerate oral intake
- Administer treatment for hyperkalemia as prescribed. There are several choices of treatment such as calcium gluconate, sodium bicarbonate, dietary restriction, loop diuretics, among others.

Chronic kidney disease/end-stage renal disease

- Interventions for client on hemodialysis
  - Ongoing monitoring of vital signs pre-during and post dialysis, expect slight elevation of temperature during dialysis due to warming of the blood coming from the dialyzer. Report persistent elevated temperature which may indicate infection. Monitor client's blood pressure during and after dialysis, noting any precipitous drop that requires treatment
  - Weigh client before and after dialysis
  - Monitor client for bleeding as heparin is used in dialysis to prevent clots
  - Monitor for fluid overload before dialysis and for hypovolemia after dialysis
  - Ensure client with femoral vein catheter sits up at less than a 45-degree angle and does not lean forward due to risk of catheter occlusion or kinking
  - Monitor graft/shunt for clotting, manifested by inability to feel a thrill and hear a bruit, and by client's complaint of tingling and discomfort in arm
- Interventions for client on peritoneal dialysis
  - Administer antibiotics for infection at catheter insertion site (common in PD) or for peritonitis
  - Apply orthopedic binders for complaint of back pain
  - Monitor dialysis fluid outflow to ensure consistency in flow. Maintain drainage bag below client's abdomen. Assess outflow for color, odor, presence of blood
  - Ongoing monitoring of protein loss to prevent loss that is too high, placing client at risk for malnutrition

Priority Potential & Actual Complications

- Cardiovascular complications, dyslipidemia, bone disease
- End-stage renal disease and dialysis, catheter site infection and peritonitis with PD
- Renal transplantation

Priority Nursing Implications

- Chronic kidney disease impacts every system in the body, so assessment must focus on all body systems. Cardiovascular disease is the most common cause of death in clients with CKD, so meticulous assessment of the cardiovascular system must be made when caring for clients with CKD
- Nurses must remember that blood pressure and venous access must never be performed in the client's arm that has a vascular access because of the risk of clotting of the vascular access
- A temporary access can be used for dialysis until a fistula or graft matures and can be used. The temporary access is made via the femoral or jugular veins. These should not be mistaken for regular intravenous lines

Priority Medications

- Several drugs are used to treat hyperkalemia associated with CKD. Below are a few of these drugs
  - sodium bicarbonate: dose is one ampule of 7.5% sodium bicarbonate administered slowly intravenously over 5 minutes. repeat at 10 to 15-minute intervals if needed. Correct acidosis
  - sodium polystyrene sulfonate: dose is 15 grams orally once daily or 30 mg rectally every 6 hours. Excretes potassium from body
  - patiromer: dose is 8.4 g orally once daily. Dose can be titrated based on potassium level. Binds potassium in gastrointestinal tract
  - calcium gluconate: dose is 500 to 3000 mg intravenous one time, rate not to exceed 0.5 to 2 mL/min. Reduce myocardial irritability from hyperkalemia
- calcium acetate
  - Used as a phosphate binder to bind phosphate and excrete it in stool
  - Initial dose is 1334 mg (2 tablets/capsules, or 10 mL), orally, taken with each meal
  - Maintenance dose is 2001 to 2668 mg (3 to 4 tablets/capsules, or 15 to 20 mL) taken with each meal
- calcitriol
  - Treat secondary hyperparathyroidism in end-stage renal disease
  - Dose is 0.25 mcg orally once daily
  - Measure serum calcium at least twice weekly during start of drug therapy
- erythropoietin
  - Treat anemia associated with chronic kidney disease
  - Dose is 50 to 100 units/kg intravenous or subcutaneous 3 times weekly
  - Monitor iron stores and administer iron if serum ferritin is below 100 ng/mL
  - Monitor hemoglobin to prevent cardiovascular complications
- atorvastatin
  - Treat dyslipidemia in CKD
  - Initial dose is 10 mg or 20 mg orally once daily
  - Maintenance dose is 10 mg to 80 mg orally once daily
- gemfibrozil
  - Use to lower triglyceride levels
  - Dose is 600 mg orally twice daily, taken 30 minutes before the morning and evening meals
  - Must be used as an adjunct to diet

Next Gen Clinical Judgment

One of the best ways to **save time studying** is to create actual lab values that would indicate a need for a certain medication or treatment. Pick 3 of the Priority Medications above and create a lab value that would indicate a need for that medication in the client with CKD.

Priority Education/Discharge Issues

> Teach client the impact of diet on the kidneys. Avoid high protein diet to decrease burden on kidneys

> Teach client to avoid eating foods with high sodium and potassium

> Teach client that daily phosphate should be no more than 1 gram

> Provide client with a list of foods that are high in potassium and phosphate

> Teach clients to read food labels in the supermarket

> Discuss barriers to dialysis with client

> Assist with information regarding resources, such as transportation to and from dialysis, if needed

> Teach client with diabetes the importance of having urine checked for albumin routinely and maintaining good glycemic control

> Teach client how to measure blood pressure and blood glucose. Have client do return demonstration

> Educate client on the PD process and have client do return demonstration, if on PD

> Provide a resource for client to call with questions or concerns

> Teach client to examine PD catheter insertion site for infection. Teach signs of peritonitis, to report cloudy outflow immediately

> Educate client on the types of PD, nightly or intermittent

> Teach client to never allow anyone to place an intravenous catheter or measure blood pressure in the arm with a graft or shunt for dialysis

> Teach the client to avoid submerging the shunt in water

> Teach client signs of shunt infection and when to contact the health care provider

> Teach importance of regular follow-up with healthcare provider

> Instruct client to organize medications by using a pill box organizer, as clients with CKD usually have several comorbidities for which they take several medications

> Assist client with seeking appropriate resources for counseling, if needed

> Educate that certain drugs worsen kidney function. These include nonsteroidal anti-inflammatory drugs (NSAIDs) and angiotensin-converting enzymes (ACE) inhibitors

> Teach client to seek advice of pharmacist before taking any over-the-counter drugs or herbal preparations as many may be nephrotoxic

> Teach client on dialysis that they may or may not produce urine

Acute kidney disease/injury

📋 Pathophysiology/Description

> Acute kidney disease (AKD) is defined as rapid loss of kidney function because of prerenal, intrarenal or postrenal damage to the kidneys. In AKD, the onset is sudden, but the condition is usually reversible once the cause is addressed

> Prerenal damage: caused by factors that occur outside of the kidneys that reduces or depletes intravascular volume such as, hemorrhage, decreased cardiac output and dehydration, among others

> Intrarenal: caused by factors that cause direct damage to the renal parenchyma, such as acute glomerulonephritis, acute tubular necrosis and effects of drugs on the kidneys, among others

> Postrenal: caused by factors that impede the flow of urine between the kidney and the urethra, such as benign prostate hyperplasia, calculi and bladder cancer, among others

> Phases associated with AKD
> - Oliguric: reduction in urine output to less than 400 mL/24 hours, occurring within 1-7 days of kidney injury is usually first sign of AKD. This phase can have a 10 to 14 days duration, but longer oliguric phase represents poorer prognosis for kidney recovery. Some clients will not experience oliguria
> - Diuretic: daily urine output starts to increase and can get a high as 5 L/day. The kidneys have not recovered but this urine output indicates that the kidneys are able to eliminate wastes from the body. The diuretic phase may last for up to 3 weeks
> - Recovery: glomerular filtration rate increases, and urine volume normalizes. Full kidney function occurs slowly, and it may take up to 1 year for kidney function to fully stabilize

> Continuous renal replacement therapy (CRRT) is sometimes done for clients with AKD
> - Double lumen catheter placed in the clients femoral or jugular vein and connected to a hemofilter where solutes are removed, and the client's blood is filtered of toxins until AKD is resolved

> Many clients with AKD recover well but if recovery does not proceed well through the phases, then the client may progress to end-stage kidney disease

✏️ Priority Assessments or Cues

> Assess for sudden decrease in urine output, manifested in oliguric phase. Perform ongoing assessment of urine output

> Assess for anorexia, nausea and vomiting, which may indicate uremia

> Assess for signs of neurological impairment, which may manifest as drowsiness, confusion, tingling of fingers and toes, to stupor

> Assess neck veins, which may be distended in oliguric phase due to fluid overload

> Assess lungs for crackles, indicating fluid in the lungs

> Assess for pericarditis, manifested by friction rub, and chest pain upon inspiration

> Assess for signs of fluid overload, which includes edema and hypertension, pulmonary edema, heart failure, among other signs

> Assessment of all body systems to identify the underlying cause of AKD

> Assess respirations, may find Kussmaul respirations because of metabolic acidosis, caused by depletion of sodium bicarbonate

> Examine electrocardiogram strips, widening of QRS complex and ST segment depression may indicate hyperkalemia

> Assess for increased urine volume to 1 liter and above. This is indicative of the diuretic phase

> Assess for hypovolemia and hypotension, tachycardia in the diuretic phase because of massive fluid loss

> Assess for stabilizing electrolytes levels, indicating client is in the diuretic phase. Assess glomerular filtration rate, expect it to be increasing

> Assess electrolytes for normalized values, indicating client is in recovery phase

> Assess for increased neurological function, indicating client is in the recovery phase

> Assess for normalized urine output, manifested in the recovery phase

> Assess for manifestations of infection such as fever, pain, malaise, as infection is common in AKD

> If client getting CRRT assess vital signs, intake and output, and hemodynamic status hourly. Assess the vascular access site for infection, and maintain patency of the CRRT system

🧪 Priority Laboratory Tests/Diagnostics

> Electrolytes: in oliguric phase, serum sodium and bicarbonate levels are decreased while potassium, blood urea nitrogen (BUN) and creatinine levels are increased

> Urinalysis showing elevated white blood cell count, casts, hematuria, pyuria and protein, indicate an intrarenal cause for AKD

> Kidney ultrasound to look for obstructions and/or other abnormalities of the urinary system

> Computed tomography (CT) scan to look for complications of the condition, such as renal masses and vascular abnormalities

> Renal scan to look at renal tubular function and kidney blood flow

> Renal biopsy is used to determine cause of the kidney injury and is considered the most definitive way to diagnose AKD caused by intrarenal factors

⚠ Priority Interventions or Actions

> Measure intake and output expect urine output below 400 mL in 24 hours in the oliguric phase. Keep careful record

> Administer diuretics as ordered, to treat fluid overload

> Weigh client daily using the same scale and at the same time. Note that weight increase 0.5 to 1-pound daily is indicative of fluid retention

> Establish intravenous line and administer quick fluid replacement in oliguric phase

> Monitor client taking nephrotoxic drugs

> Use aseptic technique where needed, as a common cause of death in AKD is infection

> Provide prescribed diet, may be a low protein diet to decrease the work on the kidneys and high carbohydrates and fats to prevent ketosis. Sodium is restricted due to edema in oliguric phase

> Provide measures to prevent blood clots from immobility, such as compression devices

> Provide measures to prevent skin breaks, since the client may be in bed for prolonged periods

> Prepare client for renal replacement therapy, if prescribed

> Administer enteral feeding if client cannot tolerate oral intake

> Administer treatment for hyperkalemia as prescribed. There are several choices of treatment such as calcium gluconate, sodium bicarbonate, dietary restriction, among others

> If client is receiving CRRT, monitor the ultrafiltrate to ensure it is clear yellow. Stop treatment if ultrafiltrate becomes bloody, as it indicates a ruptured filter membrane

⚑ Priority Potential & Actual Complications

> Infection
> Hyperkalemia
> Chronic kidney disease
> Dialysis
> Renal transplantation

⟳ Priority Nursing Implications

> When caring for clients who are older adults, it is important to know that they may not recover from AKD as do younger clients. They may not regain full function of their kidneys after AKD

> Be mindful that for clients on dialysis who are in AKD, their response to fever is blunted so they may not respond to an infection with a fever.

> Contrast media must not be used in tests for clients with AKD as they are very toxic to the kidneys and will worsen AKD

◊ Priority Medications

> furosemide
  • Loop diuretic to treat fluid overload in oliguric phase
  • Potassium-wasting drug so monitor potassium
  • Usual dose is 20 to 40 mg intravenous administered slowly over 1 to 2 minutes or may be given intramuscularly once.

> Several drugs are used to treat hyperkalemia associated with AKD. Below are a few of these drugs
  • sodium bicarbonate: dose is one ampule of 7.5% sodium bicarbonate administered slowly intravenously over 5 minutes. repeat at 10 to 15-minute intervals if needed
  • sodium polystyrene sulfonate: dose is 15 grams orally once daily or 30 mg rectally every 6 hours
  • patiromer: dose is 8.4 g orally once daily. Dose can be titrated based on potassium level
  • calcium gluconate: dose is 500 to 3000 mg intravenous one time, rate not to exceed 0.5 to 2 mL/min

👤 Priority Education/Discharge Issues

> Teach client to monitor urinary output and to seek medical care at the first sign of significantly decreased output

> Teach importance of monitoring urinary status if taking nephrotoxic drugs or working with chemicals that are potentially toxic to kidneys

> Teach client the impact of diet on the kidneys

> Educate on proper taking of medications that control possible causes of kidney disease

> Teach importance of regular follow-up with healthcare provider to assess kidney function

> Teach client the indicators of recurrent kidney disease and when to contact healthcare provider

> Teach client that full recovery after AKD may take several months

> Discuss with client possibilities if kidneys do not fully recover, such as dialysis or kidney transplantation

> Assist client with seeking appropriate resources for counseling, if needed

> Educate that certain drugs worsen kidney function. These include nonsteroidal anti-inflammatory drugs (NSAIDs) and angiotensin-converting enzyme (ACE) inhibitors

1. A nurse is assessing a 41-year-old client in an outpatient clinic. Which indication of a risk factor for bowel disease requires follow-up by the nurse?
   1. The client's 62-year-old father was diagnosed with colorectal cancer 4 years ago.
   2. The client's cousin has inflammatory bowel disease and frequent diarrhea.
   3. The client reports eating red meat 2 days a week and fish twice a week.
   4. BMI of 24.8 kg/m² and has less than optimal nutritional patterns.

2. A home health nurse is visiting a client who had a transurethral resection of the prostate (TURP) one week ago following a diagnosis of prostate cancer. The client needs to perform intermittent self-catheterization because of the surgery. What assessment data requires the nurse to follow-up during the home visit?
   1. The client uses aseptic technique when inserting the catheter.
   2. Ranks pain as a 1 on a 0-10 scale.
   3. Urine output is 200 mL following catheterization.
   4. The client states he has needed to take a stool softener.

3. The nurse is caring for a client who is having difficulty urinating following a recent diagnosis of prostate cancer. What nursing activities are a priority based on this data? Select all that apply.
   1. Ask the client if he would like someone from pastoral care to come visit him.
   2. Ask visitors to leave the room when he needs to use the toilet.
   3. Integrate the client's elimination habits into the care plan.
   4. Encourage the client to increase high-fluid foods such as fruits and drink small amounts of fluids frequently.
   5. Put the client's hand in warm water when he voids.

4. A client with a medical diagnosis of cirrhosis has been admitted to a medical unit, and the nurse is doing an assessment. What complaint from the client requires immediate follow-up?
   1. Bloody expectorant with coughing episodes.
   2. Jeans cannot zip because of enlarged abdomen.
   3. Swelling in the feet and lower legs.
   4. Yellowing of the eyes and mucous membranes.

5. Emergency Medical Services transports a known intravenous drug user to the Emergency Department. The client reports flu-like symptoms for the last week, jaundice, and inability to keep food down. What safety precautions should the nurse utilize?
   1. Droplet precautions only.
   2. Full gown, gloves, mask with shield.
   3. Report the client to the CDC.
   4. Standard precautions of gloves and handwashing.

6. The nurse has completed discharge teaching for a young client being discharged with a new diagnosis of inflammatory bowel disease after treatment for an exacerbation. Which statement by the client indicates further clarification needs to be done?
   1. "I need to decrease my stress by not taking on so much at work."
   2. "I need to get plenty of sleep, which is good, because I like to sleep."
   3. "I will need to eat a high calorie, high protein diet."
   4. "I'm glad I don't have to stay on steroids and antibiotics long-term."

7. A home health nurse is making a visit on an older client with long-standing diverticular disease. The client has been taking dietary fiber supplements, stool softeners, and oral antibiotics, along with increased fluids and a high-fiber diet. What additional assessment should the nurse make?
   1. Ask why the client takes 2 drugs to stimulate the already inflamed bowel.
   2. Palpate and percuss the abdomen immediately.
   3. Question about any possible side effects of the antibiotics.
   4. Quiz the client about what is considered "high-fiber" in the diet.

8. A client on the surgical unit is preparing to be discharged after a colectomy for an intestinal obstruction. The nurse finds the client passed out on the bathroom floor. Which response by the nurse would be most appropriate?
   1. Call another nurse to help get the client back to bed.
   2. Call the client's healthcare provider from the room.
   3. Check the client's abdominal wound for bleeding.
   4. Determine if the client is breathing and has a pulse.

9. A client in the clinic returns for a follow-up visit complaining of recurrent irritable bowel syndrome with such symptoms as nausea, bloating, flatulence, abdominal distention, and severe headache. What does the nurse further assess to help determine the next course of action?
   1. Complaints of constipation and straining at stool.
   2. Compliance with a high fiber diet, including green leafy vegetables.
   3. Share that they went out to eat Mexican food the evening before.
   4. Stated took an opioid twice in the last 12 hours for the severe headache.

10. A client in end-stage renal failure has orders for sodium polystyrene sulfonate 15 grams PO in 90 mL. water 3 times daily. What would be the total daily dose of sodium polystyrene sulfonate?

11. The clinic nurse is preparing to teach an obese client about a new weight loss program. What would be the most appropriate preface to the teaching plan?
    1. "Even with a loss of 3-5% of your current weight would reduce complications risks."
    2. "My advice is to adhere strictly to this diet plan for the next year."
    3. "We cannot continue to treat your hypertension if you don't lose some weight."
    4. "You must lose 40 pounds in the next six months or die from a heart attack or stroke."

12. The clinic nurse is interviewing a new client, who presents with increasing frequency of stools and says the last healthcare provider gave a diagnosis of ulcerative colitis. What statement by the client requires immediate follow-up?
    1. "I'm having more frequent loose stools than I did last week."
    2. "I've developed a high fever and severe abdominal pain since yesterday."
    3. "My last healthcare provider said I have a genetic link for developing this disease."
    4. "This is a depressing disease to have."

13. A nursery nurse is administering an ordered bottle feeding for an infant born with a cleft lip and palate. What action should the nurse take first to prevent complications?
    1. Assess the infant's ability to suck.
    2. Give only small volumes of feedings.
    3. Hold the infant at a 45-60 degree angle.
    4. Warm the formula.

14. The nurse is implementing teaching with a client with gastroesophageal reflux (GER). Which statement by the client demonstrates a further need for teaching?
    1. "I'll be sleeping on 2-3 pillows."
    2. "I'll take my medication to prevent reflux before my evening meal."
    3. "Reflux can cause erosion of my stomach lining."
    4. "We like to eat Mexican food at least once per week."

15. The nurse is assessing a client who has been admitted with a diagnosis of peptic ulcer disease (PUD). What assessment findings would be consistent with a psycho-emotional component to possible causes?
    1. Infection with Helicobacter pylori.
    2. Recent increase in responsibilities at work.
    3. Surgery 6 months ago secondary to a sports injury.
    4. Taking aspirin or non-steroidal anti-inflammatory drugs for chronic headaches.

16. The nurse is caring for a young client who reports being beaten in a street fight, with resultant acute kidney injury. What nursing actions would be appropriate? Select all that apply.
    1. A thorough assessment to determine the extent of the client's injuries.
    2. Dietary restrictions of potassium, phosphate, and sodium.
    3. Fluid restriction of 600 mL plus previous 24-hour fluid loss.
    4. Hourly serum BUN and creatinine levels.
    5. Schedule a renal ultrasound as ordered.

17. The nurse has planned care for a client admitted with acute gastritis and diarrhea from non-steroid anti-inflammatory drug overuse due to arthritis. In planning care for this client, in what order would the nurse perform these actions? Rank order the responses.
    1. Administer antiemetics as needed.
    2. Explore with client and healthcare provider other therapies for arthritis.
    3. Keep NPO initially.
    4. Monitor for signs/symptoms of dehydration.
    5. Ensure that the client's perineal area is clean.

18. The nurse in a dialysis unit is monitoring the client with chronic kidney disease (CKD). In what order would the nurse assess signs/symptoms and act to keep the client as comfortable as possible during peritoneal dialysis (PD)? Rank order the responses.
    1. Development of crackles in the bases of both lungs.
    2. Headache.
    3. Itching and scratching of the lower extremities.
    4. Nausea and vomiting.
    5. Spreading hematoma around the peritoneal catheter.

19. A 7-year-old client undergoes a laparotomy in the epigastric region for a small bowel obstruction. Which nursing intervention is indicated to prevent the most concerning complication of this surgery?
    1. Sterile dressing changes and intravenous antibiotics.
    2. A high fiber diet with adequate oral and intravenous hydration.
    3. Coughing and using an incentive spirometer every two hours.
    4. Turning every two hours and padding under bony prominences.

20. The nurse is discussing the plan of care with a client receiving dialysis. The nurse understands what aspect of care is a priority for this client?
    1. Eating fruits and vegetables.
    2. Monitoring fluid intake.
    3. Daily exercise.
    4. Monitoring output.

21. A client returns from surgery for placement of a colostomy secondary to ulcerative colitis. Two hours after the surgery the nurse is most concerned about which assessment?
    1. Hypoactive bowel sounds in all four quadrants.
    2. Decreased breath sounds in the bases of the lungs.
    3. Slight distension of the bladder.
    4. A blood pressure below the baseline value.

22. A 13-year-old client is receiving total parental nutrition as a treatment for Crohn's disease. The client asks the rationale for this treatment. Which statement by the nurse accurately describes the reason for this treatment?
    1. "The nutrition in your intravenous line is more complete than what you can eat."
    2. "Total parenteral nutrition allows your intestines to rest and heal for a while."
    3. "This treatment assists you in getting the nutrients you need without the allergies."
    4. "With this treatment you do not need to eat by mouth so you can get the rest you need."

23. The nurse is planning to make a home visit for a client with hepatitis C. What documentation should the nurse include in the chart concerning client/family teaching?
    1. Family and client should not share eating utensils and dishes.
    2. Eating utensils and dishes should be washed in hot water above 180°F.
    3. Proper universal precautions should be observed when cleaning up blood from the client.
    4. Family members should not come in contact with the client's medications.

24. The nurse is caring for a toddler who is postoperative day 1 after a revision of pyloric stenosis repair done when the client was an infant. The nurse's 8am assessment included blood pressure of 90/54 and heart rate of 92. At 11am the vitals included blood pressure of 102/64 and heart rate of 118. The mother reports that the child has been irritable for the past hour. What action does the nurse take?
    1. Notify the provider of the change in vital signs.
    2. Administer oral analgesics as ordered.
    3. Obtain a hemoglobin and hematocrit.
    4. Provide oxygen via a nasal cannula.

25. A nurse is caring for a client with colorectal cancer who is receiving total parenteral nutrition (TPN). The physician has prescribed the TPN to infuse at 150 mL/hr. The TPN bag holds 2400 mL. How long will it take for the TPN to infuse to the nearest whole hour? Fill in the blank.

    _____

26. A nurse is caring for these four clients. Which client would the nurse provide care to first?
    1. 25-year-old who had a splenectomy four hours ago and is reporting pain at the incisional site with movement.
    2. 75-year-old who had surgery three days ago for a bowel obstruction and has a fever, chills and purulent drainage from the wound.
    3. 18-year-old diagnosed with an infection who is receiving an intravenous antibiotic and reports tingling around the mouth and itching to the body.
    4. 68-year-old who had a unit of packed red blood cells an hour ago and reports feeling fatigued and flushed.

27. The nurse is caring for a client with renal failure. The client is on a special diet and strict intake and output. What nursing assessments would the nurse do for this client? Select all that apply.
    1. Daily weights.
    2. Monitor appetite.
    3. Monitor edema in the extremities.
    4. Monitor bowel movements.
    5. Monitor urine volume and characteristics.

28. A client is admitted with ascites from liver failure. Spironolactone 100 mg is administered. Which sign or symptom would designate a serious complication for the client?
    1. Blurry vision.
    2. Low potassium.
    3. Increased thirst.
    4. Leg pain.

29. A client diagnosed with morbid obesity is at high risk for impaired skin integrity. When the nurse is developing a plan of care for this client which nursing action is a priority?
    1. Keep the skin clean and dry.
    2. Educate the client about sun exposure.
    3. Suggest wearing loose clothing.
    4. Inspect skin daily.

30. A client has chronic diarrhea, bloating, and abdominal pain. The healthcare provider is ruling out celiac disease. The client asks the nurse about dietary guidelines. What would be the best answer from the nurse?
    1. "You will need to eat foods that bind the bowels like bananas, rice, toast, and applesauce."
    2. "You should eat a low fiber diet that limits fibers including stems, seeds, and skins."
    3. "Foods that you cannot eat include wheat proteins or gluten-based starches or fillers."
    4. "You will need to discuss your dietary needs with a nutritionist to develop a meal plan."

1. **A nurse is assessing a 41-year-old client in an outpatient clinic. Which indication of a risk factor for bowel disease requires follow-up by the nurse?**
   1. ⚲ The client's 62-year-old father was diagnosed with colorectal cancer 4 years ago.
   2. The client's cousin has inflammatory bowel disease and frequent diarrhea. *A family member with IBD is a risk factor but a cousin is not a first-degree relative.*
   3. The client reports eating red meat 2 days a week and fish twice a week. *Not risk factor concerns.*
   4. BMI of 24.8 kg/m² and has less than optimal nutritional patterns. *Not a risk factor.*

   Rationale: Persons who have a first-degree relative diagnosed with colorectal cancer before age 60, should have a colonoscopy every 5 years beginning at age 40. The nurse needs to ask this client if he or she has had a colonoscopy recently and make a referral for a colonoscopy if the client has not had one yet. The other findings do not contribute to the risk of developing colon cancer or other health concerns as significant.

   THIN Thinking: Identify Risk to Safety – *The nurse should recognize risks for bowel disease based on lifestyle and family history.* **NCLEX®:** Reduction of Risk Potential **QSEN:** Evidence-based Practice

2. **A home health nurse is visiting a client who had a transurethral resection of the prostate (TURP) one week ago following a diagnosis of prostate cancer. The client needs to perform intermittent self-catheterization because of the surgery. What assessment data requires the nurse to follow-up during the home visit?**
   1. The client uses aseptic technique when inserting the catheter. *Aseptic technique acceptable for home insertions.*
   2. Ranks pain as a 1 on a 0-10 scale. *Expected finding postoperatively.*
   3. ⚲ Urine output is 200 mL following catheterization.
   4. The client states he has needed to take a stool softener. *Not a concerning factor considering he's postoperative, less active, and may be on pain medications.*

   Rationale: When a client needs to perform self-catheterization, the goal for intermittent catheterization is to individualize the frequency of catheterization to obtain 400 mL of urine on average. The nurse needs to investigate why the client is only getting 200 mL following self-catheterization. The client may not be taking in enough fluid or he may be catheterizing himself too frequently.

   The nurse may need to provide further client education or change the plan of care based on analysis of assessment findings. The client should be using aseptic technique when inserting an intermittent catheter. This client's pain level is expected following surgery. Clients need to avoid activities that increase abdominal pressure following surgery. Taking a stool softener prevents clients from having to use the Valsalva maneuver, reducing abdominal pressure during bowel elimination.

   THIN Thinking: Top Three – Monitoring output is a priority for frequent catheterizations. **NCLEX®:** Basic Care and Comfort **QSEN:** Safety

3. **The nurse is caring for a client who is having difficulty urinating following a recent diagnosis of prostate cancer. What nursing activities are a priority based on this data? Select all that apply.**
   1. Ask the client if he would like someone from pastoral care to come visit him. *Psychosocial needs would not be a priority at this time.*
   2. ⚲ Ask visitors to leave the room when he needs to use the toilet.
   3. ⚲ Integrate the client's elimination habits into the care plan.
   4. ⚲ Encourage the client to increase high-fluid foods such as fruits and drink small amounts of fluids frequently.
   5. ⚲ Put the client's hand in warm water when he voids.

   Rationale: Clients with prostate cancer often have difficulties with urinary elimination. Nursing interventions need to focus on providing privacy and integrating the client's habits into elimination routines to promote more normal voiding patterns. Increasing fluid intake helps increase urine production and flush out solutes that collect in the urinary system. Using sensory stimuli, such as putting the client's hand in warm water during elimination, promotes relaxation and stimulates bladder contractions. A pastoral care consult will not address the client's elimination needs.

   THIN Thinking: Help Quick – *Providing an environment that is supportive of privacy and normal behaviors are most like to remedy the situation to prevent the need for a catheter.* **NCLEX®:** Basic Comfort and Care **QSEN:** Patient-centered Care

4. A client with a medical diagnosis of cirrhosis has been admitted to a medical unit, and the nurse is doing an assessment. What complaint from the client requires immediate follow-up?
   1. 🔵 Bloody expectorant with coughing episodes.
   2. Jeans cannot zip because of enlarged abdomen. *Ascites is commonly seen in cases of cirrhosis from the low protein levels in the blood.*
   3. Swelling in the feet and lower legs. *Edema is a common finding from the low serum protein levels.*
   4. Yellowing of the eyes and mucous membranes. *This is anticipated with the high bilirubin levels in the blood.*

   Rationale: All signs listed may occur with cirrhosis, as well as anorexia, nausea, and vomiting due to the enlarging abdomen. However, bleeding esophageal varices are a result of hepatoportal hypertension. Active bleeding may result in melena and hematemesis, and if not treated hemorrhage and shock.

   THIN Thinking: Help Quick – *The client with cirrhosis has a high-risk for hemorrhage and any bleeding needs to be addressed immediately.* **NCLEX®:** Physiological Adaptation **QSEN:** Patient-centered Care

5. Emergency Medical Services transports a known intravenous drug user to the Emergency Department. The client reports flu-like symptoms for the last week, jaundice, and inability to keep food down. What safety precautions should the nurse utilize?
   1. Droplet precautions only. *Droplet precautions would be implemented for coughing.*
   2. Full gown, gloves, mask with shield. *No indications for this.*
   3. Report the client to the CDC. *Not a reportable disease.*
   4. 🔵 Standard precautions of gloves and handwashing.

   Rationale: If the client is suffering from Hepatitis A, it is a self-limiting infection that can cause mild flu-like symptoms and jaundice up to acute liver failure in more severe cases. Individuals at increased risk for hepatitis A include intravenous drug users, men who have sex with men, persons traveling to foreign countries, institutionalized individuals, children in day care centers, and their family members from improper handling of food, poor hygiene, crowded living conditions, and inadequate sanitation. A vaccine and thorough hand washing are the best measures to prevent transmission and outbreaks.

   THIN Thinking: Help Quick – *Concerns for infection control would include standard precautions unless there is a concern for other illness spread.* **NCLEX®:** Safety and Infection Control **QSEN:** Evidence-based Practice

6. The nurse has completed discharge teaching for a young client being discharged with a new diagnosis of inflammatory bowel disease after treatment for an exacerbation. Which statement by the client indicates further clarification needs to be done?
   1. "I need to decrease my stress by not taking on so much at work." *Decreasing stress can help IBD exacerbation.*
   2. "I need to get plenty of sleep, which is good, because I like to sleep." *Sleep decreases stress and exacerbations.*
   3. "I will need to eat a high calorie, high protein diet." *Correct. This is a recommended choice for IBD because of decreased absorption of nutrients.*
   4. 🔵 "I'm glad I don't have to stay on steroids and antibiotics long-term."

   Rationale: The goals of treatment of Inflammatory Bowel Disease are to: 1) rest the bowel, 2) control the current inflammation, 3) combat infection, 4) correct malnutrition, 5) alleviate stress, 6) provide symptomatic relief, 7) improve quality of life. Because the cause is unknown, treatment relies solely on medications to treat inflammation and maintain remission, e.g. corticosteroids, aminosalicylates, antimicrobials, immunosuppressants and immunomodulators.

   THIN Thinking: Nursing Process – *When teaching, an important intervention is for the nurse to clarify misunderstandings about their disease or condition.* **NCLEX®:** Reduction of Risk Potential **QSEN:** Patient-centered Care

7. A home health nurse is making a visit on an older client with long-standing diverticular disease. The client has been taking dietary fiber supplements, stool softeners, and oral antibiotics, along with increased fluids and a high-fiber diet. What additional assessment should the nurse make?
   1. Ask why the client takes 2 drugs to stimulate the already inflamed bowel. *Common treatment measure. There is no reason to question this further.*
   2. Palpate and percuss the abdomen immediately. *Unnecessary.*
   3. 🔵 Question about any possible side effects of the antibiotics.
   4. Quiz the client about what is considered "high-fiber" in the diet. *No indication client doesn't understand high fiber diet.*

   Rationale: Conservative management of diverticulosis and diverticulitis includes high-fiber diet from mainly fruits and vegetables, dietary fiber supplements, stool softeners, anticholinergics, clear liquid diet (and increased liquids) in exacerbations, increased activity, oral antibiotics, mineral oil, bulk laxatives, and weight reduction if overweight. It is important that the client understand to watch for any abnormalities or side effects related to the medications ordered.

THIN Thinking: Identify Risk to Safety – *Assessing the side effects of medications can prevent additional complications.* **NCLEX®**: Pharmacological and Parenteral Therapies **QSEN**: Patient-centered Care

8. **A client on the surgical unit is preparing to be discharged after a colectomy for an intestinal obstruction. The nurse finds the client passed out on the bathroom floor. Which response by the nurse would be most appropriate?**
   1. Call another nurse to help get the client back to bed. *Assessment needs to be performed first to be sure it's safe to get the client off of the floor.*
   2. Call the client's healthcare provider from the room. *Assessment needs to occur first.*
   3. Check the client's abdominal wound for bleeding. *Not first action- ABC's should come first.*
   4. 🔵 Determine if the client is breathing and has a pulse.

   Rationale: The first order of business would be to see if the client is breathing and has a pulse, then the nurse can proceed. The fainting episode could have been because of rising to quickly off the toilet after having a stool, possible bleeding internally or externally (thus blood on the abdominal dressing), or other causes. The client needs to be put back in bed, a thorough assessment done, and the healthcare provider notified.

   THIN Thinking: Help Quick – *Airway, breathing, circulation first.* **NCLEX®**: Physiological Adaptation **QSEN**: Safety

9. **A client in the clinic returns for a follow-up visit complaining of recurrent irritable bowel syndrome with such symptoms as nausea, bloating, flatulence, abdominal distention, and severe headache. What does the nurse further assess to help determine the next course of action?**
   1. 🔵 Complaints of constipation and straining at stool.
   2. Compliance with a high fiber diet, including green leafy vegetables. *Green leafy vegetables like broccoli are not recommended since they are gas producing.*
   3. Share that they went out to eat Mexican food the evening before. *Spicy food not usually a contributor.*
   4. Stated took an opioid twice in the last 12 hours for the severe headache. *Would be looked at along with complaints of constipation and straining.*

   Rationale: Clients with irritable bowel syndrome (IBS) usually have changes in bowel patterns that quite often include diarrhea or constipation. Other symptoms include bloating, abdominal distention, cramping, excessive flatulence and abdominal pain, some of which are reported by the client. While most people with IBS engage in lifestyle changes to manage their symptoms, there are times when they may experience exacerbations, requiring careful assessment by the nurse to ensure the appropriate plan of care.

THIN Thinking: Nursing Process – *Further assessment of symptoms will allow the nurse to determine a plan of care.* **NCLEX®**: Reduction of Risk Potential **QSEN**: Patient-centered Care

10. **A client in end-stage renal failure has orders for sodium polystyrene sulfonate 15 grams PO in 90 mL. water 3 times daily. What would be the total daily dose of sodium polystyrene sulfonate?**

    Answer: 45 grams in 270 mL.

    Rationale: Multiple strategies are used to manage hyperkalemia in the client in end-stage renal failure, including restriction of high potassium foods and drugs. Acute hyperkalemia may require treatment with IV glucose and insulin or IV 10% calcium gluconate. Sodium polystyrene sulfonate, a cation-exchange resin, is commonly used to lower potassium levels and can be administered on an outpatient basis. 15 grams X 3 = 45 grams.

    THIN Thinking: Identify Risk to Safety – *Medication administration calculations are a safety concern.* **NCLEX®**: Pharmacological and Parenteral Therapies **QSEN**: Patient-centered Care

11. **The clinic nurse is preparing to teach an obese client about a new weight loss program. What would be the most appropriate preface to the teaching plan?**
    1. 🔵 "Even with a loss of 3-5% of your current weight would reduce complications risks."
    2. "My advice is to adhere strictly to this diet plan for the next year." *This comment doesn't inspire or provide hope for client. Short-term goals are more effective.*
    3. "We cannot continue to treat your hypertension if you don't lose some weight." *Inaccurate and threatening to client.*
    4. "You must lose 40 pounds in the next six months or die from a heart attack or stroke." *Inaccurate and threatening to client.*

    Rationale: Despite the known benefits of weight loss, it is a difficult process for most individuals. Achieving an "ideal" BMI isn't necessary and may not be realistic. Modest weight loss of even 3-5% of starting weight can have clinical benefits (e.g. decreased joint pain, lower blood pressure and blood glucose), and greater weight loss produces greater benefits.

    THIN Thinking: Nursing Process – *Determining short-term, manageable goals that best support a successful plan for care.* **NCLEX®**: Reduction of Risk Potential **QSEN**: Evidence-based Practice

12. The clinic nurse is interviewing a new client, who presents with increasing frequency of stools and says the last healthcare provider gave a diagnosis of ulcerative colitis. What statement by the client requires immediate follow-up?
    1. "I'm having more frequent loose stools than I did last week." *Needs to be checked, but not as immediate as elevated temperature and severe pain which could indicate infection and perforation.*
    2. 🞷 "I've developed a high fever and severe abdominal pain since yesterday."
    3. "My last healthcare provider said I have a genetic link for developing this disease." *Doesn't require an immediate follow-up.*
    4. "This is a depressing disease to have." *Needs to be addressed, but not immediately. Physiological needs are first.*

    Rationale: As one of the diseases of inflammatory bowel disease, ulcerative colitis is usually limited to the colon. As an autoimmune disease, some agent or combination of agents triggers an overactive, inappropriate, sustained immune response, e.g. frequent stools or diarrhea, abdominal pain, weight loss, and rectal bleeding. Although a mild fever can occur from the inflammatory response, a high fever and severe abdominal pain could be indicative of an infection or other complication, e.g. perforation of the bowel.

    THIN Thinking: Help Quick – *Identification of signs of perforation need to occur quickly since it can quickly lead to sepsis.* **NCLEX®**: Safety and Infection Control **QSEN**: Patient-centered Care

13. A nursery nurse is administering an ordered bottle feeding for an infant born with a cleft lip and palate. What action should the nurse take first to prevent complications?
    1. 🞷 Assess the infant's ability to suck.
    2. Give only small volumes of feedings. *This infant does not require smaller sized feedings than normal.*
    3. Hold the infant at a 45-60 degree angle. *This would be appropriate, but not first action.*
    4. Warm the formula. *This would not prevent complications.*

    Rationale: A cleft lip or palate results if the lip or palate fails to close. Cleft palate may involve both hard and soft palates or may just involve one. A cleft lip might also be involved with a cleft palate. It is important to do a visual examination of the palate as well as insertion of a finger into the mouth to feel the palate. A good time to inspect the palate is when the infant's mouth is opened during a crying episode. To feel the palate, the nurse places a gloved finger into the infant's mouth. Prevention of aspiration is imperative in these infants.

    THIN Thinking: Top Three – *Sucking and swallow assessment will prevent aspiration and is a priority.* **NCLEX®**: Reduction of Risk Potential **QSEN**: Safety

14. The nurse is implementing teaching with a client with gastroesophageal reflux (GER). Which statement by the client demonstrates a further need for teaching?
    1. "I'll be sleeping on 2-3 pillows." *This would be appropriate and can reduce reflux into the esophagus.*
    2. "I'll take my medication to prevent reflux before my evening meal." *This would be appropriate.*
    3. "Reflux can cause erosion of my stomach lining." *This is accurate.*
    4. 🞷 "We like to eat Mexican food at least once per week."

    Rationale: This client needs to know more about the risk of the Mexican food meal—high-fat and spicy—both contributors to the GER. Sleeping with the head of bed elevated and taking the proton-pump inhibitors as ordered can decrease the episodes. Frequent GER can and does cause erosion of the stomach and esophagus linings, leading to other complications.

    THIN Thinking: Nursing Process – *Evaluation of risk factors can prevent further injury.* **NCLEX®**: Health Promotion and Maintenance **QSEN**: Patient-centered Care

15. The nurse is assessing a client who has been admitted with a diagnosis of peptic ulcer disease (PUD). What assessment findings would be consistent with a psycho-emotional component to possible causes?
    1. Infection with Helicobacter pylori. *H. pylori. Bacterial, not psycho-emotional.*
    2. 🞷 Recent increase in responsibilities at work.
    3. Surgery 6 months ago secondary to a sports injury. *Stressful, but not a current concern psycho-emotional.*
    4. Taking aspirin or non-steroidal anti-inflammatory drugs for chronic headaches. *Not psycho-emotional, but physiological.*

    Rationale: Nursing assessment for the client with PUD should include assessment of coping-stress tolerance because acute or chronic stress is a risk factor, causing increase in production of hydrochloric acid in the stomach and duodenum. With stress, many individuals may increase their smoking or alcohol consumption, also risk factors for PUD.

    THIN Thinking: Nursing Process – *Assessment for risk is important for the nurse to identify in order to determine the best plan for prevention and resolve of the illness.* **NCLEX®**: Psychosocial Integrity **QSEN**: Patient-centered Care

16. **The nurse is caring for a young client who reports being beaten in a street fight, with resultant acute kidney injury. What nursing actions would be appropriate? Select all that apply.**
    1. ⓦ A thorough assessment to determine the extent of the client's injuries.
    2. ⓦ Dietary restrictions of potassium, phosphate, and sodium.
    3. ⓦ Fluid restriction of 600 mL plus previous 24-hour fluid loss.
    4. Hourly serum BUN and creatinine levels. *This frequency is not warranted.*
    5. ⓦ Schedule a renal ultrasound as ordered.

    Rationale: Because acute kidney injury is potentially reversible, the primary goals of treatment are to eliminate the cause, manage the signs and symptoms, and prevent complications while the kidneys heal and recover. If acute kidney injury is already established, forcing fluids and diuretics will not be effective and may be harmful. Hourly blood tests are not warranted. Closely monitor fluid intake during the oliguric phase of the kidney injury.

    THIN Thinking: Top Three – *During acute kidney injury, the nurse should anticipate assessment, with fluid and electrolyte restrictions.* **NCLEX®:** Physiological Adaptation **QSEN:** Patient-centered Care

17. **The nurse has planned care for a client admitted with acute gastritis and diarrhea from non-steroid anti-inflammatory drug overuse due to arthritis. In planning care for this client, in what order would the nurse perform these actions? Rank order the responses.**
    1. Keep NPO initially.
    2. Administer antiemetics as needed.
    3. Monitor for signs/symptoms of dehydration.
    4. Ensure that the client's perineal area is clean.
    5. Explore with client and healthcare provider other therapies for arthritis.

    Rationale: Eliminating the cause and preventing or avoiding potential cause(s) in the future are generally all that is needed to treat acute gastritis. Plan of care is supportive and like that of nausea and vomiting. If vomiting occurs, rest, NPO, antiemetics, and IV fluids are prescribed. Monitor for dehydration, as it can occur rapidly with vomiting. An N/G tube may have to be inserted to monitor for bleeding, lavage the precipitating agent, or keep the stomach empty of noxious stimuli. These must be addressed, followed by hygiene and then teaching and discussion about the plan of care.

    THIN Thinking: Top Three –*Prevention of injury due to vomiting blood is the priority.* **NCLEX®:** Physiological Adaptation **QSEN:** Safety

18. **The nurse in a dialysis unit is monitoring the client with chronic kidney disease (CKD). In what order would the nurse assess signs/symptoms and act to keep the client as comfortable as possible during peritoneal dialysis (PD)? Rank order the responses.**
    1. Spreading hematoma around the peritoneal catheter.
    2. Development of crackles in the bases of both lungs.
    3. Nausea and vomiting.
    4. Headache.
    5. Itching and scratching of the lower extremities.

    Rationale: As kidney function deteriorates, all body systems become affected, with many symptoms in each body system. Individuals on peritoneal dialysis (PD) may have severe complications during initial institution of the treatment. A spreading hematoma at the PD catheter insertion site could denote a severe bleeding/hemorrhage and should be addressed first, with vomiting treated next to prevent dislodgement of the PD catheter or rapid dehydration. Clients with CKD often have signs/symptoms of heart failure, pulmonary edema, itchy/dry skin, and other ailments.

    THIN Thinking: Top Three – *Priorities are based on ABCs.* **NCLEX®:** Physiological Adaptation **QSEN:** Patient-centered Care

19. **A 7-year-old client undergoes a laparotomy in the epigastric region for a small bowel obstruction. Which nursing intervention is indicated to prevent the most concerning complication of this surgery?**
    1. Sterile dressing changes and intravenous antibiotics *Respiratory issues more concerning.*
    2. A high fiber diet with adequate oral and intravenous hydration *Respiratory issues more concerning.*
    3. ⓦ Coughing and using an incentive spirometer every two hours.
    4. Turning every two hours and padding under bony prominences *Respiratory issues more concerning.*

    Rationale: Because of the location of the incision, clients having the surgery are prone to shallow breathes and pneumonia. Using the incentive spirometer and coughing are important preventative strategies. Although skin breakdown, infection, and constipation are known complications, they are not more critical than respiratory complications.

    THIN Thinking: Top Three – *Aggressive pulmonary toileting is important to the prevention of pneumonia. Given the age of the client and the location of the surgery, the risk is greater.* **NCLEX®:** Reduction of Risk Potential **QSEN:** Evidence-based Practice

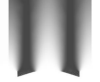

20. The nurse is discussing the plan of care with a client receiving dialysis. The nurse understands what aspect of care is a priority for this client?
    1. Eating fruits and vegetables. *May need to limit due to the vitamins and electrolytes within foods.*
    2. 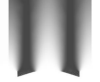 Monitoring fluid intake.
    3. Daily exercise. *Not a priority.*
    4. Monitoring output. *Client may not have urine output.*

    Rationale: Of all the choices, monitoring fluid intake is the most important for the client. The intake of too much fluid can cause a fluid overload for the body since the kidneys are not working as they should and dialysis is only several times per week. Clients who are on dialysis need to monitor the intake of fruits and vegetables that are high in potassium and sodium. Due to the kidney being impaired, there may be a dangerous buildup of potassium or sodium if the intake of fruits and vegetables are not monitored, but fluid intake is more important. Daily exercise is good for the client but this is not a priority action of care at this time. Monitoring the output for a dialysis client is not a priority due to the fact that output is little to none since kidney function is impaired.

    THIN Thinking: Nursing Process – *Understanding the needs of client that is on dialysis is important to planning care.* **NCLEX®:** Physiological Adaptation **QSEN:** Patient-centered Care

21. A client returns from surgery for placement of a colostomy secondary to ulcerative colitis. Two hours after the surgery the nurse is most concerned about which assessment?
    1. Hypoactive bowel sounds in all four quadrants *Expected finding after general surgery.*
    2. Decreased breath sounds in the bases of the lungs *Expected findings in the initial postoperative client due to sedation.*
    3. Slight distension of the bladder *Expected finding.*
    4. A blood pressure below the baseline value.

    Rationale: Although all of these findings cause concern, the lowering of the blood pressure could indicate hypovolemia and shock. Fluids would be needed to ensure perfusion. Decreased breath sounds would require intervention, but are not unexpected two hours post-op. Decreased bowel sounds and distension of the bladder are also not unexpected and would require intervention if they did not resolve in two to four hours post-op.

    THIN Thinking: Identify Risk to Safety – *Low blood pressure could indicate bleeding and a state of low perfusion.* **NCLEX®:** Physiological Adaptation **QSEN:** Evidence-based Practice

22. A 13-year-old client is receiving total parental nutrition as a treatment for Crohn's disease. The client asks the rationale for this treatment. Which statement by the nurse accurately describes the reason for this treatment?
    1. "The nutrition in your intravenous line is more complete than what you can eat." *TPN and enteral feedings can both complete nutrition with adequate absorption.*
    2. 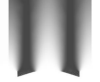 "Total parenteral nutrition allows your intestines to rest and heal for a while."
    3. "This treatment assists you in getting the nutrients you need without the allergies." *No evidence of allergies.*
    4. "With this treatment you do not need to eat by mouth so you can get the rest you need." *Client does not require rest, but bowel does.*

    Rationale: Crohn's disease is characterized by erosion of the intestinal lining, with significant diarrhea, pain, and weight loss. TPN allows for the bowel to rest while it provides complete nutrition to replace losses. It is not about generalized rest needed, but about the gut. TPN actually may stimulate allergies, but Crohn's is not about allergies. Although eating by mouth is preferable, TPN offers a viable option for clients.

    THIN Thinking: Top Three – *Providing nutrition is important to sustain muscle and cell strength.* **NCLEX®:** Pharmacological and Parenteral Therapies **QSEN:** Evidence-based Practice

23. The nurse is planning to make a home visit for a client with hepatitis C. What documentation should the nurse include in the chart concerning client/family teaching?
    1. Family and client should not share eating utensils and dishes. *Hepatitis is blood borne, not oral. Not a risk factor.*
    2. Eating utensils and dishes should be washed in hot water above 180°F. *Oral transfer of virus not a concern. Not a risk factor.*
    3. 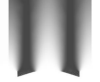 Proper universal precautions should be observed when cleaning up blood from the client.
    4. Family members should not come in contact with the client's medications *Not a risk factor.*

    Rationale: Coming into contact with blood from a person infected with hepatitis C can put all in danger of contracting the disease if they have an open cut or sore. Mixing open areas with infected blood increases the chances of contracting the disease.

    THIN Thinking: Top Three – *The nurse needs to understand the transfer of infection via blood and oral body fluids in order to use proper instructions.* **NCLEX®:** Safety and Infection Control **QSEN:** Safety.

24. The nurse is caring for a toddler who is postoperative day 1 after a revision of pyloric stenosis repair done when the client was an infant. The nurse's 8am assessment included blood pressure of 90/54 and heart rate of 92. At 11am the vitals included blood pressure of 102/64 and heart rate of 118. The mother reports that the child has been irritable for the past hour. What action does the nurse take?
    1. Notify the provider of the change in vital signs. *Unnecessary if there is an action the nurse can take to help client.*
    2. 🔘 Administer oral analgesics as ordered.
    3. Obtain a hemoglobin and hematocrit. *Unnecessary- no reason to believe there is bleeding.*
    4. Provide oxygen via a nasal cannula. *No indication this is needed.*

    Rationale: Restlessness, tachycardia and an increased blood pressure are signs of pain in a toddler. The least invasive route of administering analgesics should be used, especially in toddlers. The child's pain should be documented using an age appropriate pain assessment scale such as FLACC (Face, Legs, Activity, Cry and Consolability).

    THIN Thinking: Nursing Process – *The vital signs and recent surgery support pain and that proper treatment should be provided.* **NCLEX®:** Basic Care and Comfort **QSEN:** Patient-centered Care

25. A nurse is caring for a client with colorectal cancer who is receiving total parental nutrition (TPN). The physician has prescribed the TPN to infuse at 150 mL/hr. The TPN bag holds 2400 mL. How long will it take for the TPN to infuse to the nearest whole hour? Fill in the blank.

    Answer: 16 hours

    Rationale: The TPN is infusing at 150 mL/hour, 2400 mL divided by 150 mL = 16 hours

    THIN Thinking: Identify Risk to Safety – *Safe medication and fluid calculation is important to prevention of injury.* **NCLEX®:** Pharmacological and Parenteral Therapies **QSEN:** Safety

26. A nurse is caring for these four clients. Which would the nurse provide care to first?
    1. 25-year-old who had a splenectomy four hours ago and is reporting pain at the incisional site with movement. *Expected finding.*
    2. 75-year-old who had surgery three days ago for a bowel obstruction and has a fever, chills and purulent drainage from the wound. *Needs to be looked at but not as life-threatening as potential anaphylactic shock.*
    3. 🔘 18-year-old diagnosed with an infection who is receiving an intravenous antibiotic and reports tingling around the mouth and itching to the body.
    4. 68-year-old who had a unit of packed red blood cells an hour ago and reports feeling fatigued and flushed. *Needs to be looked at, but not as life-threatening as potential anaphylactic shock.*

    Rationale: The nurse would immediately stop the infusion. The client's signs and symptoms point to a negative reaction toward the antibiotic potentially leading to airway collapse and anaphylaxis. The client's airway needs to be supported immediately. The nurse would notify the client's healthcare provider. Although pain, a fever with infection, and flushing after a transfusion is important, they are not the highest priority when faced with a potential adverse reaction to a medication.

    THIN Thinking: Identify Risk to Safety – *Identifying the risk for anaphylaxis is the priority. Difficulty speaking can indicate an airway issue.* **NCLEX®:** Physiological Adaptation **QSEN:** Safety

27. The nurse is caring for a client with renal failure. The client is on a special diet and strict intake and output. What nursing assessments would the nurse do for this client? Select all that apply.
    1. 🔘 Daily weights.
    2. Monitor appetite *Not as important as monitoring fluid balance.*
    3. 🔘 Monitor edema in the extremities.
    4. Monitor bowel movements *Not as important as monitoring fluid balance.*
    5. 🔘 Monitor urine volume and characteristics.

    Rationale: Daily weights should be done to assess for retained fluid. 1 kg of body weight is equivalent to 1 liter of fluid. Edema in the extremities could be indicative of fluid retention which may be indicative of renal failure. Assessing urine output and characteristics of urine would be a correct assessment as urine output would certainly provide information regarding kidney function and/or renal failure. The color, odor and consistency of the urine would be an important assessment for the nurse to make in client care. Although monitoring nutrition and monitoring bowel movements are important to assess, they are not critical in the assessment of renal function.

    THIN Thinking: Nursing Process – *For this client, monitoring fluid status is a priority.* **NCLEX®:** Reduction of Risk Potential **QSEN:** Patient-centered Care

28. A client is admitted with ascites from liver failure. Spironolactone 100 mg is administered. Which sign or symptom would designate a serious complication for the client?
   1. Blurry vision *Incorrect, not related to medication.*
   2. Low potassium *Incorrect, spironolactone is potassium sparing.*
   3. ⑨ Increased thirst.
   4. Leg pain – *Incorrect, not related to medication.*

   Rationale: Increased thirst is a potentially serious side effect since the signaling of thirst means the body is moderately dehydrated. This symptom may signal the drug is forcing out too much fluid from the body and drug dose modifications may be needed. Blurry vision is not usually associated with this medication, the medication is a potassium sparing diuretic and will not bring down potassium levels and leg pain is not a sign or symptom of this drug. Usually with low potassium, leg cramps could happen but since this drug is potassium sparing, the leg cramps should not be seen.

   THIN Thinking: Identify Risk to Safety – *The nurse must be aware of all complications of medications to properly evaluate the care.* **NCLEX®**: Reduction of Risk Potential **QSEN**: Safety

29. A client diagnosed with morbid obesity is at high risk for impaired skin integrity. When the nurse is developing a plan of care for this client which nursing action is a priority?
   1. Keep the skin clean and dry *Important, but priority is skin inspection (assessment first).*
   2. Educate the client about sun exposure *Not a priority for impaired skin integrity.*
   3. Suggest wearing loose clothing *Not a priority for impaired skin integrity.*
   4. ⑨ Inspect skin daily.

   Rationale: Inspection of the skin daily is the priority action because with obesity, new breakdown can occur rapidly. Skin should be inspected daily to monitor healing of existing breakdown and identify new breakdown, so treatment can occur in a timely manner. It is important to keep the skin clean and dry as this helps to prevent breakdown but for this client, it is not the priority nursing action. Monitoring sun exposure is important for any client as no one should be exposed to the sun for prolonged periods, but it is not the priority action for this client. Loose clothing prevents chafing for the client who is obese, and this will certainly help with protecting the skin; however, it is not the priority action for this client.

   THIN Thinking: Nursing Process – *Assessment before intervention.* **NCLEX®**: Basic Comfort and Care **QSEN**: Patient-centered Care

30. A client has chronic diarrhea, bloating, and abdominal pain. The healthcare provider is ruling out celiac disease. The client asks the nurse about dietary guidelines. What would be the best answer from the nurse?
   1. "You will need to eat foods that bind the bowels like bananas, rice, toast, and applesauce." *Inaccurate. These foods (BRAT diet) are for diarrhea.*
   2. "You should eat a low fiber diet that limits fibers including stems, seeds, and skins." *Inaccurate. This would be a recommendation for someone with diverticular disease.*
   3. ⑨ "Foods that you cannot eat include wheat proteins or gluten-based starches or fillers."
   4. "You will need to discuss your dietary needs with a nutritionist to develop a meal plan." *The nurse is able to answer client's question.*

   Rationale: Celiac disease leads to an inability to metabolize and absorb gluten which is a protein from wheat, barley, and rye products. It is found in many sauces, prepared, and processed foods, in addition to breads, pasta, baked goods, and whet products. Low fiber diet is indicated for diverticulitis or diverticulosis. The BRAT diet is indicated for diarrhea, this diarrhea and symptoms are not responsive to this diet. The nurse is capable of beginning teaching with the client and providing brief instruction. A more comprehensive referral to a nutritionist may be indicated, but the nurse can begin the teaching.

   THIN Thinking: Nursing Process – *Understanding proper diets can help the nurse provide high-quality client care.* **NCLEX®**: Health Promotion and Maintenance **QSEN**: Evidence-based Practice

Hormonal

Neuroendocrine / Glucose Regulation

This chapter addresses conditions that impact the body's hormonal processes. The neuroendocrine system is an intricate design of interwoven processes that involve the nervous and endocrine systems. The nervous and endocrine systems often function perfectly in a process called neuroendocrine integration to ensure that the body's physiological processes regulate effectively. The interaction between the endocrine system and the nervous system is made possible because of the hypothalamus and the significant role it plays in controlling endocrine glands such as the pituitary gland.

The functions regulated by the various glands in the body manage life and so when there is impairment in any aspect of neuroendocrine function, the threat to life is significant. Therefore, nurses must understand the pathophysiological processes that affect the effective functioning of each gland in the system but more importantly, they must be knowledgeable and prepared to provide quality care to clients who present to their facilities with neuroendocrine disorders.

Priority Exemplars:

> Diabetic ketoacidosis
> Diabetes mellitus–type 2
> Diabetes mellitus–type 1
> Gestational diabetes
> Hyperglycemic hyperosmolar syndrome
> Hyperparathyroidism
> Hypoparathyroidism
> Hyperthyroidism
> Hypothyroidism
> Addison's disease
> Cushing's syndrome
> Syndrome of inappropriate antidiuretic hormone (SIADH)
> Diabetes insipidus
> Wilms tumor
> Metabolic syndrome

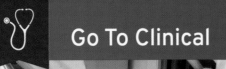

Go To Clinical

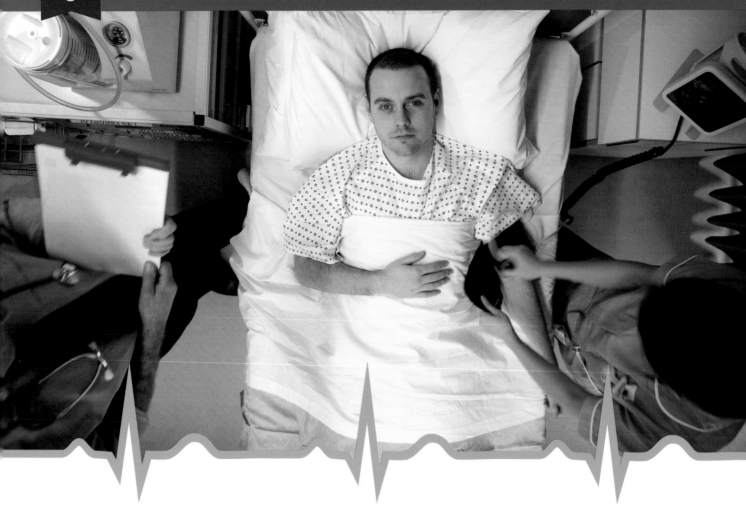

Go To Clinical Case 1

A 36-year-old man presents to the emergency department with complaints of abdominal pain, nausea, vomiting and fatigue. He reports urinating frequently over the past two days and has been drinking a lot of water because of excessive thirst.

Health history reveals hypertension and high cholesterol. Vital signs are as follows: Blood pressure 102/66, heart rate 132, temperature 99.8°F and respirations 32. As he speaks with the nurse, his breath has a strong smell of acetone and he is observed to be somewhat lethargic.

Lab are drawn, and results reveal the following: Blood glucose 360 mg/dL, pH 7.20, bicarbonate 10 mEq/l, pCO_2 18 mmHg, potassium 4.8 mEq/L and sodium 142 mEq/L. Urinalysis shows 4+ ketones and 5+ glucose. The client is admitted to your unit for care.

NurseThink® Time

Using the NurseThink® system, complete the priorities. Check your answers designated by 💡 in the Diabetic ketoacidosis Priority Exemplar.

Clinical Hint

Remember hyperglycemia is the "dry one" characterized by dehydration. Hypoglycemia is the "wet one" often manifested by diaphoresis.

NurseThink® Time

✎ Priority Assessments or Cues

1.

2.

3.

⚗ Priority Laboratory Tests/Diagnostics

1.

2.

3.

⚠ Priority Interventions or Actions

1.

2.

3.

⚑ Priority Potential & Actual Complications

1.

2.

3.

⚕ Priority Nursing Implications

1.

2.

3.

◉ Priority Medications

1.

2.

3.

● Priority Education/Discharge Issues

1.

2.

3.

Diabetic ketoacidosis

Pathophysiology/Description

> Diabetic ketoacidosis (DKA) results when cells of the body cannot get the insulin they need for energy because there is profound insulin deficiency

> Usually occurs when the pancreas is unable to adjust to the extra need for insulin brought on by conditions such as significant stress or severe illness

> The condition occurs most often in individuals with type 1 diabetes, but can also occur with type 2 diabetes, even though rare

> Contributing factors to DKA
  - Type 1 diabetes not diagnosed
  - Illness
  - Infection
  - Poor management of diabetes
  - Dosage of insulin inadequate
  - Insulin pump malfunction

> How diabetic ketoacidosis occurs
  - Glucose gets to a very high level because there is no insulin to break it down to usable energy
  - The body needs energy, so it breaks down fats to use as fuel
  - When fats breakdown, ketone acids are produced
  - If the process is sustained, then ketones accumulate in the blood causing major problems on systems of the body

> Diabetic ketoacidosis progresses rapidly and is life-threatening if the individual does not get treatment readily. Fluid imbalance is a major factor in this disease

Priority Assessments or Cues

- Assess for patent airway and determine oxygen level. Assess level of consciousness and cardiac status. Confusion and cardiac dysrhythmias can occur with DKA

- Assess glucose levels. Expect blood glucose levels of 250 mg/dL or higher

- Assess urine output and signs and symptoms of dehydration. Assess for fluid overload as fluid resuscitation is initiated. Assess ongoing results of electrolyte levels to determine effect of therapy

> Complete a history to include time of last food intake and insulin administration as well as overall self-management of diabetes

> Assess all body systems as DKA impacts functions in all systems

> Assess vital signs frequently to identify problems such as Kussmaul respirations, hypovolemic shock and fever

Priority Laboratory Tests/Diagnostics

- Blood glucose level, expected greater than 250 mg/dL

- Urinalysis positive for ketones

- Blood pH shows acidity. With excess ketone acids, expect the pH of blood to be below 7.30

> Electrolytes levels expected to be low because of the changing pH, acidosis and dehydration
  - Hyponatremia, hypokalemia, hypomagnesemia, hypocalcemia, hypophosphatemia

> Bicarbonate (HCO_3) expected to be low, less than 15 mEq/L

> Blood urea nitrogen (BUN) level expected to be high, greater than 20 mg/dL due to dehydration

> Creatinine expected to be high, greater than 1.5 mg/dL due to dehydration

> Urinalysis positive for ketones

Priority Interventions or Actions

- Ensure airway is patent and start oxygen therapy. Establish a functional intravenous access

- Initiate IV fluid with 0.9% NaCL at 1 L per hour. The goal is to stabilize the blood pressure and achieve a urine output that is 30 – 60 mL/hr. Add 5% to 10% dextrose to the fluid therapy when blood glucose reaches 250 mg/dL or lower. This prevents a quick drop in the blood glucose level

- Start an insulin drip with regular insulin at 0.1 U/kg/hr. Monitor fluid balance and potassium levels as insulin causes potassium to enter the cells. This creates a depletion of potassium in the extracellular fluid

> If acidosis is severe, with pH less than 7.0, administer sodium bicarbonate. This works as a buffer to increase the pH

> Administer potassium to correct issue of hypokalemia

Priority Potential & Actual Complications

- Cerebral edema from rapid lowering of the glucose, rapid administering IV fluids or administering the wrong IV fluid
- Coma
- May be fatal

Priority Nursing Implications

- Administration of insulin causes potassium to decrease. This occurs because insulin moves potassium into the cells, causing detrimental hypokalemia levels. It is important to start potassium replacement early during treatment

It is important to involve willing family members in the education regarding diabetes management of their loved one, as all persons living in the home with the individual will be impacted in some way by the individual's diagnosis of diabetes

⬤ Priority Medications

regular insulin

- Administered via continuous intravenous route

- Watch for hypoglycemia

sodium bicarbonate

- Reverses metabolic acidosis. Dosage dependent on the client's weight, age, health condition and lab data

- Mild acidosis, usual dose is 1 to 2 mEq per kg of body weight

- Severe acidosis, usual dose is 2 to 5 mEq per kg of body weight that may be administered over a 4 to 8-hour period. Can be administered more rapidly in an emergency

potassium

- Replaces potassium loss

- Administered intravenously

- Suggested dosage is 30 -60 mEq every 24 hours. However, the dosage can be adjusted based on the client's needs

Priority Education/Discharge Issues

> Insulin therapy
  - Storage and expiration date
  - Preparation
  - Administration and site rotation
> Measure blood glucose regularly
> Adhere to exercise and meal plan
> Teach about signs and symptoms of hypo and hyperglycemia
> Managing insulin when sick
> Meal consumption in relationship to insulin administration
> Wear diabetes identification

Go To Clinical Answers

Text designated by 💡 are the top answers for the Go To Clinical related to Diabetic ketoacidosis.

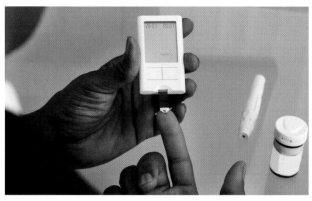

Image 12-1: When patients manage their own diabetic regimen, they often have to ensure they are using appropriate technique to assess their blood glucose levels. List 3 statements by a client that would indicate further need for teaching related to self-monitoring of blood glucose levels.

_____

_____

_____

_____

_____

_____

Next Gen Clinical Judgment

Compare and Contrast

1. How are diabetic ketoacidosis and hyperglycemic hyperosmolar syndrome the same? How is the nursing care the same?

2. How are diabetic ketoacidosis and hyperglycemic hyperosmolar syndrome different? How is the nursing care different?

_____

_____

_____

_____

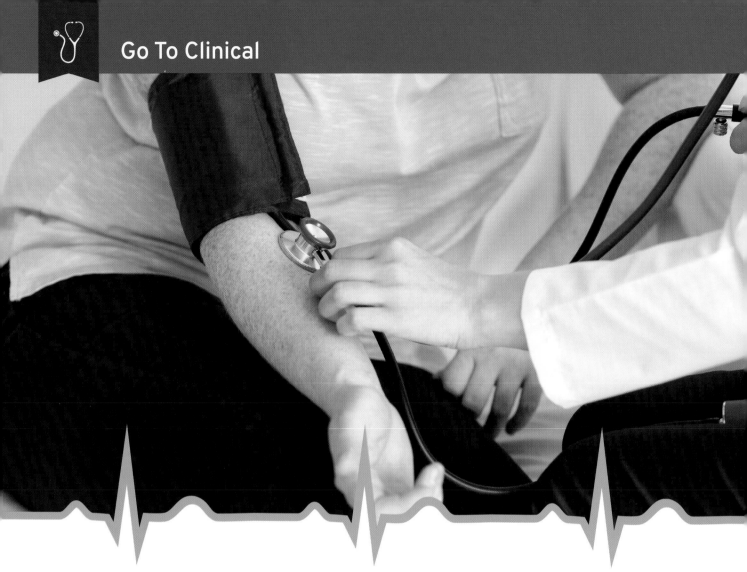

Go To Clinical Case 2

W. T. is a 60-year-old woman with type 2 diabetes, who has had the disease for many years. Her health history is also significant for hypertension, high cholesterol and obesity. She presents to the emergency department complaining of repeated vaginal infections and states that she is starting to experience "decreased sensation" in her feet.

Vital signs are as follows: Temperature 98.2°F, blood pressure 136/90, heart rate 102, respirations 22. Assessment reveals a 2 cm by 3 cm stage 2 wound to the sole of her left foot that she denies knowing that she has. Pedal pulses are not palpable.

W.T. states that she has been taking metformin and glyburide to control her blood glucose but that with the loss of her job and health insurance recently, she has not been able to buy the pills readily, so she cuts her pills in half to make them last.

Lab findings reveal the following: Blood glucose of 210 mg/dL, hemoglobin A1c (HgbA1c)12, and +4 ketones. You are the nurse caring for W.T. today

NurseThink® Time

Using the NurseThink® system, complete the priorities. Check your answers designated by 💡 in the Diabetes type 2 Priority Exemplar.

✏ Priority Assessments or Cues

1.

2.

3.

⚗ Priority Laboratory Tests/Diagnostics

1.

2.

3.

⚠ Priority Interventions or Actions

1.

2.

3.

⚑ Priority Potential & Actual Complications

1.

2.

3.

⚕ Priority Nursing Implications

1.

2.

3.

◌ Priority Medications

1.

2.

3.

◌ Priority Education/Discharge Issues

1.

2.

3.

Diabetes mellitus – type 2

Pathophysiology/Description

> Diabetes is a multisystem disease of glucose metabolism that is marked by hyperglycemia

> It relates to impaired usage of insulin, abnormal production of insulin or both occurring at the same time

> Two most common types of diabetes mellitus are types 1 and 2. Type 2 diabetes is the most prevalent

> Type 2 is marked by insulin resistance, inadequate insulin secretion or a combination of both

  • Insulin resistance: Body tissues do not respond to insulin's action due to unresponsive or insufficient numbers of insulin receptors

  • Inadequate insulin secretion: Cells of the pancreas become fatigued and so insulin production is decreased

> Risk factors

  • Family history. More likely to get the condition if there are first degree relatives with it

  • Obesity or overweight. Fat cells are resistant to insulin

  • Certain ethnicities. It is more prevalent in Asian Americans, African Americans, Hispanics, Pacific Islanders and Native Americans

  • Being older than 40 years of age

> Type 2 diabetes has a gradual onset. Many persons do not know they have the condition until it is detected on routine lab testing

> Diabetes is a life-altering condition

Priority Assessments or Cues

• Ask about symptoms such as polydipsia, polyuria, polyphagia, fatigue, recurrent infections, visual changes and poor wound healing. Determine blood glucose level

• Ask about management of the condition such as meal planning and medication administration

> Measure vital signs

• Perform skin assessment, focusing on feet. Diabetes causes neuropathy and individuals with the disease can have wounds on their soles without knowing it. Untreated wounds can lead to amputations

> Perform neurological assessment, focus on the eyes. Blindness is a major complication of diabetes

> Review labs, including kidney function tests. Nephropathy is a major complication of diabetes

> Determine social support

> Assess client's understanding of disease management

Priority Laboratory Tests/Diagnostics

• Diagnosis made with one of the following

  • Fasting blood glucose 126 mg/dL or higher

  • A1C of 6.5% or higher

  • Using a glucose load of 75 g during an oral glucose tolerance test, a two-hour plasma level that is equal to or greater than 200 mg/dL

  • Random blood glucose greater than or equal to 200 mg/dL in a client who has the classic symptoms of hyperglycemia or is in a hyperglycemic crisis

  • The first 3 items above must be repeated to confirm the diagnosis. However, the fourth does not need to be repeated

Priority Interventions or Actions

• Administer medications and monitor blood glucose for effectiveness of dosage

• Monitor meal intake

• Schedule meeting with dietician to talk with client about nutrition planning

> Schedule meeting with diabetic educator to ensure client's knowledge needs are met

Priority Potential & Actual Complications

• Nephropathy, leading to kidney failure, neuropathy, leading to sores and amputations and retinopathy, leading to blindness

• Hyperglycemic hyperosmolar syndrome, hypoglycemia

• Conditions related to the heart, brain and blood vessels

> Gastroparesis

> Fungal infections

Priority Nursing Implications

• Understand that most people with diabetes, even if the condition is controlled without medications, will require medicines at some point because of the progressive nature of the condition

• Persons with type 2 diabetes who take oral medications can require insulin in times of stress, as in acute illness

• Metformin must be stopped for surgery or if having a procedure that uses a contrast medium. Resume 48 hours post procedure but get creatinine level first. Not stopping the drug will increase the risk of metformin-induced lactic acidosis

> The thiazolidinediones can only be had through a restricted access program because of their serious cardiac adverse effects

> exenatide causes acute pancreatitis and kidney problems and liraglutide should not be used in clients with family or personal history of medullary thyroid cancer

◆ Priority Medications

💡 biguanides

- metformin, the most effective first line treatment for type 2 diabetes

- Decrease production of glucose in liver and enhances transport of glucose into cells

- Must not be used if kidney or liver disease, or heart failure. Major side effect is lactic acidosis

💡 sulfonylureas

- glipizide, glyburide, glimepiride

- Increase production of insulin by the pancreas

- Major side effect is hypoglycemia

💡 thiazolidinediones

- Pioglitazone, rosiglitazone

- Increase uptake of glucose in muscle and decrease endogenous production of glucose

- Major side effect is adverse cardiovascular events

> a-Glucosidase inhibitors

- acarbose, miglitol

- Cause absorption of starches from the gastrointestinal tract to be delayed

- Must be taken with the first bite of food, most effective in lowering postprandial blood glucose

> dipeptidyl peptidase-4

- linagliptin, saxagliptin, sitagliptin, alogliptin

- Increase the activity of incretin. Stimulate insulin release from pancreatic B-cells and decrease the liver's production of glucose

- Does not cause weight gain as the other classes of drugs do

> sodium-Glucose Co-Transporter 2

- canagliflozin, dapagliflozin

- Decrease reabsorption of glucose in the kidneys and increase its excretion through urine

- Causes urinary tract and genital infections

> glucagon-like Peptide-1 Receptor Agonists

- exenatide, exenatide extended-release, dulaglutide, albiglutide, lixisenatide, liraglutide

- Decrease secretion of glucagon, stimulate release of insulin and slow gastric emptying, thus causing a feeling of fullness and satiety

> Combination oral therapy

- Combination of two different classes of medications into one pill

- Advantageous, as only 1 pill is taken instead of two different pills, thus increasing medication compliance

👤 Priority Education/Discharge Issues

💡 Measure blood glucose regularly

> Adhere to exercise and meal plan

💡 Teach about signs and symptoms of hypo and hyperglycemia

💡 Teach proper administration as well as adverse effects of medications. Ensure understanding of adherence to exercise and meal planning

> Meal consumption in relationship to insulin administration

> Wear diabetes identification

> Educate on the importance of having A1C measured regularly to determine effectiveness of treatment protocol

> Teach proper foot care

> Teach the importance of getting eye exams

> Teach importance of getting annual physicals, ensuring kidney function is assessed

Go To Clinical Answers

Text designated by 💡 are the top answers for the Go To Clinical related to Diabetes type 2.

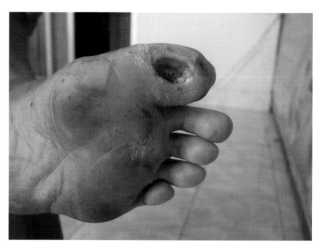

Image 12-2: What are the top 3 instructions for the client with this diabetic foot ulcer?

Diabetes mellitus – type 1

📋 Pathophysiology/Description

> Diabetes is a multisystem disease of glucose metabolism that is marked by hyperglycemia

> Two most common types of diabetes mellitus are types 1 and 2. Type 1 is less prevalent than type 2 and usually affects younger individuals

> Type 1 is an autoimmune disorder where antibodies are developed against the pancreas B-cells or against insulin.

> Has a genetic link

> Has a sudden onset once the pancreas can no longer produce insulin. Some individuals are diagnosed initially when they are in diabetic ketoacidosis

> Classic symptoms, known as the 3 Ps
> • Polyuria (frequent voiding), because of the osmotic effect of glucose
> • Polydipsia (excessive thirst), because of the osmotic effect of glucose
> • Polyphagia (excessive hunger), because of lack of glucose usage for energy

> Exogenous insulin is required for life

> Diabetes is a life-altering condition

✏️ Priority Assessments or Cues

> Ask about symptoms such as polydipsia, polyuria, polyphagia, fatigue, weight loss. Determine blood glucose level

> Ask about management of the condition such as meal planning and medication administration

> Assess knowledge of insulin preparation and administration

> Assess ability to manage diabetes at home

> Measure vital signs

> Perform skin assessment, focusing on feet
> • Diabetes causes neuropathy and individuals with the disease can have wounds on their soles without knowing it
> • Untreated wounds can lead to amputations

> Perform neurological assessment, focus on the eyes. Blindness is a major complication of diabetes

> Review labs, including kidney function tests. Nephropathy is a major complication of diabetes

> Determine social support

> Assess client's understanding of disease management and physical ability to prepare and administer insulin injections

🧪 Priority Laboratory Tests/Diagnostics

> Diagnosis made with one of the following
> • Fasting blood glucose 126 mg/dL or higher
> • A1C of 6.5% or higher
> • Using a glucose load of 75 g during an oral glucose tolerance test, a two-hour plasma level that is equal to or greater than 200 mg/dL

• Random blood glucose greater than or equal to 200 mg/dL in a client who has the classic symptoms of hyperglycemia or is in a hyperglycemic crisis

• The first 3 items above must be repeated to confirm the diagnosis. However, the fourth does not need to be repeated

⚠️ Priority Interventions or Actions

> Administer insulin and monitor blood glucose for effectiveness of dosage

> Monitor meal intake

> Schedule meeting with dietician to talk with client about nutrition planning

> Schedule meeting with diabetic educator to ensure client's knowledge needs are met

> Have newly diagnosed client teach back on blood glucose checks and insulin preparation and injection

🚩 Priority Potential & Actual Complications

> Nephropathy, leading to kidney failure. Neuropathy, leading to sores and amputations. Retinopathy, leading to blindness

> Hypoglycemia

> Somogyi Effect, caused by high dose of insulin that causes some counter regulatory hormones to be released, which then causes rebound hyperglycemia in the morning

> Dawn phenomenon occurs similar to the Somogyi effect but the treatment for both is different

> Diabetic ketoacidosis, hypoglycemia

> Atrophy or hypertrophy of tissue at injection site

> Conditions related to the heart, brain and blood vessels

> Gastroparesis

🩺 Priority Nursing Implications

> Timing of a meal is crucial based on the type of insulin being administered

> It is important to involve willing family members in the education regarding diabetes management of their loved one, as all persons living in the home with the individual will be impacted in some way by the individual's diagnosis of diabetes

> Knowing that with type 1 diabetes the individual will need to take exogenous insulin to sustain life

> Premix insulin formulas are better for individuals who lack the ability to prepare insulin for themselves. These might be individuals with cognitive, physical or visual impairments

> Insulin pumps must be used only if the individual is capable to manage the pump

Priority Medications

> Rapid-acting insulin
> - lispro, aspart, glulisine
> - Onset 10-30 minutes, peak 30 minutes - 3 hours, duration 3-5 hours
> - Administered via subcutaneous route but can be given intravenous in a monitored setting

> Short-acting insulin
> - regular
> - Onset 30 minutes- 1 hour, peak 2-5 hours, duration 5-8 hours
> - Administered via subcutaneous route

> Intermediate-acting insulin
> - NPH
> - Onset 1.5-4 hours, peak 4-12 hours, duration 12-18 hours
> - Administered via subcutaneous route

> Long-acting insulin
> - glargine, detemir, degludec
> - Onset 0.8-4 hours, peak no identified/pronounced peak, duration 16-24 hours
> - Administered via subcutaneous route

> Inhaled insulin
> - afrezza
> - Onset 12-15 minutes, peak 60 minutes, duration 2.5-3 hours

> Combination therapy
> - Several combinations of premixed insulins (2 insulins combined)

> More concentrated insulin
> - humulin R U-500, toujeo U-300

Priority Education/Discharge Issues

> Measure blood glucose regularly
> Insulin
> - Storage
> - Care of insulin container
> - Preparation and administration
> - Appropriate injection sites and injection site rotation
> - Side effects
> Client teach back on insulin administration and blood glucose checks
> Teach about signs and symptoms of hypo and hyperglycemia
> Teach proper administration as well as adverse effects of medications
> Meal consumption in relationship to insulin administration

> Educate on the complications of insulin therapy
> Wear diabetes identification
> Educate on the importance of having A1C measured regularly to determine effectiveness of treatment protocol
> Teach proper foot care
> Teach the importance of getting eye exams
> Teach importance of getting annual physicals, ensuring kidney function is assessed
> Teach about options for insulin administration, like insulin pen and insulin pump

TYPES OF INSULIN

	Types/Brand	Onset/Peak/Duration
Rapid-acting	Aspart-Novolog	
	Lispro-Humalog	> Onset: 10 - 30m
	Glulisine-Apidra	> Peak: 30m - 3hr > Duration: 3 - 5hr
	Inhaled insulin-Afrezza	
Short-acting	Regular-Humulin R	> Onset: 30 - 60m > Peak: 2 - 5hr
	Regular-Novolin R	> Duration: 6 - 8hr
Intermediate-acting	NPH-Humulin N	> Onset: 2 - 4hr > Peak: 5 - 12hr
	NPH-Novolin N	> Duration: 10 - 18hr
Long-acting	Detemir-Levemir	> Onset: 1 - 2hr > Peak: None
	Gargine-Lantus	> Duration: 20 - 24hr
Intermediate + Rapid	Novolog Mix 70/30	> Onset: 10 - 30m > Peak: 1 - 6hr
	Humalog Mix 70/25	> Duration: 18 - 20hr
Intermediate + Short	NPH+ Regular 70/30	> Onset: 30m > Peak: 2 - 12hr > Duration: 10 - 16hr

Table 12-1

Gestational diabetes

Pathophysiology/Description

> Diabetes that develops during pregnancy

> Usually resolves after pregnancy

> In pregnancy, the placenta makes hormones that make it more difficult for insulin to work

> Women at high-risk
- Family history of diabetes
- Pregnancy at advanced maternal age
- Obesity
- Given birth to a large baby previously

> Impact of gestational diabetes
- Birth injury to the infant
- Perinatal death of the infant
- Mother giving birth via cesarean section

> Women with high-risk for the condition are screened on their first prenatal visit

> Women with moderate risk are screened at 24-28 weeks using the oral glucose tolerance test (OGTT)

> Gestational diabetes is mostly controlled with diet, but some women may require insulin

Priority Assessments or Cues

> Assess status of baby in utero; assess for macrosomia

> Ask about symptoms such as polydipsia, polyuria, polyphagia. Determine blood glucose level

> Ask about diet and exercise habits

> Assess knowledge of insulin preparation and administration

> Assess ability to manage diabetes at home

> Measure vital signs

> Assess client's understanding of disease management and physical ability to prepare and administer insulin injections

Priority Laboratory Tests/Diagnostics

> Glucose challenge test is performed. One hour after drinking a glucose solution, blood sample is taken to measure glucose level. If result is greater than 140 mg/dL, a second test called an oral glucose tolerance test (OGTT) is done. The OGTT is a fasting test

> Follow-up oral glucose tolerance test (OGTT) is performed. Blood glucose is tested every hour for three hours. The diagnosis of gestational diabetes is made if two of the three blood glucose levels are higher than normal

Priority Interventions or Actions

> Monitor blood glucose with expectation of the following results
- Before a meal (preprandial) should be 95 mg/dL or less
- 1-hour after a meal (postprandial) should be 140 mg/dL or less
- 2-hours after a meal (postprandial) should be 120 mg/dL or less

> Administer insulin and monitor for adverse effects

> Monitor meal intake

> Schedule meeting with dietician to talk with client about nutrition planning and ensure client's knowledge needs are met

Priority Potential & Actual Complications

> Complications in the infant
- Birth defects
- Very high birth weight
- Hypoglycemia

> Complications in the mother
- Having cesarean section
- Development of type 2 diabetes in future years

> Hypoglycemia, if on insulin

> Atrophy or hypertrophy of tissue at injection site

Priority Nursing Implications

> There is a 63% likelihood of developing type 2 diabetes within 16 years for women with a history of gestational diabetes

> It is important to involve the woman's partner or other willing family members in the education regarding diabetes management of their loved one, as all persons living in the home with the individual will be impacted in some way by the individual's diagnosis of gestational diabetes

Priority Medications

> Rapid-acting insulin
- lispro, aspart
- Onset 10-30 minutes, peak 30 minutes - 3 hours, duration 3-5 hours
- Administered via subcutaneous route but can be given intravenous in a monitored setting

> Short-acting insulin
- regular
- Onset 30 minutes- 1 hour, peak 2-5 hours, duration 5-8 hours
- Administered via subcutaneous route

- › Intermediate-acting insulin
  - NPH
  - Onset 1.5-4 hours, peak 4-12 hours, duration 12-18 hours
  - Administered via subcutaneous route
- › Combination therapy
  - Several combinations of premixed insulins (2 insulins combined)

Priority Education/Discharge Issues

- › Measure blood glucose regularly
- › Adhere to prescribed diet
- › If controlled with insulin
  - Storage
  - Care of insulin container
  - Preparation and administration
  - Appropriate injection sites and injection site rotation
  - Side effects
- › Client teach back on insulin administration and blood glucose checks
- › Teach about signs and symptoms of hypo and hyperglycemia
- › Meal consumption in relationship to insulin administration
- › Educate on the complications of insulin therapy
- › Remind client that gestational diabetes usually goes away after the baby is born
- › Teach about the likelihood of developing type 2 diabetes in the future
- › Teach impact of gestational diabetes on the baby

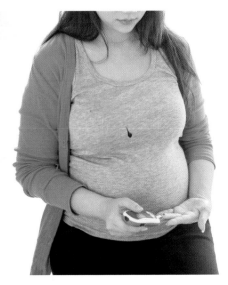

Image 12-3: Gestational diabetes is difficult to manage for many reasons. What are the 3 priority concerns for a baby born to a mom suffering from gestational diabetes?

Hyperglycemic hyperosmolar syndrome

Pathophysiology/Description

> The syndrome of hyperglycemic hyperosmolar syndrome (HHS) results when clients with diabetes whose pancreas still make some insulin, have severely high blood glucose levels

> Enough insulin is produced to prevent the breakdown of fats for energy that would result in DKA, but insulin is not produced in enough quantity to prevent hyperglycemia

> Contributing factors to HHS
  - Sepsis
  - Urinary tract infection
  - Type 2 diabetes that is newly diagnosed or poorly controlled
  - Pneumonia
  - Just about any acute illness
  - Impaired sensation of thirst
  - Not being able to replace fluids

> Results of severely high glucose levels in HHS
  - Increase in serum osmolality
  - Lethargy
  - Sleepiness
  - Seizures
  - Aphasia
  - Hemiparesis
  - Coma

> Hyperglycemic hyperosmolar syndrome is potentially fatal if the individual does not get treatment readily

Priority Assessments or Cues

> Assess for patent airway and determine oxygen level

> Determine glucose level and dehydration. Profound dehydration is classic of HHS

> Assess neurological status. Neurological deficits are prominent in HHS

> Complete a health history to include diet, medications and overall self-management of diabetes

> Measure vital signs (tachycardia and hypotension seen due to dehydration and fluid depletion)

> Determine efficacy of therapy by performing ongoing assessment of the following
  - Lab values (show electrolytes and dehydration status)
  - Cardiac and respiratory systems
  - Renal system (shows intake and output issues)
  - Integumentary system (shows skin turgor status)
  - Neurologic system (shows changes in neurologic symptoms)

Priority Laboratory Tests/Diagnostics

> Blood glucose level expected to be greater than 600 mg/dL

> Serum osmolality expected to be 350 mOsm/kg or greater

> Serum pH expected to be less than 7.30

> Bicarbonate expected to be greater than 20 mEq/L

> Sodium expected to be normal to low

> Potassium expected to be normal to low

> Creatinine expected to be elevated, greater than 1.5 mg/dL, due to dehydration

> Blood urea nitrogen (BUN) expected to be elevated, greater than 20 mg/dL, due to dehydration

Priority Interventions or Actions

> Ensure airway is patent and start oxygen therapy. Establish a large bore intravenous access

> Initiate IV fluid with 0.9% or 0.45% NaCL
  - Large volumes of fluid are required but must be administered slowly due to age of clients (usually older), and likelihood that they have co-morbidities and increased risk of cardiac events from fluid overload
  - Add 5% to 10% dextrose to the fluid therapy when blood glucose reaches 250 mg/dL or lower
  - This prevents a quick drop in the blood glucose level

> Start insulin drip with low dose regular insulin at 0.05 U/kg/hour if HHS is not corrected with fluid therapy alone

> Monitor electrolyte levels and correct as needed

> Monitor intake and output carefully. Have client drink fluids when safe to do so

> Once the immediacy of the client's status is managed, the underlying cause must be treated

Priority Medications

> Regular insulin
  - Administered via continuous intravenous route
  - Starting dose is 0.05U/kg/hour
  - Monitor for decrease in blood glucose level

> Electrolyte replacement only if indicated

Priority Potential & Actual Complications

> Shock

> Seizures

> Stroke

> Coma

> May be fatal

Priority Nursing Implications

> The outstanding difference between DKA and HHS is that with HHS, the individual has some insulin production to prevent the breakdown of fats, so ketoacidosis does not become a factor

> Blood glucose can progress to very high levels before the issue is recognized. This is because fewer symptoms are seen in the early stages of the condition

> Symptoms of HHS are similar to those seen in a stroke. Therefore, it is imperative to determine the glucose level so a diagnosis can be made, affording correct treatment

> With HHS, the role of insulin is less important because ketoacidosis does not occur. Rehydration may be all that is needed to correct the problem

> Understand that HHS is a medical emergency that must be treated immediately. It has a high mortality rate

Priority Education/Discharge Issues

> Insulin therapy
  - Storage/care of insulin
  - Preparation and administration
  - Appropriate injection sites and injection site rotation
  - Side effects

> Measure blood glucose regularly

> Adhere to exercise and meal plan

> Teach signs/symptoms of hypo/hyperglycemia

> Discuss social/community support to assist in preventing recurrence of HHS

> Wear diabetes identification

> Teach what to do when physiological and psychosocial stressors for HHS occur and the importance of seeking medical care immediately

> Discuss adequate daily fluid intake

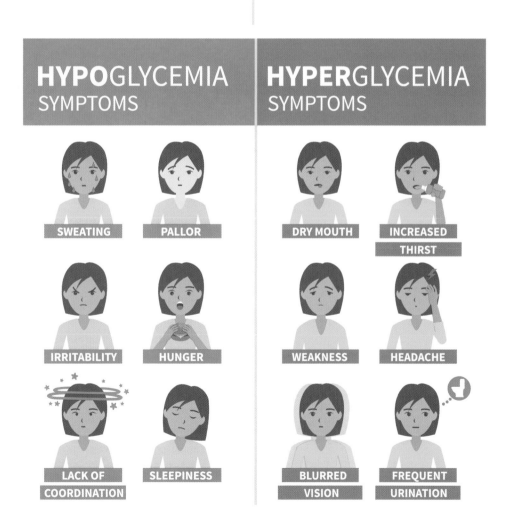

HYPOGLYCEMIA SYMPTOMS

SWEATING | PALLOR
IRRITABILITY | HUNGER
LACK OF COORDINATION | SLEEPINESS

HYPERGLYCEMIA SYMPTOMS

DRY MOUTH | INCREASED THIRST
WEAKNESS | HEADACHE
BLURRED VISION | FREQUENT URINATION

Image 12-4: Understanding the concepts of glucose regulation, it is vital to help quickly assess and intervene even if you don't know the client's serum glucose levels. Can you quickly identify hyper/hypoglycemia even if you don't know anything about the client?

Hyperparathyroidism

Pathophysiology/Description

> Hyperparathyroidism occurs when secretion of the parathyroid hormone is increased

> Parathyroid hormone (PTH) is needed to regulate phosphate and calcium levels and it acts in the following manner

- Stimulates reabsorption of calcium in the renal tubule, stimulates reabsorption of calcium in the bone and activates vitamin D

> Three classifications of hyperparathyroidism, primary, secondary and tertiary

- Primary hyperparathyroidism is increased secretion of PTH resulting in conditions related to phosphate, calcium and bone metabolism. A benign tumor in the parathyroid gland is the most common cause of primary hyperparathyroidism

- Secondary hyperparathyroidism occurs when there is a response that compensates for conditions that cause or induce hypocalcemia, since hypocalcemia is the primary stimulus for the secretion of PTH. A few of these conditions are chronic kidney disease, vitamin D deficiency, hypophosphatemia, malabsorption

- Tertiary hyperparathyroidism is due to the parathyroid glands experiencing hyperplasia. This results in loss of negative feedback from circulating calcium so even with normal calcium levels, there is secretion of PTH. Tertiary hyperparathyroidism is usually seen in kidney transplant clients who have had long duration of dialysis

> Most effective treatment for primary and secondary disease is surgery to partially or completely remove the parathyroid gland. Surgery has a high cure rate

Priority Assessments or Cues

> Conduct a complete health history

> Assess for hypophosphatemia and hypercalcemia

> Ask about fatigue, skeletal pain, and muscle weakness. Assess for pathological fractures and bone deformities

> Assess for cardiac and renal issues. Measure vital signs, particularly blood pressure, as high serum calcium levels can cause hypotension

> Assess client's knowledge of surgery and follow-up care. Assess for hemorrhage after surgery

> Examine post-surgery electrolytes levels and assess for electrolyte disturbances

> Assess for tetany, which occurs when there is sudden decrease in calcium levels

- Mild tetany includes tingling around the mouth and hands and resolves over time

- Severe tetany includes muscular spasms and is treated with medications

> Ongoing assessment of potassium, calcium, phosphate and magnesium levels

> Assess Chvostek' sign, seen when the facial nerve is tapped in front of the ear. The muscle will contract, due to excitability of the nerve that occurs from hypocalcemia

> Assess Trousseau's sign, seen as spasm of the muscles in the hand and forearm when a blood pressure cuff is inflated on the arm for 3 minutes and the brachial artery is occluded. The fingers adduct, wrist flex and joints extend. These result from hypocalcemia and neuromuscular irritability

Priority Laboratory Tests/Diagnostics

> Serum calcium expected to exceed 10 mg/dL

> Serum phosphorus, expected to be less than 3 mg/dL (There is an inverse relationship between calcium and phosphorus)

> A 24-hour urine test can provide information on kidney function and how much calcium is excreted in your urine

> Bone mineral density test, using dual energy X-ray absorptiometry (DXA) scan. This measures amounts of bone minerals and calcium that are in a segment of bone

> Magnetic resonance imaging (MRI) and computed tomography (CT) scan to look for an adenoma

> X-rays or other imaging tests of the abdomen to detect kidney stones or other kidney abnormalities

Priority Interventions or Actions

> Prepare client for parathyroidectomy and autotransplantation of normal parathyroid tissue (if this is a choice)

> Monitor intake and output, looking for signs of renal stones and determining fluid status

> Monitor for dysrhythmias

> Ensure ordered labs are drawn and review results

> Encourage mobility as it fosters calcification of bone

> Ongoing care if no surgical intervention

- Conduct regular physical exams

- Ongoing measurements of calcium, PTH, phosphorus and phosphatase

- Ongoing measurement of blood urea nitrogen (BUN) and creatinine to determine function of renal system

- Ongoing measurement of urinary excretion of calcium

- Annual dual energy X-ray absorptiometry (DXA) scan to assess bone loss

> Encourage moderate dietary intake of calcium and high fluid

> Administer medications and monitor side effects

> Administer IV fluids for hydration

Priority Potential & Actual Complications

> Sustained low calcium levels, necessitating the intake of calcium and vitamin D supplements

> Impairment in speech due to damage to nerves controlling the vocal cords

Priority Nursing Implications

> Understand that surgery is indicated with the following criteria

- Hypercalciuria above 400 mg/day

- Calcium levels greater than 1 mg/dL above the upper limit of normal

- Bone mineral density that is significantly reduced

- Obvious symptoms such as kidney stones

> With multiple removal of parathyroid glands, client may opt to autotransplant normal parathyroid tissue in the arm close to the sternocleidomastoid muscle so that secretion of PTH can continue. If no autotransplant, or if the transplant fails, calcium will be needed for life

> Monitor potassium with furosemide, as it is potassium-wasting

Priority Medications

> Calcium gluconate

- Administered via intravenous route

- Must be readily available after parathyroidectomy surgery

> Loop diuretic

- furosemide (common drug used)

- Administered intravenous or oral. Dosage is 20-40 mg/dose and oral 20-120 mg/day

- Increase calcium excretion in urine

- Inhibit calcium reabsorption in the renal tubule

> Bisphosphonates

- alendronate, most common drug in class

- Inhibit resorption of osteoblastic bone, brings normalcy to serum calcium levels, improve mineral density of bone

- Administered orally. Dosage is 5-10 mg/day

> Calcimimetic agents

- cinacalcet

- Administered orally based on titration. Start with 30 mg daily and increase by 30 mg every 2 to 4 weeks. Target is to get parathyroid hormone to the level of 150-300 pg/mL. The maximum dose is 180 mg daily

- Cause sensitivity of calcium receptors on parathyroid gland to be magnified. It tricks the parathyroid gland into the release of less parathyroid hormone fostering lowered calcium levels and PTH

> calcitonin

- Inhibits osteoclast activity of bones

- Administered intramuscular, intravenous or via nasal spray

- Should not be taken if allergic to salmon (it is a salmon-based drug)

Priority Education/Discharge Issues

> Teach client about side effects of medications

> Teach about symptoms of hypo and hypercalcemia

> Teach about expectations of parathyroid surgery

> Teach about expectations of parathyroid tissue autotransplantation

> Refrain from sedentary lifestyle, walk frequently

> Assist with adaption to meal plan. Make referral to dietitian

> Teach importance of an exercise program as immobility can worsen bone loss

> Teach importance of keeping physician's appointments

> Teach that alendronate must be taken alone on an empty stomach, and with a full glass of water. Remain in sitting position for 30 minutes as it has a risk of causing ulcers in the esophagus

Next Gen Clinical Judgment

Find a Mnemonic for Hyperparathyroidism on the internet and write it here.

_____

_____

_____

_____

_____

_____

_____

_____

Hypoparathyroidism

Pathophysiology/Description

> Hypoparathyroidism occurs when circulating parathyroid hormone (PTH) is inadequate

> Parathyroid hormone (PTH) is needed to regulate phosphate and calcium levels and it acts in the following manner

- Stimulates reabsorption of calcium in the renal tubule, stimulates reabsorption of calcium in the bone and activates vitamin D

> Lack of PTH causes hypocalcemia because serum calcium levels cannot be maintained

> Common causes of hypoparathyroidism

- Thyroidectomy, where the parathyroid gland is damaged accidentally

- Autoimmune where the immune system develops antibodies against the parathyroid gland

> Treatment is focused on addressing the acute condition, such as managing tetany and normalizing calcium levels. Long-term goal is to prevent complications

Priority Assessments or Cues

> Assess airway, breathing and circulation. Acute condition with sudden decrease in calcium level can cause painful spasms to smooth and skeletal muscles, including laryngospasms and respiratory compromise

> Conduct a complete health history

> Assess neurological status as anxiety and lethargy can occur with hypoparathyroidism

> Assess for tetany, which occurs when there is sudden decrease in calcium levels

- Mild tetany includes tingling around the mouth and hands, and resolves over time

- Severe tetany includes muscular spasms and may be treated with medications

> Ongoing assessment of potassium, calcium, phosphate and magnesium levels

> Assess Chvostek' sign, seen when the facial nerve is tapped in front of the ear. The muscle will contract, due to excitability of the nerve that occurs from hypocalcemia

> Assess Trousseau's sign, seen as spasm of the muscles in the hand and forearm when a blood pressure cuff is inflated on the arm for 3 minutes and the brachial artery is occluded. The fingers adduct, wrist flex and joints extend. These result from hypocalcemia and neuromuscular irritability

Priority Laboratory Tests/Diagnostics

> Serum calcium expected to be low

> Serum phosphorus, expected to be high (There is an inverse relationship between calcium and phosphorus)

> Parathyroid level expected to be low

> Serum magnesium expected to be low

Priority Interventions or Actions

> Administer calcium and monitor serum calcium levels

> Ensure electrocardiogram monitoring during acute IV calcium administration as cardiac dysrhythmias or arrest are adverse effects of high calcium levels

> Place oxygen, tracheostomy set and suction supplies at the bedside in the event of a cardiac event

> Ensure a patent intravenous line before starting calcium therapy

> Ensure intake of high calcium low phosphorus diet

> Teach rebreathing exercises, such as breathing in a paper bag. This helps to excrete CO_2 from the lungs and lower the pH. The decrease in pH helps with the ionization of calcium, resulting in increased available body calcium

> Ensure ordered labs are drawn and review results to determine efficacy of treatment

> Administer medications and monitor side effects. Administer IV fluids for hydration

Priority Potential & Actual Complications

> Long-term low calcium levels, necessitating the intake of calcium and vitamin D supplements

> Paresthesia

> Tetany

> Heart arrhythmias

> Heart failure

> Slowed mental development

> Stunted growth

> Calcium deposits in brain

Priority Nursing Implications

> Calcium chloride is irritating to veins and can cause inflammation. Extravasation can result in tissue necrosis, so the intravenous line must be monitored to ensure patency

Priority Medications

> calcium (for acute use)
  - Administered slowly via intravenous route
  - Electrocardiogram monitoring must occur (See rationale stated in priority interventions above)
  - Administered in the acute phase only. Client will be discharged with oral calcium as calcium carbonate supplements 1.5-3 g/day in divided doses

> vitamin D
  - calcitriol
  - Administered orally. Dose is 0.2-2 mcg/day
  - Regulates serum calcium levels

> Parathyroid hormone
  - natpara
  - Administered via injection once daily
  - Restricted use due to potential risk of getting bone cancer. Availability only via a restricted program and used when levels of calcium cannot be controlled with vitamin D and calcium

Priority Education/Discharge Issues

> Teach client about side effects of medications. Teach about symptoms of hypo and hypercalcemia

> Instruct on the administration of calcium and vitamin D supplements as prescribed

> Teach management of long-term dietary needs, foods that are low in phosphorus and rich in calcium. Make referral to dietitian

> Teach importance of keeping physician's appointments and monitoring of calcium levels

Next Gen Clinical Judgment

Compare and Contrast

1. How are hyperparathyroidism and hypoparathyroidism the same?

2. How are hyperparathyroidism and hypoparathyroidism different?

3. How is the nursing care for hyperparathyroidism and hypoparathyroidism the same?

4. How is the nursing care for hyperparathyroidism and hypoparathyroidism different?

Signs of Hypocalcemia

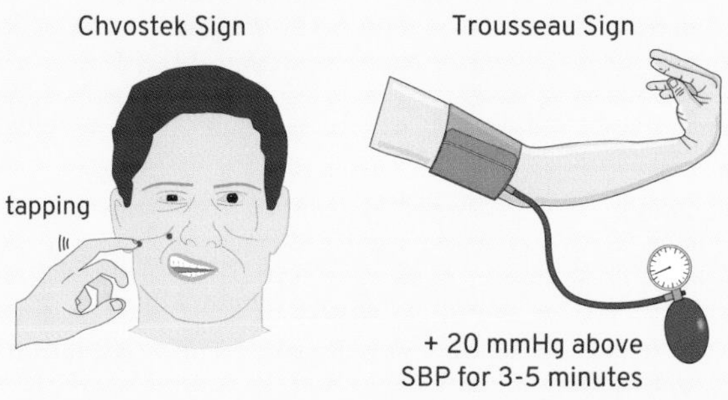

Chvostek Sign

Trousseau Sign

tapping

+ 20 mmHg above SBP for 3-5 minutes

Image 12-5: In addition to the Chvostek's and Trousseau's sign, what are other signs of hypocalcemia?

_____

_____

_____

_____

_____

_____

_____

_____

_____

_____

_____

_____

_____

_____

Hyperthyroidism

Pathophysiology/Description

> Hyperthyroidism occurs when the thyroid gland is hyperactive, causing continuous increase in the production and release of thyroid hormones (T3 and T4)

> Commonly seen in the 20 to 40 age range and occurs most often in women than men

> Common causes of hyperthyroidism

  • Graves' disease, thyroiditis, excess iodine intake, thyroid cancer, toxic nodular goiter, and pituitary tumor

> The clinical manifestations of hyperthyroidism are termed thyrotoxicosis

> Hyperthyroidism causes functions of the body to speed up

> The goal of hyperthyroidism management is to prevent complications, suppress over production of thyroid hormone and prevent adverse effects

Priority Assessments or Cues

> Assess for symptoms of acute thyrotoxicosis

> Assess vital signs (heart rate likely to be greater than 100 beats per minute, hypertension)

> Complete history and physical

> Assess cardiac system (arrhythmias, palpations, angina and systolic murmurs are common)

> Ask about appetite and meal consumption (causes increased appetite)

> Ask about sudden weight loss pattern (weight loss is likely)

> Ask about heat tolerance (increased heat sensitivity is likely)

> Determine sleep pattern (difficulty sleeping is an expectation)

> Assess the integumentary system (likely to find thinning skin and hair that is fine and brittle)

> Examine the neck (a swelling at the base of the neck, called a goiter, is common)

> Assess for bulging eyes, called exopthalmos (common with the disease)

> Ask about bowel elimination (likely to have increased number of bowel movements)

> Assess the neurologic system (irritability, fine tremors of the hands and fingers, anxiety, depression and nervousness are common)

> Ask about menstrual changes, decreased libido and impotence (common occurrences)

> Assess for activity intolerance due to fatigue

> Assess knowledge regarding treatment plan such as iodine therapy and thyroidectomy

> After thyroidectomy

  • Assess respiratory status as breathing may be affected by neck swelling

  • Assess client for tracheal compression and damage, frequent swallowing, choking, hemorrhage, sensation of fullness at insertion site

  • Assess for tetany which can occur if the pituitary gland is damaged in surgery

Priority Laboratory Tests/Diagnostics

> Thyroid stimulating hormone (TSH) will be low or not detectable, with level of less than 0.4 mU/L and free thyroxine (free T4) will be elevated

> Radioactive iodine uptake (RAIU) test. Client swallows radioactive iodine in the form of a capsule or liquid and radioactivity of the thyroid gland is measured 6-24 hours after ingestion. Level is expected to be elevated, greater than 35%. Normal level at 24 hours is 8-25%

> Electrocardiogram, showing tachycardia and atrial fibrillation

Priority Interventions or Actions

> Provide oxygenation in thyrotoxicosis crisis

> Assist with process of radioactive iodine uptake test and iodine therapy

> Encourage adequate rest in a quiet, calm and cool environment

> Place light covering on client and change frequently if diaphoretic

> Administer antithyroid medications as prescribed

> Administer medications as prescribed, to treat the symptoms

> Prepare client for subtotal thyroidectomy, if indicated. Administer pre-surgery medications as prescribed

> Apply artificial tears to moisten conjunctiva and prevent corneal injury and eye discomfort, if exophthalmos is present

> Monitor daily weights

> Monitor nutritional status due to increased rate of metabolism. Provide increased carbohydrate diet. Calories should be increased to 4,000 to 5,000 cal/day

> Help client with coping strategies for altered body image (mainly due to bulging eyes)

> Interventions after thyroidectomy

  • Maintain patent airway

  • Position client in the semi-Fowler's position

  • Use pillows to support client's head

  • Administer pain medications

Priority Potential & Actual Complications

> Cardiac problems, thyrotoxicosis, thyroid storm, eye problems, brittle bones, accidental removal of thyroid gland, hemorrhage and injury to laryngeal nerve resulting in vocal cord paralysis

Priority Nursing Implications

> Individuals at risk for hyperthyroidism must be closely monitored if they have a procedure that involves the use of iodinated contrast medium, since iodine is a causative factor for the condition

> Understand that thyrotoxicosis is a medical emergency that must be treated quickly. Symptoms include hyperthermia (temperature as high as 106°F), tachycardia, irritability, heart failure, shock, diarrhea, vomiting and pain in the abdomen. Coma is also likely

> Client may be distressed looking at the scar after surgery, Encourage the wearing of a scarf and let client know that the scar will fade over time

> Assess for thyroid storm when using methimazole and propylthiouracil

> Black box warning with beta blockers, used to treat the cardiac symptoms, indicate that they must be tapered over 1-2 weeks and not withdrawn abruptly. Sudden withdrawal may exacerbate cardiac symptoms

Priority Medications

> Antithyroid medication
  - methimazole 5-15 mg/day, administered orally
  - propylthiouracil 100-150 mg/day administered orally
  - Both medications impede formation of thyroid hormone.

> Beta Blockers
  - propranolol, atenolol and metoprolol. Dose ranges vary for each
  - Used to treat the cardiac symptoms associated with hyperthyroidism
  - A common adverse effect is bradycardia

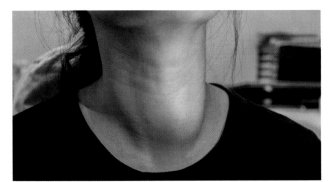

Image 12-6: When is treatment indicated for a Goiter?

Priority Education/Discharge Issues

> Educate client and family members about the signs and symptoms of hyperthyroidism

> Educate about the radioactive iodine uptake test and how soon after ingestion of the medication to return for measurement

> Teach the prevention of overly seasoned foods as well as foods with high fiber. These exacerbate hyperactivity of the gastrointestinal system

> Assist with referral to dietician

> Educate on avoidance of caffeinated beverages as these will add to the problem of sleep disturbance

> Preoperatively, teach client post-surgery activities, such as range of motion exercises and positioning of head

> Reinforce the importance of following up with physician's visits

> Teach the importance of taking lifelong thyroid hormone if surgery was complete thyroidectomy

> Teach importance of monitoring heart rate when taking beta blockers

Next Gen Clinical Judgment

1. How are hyperthyroidism and hypothyroidism the same?

2. How are hyperthyroidism and hypothyroidism different?

3. How is the nursing care for hyperthyroidism and hypothyroidism the same?

4. How is the nursing care for hyperthyroidism and hypothyroidism different?

_____

_____

_____

_____

_____

_____

_____

Hypothyroidism

Pathophysiology/Description

> Hypothyroidism occurs when there is not enough thyroid hormone (deficiency), causing a slowing of the body's metabolic rate. The condition is more commonly seen in women than men

> There are two classifications to the condition, primary and secondary

  • In primary hypothyroidism the thyroid tissue is destroyed, or synthesis of the hormone is defective. Atrophy of the thyroid gland is the most common cause of hypothyroidism in the United States. This is as a result of Graves' disease or Hashimoto's disease, both autoimmune conditions

  • Secondary hypothyroidism results when there is a disease of the pituitary gland

> Risk factors for hypothyroidism are family history, female and Caucasian, type 1 diabetes, Down syndrome, previous hyperthyroidism, radiation to neck and head, and goiter

> When an individual has a thyroidectomy or when iodine is used to destroy the thyroid gland in treating hyperthyroidism, hypothyroidism can occur. Certain drugs that contain iodine can also cause hypothyroidism. Hypothyroidism can also develop at birth (called cretinism). Screening for the condition in all infants occurs in the United States

> Hypothyroidism causes functions of the body to slow down. Clinical manifestations of hypothyroidism impact all body systems

  • Cardiac (decreased heart rate and contractibility, heart failure, heart hypertrophy, anemia)

  • Respiratory (decreased breathing, difficulty breathing)

  • Neurologic (slowed speech, slowed mental processing, depression, lethargy, hoarseness)

  • Gastrointestinal (weight gain, constipation, distended abdomen, enlarged tongue)

  • Musculoskeletal (weakness, slow movements, muscle aches, fatigue)

  • Integumentary (poor skin turgor, decreased sweating, dry and sparse hair, thick brittle nails, puffy face, cold skin, cold intolerance, goiter)

  • Reproductive (decreased libido, infertility and prolonged menstruation)

> Myxedema occurs with longstanding hypothyroidism. It is the result of accumulated hydrophilic mucopolysaccharides in the dermis of the skin as well as other tissues. Causes puffiness to skin, edema around the eyes (periorbital edema), facial edema, and a flat or masklike affect

> Myxedema coma results if myxedema is not treated early. Survival depends on support of vital functions and intravenous hormone replacement

> Symptoms of myxedema coma are hypotension, subnormal body temperature, hypoventilation and complete collapse of the cardiovascular system

Priority Assessments or Cues

> Ask about past treatment for hyperthyroidism, antithyroid or iodine intake

> Assess all body systems (looking for system manifestations stated above in pathophysiology)

> Assess for myxedema (looking for manifestations stated above in pathophysiology)

> Assess oxygen saturation level

> Complete history and physical

> In acute situation (myxedema or myxedema coma)

  • Ongoing assessment of cardiac system. Medication regimen is determined by the cardiovascular response

  • Assessment of vital signs, looking for gradual increase

  • Skin assessment, to determine skin breakdown

> Assess response to treatment

> Assess need for psychological referral due to depression and body image disturbances

Priority Laboratory Tests/Diagnostics

> Thyroid stimulating hormone (TSH) will be low in secondary hypothyroidism and high in primary hypothyroidism. Repeated tests with consistent levels of greater than 5.0 mU/L indicate the condition. Thyroxine (T4) will be low in both primary and secondary hypothyroidism. Thyroid antibodies will be positive in Hashimoto's disease

Priority Interventions or Actions

> In acute situation

  • Initiate intravenous line

  • Provide cardiac monitoring and mechanical respiratory support in myxedema crisis

  • Administer medications intravenously in myxedema coma as poor gastric motility may prevent absorption if administered orally

  • Monitor body temperature as severe hypothermia occurs in myxedema coma

  • Position client frequently to minimize risk of skin breakdown. Use pressure relief mattress

> Encourage exercise but space activities to conserve energy, activity intolerance is an issue

> Administer medications to treat symptoms as indicated

> Administer thyroid hormone

> Monitor environmental temperature to ensure it is not too cold

> Orient to environment, since mental processing is slowed

> Allow client time to verbalize feelings about body image issues

Priority Potential & Actual Complications

> Unconsciousness, mental sluggishness, myxedema coma, collapse of cardiovascular system

Priority Nursing Implications

> Altered self-image is a significant problem. Devise strategies to assist client with coping skills

> Understand that if a client has diabetes mellitus, blood glucose must be checked daily as return to a euthyroid state often causes an increase in insulin requirement

Priority Medications

> Thyroid hormone (intravenous)

  • levothyroxine

  • Administered in acute phase (myxedema coma)

  • Intravenous dosage 200-500 mcg single dose, 100-300 mcg given second day if needed, continue with 75-100 mcg/day until switch is made to oral administration

> Thyroid hormone (oral)

  • levothyroxine

  • Administered as long-term therapy

  • Oral dosage 25-200 mcg/day

Priority Education/Discharge Issues

> Educate client and family members about the signs and symptoms of hypothyroidism

> Educate about avoidance of extreme cold temperatures

> Teach weight reduction measures. Inform about low-calorie meal plans

> Educate on importance of high-fiber diet, and fluid intake to prevent constipation

> Assist with referral to dietician

> Assist with psychological referral if needed to manage depression and body image disturbance

> Teach that mental alertness and energy level is expected to improve in 2 -14 days

> Reinforce the importance of following up with healthcare provider visits

> Teach the importance of lifelong drug therapy

> Educate on the side effects of medication therapy

> Educate not to switch brand of hypothyroid medication as it may alter the body's response to the drug

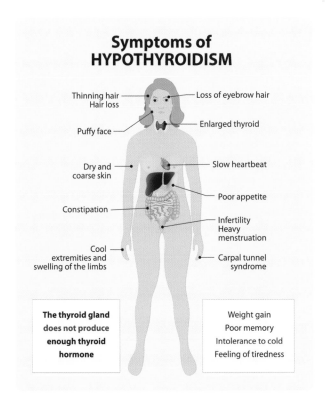

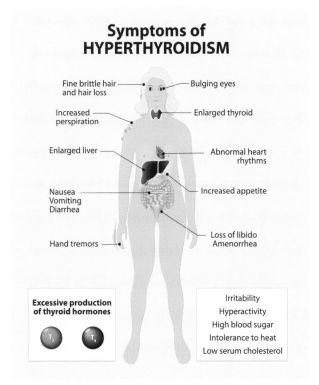

Images 12-7a (left) and 12-7b (right): How might a client with no medical background/knowledge, describe these symptoms?

Cushing's syndrome

Pathophysiology/Description

> Cushing's syndrome results when an individual experiences chronic exposure to corticosteroids

> Common causes

- Exogenous administration of corticosteroids

- Pituitary tumor that secretes adrenocorticotropic hormone (Cushing's disease)

- More common in women than men and occur mostly in ages 20-40

> Common clinical manifestations include lower extremities edema, hypertension, fatigue, muscle wasting in extremities, weakness, osteoporosis resulting in compression fractures, inhibition of immune and allergic responses, petechial hemorrhage, thin and fragile skin, bruises, purplish striae, problems with wound healing

Priority Assessments or Cues

> Conduct detailed history and physical

> Assess for muscle wasting and weakness

> Assess for classic appearance of hump to back, called buffalo hump. Assess face for moon shaped appearance from fatty deposits

> Assess for classic obesity to trunk with thin extremities and fatty deposits to supraclavicular area

> Assess skin for reddish-purple stretch marks (called striae) on abdomen and thighs, resulting from inflamed and ruptured dermal tissue because of the weight gain associated with Cushing's syndrome

> Assess for facial hair in women (called hirsutism) and gynecomastia in men

> Assess blood pressure, blood glucose and sodium levels, all elevated with Cushing's syndrome

> Assess potassium and calcium levels, both decreased with Cushing's syndrome

> Assess response to treatment

> Assess need for psychological referral due to depression and body image disturbances

> Assess for hemorrhage postoperatively

> Assess for subtle signs of infection postoperatively (important as the inflammatory response is decreased)

> Assess for adverse effects of corticosteroid therapy

Priority Laboratory Tests/Diagnostics

> Late night salivary cortisol is expected to be elevated above the normal range of 0.10-0.15 ug/dL with Cushing's syndrome. Normally, cortisol secretion is very low at late night

> Low dose dexamethasone suppression test. A serum cortisol level >1.7 µg/dL after the single dose dexamethasone is a positive test

> Urine free cortisol, levels higher than 80 -120 mcg/24 hour is positive for Cushing's syndrome

> ACH test to determine cause with results that may be normal, elevated or low depending on the cause of the condition

> Computed tomography (CT) scan and magnetic resonance imaging (MRI) to examine pituitary and adrenal glands for tumors

Priority Interventions or Actions

> Initiate intravenous line, anticipate administration of fluid and medications

> Prepare client for surgery, radiation or chemotherapy based on the cause

- Adrenalectomy if adrenal adenoma, along with drug therapy

- Radiation and surgery if cause is a pituitary adenoma

- Surgery or radiation if cause is related to a tumor that is secreting ACTH

- Chemotherapy if cause is from adrenal tumor that is inoperable

> Preoperatively, provide expectations regarding postoperative care

> Discontinue corticosteroid medications if cause of Cushing's syndrome is from exogenous intake of corticosteroids

> Postoperative interventions

- Monitor urinary catheter, and nasogastric tube (often used) postoperatively

- Ensure placement of sequential leg compression device to minimize risk of blood clot formation

- Monitor vital signs, particularly blood pressure, since hypertension is a manifestation

- Monitor for hemorrhage (common because of vascularity of adrenal glands)

- Monitor central venous pressure

- During first 24-48 hours postoperative, constant monitoring for corticosteroid imbalance

Priority Potential & Actual Complications

> Osteoporosis resulting in fractures, hypertension, type 2 diabetes and infections, hemorrhage from surgery

Priority Nursing Implications

> If client is having surgery, ensure hypertension, hyperglycemia, and hypokalemia are controlled before surgery

> Keep in mind that the adrenal glands are very vascular so postoperatively, surgery presents a significant risk of bleeding

> Do not taper corticosteroid dosage too rapidly as adrenal insufficiency may occur, manifested by increased weakness, vomiting, hypotension dehydration, peeling skin, joint pain, and pruritus

> It is normal for cortisol levels in the blood to drop after taking dexamethasone. If the level does not drop, it suggests Cushing's syndrome

Priority Medications

> ketoconazole
  - Used to control cortisol production by decreasing steroid hormone production in the adrenal gland
  - Dose range is 600-800 mg/day orally
  - Causes liver toxicity at high doses

> aminoglutethimide
  - Used to control the production of excess cortisol
  - Dose 250 mg orally every 6 hours. If inadequate, then dose is titrated in 250 mg increments every 1-2 weeks. Dose should not exceed 2 grams
  - May cause drowsiness and dizziness

> mitotane
  - Initial dosage is 1.5 grams orally divided every 6-8 hours, not to exceed 3 grams every 8 hours.
  - Maintenance dose is 500 mg 2 times week
  - Increases clearance of warfarin and phenytoin from body, which deceases their effectiveness.

> mifepristone
  - Used to treat high blood glucose associated with Cushing's syndrome in clients with type 2 diabetes (not used to treat diabetes outside of Cushing's syndrome)
  - Blocks effect of excess cortisol
  - Initial dose is 300 mg orally once a day. Maximum dose is 1200 mg or 20 mg/kg once a day

> Corticosteroids (hydrocortisone most common drug in class)
  - High doses administered intravenously in surgery and days following to ensure stress that is caused by surgery is adequately managed
  - Administered intravenous 100-500 mg every 2-6 hrs. Range is 100-800 mg/day
  - Do not taper too quickly after surgery as acute adrenal insufficiency may occur

Priority Education/Discharge Issues

> Educate client and family members about the signs and symptoms of corticosteroid therapy

> Recommend and assist client to schedule a home health nurse for ongoing teaching and evaluation

> Teach proper administration of drug therapy

> Assist with psychological referral if needed to manage depression and body image disturbance

> Reinforce the importance of following up with healthcare provider visits

> Teach the importance of lifelong drug therapy

> Educate on the side effects of medication therapy

> Teach stress reduction strategies

> Encourage client to wear a MedicAlert identification

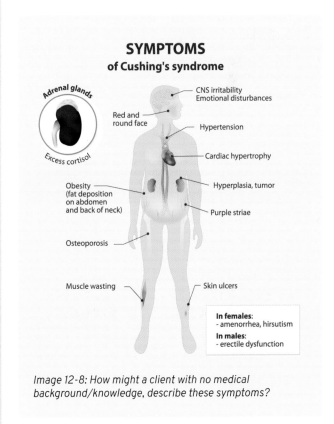

SYMPTOMS
of Cushing's syndrome

Adrenal glands

Excess cortisol

- CNS irritability / Emotional disturbances
- Red and round face
- Hypertension
- Cardiac hypertrophy
- Obesity (fat deposition on abdomen and back of neck)
- Hyperplasia, tumor
- Purple striae
- Osteoporosis
- Muscle wasting
- Skin ulcers

In females:
- amenorrhea, hirsutism
In males:
- erectile dysfunction

Image 12-8: How might a client with no medical background/knowledge, describe these symptoms?

Addison's disease

Pathophysiology/Description

> Addison's disease results when there is hypofunction of the adrenal glands causing corticosteroids (mineralocorticoids, glucocorticoids and androgens) to be insufficient. This is primary adrenal insufficiency. Adrenal insufficiency may also occur from insufficient pituitary adrenocorticotropic hormone as a secondary cause

> Majority of Addison's disease in the United States result from an autoimmune response which causes destruction to the adrenal cortex by antibodies

> Common clinical manifestations are many
  - Bronzed hyperpigmentation of skin
  - Hypotension, lethargy, hypovolemia, decreased cardiac output
  - Anorexia, weight loss, abdominal cramping, depression, confusion delusions
  - Hyperkalemia, sodium loss, salt craving,
  - Decreased pubic and axillary hair in women, decreased libido, decreased muscle size and tone

> Occurs most often in adults younger than age 60 and is not gender specific

Priority Assessments or Cues

> Assess for the clinical manifestations of Addison's disease (as stated in pathophysiology above)

> Assess for Addisonian crisis, a life-threatening condition, which have added manifestations of severe abdominal and lower back pain, severe headache, severe hypotension, tachycardia, generalized weakness and shock

> Conduct a complete medical history

> Assess response to treatment

> Assess need for psychological referral due to depression

> Ongoing assessment of labs and vital signs

Can you Complete this table? Are these up or down?

	Addison's	Cushing's
Serum		
Calcium		
Glucose		
Potassium		
Sodium		
Blood pressure		
Weight		

Table 12-2: Be sure to make a note card with this table and keep it nearby. Compare and Contrast is a way to SAVE TIME STUDYING.

Priority Laboratory Tests/Diagnostics

> Adrenocorticotropic(ACTH) stimulation test
  - Baseline cortisol and ACTH are measured. Intravenous ACTH is administered, and cortisol and ACTH levels are re-measured at 30 and 60-minute intervals. Addison's disease is indicated if cortisol level is increased minimally or not increased at all

> Corticotropin-releasing hormone (CRH) stimulation test (measured when ACTH test is abnormal)
  - CRH is administered intravenously and ACTH and cortisol levels are checked at 30 and 60 minutes. Addison's disease is indicated if ACTH level is high, but cortisol level is absent

> Blood tests will show increased potassium and deceased blood glucose, sodium and chloride

> Electrocardiogram will show peaked T waves from hyperkalemia

> Computed tomography (CT) scan and magnetic resonance imaging (MRI) will show other non-autoimmune causes

Priority Interventions or Actions

> Assist with labs and diagnostic tests

> In acute Addisonian crisis
  - Initiate intravenous line
  - Administer large volumes of 5% and 0.9% saline solutions. These offer quick treatment of hypotension and electrolyte imbalances
  - Administer high dose hydrocortisone replacement as prescribed
  - Monitor vital signs, focus on blood pressure which is severely low with Addison's crisis
  - Monitor neurologic status, due to confusion and irritability
  - Administer intravenous fluid to restore fluid and electrolyte balance
  - Monitor lab values to determine effectiveness of treatment
  - Monitor intake and output
  - Administer mineralocorticoids and glucocorticoids orally when crisis has resolved
  - Ensure bedrest in a quiet environment away from stressors

> Monitor weight, as unexplained weight loss is an issue

> Administer medications replacement hormones as prescribed

> Allow client time to verbalize feelings about the disease

Priority Potential & Actual Complications

> Addisonian crisis
> Depression

Priority Nursing Implications

> It is crucial for individuals with Addison's disease to determine a clear plan with their health care provider on how hormone replacement will be managed during times of added stress

> Understand the importance of carrying medications at all times in the event an emergency occurs. Clients must teach someone else how to administer hydrocortisone injections

Priority Medications

> hydrocortisone
  - Used in Addisonian crisis to replace hormone: dosage is 100 mg IV, immediately followed by infusion of 200 mg over 24 hours or 50 mg IV every 6 hours. An IV dose of 100 mg is administered the next day
  - Used as maintenance hormone replacement: common oral dosage is 15-20 mg divided over two to three times daily
  - hydrocortisone (has both mineralocorticoid and glucocorticoid properties and is the most commonly used in Addisonian crisis)

> fludrocortisone (most commonly prescribed mineralocorticoid)
  - Used as partial replacement therapy for Addison's disease
  - Administered orally, dosage 0.05-0.2 mg every 24 hours
  - Adverse effects include fluid retention, hypertension and potential heart failure

> dehydroepiandrosterone (DHEA)
  - Given to women as androgen replacement
  - 25-200 mg a day
  - Alert to the fact that DHEA can cause acne and unwanted, male-pattern hair growth in women (hirsutism)

Priority Education/Discharge Issues

> Educate client and family members about the signs and symptoms of Addisonian crisis

> Teach importance of wearing MedicAlert identification or carrying a MedicAlert card

> Educate on proper time of day to take prescribed glucocorticoids and mineralocorticoids to mimic the normal pattern of the body's endogenous hormone secretion

> Educate on importance of carrying a kit at all times to include, 100 mg of hydrocortisone with a syringe and clear instructions for use

> Reinforce the importance of following up with healthcare provider visits

> Teach the importance of lifelong hormone drug therapy

> Reinforce that in times of stress, such as illness, corticosteroid dosage will need to be increased

> Educate on the side effects of medication therapy and signs and symptoms of corticosteroid deficiency

> Teach to avoid the stress of strenuous exercise

> Teach the importance of adhering to a prescribed diet of high protein and carbohydrate. Take calcium and vitamin D if glucocorticoid is being replaced. This prevents the condition of glucocorticoid-induced osteoporosis. May need a high sodium diet if taking mineralocorticoid

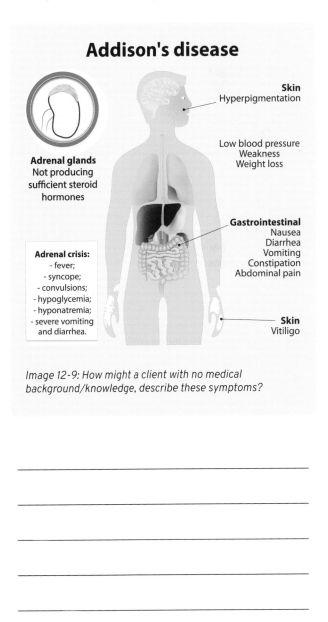

Image 12-9: How might a client with no medical background/knowledge, describe these symptoms?

_____

_____

_____

_____

_____

Syndrome of inappropriate antidiuretic hormone (SIADH)

Pathophysiology/Description

- Occurs when there is release of antidiuretic hormone without the body signaling a need for it
- Pathophysiology
  - Renal tubules and collecting ducts suffer increased permeability which causes fluid to be reabsorbed into the body's circulation. There is expansion of extracellular fluid volume. The overall result is increased glomerular filtration rate, expansion of extracellular fluid volume, decrease of plasma osmolality and decrease in sodium levels
- The pathophysiology results in
  - Fluid retention
  - Dilutional hyponatremia
  - Urine that is concentrated when intravascular fluid volume is increased or normal
  - Low serum osmolality
  - Hypochloremia
- Clinical manifestations
  - Increased body weight, decreased urine output and signs of fluid overload
  - Fatigue and exertional dyspnea, headache, muscle cramping
  - Nausea, vomiting and loss of appetite
  - When the sodium level decreases drastically (below 120 mEq/L), manifestations are more severe and include muscle twitching, cerebral edema, seizures and coma

Priority Assessments or Cues

- Assess for low urine output coupled with a high urine specific gravity
- Assess electrolyte level, be alert for low sodium level
- Assess for weight gain in the absence of edema
- Assess for signs of low sodium, which manifest as headache, vomiting, seizures and impaired neurological functioning
- Complete history and physical
- Assess response to treatment
- Assess for neurologic impairment

Priority Laboratory Tests/Diagnostics

- Serum sodium, less than 134 mEq/L, serum osmolality less than 280 mOsm/kg and urine specific gravity that is greater than 1.025, indicate dilutional hyponatremia

Priority Interventions or Actions

- Administer intravenous fluid with normal saline. Monitor intake and output carefully due to risk of fluid overload
- Obtain weights daily to monitor gain or loss
- Treat underlying cause
- Monitor for signs of intracranial pressure due to neurological manifestations
- Elevate head of bed no higher than 10 degrees This promotes venous return to the heart and increases the pressure at which the left atrium fills, fostering reduction in the release of ADH
- Implement precautions against seizures
- Conduct ongoing monitoring of electrolyte levels, serum and urine osmolality
- Administer small amounts of 3% sodium chloride if severe hyponatremia (less than 120 mEQ/dL) to increase the sodium level slowly. Rapid increase in sodium level can cause permanent injury to brain cells
- Manage fluid restriction

Priority Potential & Actual Complications

- Seizures
- Cerebral edema
- Pulmonary edema

Priority Nursing Implications

- Understand that with severe hyponatremia, fluid must be managed carefully. Usually no more than 500 mL/day is given
- Must replace potassium with furosemide administration as it is potassium-wasting

Priority Medications

- Loop diuretic
  - furosemide (most commonly used) to promote diuresis
  - Carefully monitor blood pressure, electrolyte levels (especially sodium and potassium), and urine output

> Vasopressin antagonist
  - conivaptan, tolvaptan (both used in acute setting)
  - conivaptan with initial loading dose of 20 mg intravenous administered over 30 minutes, then 20 mg continuous intravenous infusion over 24 hrs. After initial day of therapy, administer 20 mg via continuous intravenous infusion over 24 hours for 1-3 days. Works by blocking the effect of ADH on the renal tubules
  - tolvaptan with initial dose of 15 mg daily administered orally. Maintenance dose is increased to 30 mg daily for 24 hours, then after 24 hours, increase to 60 mg daily. Therapy should last no more than 30 days
  - Administer vasopressin antagonists with caution in liver disease, may worsen liver function

Priority Education/Discharge Issues

> Educate client and family members about the signs and symptoms of SIADH

> Educate about avoiding common medications that stimulate the release of antidiuretic hormone such as thiazide diuretics, some chemotherapy drugs and opioids, to name just a few

> Teach importance of fluid restriction in chronic SIADH. Drink no more than 800-1000 mL/day

> Teach alternative to fluids to minimize thirst, such as sugarless gum and ice chips

> Assist with referral to dietician

> Teach client to weigh daily

> Teach about foods that contain potassium if taking furosemide

> Teach about signs and symptoms of electrolyte imbalance and reinforce the importance of following up with healthcare provider visit

Next Gen Clinical Judgment

Compare and Contrast

1. How are diabetes insipidus and syndrome of inappropriate antidiuretic hormone the same?

2. How are diabetes insipidus and syndrome of inappropriate antidiuretic hormone different?

3. How is the nursing care for diabetes insipidus and syndrome of inappropriate antidiuretic hormone the same?

4. How is the nursing care for diabetes insipidus and syndrome of inappropriate antidiuretic hormone different?

Diabetes insipidus

Pathophysiology/Description

> Diabetes insipidus (DI) occurs when there is hyposecretion of antidiuretic hormone (ADH). This is caused by a deficit in secretion or production of ADH or the kidney's inability to respond appropriately to ADH, in the presence of adequate production of the hormone. There are three types of DI
> - Central DI, occurring when there is a problem with the production of ADH. This is the most common type of DI
> - Nephrogenic DI, occurring when there is inadequate response of renal system to ADH
> - Primary DI, occurring from excessive intake of water
> Clinical manifestations
> - Polyuria and polydipsia, excretion of significantly large amounts of urine, up to 20 L/day
> - Fatigue and exertional dyspnea, headache, muscle cramping
> - Nausea, vomiting and loss of appetite
> - When the sodium level decreases drastically (below 120 mEq/L), manifestations are more severe and include muscle twitching, cerebral edema, seizures and coma

Priority Assessments or Cues

> Assess urine output, expect large amounts of dilute urine
> Assess skin and mucous membranes for dehydration, expected to be dry with poor turgor from loss of water
> Assess for fatigue, muscle weakness and headache
> Assess for postural hypotension as a result of significant fluid loss
> Assess for collapse of the vascular system
> Assess cardiovascular and neurological systems as several manifestations relate to these systems
> Assess vital signs, likely to see tachycardia, and hypotension
> Complete history and physical
> Assess response to treatment
> Assess for neurologic impairment
> Ongoing assessment of heart rate, and blood pressure to determine their return to normal

Priority Laboratory Tests/Diagnostics

> Urine specific gravity expected to be less than 1.005
> Water deprivation test (if identified as central DI): Urine osmolality, volume, body weight and urine specific gravity are measured pretest then water deprivation occurs for 8- 12 hours. Desmopressin is then administered via subcutaneous or nasal routes. With central DI a dramatic increase in urine osmolality, to 600 mOsm/kg, will be seen along with decrease in volume of urine. If neurogenic DI, urine osmolality will not be greater than 300 mOsm/kg
> Test with ADH analog (if identified as central DI): Desmopressin is given. If cause is central DI, urine will be concentrated by the kidneys. If the cause is neurogenic, the kidneys will not concentrate urine

Priority Interventions or Actions

> Administer intravenous or oral fluids as the client tolerates
> Administer intravenous dextrose 5% or hypotonic saline solution to replace urine loss, in acute DI cases
> Monitor blood glucose as glycosuria and hyperglycemia can cause osmotic diuresis
> Monitor intake and output carefully
> Monitor urine specific gravity as treatment starts, to determine an increase back to normal level
> Monitor neurologic status to determine resolution of neurologic symptoms
> Ensure accurate documentation of daily weights
> Administer medications to relieve thirst
> Administer thiazide diuretics as ordered for nephrogenic DI

Priority Potential & Actual Complications

> Severe dehydration, seizures, and brain damage

Priority Nursing Implications

> chlorpropamide can cause significant hypoglycemia so blood glucose must be checked when taking this drug

Priority Medications

> carbamazepine and chlorpropamide
> - Used to help control thirst that results from central DI
> - chlorpropamide is 3 to 5 mg/kg PO once or twice daily
> - carbamazepine 100 to 400 mg orally, twice daily is recommended for adults

> desmopressin
  - Used with severe ADH deficiency
  - Administered orally, intranasally, subcutaneously and intravenously. Usual dose range is 10 to 40 mcg, with most adults requiring 10 mcg two times daily
  - Water intoxication is a serious adverse effect
> Thiazide diuretics
  - Reduce volume of urine in central DI and nephrogenic DI. Reduced volume results from reduction in extracellular volume and proximal tubule reabsorption.
  - With 15 to 25 mg/kg of chlorothiazide, there can be a drop-in urine volume of 25-50%
> indomethacin
  - Prostaglandin inhibitor that helps to increase responsiveness of renal system to ADH
  - Administered 0.5 to 1.0 mg/kg orally three times daily

Priority Education/Discharge Issues

> Teach proper administration of medications
> Teach limiting of sodium intake to decrease in urine output
> Teach avoidance of foods that produce diuresis
> Instruct on the wearing of a MedicAlert bracelet and carrying a MedicAlert card
> Teach about signs and symptoms of DI and reinforce the importance of following up with healthcare provider visit

Can you complete this table? Are these up or down?		
	SIADH	D. INSIPIDUS
Serum		
Sodium		
Osmolality		
Hematocrit		
Urine output		
Blood pressure		
Pulse		

Table 12-3: Be sure to make a note card with this table and keep it nearby. Compare and contrast is a way to SAVE TIME STUDYING.

Wilms tumor

Pathophysiology/Description

> Wilms tumor is a rare solid malignant tumor that affects children. It occurs in the abdomen and kidney and is initiated from immature cells in the kidney

> It usually occurs unilaterally but can be bilateral

> The tumor may spread to the blood vessels that immediately surround the kidney in the form of a clot. Another common site of metastasis is the lungs

> Wilms tumor has a genetic predisposition, but certain congenital conditions are also associated with the disease. The incidence of Wilms tumor peaks at age 3

> About 15% of children with Wilms tumor have someone in the family with the disease

> Treatment is surgery, chemotherapy and/or radiation

> Clinical manifestations
> - Abdominal swelling (usually described as an area of firmness or a lump) with, or without pain
> - Fever
> - Hypertension, resulting from secretion of renin by the tumor
> - Hematuria and urinary retention
> - Anemia because of bleeding in the tumor
> - Lethargy and anorexia, resulting from anemia
> - With lung metastasis, dyspnea and chest pain can occur

> Treatment is based on the stage of the disease and the condition. Condition is termed favorable or unfavorable. If favorable, the prognosis is good. If unfavorable, the tumor is aggressive, and cure is difficult

Priority Assessments or Cues

> Assess abdomen for a firm mass, usually to one side but can be on both sides; avoid palpation of abdomen

> Measure vital signs, blood pressure and temperature are expected to be elevated due to fever and renin excess

> Assess urine for presence of blood. Measure urine output to monitor urinary retention

> Assess results of blood test, looking for anemia

> Ask caregiver about meal intake and appetite

> Assess neurologic system as lethargy is an issue

> Assess respiratory system to determine lung involvement, evidenced by dyspnea and chest pain

> Complete history and physical

> Assess response to treatment

> Assess caregiver's knowledge about treatment plan

> Assess surgical site for signs and symptoms of hemorrhage and infection

Priority Laboratory Tests/Diagnostics

> Ultrasound, computed tomography (CT) scan, magnetic resonance imaging (MRI) used to identify the tumor and determine its exact location

> Chest X-ray looks for metastasis to the lungs (a common organ of metastasis for this tumor)

> Lab tests (blood count and metabolic profile) to examine blood levels such as anemia, white blood cells and certain electrolytes that might be abnormal with cancerous processes in the body

> Kidney biopsy, looking at a piece of tumor tissue under a microscope, should show cancer cells

Priority Interventions or Actions

> Prepare client for nephrectomy

> Prepare client for chemotherapy and radiation after surgery

> Instruct caregiver on expectations postoperatively

> Initiate intravenous line

> Place sign at head of client's bed indicating that abdomen is not to be palpated

> Measure client's abdominal girth daily

> Monitor for hemorrhage and infection at surgery site

> Monitor gastrointestinal system (high-risk of intestinal obstruction)

> Monitor intake and output

> Administer chemotherapy and monitor side effects

> Treat side effects of chemotherapy

> Allow caregiver time to verbalize feelings about child's disease

Priority Potential & Actual Complications

> Hemorrhage, intestinal injury bowel obstruction

> If both kidneys are affected, there will be complication of kidney function

> Spread of tumor to lungs, bone, liver or brain

> High blood pressure may occur due to the tumor or treatment

Priority Nursing Implications

> Never palpate the abdomen as it might cause the encapsulated tumor cells to spread in the abdomen and move into bloodstream and lymph system. The child must be moved and positioned with care

> Allow caregiver the opportunity to be involved in care of child

Priority Medications

> dactinomycin, doxorubicin, vincristine, etoposide, cyclophosphamide, irinotecan

- Several chemotherapy agents used in various combination therapies
- Administered via intravenous infusion, injection or orally
- Chemotherapy drugs are high alert medications. Administer cautiously
- Increased risk of infection, anemia and bleeding due to decreased platelets red and white blood cells

Priority Education/Discharge Issues

> Educate client and family members about the signs and symptoms of postoperative infection. Report fever to provider immediately

> Reinforce the importance of following up with healthcare provider visits

> Teach caregiver how to care for surgery site at home and how to assess for hemorrhage

> Teach about side effects of chemotherapy and ensure caregiver understand how to manage side effects

> Educate caregivers to call health care provider if a lump is felt in their child's abdomen, blood is seen in the urine, or other symptoms associated with Wilms tumor are observed

Next Gen Clinical Judgment

You are caring for a 3-year-old client recently diagnosed with a Wilms tumor. You are assisting the unlicensed assistive personnel (UAP) in the care of the client, including vital signs. You instruct the client not to palpate or press on the abdomen.

1. What reasons/rationale do you provide to explain your instruction?

2. How can the UAP ensure developmentally appropriate care for this client?

3. How can you, as a registered nurse, provide age-appropriate preoperative teaching to this client and the family?

Metabolic syndrome

Pathophysiology/Description

> Metabolic syndrome is not one disease but a group of metabolic risk factors that cause an increase in the likelihood that a person will develop diabetes mellitus, heart disease and stroke

> Risk factor is insulin resistance because of too much visceral fat. Insulin resistance causes the cells of the body to have decreased ability to respond to the action of insulin. The pancreas secretes more insulin in an attempt to compensate and this compounds the issue by causing hyperinsulinemia.

> Cluster of health conditions associated with metabolic syndrome
> - Hypertension
> - Abnormal lipid levels
> - Obesity
> - High blood glucose

> More prevalent in adults, 60 years and older

> Untreated metabolic syndrome places the individual at risk for a myriad of conditions

Priority Assessments or Cues

> Complete a thorough health history

> Determine presence of diagnostic measures

> Measure vital signs

> Assess barriers to lifestyle modification

Priority Laboratory Tests/Diagnostics

> Diagnosis is made if individual has 3 or more of the following
> - Fasting blood glucose greater than or equal to 110 mg/dL or drug treatment for high blood glucose
> - Waist circumference greater than or equal to 40 inches in men and greater than or equal to 35 inches in women
> - Triglycerides greater than 150 mg/dL or drug treatment for high triglycerides
> - Blood pressure greater than or equal to 130 mmHg systolic or 85 mmHg diastolic or drug treatment for hypertension
> - High-density lipoprotein cholesterol less than 40 mg/dL in men and less than 50 mg/dL in women or drug treatment for high cholesterol

Priority Interventions or Actions

> Schedule dietary consult

> Treat symptoms

> Treat conditions that predispose to metabolic syndrome, like high blood pressure and high cholesterol

> Provide resources for community support to reduce risk factors

Priority Potential & Actual Complications

> If metabolic syndrome is not addressed
> - Cardiovascular events
> - Diabetes
> - Stroke
> - Polycystic ovary syndrome
> - Renal disease

Priority Nursing Implications

> Individuals who have metabolic syndrome and smoke are at a much higher risk of getting serious complications

Priority Medications

> Drugs are not usually used to treat metabolic syndrome but if the individual is unable to lower risks with using lifestyle modification, or if there is a high-risk for diabetes mellitus or cardiac events, then blood pressure, cholesterol and diabetes medications may be given

Priority Education/Discharge Issues

> Teach proper lifestyle modification. This is first line intervention

> Teach importance of physical activity and assist with plans to engage in exercise

> Teach strategies to maintain a healthy weight

Next Gen Clinical Judgment

You are caring for a 64-year-old with metabolic syndrome. He would like to begin an exercise program. The client has not exercised since high school. What recommendations do you have for this client?

1. A nurse enters the room of a client with type 1 diabetes. The client is lethargic, diaphoretic, and has a decreased level of consciousness. Which assessment assists the nurse to plan the next nursing action?
   1. The client ate a high carbohydrate breakfast.
   2. The client's insulin is peaking at the time of this encounter.
   3. The client's Hgb A1c is 10%.
   4. The client receives insulin glargine every evening.

2. The nurse is planning discharge teaching for a client with a new diagnosis of Addison's disease. This nurse is addressing home medications. What statement by the client shows an understanding of the material that's been taught?
   1. "I should be able to go care for my grandchildren with chicken pox this weekend."
   2. "I should carry this card in my wallet, with my healthcare provider and my medications listed."
   3. "I will order my MedicAlert bracelet at the end of the month when I get paid."
   4. "I will need to limit my salt and water intake."

3. A client in the clinic has been diagnosed with Cushing's syndrome for several years and comes into the clinic today complaining that "Nobody wants to be around me. I'm fat and ugly, and I smell." Which response by the nurse will be most appropriate?
   1. "Have you been taking all of your medications correctly?"
   2. "I'm sure you just feel that way because you've gained a little weight since last clinic appointment."
   3. "I understand that you feel unattractive right now, but it will get better when your medications stabilize."
   4. "You're not fat and ugly! You look fine to me."

4. A middle-aged client with metabolic syndrome presents to the clinic for help with elevated blood pressure and slight hyperglycemia. What would be the first action taken by the nurse?
   1. Ask the healthcare provider to order a blood pressure lowering medication.
   2. Do dietary teaching for weight loss and control of blood glucose.
   3. Instruct the client to eat a low saturated fat diet.
   4. Work with the client for an overall plan for lifestyle modifications to reduce risks.

5. A client sustains a brain injury subsequent to a motor vehicle accident. The client is being treated with vasopressin. Which would indicate that the medication is effective?
   1. Decreased reabsorption of water in the renal tubules.
   2. A reduction in urine output.
   3. A change in the serum potassium levels.
   4. A specific gravity of 1.035.

6. A teenager was diagnosed with type 1 diabetes mellitus after collapsing during a tennis match. Parents attributed recent complaints of fatigue, frequent urination, hunger, and weight loss to an active schedule. The teen is fearful that competitive tennis will have to be eliminated from her lifestyle. In developing a teaching plan for this teen, what should be the nurse's priority?
   1. Assure the teen that physical activities can be resumed but may have to be modified for a while until the blood glucose/insulin needs are adjusted.
   2. Do dietary teaching to help increase calories during times of physical activity and stress from competition.
   3. Show the insulin pump that can be attached to take care of insulin needs during tennis matches and other strenuous activities.
   4. Tell the teen that all extreme activities, such as tennis and soccer, will have to be permanently curtailed.

7. The nurse is doing discharge teaching with a client who is newly diagnosed with type 2 diabetes. What instructions should the nurse to the client give first?
   1. Be aware that excessive amounts of alcohol intake may lead to unpredictable low glucose reactions.
   2. Examine your feet at home, avoid going barefoot, and avoid applying heat or cold directly to your feet.
   3. Monitor your blood glucose at home and record in a daily log, while demonstrating glucose meter.
   4. Work with the dietician to create an individualized meal plan with healthy food choices at regular times.

8. A nurse is caring for a client with hypothyroidism. The nurse is teaching him the signs he needs to watch for in monitoring his response to levothyroxine sodium. What symptoms would the nurse teach the client to watch for that would indicate a need to decrease the dosage?
   1. Dry mouth and lack of ability to urinate.
   2. Rapid or racing heart rate.
   3. Lethargy and fatigue.
   4. Nausea and a headache.

9. The nurse visits a client who is taking thyroid medication and is having trouble sleeping. The client asks for a "sleeping pill." Which is an appropriate first response by the nurse?
   1. "Do you have any allergies to medications?"
   2. "Have you ever taken medications to help you sleep before?"
   3. "What time of day are you taking your thyroid medication?"
   4. "Have you tried over-the-counter sleeping medication?"

10. A client is hospitalized with diabetic ketoacidosis (DKA), given insulin, and started on intravenous fluids. The nurse completes an assessment and finds the client breathing rapidly, has a rapid pulse, and poor skin turgor. His breath has a fruity odor. What priority action should the nurse next make?
    1. Check the client's blood glucose.
    2. Check to see that the IV fluids are running as prescribed.
    3. Give more insulin per sliding scale.
    4. Send a blood sample for electrolytes to the lab.

11. The client with type 2 diabetes mellitus is admitted to the emergency department with a blood glucose of 650 mg/dL and confusion. A diagnosis of hyperosmolar hyperglycemic nonketotic syndrome (HHNS) is made by the emergency department healthcare provider. What other lab values would be consistent with this syndrome?
    1. Elevated sodium levels.
    2. Ketosis.
    3. Low potassium levels.
    4. Normal phosphorus levels.

12. A client is receiving steroids to manage Addison's disease. Which side effects of this medication would the nurse assess for in this client?
    1. Weight loss and dehydration.
    2. Hyperkalemia and dysrhythmias.
    3. Hyperglycemia and hyperosmolarity.
    4. Alopecia and dry, scaly skin.

13. The nurse plans to teach the client about a diagnosis of hypoparathyroidism, secondary to a thyroidectomy 6 weeks ago. What would be important to teach the client to prevent complications?
    1. Avoid foods high in vitamin D, such as milk and cheese.
    2. Try to minimize stress in your life to prevent complications.
    3. Rebreathe in a paper bag any time you feel numb or tingly around the mouth.
    4. Report any painful spasms in smooth and skeletal muscles.

14. The clinic nurse has assessed a new client with a diagnosis of hypothyroidism after having three large babies over the last five years. The assessment shows insidious weight gain, sluggish thought processes, dry skin and hair, and constipation. What action should the nurse take first?
    1. Avoid allowing the client to get chilled because of cold intolerance.
    2. Discuss the thyroid hormone drug, actions, side effects, when to take it.
    3. Minimize constipation by increased dietary fiber, increased activity, regular elimination time.
    4. Prevent skin breakdown and use soap sparingly.

15. A child who is 7-years-old and is being treated for enuresis. After several other treatments, the child is prescribed desmopressin acetate. The nurse plans to teach the parents that this medication is administrated for which reason?
    1. It decreases stimulation to the bladder.
    2. The child is overhydrated.
    3. It provides antidiuretic hormone.
    4. The medication stimulates pituitary function.

16. A young client was admitted through the emergency department, after collapsing at a high school soccer game. She was diagnosed as having type 1 diabetes mellitus. What assessment findings by the nurse would be consistent with this diagnosis? Select all that apply.
    1. Poor appetite.
    2. Recent history of amenorrhea managed with oral contraceptives.
    3. Recent weight loss, thought by friends to be from dieting.
    4. Drinking frequently throughout the day.
    5. Sudden onset of symptoms, evidenced by the collapse from a hypoglycemic episode.

17. The nurse working in a long-term care facility is teaching a class for the unlicensed assistive personnel about type 2 diabetes mellitus. Which care and comfort needs for the residents should be included in the discussion? Select all that apply.
    1. Frequent skin inspection and position changes.
    2. Inspection and care of the residents' feet.
    3. Limiting visitors to the residents to prevent infections.
    4. Restricting access to television to 3 hours/day.
    5. Showers for residents every other day with emollient cleansers.

18. A client admitted to the intensive care unit was diagnosed with Diabetes Insipidus (DI). The healthcare provider orders intravenous replacement fluids of D5 ½ NS to match each urine output per hour plus one-half of the previous hour's output. Urine output from 0900-1000 was 300 mL. What would be the intravenous volume for 1000-1100? _____ mL

19. The nurse is caring for a client in intensive care with a head injury from a fall. The healthcare provider suspects possible syndrome of inappropriate antidiuretic hormone (SIADH). What factors are important to include in the physical assessment? Select all that apply.
    1. Daily weights on same scales in hospital gown.
    2. Decrease in mental function.
    3. Levels of edema with increased pitting.
    4. Monitor daily protein levels.
    5. Twitching in muscle groups or seizures.

20. A homebound client with type 2 diabetes mellitus calls the nurse to report nausea and flu-like symptoms for two days. What advice should the nurse give the client?
    1. "Be sure to check your blood glucose level every four hours or when you feel symptoms."
    2. "Only take half of your regular dose of insulin or hypoglycemic agent."
    3. "Limit fluid intake to 8 ounces every 4 hours and only eat when you feel hungry."
    4. "Stop taking your oral hypoglycemic since you are not eating or taking in carbohydrates."

21. The nurse is preparing to teach a client who's been recently diagnosed with hyperthyroidism. What instructions should the nurse tell the client? Select all that apply.
    1. Eat a high calorie, high protein diet.
    2. Keep hair and skin clean and well groomed.
    3. Pace activities to keep exertion minimized.
    4. Try to stay calm when in a stressful situation.
    5. Use ordered moisturizing eye drops regularly.

22. A client is taking a thiazide diuretic and has type 2 diabetes. The nurse assesses the client's serum glucose level. Her fasting blood glucose level is 150 mg/dL. Which is an appropriate recommendation by the nurse?
    1. Inform the client to discontinue taking hydrochlorothiazide.
    2. Inform the health care provider of the client's blood glucose and the possible need for a different diuretic.
    3. Instruct the client to take hydrochlorothiazide every other day.
    4. Instruct the client that her fasting blood glucose is elevated and should take an additional antidiabetic drug with the diuretic.

23. A 13-year-old with a body mass index (BMI) of 30 kg/m² enters the clinic with a four-week history of fatigue, frequent urination, and weight loss. Which laboratory study is most critical at this time?
    1. Complete blood count.
    2. Serum electrolytes.
    3. Serum albumin levels.
    4. Random blood glucose.

24. A child newly diagnosed with Wilms tumor is scheduled for surgery. In planning care for the child, which outcome would the nurse deem most important?

Chart Exhibit Nursing Care of the Child with Wilms Tumor—Outcome Planning
EXPECTED OUTCOME
1. Child and caregivers will express decreased anxiety about the outcome of the surgery.
2. Child and caregivers will describe the disease process and treatment plan.
3. Child will maintain normal fluid balance postoperatively.
4. Child will rank pain <3 on a scale of 1-10.

25. The nurse is reviewing discharge education with an adolescent newly diagnosed with diabetes mellitus. Which strategies should the nurse implement when creating a discharge plan of care for monitoring blood glucose levels. Select all that apply.
    1. Maintain the same schedule the adolescent was on during his hospitalization.
    2. Determine the schedule the adolescent is likely to follow at home.
    3. Allow the parents to decide together what the best schedule is for the adolescent.
    4. Tell the parents to always remind the adolescent 15 minutes before a fingerstick.
    5. Gradually allow the adolescent increasing independence in monitoring his blood glucose.

26. The parent of a child with type 1 diabetes mellitus calls the primary care provider about the management of her child who is sick with a fever. Which instructions should the nurse provide?
    1. Do not administer the insulin injections.
    2. Obtain a blood glucose every 8 hours.
    3. Provide only clear liquids for 24 hours.
    4. Test urine for ketones.

27. A client is found unconscious in a park with a MedicAlert bracelet indicating Type I diabetes mellitus. What emergency treatment is indicated if blood glucose monitoring equipment is unavailable?
    1. Administer insulin according to the client's body weight and appearance.
    2. Give the client an oral feeding of juice or sugared soda drink.
    3. Administer glucagon intramuscularly in the client's thigh.
    4. Administer fluids intravenously as soon as access is established.

28. An older adult client is prescribed to receive prednisone to treat an acute exacerbation of rheumatoid arthritis. Which would the nurse include in the teaching plan?
    1. Instruct the client to lower the prednisone dose as the pain decreases.
    2. Advise the client to avoid foods rich in potassium.
    3. Inform the client that prednisone should be taken between meals and without food.
    4. Teach the client about the potential side effects of steroids.

29. A nurse working in an obstetrical practice is identifying those women who are at risk for gestational diabetes during their pregnancy. Which represent risk factors for gestational diabetes? Select all that apply.
    1. Women who are in their teens when they become pregnant.
    2. Clients who have a family history of glucose intolerance.
    3. Women who have a body mass index >30 kg/m^2.
    4. Women with advanced maternal age.
    5. Women who drink alcohol during their pregnancy.
    6. Women with a body mass index of < 18.5 kg/m^2.

30. A nurse is planning the teaching for a young client with type 1 diabetes to test her blood glucose at home. In what order should these steps be conducted? Rank order the responses.
    1. Massage finger and keep hand dependent.
    2. Use lancet to puncture the lateral side of a finger.
    3. Wash hands thoroughly with soap and water.
    4. Calibrate the glucometer.
    5. Record the blood glucose with time and date.

1. **A nurse enters the room of a client with type 1 diabetes. The client is lethargic, diaphoretic, and has a decreased level of consciousness. Which assessment assists the nurse to plan the next nursing action?**
   1. The client ate a high carbohydrate breakfast. *This would increase blood glucose level and signs and symptoms are of low blood glucose.*
   2. ⦿ The client's insulin is peaking at the time of this encounter.
   3. The client's Hgb A1c is 10% *This is a measure of average sugar levels over time and is not pertinent to current signs and symptoms.*
   4. The client receives insulin glargine every evening. *This is a basal dose, and not as significant.*

   Rationale: The insulin peaking indicates that the client's blood glucose is dropping and requires a snack. It may also require monitoring to reduce the dose of the insulin or increase the client's intake. Insulin glargine functions as a basal dose of insulin throughout the 24-hour period and does not peak. Although the dosage may need to be decreased, it is not the priority concern. The glycosylated hemoglobin is elevated but is not a priority at this time.

   THIN Thinking: Help Quick - *It is important for the nurse to quickly determine the problem and act quickly when the client is hypoglycemic.* **NCLEX®:** Physiological Adaptation **QSEN:** Evidence-based Practice

2. **The nurse is planning discharge teaching for a client with a new diagnosis of Addison's disease. This nurse is addressing home medications. What statement by the client shows an understanding of the material that's been taught?**
   1. "I should be able to go care for my grandchildren with chicken pox this weekend." *Clients with this disease should avoid infections.*
   2. ⦿ "I should carry this card in my wallet, with my healthcare provider and my medications listed."
   3. "I will order my MedicAlert bracelet at the end of the month when I get paid." *It would be important for client to obtain this ASAP.*
   4. "I will need to limit my salt and water intake." *Clients with this disease need to increase salt.*

   Rationale: Treatment of Addison's disease (adrenocortical insufficiency) focuses on managing the underlying cause when possible. The nurse plays a key role in the long-term management of the client. The seriousness of the disease and the need for lifelong hormone therapy necessitate a comprehensive teaching plan, including the medications, side effects, symptoms of Addisonian crisis, dietary restrictions, prevention of infection and falls, medical identification, and any additional instructions for the client with secondary diabetes mellitus.

   THIN Thinking: Identify Risk to Safety – *Adrenal crisis is a life-threatening situation and the client needs to be sure that others are alerted, should it occur.* **NCLEX®:** Reduction of Risk Potential **QSEN:** Safety

3. **A client in the clinic has been diagnosed with Cushing's syndrome for several years and comes into the clinic today complaining that "Nobody wants to be around me. I'm fat and ugly, and I smell." Which response by the nurse will be most appropriate?**
   1. "Have you been taking all of your medications correctly?" *This statement would not be helpful as it does not address the verbalized concerns.*
   2. "I'm sure you just feel that way because you've gained a little weight since last clinic appointment." *This statement would not be helpful since it supports the negative feelings.*
   3. ⦿ "I understand that you feel unattractive right now, but it will get better when your medications stabilize."
   4. "You're not fat and ugly! You look fine to me." *False reassurance.*

   Rationale: Emotional support is an important focus of nursing care of the client with Cushing's syndrome. Changes in appearance, such as truncal obesity, multiple bruises, hirsutism in women, and gynecomastia in men, can be distressing. Other symptoms such as acne, striae, and thinning of the hair may occur. The client may feel unattractive or unwanted. The nurse should remain sensitive to the client's feelings and offer respect and unconditional acceptance, giving reassurance that the physical changes and emotional lability will resolve when levels are controlled.

   THIN Thinking: Top Three – *Supporting the client with negative self-perception can provide for hope.* **NCLEX®:** Psychosocial Integrity **QSEN:** Patient-centered Care

4. **A middle-aged client with metabolic syndrome presents to the clinic for help with elevated blood pressure and slight hyperglycemia. What would be the first action taken by the nurse?**
   1. Ask the healthcare provider to order a blood pressure lowering medication. *Not the first intervention. Item does not demonstrate an urgent need for blood pressure.*
   2. Do dietary teaching for weight loss and control of blood glucose. *Not the first intervention. Item does not demonstrate an urgent need for glucose control.*
   3. Instruct the client to eat a low saturated fat diet. *Not the first intervention. Assessment and planning need to occur first.*
   4. ⦿ Work with the client for an overall plan for lifestyle modifications to reduce risks.

Rationale: Lifestyle modifications are the first line interventions to reduce risk factors associated with metabolic syndrome and reducing risk factors for cardiovascular disease. There is no specific management of metabolic syndrome, but information on healthy diets to lower LDL cholesterol, control blood pressure and blood glucose, activity/exercise, weight loss, and other positive lifestyle changes may be effective.

THIN Thinking: Nursing Process – *Once the nurse identified a problem it is important to create a success plan that the client can be involved in.* **NCLEX®:** Health Promotion and Maintenance **QSEN:** Quality improvement

5. **A client sustains a brain injury subsequent to a motor vehicle accident. The client is being treated with vasopressin. Which would indicate that the medication is effective?**
   1. Decreased reabsorption of water in the renal tubules. *Inaccurate. Vasopressin increases reabsorption of water.*
   2. A reduction in urine output.
   3. A change in the serum potassium levels. *Inaccurate. The goal of the medication is not to change potassium levels.*
   4. A specific gravity of 1.035. *This is too high and indicated dehydration.*

   Rationale: Clients with a brain injury may have pituitary gland involvement. Vasopressin is antidiuretic hormone and indicated for diabetes insipidus (DI), which results in a large amount of urine output. The client is at risk of dehydration and electrolyte imbalance if this medication is not given. The medication decreases the urine output and is used for treatment of DI.

   THIN Thinking: Nursing Process – *The nurse needs to understand how to evaluate a client's status to determine effectiveness of a medication.* **NCLEX®:** Pharmacological and Parenteral Therapies **QSEN:** Patient-centered Care

6. **A teenager was diagnosed with type 1 diabetes mellitus after collapsing during a tennis match. Parents attributed recent complaints of fatigue, frequent urination, hunger, and weight loss to an active schedule. The teen is fearful that competitive tennis will have to be eliminated from her lifestyle. In developing a teaching plan for this teen, what should be the nurse's priority?**
   1. Assure the teen that physical activities can be resumed but may have to be modified for a while until the blood glucose/insulin needs are adjusted.
   2. Do dietary teaching to help increase calories during times of physical activity and stress from competition. *Doesn't address client's fears.*
   3. Show the insulin pump that can be attached to take care of insulin needs during tennis matches and other strenuous activities. *Doesn't address client's fears.*
   4. Tell the teen that all extreme activities, such as tennis and soccer, will have to be permanently curtailed. *Untrue statement.*

Rationale: Overall goals for the client with type 1 diabetes are to: 1) engage in self-care behaviors to actively manage diabetes, 2) experience few or no hyperglycemic or hypoglycemic emergencies, 3) maintain blood glucose levels at normal or new-normal levels, 4) prevent or minimize long-term complications related to diabetes, and 5) adjust lifestyle to accommodate the diabetes plan with minimum stress. Clients with diabetes have high rates of depression, anxiety, and eating disorders, contributing to diminished diabetes self-care, feelings of helplessness, and poor outcomes. In a teen whose body and body image are changing, some of these feelings may be pronounced so, it is important to understand a teen's development. Nursing activities and teaching should promote healthy development, along with teaching for self-care of one's disease process. Being like one's peers is extremely important for adolescents, and any deviation from that "norm" is extremely difficult for them to accept.

THIN Thinking: Nursing Process – *It is important for the nurse to reassure the client that a normal lifestyle with some modifications can be achieved.* **NCLEX®:** Psychosocial Integrity **QSEN:** Patient-centered Care

7. **The nurse is doing discharge teaching with a client who is newly diagnosed with type 2 diabetes. What instructions should the nurse to the client give first?**
   1. Be aware that excessive amounts of alcohol intake may lead to unpredictable low glucose reactions. *Not the priority at this time.*
   2. Examine your feet at home, avoid going barefoot, and avoid applying heat or cold directly to your feet. *Important, but not the priority.*
   3. Monitor your blood glucose at home and record in a daily log, while demonstrating glucose meter.
   4. Work with the dietician to create an individualized meal plan with healthy food choices at regular times. *Important, but not the priority.*

Rationale: The goals of diabetes self-management education are to match the level of self-management to the individual's ability to promote the most active participant possible. Diabetes self-management teaching is a multi-faceted approach, including checking one's blood glucose levels, exercise/activity, dietary, foot care/cleanliness, and complication prevention and recognition. Many resources are available for teaching clients. Blood glucose monitoring is an essential component of initial teaching about diabetes management.

THIN Thinking: Top Three – *The priority for diabetic teaching is to monitor and control glucose levels to prevent urgent life-threatening complications.* **NCLEX®:** Physiological Adaptation **QSEN:** Patient-centered Care

8. A nurse is caring for a client with hypothyroidism. The nurse is teaching him the signs he needs to watch for in monitoring his response to levothyroxine sodium. What symptoms would the nurse teach the client to watch for that would indicate a need to decrease the dosage?
   1. Dry mouth and lack of ability to urinate. *Inaccurate. Not related to the medication.*
   2. 💡 Rapid or racing heart rate.
   3. Lethargy and fatigue. *This is an indication of too little medication.*
   4. Nausea and a headache. *May not be related to the medication.*

   Rationale: Hypothyroidism is characterized by a hypometabolic state. Levothyroxine is a medication to manage symptoms and elevate the metabolic rate. If too much medication is given, the client becomes hypermetabolic and experiences hypermetabolism symptoms, such as tachycardia and palpitations. Clients are taught to monitor their heart rate and report tachycardia to the healthcare provider and the dose may need to be reduced. The other symptoms are not correct.

   THIN Thinking: Top Three – *Excess intake of levothyroxine is exhibited by signs on hypermetabolism. The rapid heart rate is the highest concern due to the stress on the heart.* **NCLEX®:** Pharmacological and Parenteral Therapies **QSEN:** Patient-centered Care

9. The nurse visits a client who is taking thyroid medication and is having trouble sleeping. The client asks for a "sleeping pill." Which is an appropriate first response by the nurse?
   1. "Do you have any allergies to medications?" *Doesn't address concern.*
   2. "Have you ever taken medications to help you sleep before?" *Not as important to know as when client is taking thyroid medication.*
   3. 💡 "What time of day are you taking your thyroid medication?"
   4. "Have you tried over-the-counter sleeping medication?" *Need to know timing of thyroid medication first.*

   Rationale: Thyroid supplementation, levothyroxine, may cause wakefulness and insomnia. The client is instructed to take their medication in the morning to avoid trouble sleeping. Experts recommend that the dose is given one-half hour prior to breakfast to ensure complete absorption and maximum effect.

   THIN Thinking: Nursing Process – *Further assessment is the priority to determine what can be causing the sleeplessness.* **NCLEX®:** Pharmacological and Parenteral Therapies **QSEN:** Patient-centered Care

10. A client is hospitalized with diabetic ketoacidosis (DKA), given insulin, and started on intravenous fluids. The nurse completes an assessment and finds the client breathing rapidly, has a rapid pulse, and poor skin turgor. His breath has a fruity odor. What priority action should the nurse next make?
    1. Check the client's blood glucose. *The glucose will be high, it's already been established that the client is in DKA.*
    2. 💡 Check to see that the IV fluids are running as prescribed.
    3. Give more insulin per sliding scale. *Fluids will help to correct the acidosis. Glucose cannot be dropped too rapidly or complications can occur.*
    4. Send a blood sample for electrolytes to the lab. *Assessment indicates fluid volume deficit, electrolytes are not the priority.*

    Rationale: The client is still showing signs of DKA. Fluid resuscitation is critical for hemodynamics stabilization and appropriate access is critical. The client has received insulin, so the nurse would make sure the intravenous line is patent and running and then double check the blood glucose and give insulin per sliding scale. On-going monitoring would include vital signs, breath sounds, blood glucose and serum potassium, and administration of other ordered medications.

    THIN Thinking: Top Three – *Rehydration is the priority, followed with glucose assessment and additional insulin per order.* **NCLEX®:** Pharmacological and Parenteral Therapies **QSEN:** Patient-centered Care

11. The client with type 2 diabetes mellitus is admitted to the emergency department with a blood glucose of 650 mg/dL and confusion. A diagnosis of hyperosmolar hyperglycemic nonketotic syndrome (HHNS) is made by the emergency department healthcare provider. What other lab values would be consistent with this syndrome?
    1. Elevated sodium levels. *Sodium is normally low.*
    2. Ketosis *No ketones with HHNS.*
    3. 💡 Low potassium levels.
    4. Normal phosphorus levels. *Phosphorus is normally low.*

    Rationale: In the pathophysiology of HHNS, the individual may have enough insulin on board to prevent DKA and ketosis, but not enough to prevent severe hyperglycemia, osmotic diuresis, and extracellular fluid deficit. HHNS also causes hyponatremia, hypokalemia, hypophosphatemia, hyperosmolality, and profound dehydration—all leading to decreased renal perfusion, hypotension, and hemoconcentration. Potentially without treatment the individual can suffer from seizures, shock, coma, and death.

    THIN Thinking: Nursing Process – *Understanding and anticipating labs is important to the care of a critical client.* **NCLEX®:** Basic Care and Comfort **QSEN:** Patient-centered Care

12. **A client is receiving steroids to manage Addison's disease. Which side effects of this medication would the nurse assess for in this client?**
    1. Weight loss and dehydration. *Side effects of corticosteroids would be increased weight.*
    2. Hyperkalemia and dysrhythmias. *Side effects would be a low potassium.*
    3. 🔘 Hyperglycemia and hyperosmolarity.
    4. Alopecia and dry, scaly skin. *These are signs of Addison's.*

    Rationale: Clients with Addison's disease are deficient in adrenal function and in endogenous corticosteroids. They are treated with steroids, usually oral doses of prednisone. Known side effects of the steroids are hyperglycemia and hyperosmolarity which may lead to edema, swelling, and water retention.

    THIN Thinking: Nursing Process – *It is important for the nurse to identify side effects of medications and differentiate them from the illness.* **NCLEX®:** Pharmacological and Parenteral Therapies **QSEN:** Patient-centered Care

13. **The nurse plans to teach the client about a diagnosis of hypoparathyroidism, secondary to a thyroidectomy 6 weeks ago. What would be important to teach the client to prevent complications?**
    1. Avoid foods high in vitamin D, such as milk and cheese. *Client should increase intake of these foods.*
    2. Try to minimize stress in your life to prevent complications. *This is not a priority.*
    3. Rebreathe in a paper bag any time you feel numb or tingly around the mouth. *This would not be indicated.*
    4. 🔘 Report any painful spasms in smooth and skeletal muscles.

    Rationale: Managing long-term complications associated with hypoparathyroidism is the overarching goal of treatment. These include ensuring calcium level is normal and preventing tetany.

    THIN Thinking: Help Quick - *The loss of the parathyroid gland can result in hypocalcemia. The nurse must quickly recognize symptoms of hypocalcemia.* **NCLEX®:** Management of Care **QSEN:** Patient-centered Care

14. **The clinic nurse has assessed a new client with a diagnosis of hypothyroidism after having three large babies over the last five years. The assessment shows insidious weight gain, sluggish thought processes, dry skin and hair, and constipation. What action should the nurse take first?**
    1. Avoid allowing the client to get chilled because of cold intolerance. *Not the first step, cold is related to comfort.*
    2. 🔘 Discuss the thyroid hormone drug, actions, side effects, when to take it.
    3. Minimize constipation by increased dietary fiber, increased activity, regular elimination time. *Not the first step, constipation is a longer-term concern.*
    4. Prevent skin breakdown and use soap sparingly. *Not the first step, this is long-term care.*

    Rationale: Most people with hypothyroidism are treated on an outpatient basis. Teaching regarding medication management and identification of complications is most essential, with the need for lifelong drug therapy and follow-up. Avoid abrupt discontinuation of meds, and caution against doubling up on or changing doses for any reason.

    THIN Thinking: Help Quick – *The goal is to prioritize the most urgent concerns for teaching.* **NCLEX®:** Safety and Infection Control **QSEN:** Safety

15. **A child who is 7-years-old and is being treated for enuresis. After several other treatments, the child is prescribed desmopressin acetate. The nurse plans to teach the parents that this medication is administrated for which reason?**
    1. It decreases stimulation to the bladder. *Inaccurate.*
    2. The child is overhydrated. *Inaccurate.*
    3. 🔘 It provides antidiuretic hormone.
    4. The medication stimulates pituitary function. *Inaccurate.*

    Rationale: After other therapies, including behavioral modification, teaching child to change self and sheets, restricting fluids (especially caffeinated beverages), conditioning therapy, and frequent toileting, medication may be indicated. Desmopressin provides synthetic antidiuretic hormone which decreases the urine output. The goal of therapy is short-term use of medication to retrain the child not to void in bed. The other answers are not correct.

    THIN Thinking: Nursing Process – *The nurse must understand medications in order to properly teach the client and family.* **NCLEX®:** Pharmacological and Parenteral Therapies **QSEN:** Evidence-based Practice

16. **A young client was admitted through the emergency department, after collapsing at a high school soccer game. She was diagnosed as having type 1 diabetes mellitus. What assessment findings by the nurse would be consistent with this diagnosis? Select all that apply.**
    1. Poor appetite. *Appetite usually increases.*
    2. Recent history of amenorrhea managed with oral contraceptives. *Not significant.*
    3. 🔘 Recent weight loss, thought by friends to be from dieting.
    4. 🔘 Drinking frequently throughout the day.
    5. 🔘 Sudden onset of symptoms, evidenced by the collapse from a hypoglycemic episode.

Rationale: With Type I diabetes mellitus, there is usually a sudden onset, a strong genetic link, and a complex interaction with autoimmune and environmental factors. The individual usually has a history of recent and sudden weight loss, excessive thirst, frequent urination, excessive hunger, and fatigue.

THIN Thinking: Nursing Process – *The nurse should be able to recognize assessment findings and risk factors of illness in order to plan care.* NCLEX®: Safety and Infection Control QSEN: Patient-centered Care

17. **The nurse working in a long-term care facility is teaching a class for the unlicensed assistive personnel about type 2 diabetes mellitus. Which care and comfort needs for the residents should be included in the discussion? Select all that apply.**
    1. 🔘 Frequent skin inspection and position changes.
    2. 🔘 Inspection and care of the residents' feet.
    3. Limiting visitors to the residents to prevent infections. *Although the diabetic is more prone to infection, visitors should not be restricted.*
    4. Restricting access to television to 3 hours/day. *Not pertinent.*
    5. 🔘 Showers for residents every other day with emollient cleansers.

Rationale: The goals of diabetes management are to reduce symptoms, promote well-being, prevent acute complications related to hyper-hypoglycemia, and prevent or delay onset and progression of long-term complications. These goals are most likely to be met when the client can maintain blood glucose levels as near to normal as possible (via glucose monitoring and medications—not within the UAP's scope of practice), decisions about (and in the case of clients in long-term care—encouragement) of appropriate food intake, positioning, and exercise, along with client teaching. Comfort measures include skin care and hygiene.

THIN Thinking: Nursing Process – *The nurse needs to be able to identify priority teaching needs while understanding the scope of practice of the assistive personnel.* NCLEX®: Basic Care and Comfort QSEN: Teamwork and Collaboration

18. **A client admitted to the intensive care unit was diagnosed with Diabetes Insipidus (DI). The healthcare provider orders intravenous replacement fluids of D5 ½ NS to match each urine output per hour plus one-half of the previous hour's output. Urine output from 0900-1000 was 300 mL. What would be the intravenous volume for 1000-1100? _____ mL**

Answer: 450 mL

Rationale: For central DI, fluid and hormone therapy is the cornerstone of treatment. Fluids are replaced orally or IV, depending on the client's condition and ability to drink copious amounts of fluids. IV hypotonic saline or dextrose 5% in water is given and titrated to replace urine output. 300 mL + ½ (300) = 450 mL.

THIN Thinking: Identify Risk to Safety – *It is important for the nurse to safely titrate IV fluids to meet the hydration needs of the client.* NCLEX®: Pharmacological and Parenteral Therapies QSEN: Patient-centered Care

19. **The nurse is caring for a client in intensive care with a head injury from a fall. The healthcare provider suspects possible syndrome of inappropriate antidiuretic hormone (SIADH). What factors are important to include in the physical assessment? Select all that apply.**
    1. 🔘 Daily weights on same scales in hospital gown.
    2. 🔘 Decrease in mental function.
    3. 🔘 Levels of edema with increased pitting.
    4. Monitor daily protein levels. *Not significant for this client.*
    5. 🔘 Twitching in muscle groups or seizures.

Rationale: Causes of SIADH can be cancer, central nervous system injuries (head injury, stroke, tumors, infections & others), drug therapy, hypothyroidism, lung infections or COPD, HIV, or adrenal insufficiency. The client may experience low urine output and increased body weight, muscle cramping, irritability, headache, thirst, edema, fatigue/lethargy, confusion, seizures, and coma. It is important that the client suspected of SIADH be monitored closely for progressing symptoms and appropriate actions taken to treat the cause and prevent a downward or irreversible cascade of symptoms.

THIN Thinking: Help Quick – *The nurse needs to recognize that because of the low sodium level and excess water in the vascular space, the client is at risk for injury.* NCLEX®: Reduction of Risk Potential QSEN: Patient-centered Care

20. **A homebound client with type 2 diabetes mellitus calls the nurse to report nausea and flu-like symptoms for two days. What advice should the nurse give the client?**
    1. 🔘 "Be sure to check your blood glucose level every four hours or when you feel symptoms."
    2. "Only take half of your regular dose of insulin or hypoglycemic agent." *Inaccurate- client may require more insulin due to infection.*
    3. "Limit fluid intake to 8 ounces every 4 hours and only eat when you feel hungry." *Client should increase fluid intake.*
    4. "Stop taking your oral hypoglycemic since you are not eating or taking in carbohydrates." *Inaccurate. The stress of illness with cause the glucose levels to rise.*

Rationale: When clients are ill, stress hormones are released throughout the body as corticosteroids. These are glucose-based and raise the blood glucose which can lead to hyperglycemia and ketosis. One of the leading precursors of diabetic ketoacidosis (DKA) is being ill and not taking insulin or oral hypoglycemics. Also, the client may experience low blood glucose due to lack of intake or losses due to diarrhea or vomiting. Therefore, the client needs to monitor blood glucose and ketone levels closely in order to avoid hyperglycemia and these sequelae. The nurse should recommend drinking water to lower blood glucose and ketones. The nurse can't recommend stopping medications or changing the dose of insulin.

THIN Thinking: Identify Risk to Safety – *Because the stress of illness can cause glucose levels to rise, the nurse should encourage more frequent glucose monitoring to prevent injury.* **NCLEX®:** Physiological Adaptation **QSEN:** Safety

21. **The nurse is preparing to teach a client who's been recently diagnosed with hyperthyroidism. What instructions should the nurse tell the client? Select all that apply.**
    1. ◉ Eat a high calorie, high protein diet.
    2. ◉ Keep hair and skin clean and well groomed.
    3. ◉ Pace activities to keep exertion minimized.
    4. Try to stay calm when in a stressful situation. *Not a concern. Stress is not regulated by the thyroid gland.*
    5. ◉ Use ordered moisturizing eye drops regularly.

Rationale: Clinical manifestations of hyperthyroidism are related to the effect of excess circulating thyroid hormone, directly increasing metabolism and tissue sensitivity to stimulation by the sympathetic nervous system. Symptoms may include exophthalmos, bounding rapid pulse, palpitations, angina, dyspnea on exertion, increased respiratory rate, heat intolerance, hair loss, thin & brittle nails, increased bowel sounds & peristalsis, warm & moist skin with diaphoresis, palmar erythema. Stress itself does not exacerbate the symptoms of hyperthyroidism. The goal of management is to block the adverse effects of excessive thyroid hormone (as with drugs, radiation, or surgery) and to prevent complications (e.g. respiratory or cardiac distress, dehydration or malnutrition, drying corneas and visual difficulties, as well as acute thyrotoxicosis—a medical emergency).

THIN Thinking: Identify Risk to Safety – *The nurse needs to create a teaching plan that reduces the client's risk of developing complications.* **NCLEX®:** Safety and Infection Control **QSEN:** Safety

22. **A client is taking a thiazide diuretic and has type 2 diabetes. The nurse assesses the client's serum glucose level. Her fasting blood glucose level is 150 mg/dL. Which is an appropriate recommendation by the nurse?**
    1. Inform the client to discontinue taking hydrochlorothiazide. *Nurse would not discontinue drug without a prescription.*
    2. ◉ Inform the health care provider of the client's blood glucose and the possible need for a different diuretic.
    3. Instruct the client to take hydrochlorothiazide every other day. *Nurse would not change dosing of drug without a prescription.*
    4. Instruct the client that her fasting blood glucose is elevated and should take an additional antidiabetic drug with the diuretic. *Nurse would not prescribe drug.*

Rationale: Thiazide diuretics are known to raise the blood glucose and are often not recommended for clients who have type 2 diabetes. The nurse cannot change the dosage of the medication but can recommend the client consult the healthcare provider. Normal serum glucose level is 80-110 mg/dL. The value of 150 mg/dL indicates an elevated value which may be caused by the thiazide diuretic.

THIN Thinking: Identify Risk to Safety – *The nurse needs to understand how medications can affect each other and to intervene when appropriate.* **NCLEX®:** Pharmacology and Parenteral Therapies **QSEN:** Patient-centered Care

23. **A 13-year-old with a body mass index (BMI) of 30 kg/m² enters the clinic with a four-week history of fatigue, frequent urination, and weight loss. Which laboratory study is most critical at this time?**
    1. Complete blood count. *A CBC includes WBCs, RBCs, and platelets. Not a priority given the symptoms.*
    2. Serum electrolytes. *The potassium level could be of concern, but a glucose level is needed first.*
    3. Serum albumin levels. *Although this can indicate malnutrition, it is not the priority.*
    4. ◉ Random blood glucose.

Rationale: The client's obesity, polyuria, fatigue, and weight loss may indicate type 1 or type 2 diabetes. Obesity is known to increase insulin resistance. A fasting blood glucose is preferable, but a random level will indicate current blood glucose levels. The other diagnostics may be important after blood glucose is determined.

THIN Thinking: Top Three – *Given the client's presenting symptoms, a random blood glucose is priority to rule out diabetes.* **NCLEX®:** Physiological Adaptation **QSEN:** Evidence-based Practice

24. A child newly diagnosed with Wilms tumor is scheduled for surgery. In planning care for the child, which outcome would the nurse deem most important?

Chart Exhibit Nursing Care of the Child with Wilms Tumor—Outcome Planning
EXPECTED OUTCOME
1. Child and caregivers will express decreased anxiety about the outcome of the surgery.
2. ⦿ Child and caregivers will describe the disease process and treatment plan.
3. Child will maintain normal fluid balance postoperatively.
4. Child will rank pain <3 on a scale of 1-10.

Rationale: The most common cancer in children is Wilms tumor or nephroblastoma. In planning care of a child with this condition, who is scheduled for surgery, the nurse must ensure that the child and caregiver(s) understand the disease process and the plan of treatment for the child. Having a firm understanding of both, will allow the child and caregiver (s) to be fully involved in the child's care after surgery.

THIN Thinking: Nursing Process – *Preoperatively, the priority is client/family teaching. In planning care, this must be a priority focus for the nurse.* **NCLEX®:** Management of Care **QSEN:** Teamwork and Collaboration

25. The nurse is reviewing discharge education with an adolescent newly diagnosed with diabetes mellitus. Which strategies should the nurse implement when creating a discharge plan of care for monitoring blood glucose levels. Select all that apply.
1. Maintain the same schedule the adolescent was on during his hospitalization. *Does not give client control.*
2. ⦿ Determine the schedule the adolescent is likely to follow at home.
3. Allow the parents to decide together what the best schedule is for the adolescent. *Does not give client input.*
4. Tell the parents to always remind the adolescent 15 minutes before a fingerstick. *Client should not require constant reminders.*
5. ⦿ Gradually allow the adolescent increasing independence in monitoring his blood glucose.

Rationale: An adolescent is more likely to follow a schedule that he or she has created based on his or her usual daily schedule. Gradually increasing independence is appropriate for an adolescent learning about the management of his care though it is still beneficial for parents to have some management in the care.

THIN Thinking: Nursing Process – *Preparing for a plan that meets the client's needs will increase the likelihood of compliance and decrease the risk of complications, including diabetic ketoacidosis.* **NCLEX®:** Management of Care **QSEN:** Patient-centered Care

26. The parent of a child with type 1 diabetes mellitus calls the primary care provider about the management of her child who is sick with a fever. Which instructions should the nurse provide?
1. Do not administer the insulin injections. *Inaccurate.*
2. Obtain a blood glucose every 8 hours. *Should be checked more frequently.*
3. Provide only clear liquids for 24 hours. *Unnecessary.*
4. ⦿ Test urine for ketones.

Rationale: Testing the urine for ketones will determine if additional insulin is needed. The parent should administer all insulin injections and test the blood glucose at least every 4 hours. Though clear liquids are encouraged, the child should try to follow their usual eating habits.

THIN Thinking: Identify Risk to Safety – *A fever in a child with diabetes increases the risk of complications.* **NCLEX®:** Physiological Adaptation **QSEN:** Safety

27. A client is found unconscious in a park with a MedicAlert bracelet indicating Type I diabetes mellitus. What emergency treatment is indicated if blood glucose monitoring equipment is unavailable?
1. Administer insulin according to the client's body weight and appearance. *Low blood glucose is more dangerous than high blood glucose.*
2. Give the client an oral feeding of juice or sugared soda drink. *Client is unconscious.*
3. ⦿ Administer glucagon intramuscularly in the client's thigh.
4. Administer fluids intravenously as soon as access is established. *Would not be the first intervention.*

Rationale: It is known that the client has type 1 diabetes but it is not known if his unconsciousness is the result of high or low blood glucose or another etiology. Because hypoglycemia occurs rapidly and blood glucose can go dangerously low, leading to seizures, coma, and death, it is recommended to suspect it is a low and treat with glucagon. This will raise the blood glucose if low but will not dramatically change a high blood glucose. If the client does not become conscious, then other interventions will be employed.

THIN Thinking: Identify Risk to Safety – *If it is unknown if the glucose is high or low in the unconscious diabetic, it is better to treat as if it is hypoglycemia.* **NCLEX®:** Physiological Adaptation **QSEN:** Safety

28. An older adult client is prescribed to receive prednisone to treat an acute exacerbation of rheumatoid arthritis. Which would the nurse include in the teaching plan?
    1. Instruct the client to lower the prednisone dose as the pain decreases. *Nurse needs a prescription to change dosing.*
    2. Advise the client to avoid foods rich in potassium. *This is irrelevant.*
    3. Inform the client that prednisone should be taken between meals and without food. *Should be taken with meals.*
    4. ☻ Teach the client about the potential side effects of steroids.

Rationale: The client needs to be taught about side effects of steroids due to the large number of potential side and adverse effects associated with this medication. Although the dose of the medication is tapered down, the tapering schedule should be part of the prescription and not only at the client's discretion. The medication can't be withdrawn too quickly to avoid adrenal insufficiency. Prednisone may lower serum potassium levels so the client is encouraged to eat normal or increased amounts of potassium and serum potassium levels should be monitored. Prednisone is irritating to the gastric lining so it should be taken with meals.

THIN Thinking: Identify Risk to Safety – *The nurse must teach the client the side effects of all new medications. Steroids offer many risks and thorough education is important.* **NCLEX®:** Pharmacology and Parenteral Therapies **QSEN:** Safety

29. A nurse working in an obstetrical practice is identifying those women who are at risk for gestational diabetes during their pregnancy. Which represent risk factors for gestational diabetes? Select all that apply.
    1. Women who are in their teens when they become pregnant. *This does not offer a greater risk.*
    2. ☻ Clients who have a family history of glucose intolerance.
    3. ☻ Women who have a body mass index >30 kg/m².
    4. ☻ Women with advanced maternal age.
    5. Women who drink alcohol during their pregnancy. *Inaccurate.*
    6. Women with a body mass index of < 18.5 kg/m². *Inaccurate.*

Rationale: Gestational diabetes is associated with family history of glucose intolerance or diabetes mellitus (Types 1 and 2), obesity, and advanced maternal age. Being a teenager and pregnant, drinking alcohol, and being underweight are not associated with gestational diabetes, although these characteristics may place the woman at risk for other complications or issues.

THIN Thinking: Identify Risk to Safety – *Identification of risk for complications is an important part of the nurse's role.* **NCLEX®:** Physiological Adaptation **QSEN:** Safety

30. A nurse is planning the teaching for a young client with type 1 diabetes to test her blood glucose at home. In what order should these steps be conducted? Rank order the responses.
    1. Wash hands thoroughly with soap and water.
    2. Calibrate the glucometer.
    3. Use lancet to puncture the lateral side of a finger.
    4. Massage finger and keep hand dependent.
    5. Record the blood glucose with time and date.

Rationale: Alcohol is no longer recommended because it dries the skin and causes skin breakdown. Therefore, handwashing is indicated. Calibration ensures the meter is working correctly, the lateral side of the finger tends to yield greater blood flow and samples, and massaging encourages blood flow and an adequate sample. Recording the reading and actions are important to determine trends and future treatment.

THIN Thinking: Identify Risk to Safety – *In order to obtain accurate information, safely the nurse must perform the actions in the proper order.* **NCLEX®:** Physiological Adaptation **QSEN:** Evidence-based Practice

CHAPTER

13

Movement

Mobility / Sensory / Nerve conduction

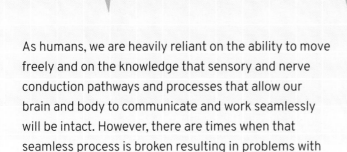

As humans, we are heavily reliant on the ability to move freely and on the knowledge that sensory and nerve conduction pathways and processes that allow our brain and body to communicate and work seamlessly will be intact. However, there are times when that seamless process is broken resulting in problems with how we move and manage our daily lives.

There are many illnesses that stem from impairment in sensory and nerve conduction and as nurses you must be knowledgeable about these illnesses and be able to apply that knowledge as you provide quality care to clients.

Priority Exemplars:

- Cerebral palsy
- Seizures
- Osteoporosis
- Osteoarthritis
- Fractures

- Peripheral neuropathy
- Trigeminal neuralgia
- Carpal tunnel
- Amputation
- Amyotrophic lateral sclerosis
- Guillain-Barré syndrome
- Multiple sclerosis
- Myasthenia gravis
- Parkinson's disease
- Cataracts
- Glaucoma
- Conjunctivitis
- Macular degeneration
- Hearing impairment
- Scoliosis
- Labyrinthitis/Meniere's disease
- Otitis media/externa
- Spina bifida
- Spinal cord injury

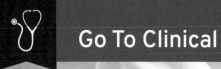

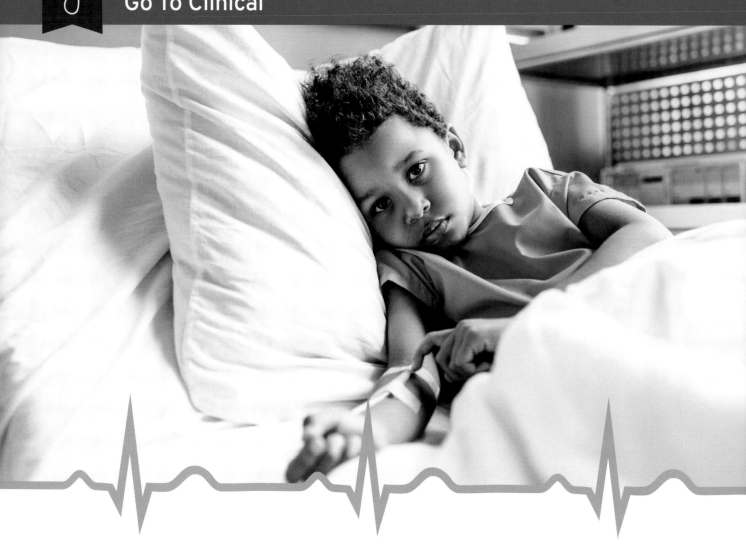

Go To Clinical Case 1

M.N. is a 3-year-old boy who has been seen by the pediatrician because his parents are concerned something is "wrong with M.N." His mother states that when M.N.'s brother was his age, he was riding a bike, dressing and undressing himself and running around the house but M.N. is not able to do those things. He walks very slowly, and they notice that his body seems somewhat "stiff." When he tries to speak, he has a hard time getting his words out and he gets very frustrated because he cannot seem to grasp small pieces of toys, like his puzzle pieces. M.N.'s parents reveal that he was very slow to roll over and sit up, but they attributed that to the fact that he was born prematurely.

Vital signs are: Temperature 99.0°F, pulse 102, respirations 22, blood pressure 98/66. The pediatrician's initial assessment suspects that M.N. has cerebral palsy and further testing is ordered. You are the nurse caring for M.N. today.

NurseThink® Time

Using the NurseThink® system, complete the priorities. Check your answers designated by 💡 in the Cerebral palsy Priority Exemplar.

Priority Assessments or Cues

1.

2.

3.

Priority Laboratory Tests/Diagnostics

1.

2.

3.

Priority Interventions or Actions

1.

2.

3.

Priority Potential & Actual Complications

1.

2.

3.

Priority Nursing Implications

1.

2.

3.

Priority Medications

1.

2.

3.

Priority Education/Discharge Issues

1.

2.

3.

Cerebral palsy

Pathophysiology/Description

> Cerebral palsy (CP) is a disorder that affects the ability of an individual to move and maintain proper posture. It results from an abnormality in the pyramidal or extrapyramidal motor system

> While some persons with cerebral palsy are not able to walk or function independently, others are able to walk and perform activities of daily living without difficulty

> Types of cerebral palsy
> - Spastic cerebral palsy, which is the most common type. With this type of CP, the person's body has increased muscle tone, causing stiffness
> - Dyskinetic cerebral palsy causes loss of control with movements of the hands and feet, making walking and sitting challenging for the person with dyskinetic CP
> - Ataxic cerebral palsy causes poor coordination and balance so persons with ataxic CP may be unsteady on their feet when they walk
> - Mixed cerebral palsy incorporates a combination of different types of CP, most common combination being dyskinetic and spastic

> Cerebral palsy has significant impact on every aspect of the individual's life and can cause a myriad of other health problems. Seizures, deafness and blindness are often seen in persons with cerebral palsy

> There are several causes and risk factor associated with CP. Here are just a few:
> - Fetal stroke due to lack of blood flow to the developing brain
> - Genetic: mutation in genes
> - Infections in infancy that affect the brain
> - Maternal infections that affect the fetus in development
> - Decreased oxygenation during labor
> - Infant involved in a traumatic head injury, such as a fall
> - Zika virus
> - Measles and chickenpox (both can cause pregnancy complications)
> - Herpes, cytomegalovirus, syphilis from mother to infant
> - Exposure to certain toxins while pregnant

Priority Assessments or Cues

> Assess for variations in muscle tone and movement, such as floppiness, stiffness, exaggerated reflexes, tremors, involuntary movements

> Determine the child's attainment of developmental milestones. Ask caregiver about child's progression to developmental milestones since birth. Lack of reaching developmental milestones is an early sign of CP

> Assess use of hands, child may favor one side of the body, using the same hand all the time and never attempting to use the other

> Assess the child's gait (if able to walk), may observe a crouched walk, wide gait, tip-toe walking or knees crossing when walking

> Assess child's mouth, may find drooling

> Assess eating, may see difficulty swallowing or difficulty with eating

> Assess child's speech, may find that there is difficulty getting words out or delayed development of speech

> Assess child's fine motor skills, may find inability to pick up objects or use objects, such as using a crayon to color

> Assess for seizure activity as these are oftentimes seen in CP

> Assess child for extreme irritability and crying

> Assess for abnormal posture such as bent sideways or exaggerated arching of the back

Priority Laboratory Tests/Diagnostics

> There are no tests to diagnose CP but some tests may be done to look at some of the symptoms related to CP
> - Cranial ultrasound to provide a first assessment of the brain
> - Magnetic resonance imaging (MRI) to detect neurological abnormalities or lesions
> - Computed tomography (CT) scan to help determine the cause and time of a brain injury that may have contributed to the cerebral palsy
> - Electroencephalogram (EEG) for assessing seizure activity

Priority Interventions or Actions

> An interprofessional, long-term intervention is needed for a child with cerebral palsy
> - Physical therapist to help with muscle strength and gait
> - Occupational therapist to help with activities of daily living and adaptive equipment
> - Speech therapist to manage speech problems and impaired swallowing
> - Mental health professional to assist child with coping skills
> - Orthopedic surgeon to diagnose and treat bone and muscle problems
> - Developmental therapist to assist with development of social skills and age-specific behaviors
> - Pediatric neurologist to manage the many neurological symptoms associated with CP
> - Special education teacher to manage special learning needs

Priority Potential & Actual Complications

> Seizures

> Cognitive impairment, difficulty with vision and hearing

> Dental diseases

> Contractures, malnutrition

> Abnormal sensory perception

> Urinary incontinence

> Mental health conditions

Priority Nursing Implications

- Cerebral palsy is a long-term, life-altering condition that will change the lives of both parents and child. It is important to discuss the long-term social support that may be required, so that caregivers can cope well with caring for a child with this condition

Priority Medications

- baclofen: muscle relaxant used to treat spasticity
  - Screening doses are given first and maintenance dose is not recommended unless screening dose criteria are met
- onabotulinum toxin A
  - Know widely under the brand name Botox
  - Used to treat when spasticity is localized to a single group of muscles

Priority Education/Discharge Issues

- Educate caregivers on importance of ensuring child keeps all appointments with the health professionals who will manage the various aspects of the child's health and development
- Teach caregiver how to use adaptive equipment/devices with child. Teach proper administration of medications
- › Teach the importance of communicating with child at the child's developmental level
- › Teach importance of reinforcing work done by the various therapists
- › Encourage caregiver to intervene early on child's behalf so that severity of symptoms might be minimized
- Educate on safety for the child, to include use of helmets, removal of sharp objects and ensuring the home is conducive to mobility of a child with CP. Teach seizure precautions and what to do if the child has a seizure
- › Provide caregiver with information on cerebral palsy support groups

Go To Clinical Answers

Text designated by 💡 are the top answers for the Go To Clinical related to Cerebral palsy.

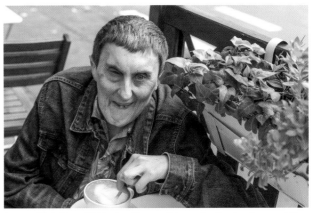

Image 13-1: Over 60% of patients with cerebral palsy live past the age of 50.

There are many disorders associated with cerebral palsy. For these 3 disorders, list 3 priority nursing concerns. Remember that a priority nursing concern can be either assessment or intervention.

SEIZURES

1. _____

2. _____

3. _____

INTELLECTUAL DISABILITIES

1. _____

2. _____

3. _____

SENSORY IMPAIRMENT

1. _____

2. _____

3. _____

Table 13-1: Disorders associated with cerebral palsy

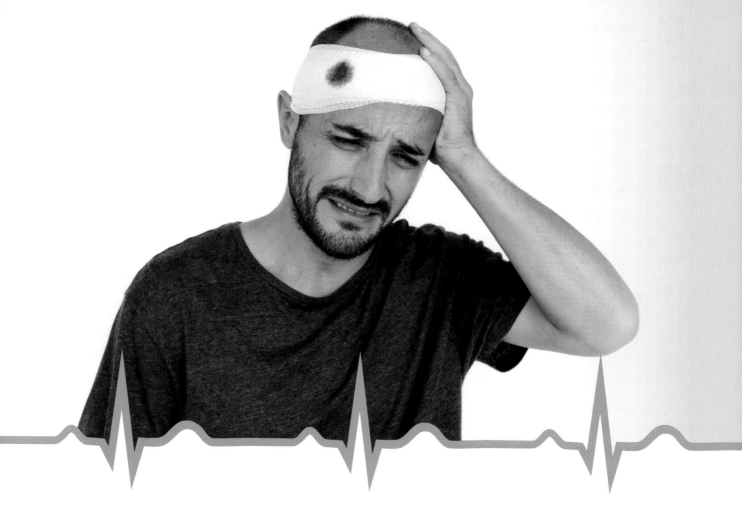

Go To Clinical Case 2

Z.A. is a 45-year-old man who is being admitted to the neurology unit from the emergency department. Z.A.'s wife reports that he has had two seizures in the past 7 days where he fell to the floor and became unconscious. She reports that on both occasions, she was at home and witnessed the seizures. With the seizure this morning he hit his head as he fell, and a bandage is now observed to the right side of his head. She reports that Z.A. lost control of his bladder during the seizure.

Health history reveals that other than the seizures, Z.A. has no other health conditions and so he and his wife are very concerned about this new health situation. His vital signs are: Blood pressure 126/84, heart rate 88, temperature 98.8°F, respirations 24. Z.A. is having a series of tests today and you are the nurse caring for him.

Next Gen Clinical Judgment

What is included in seizure precautions in a clinical agency?

How are these adapted for a client's home?

NurseThink® Time

Using the NurseThink® system, complete the priorities. Check your answers designated by 💡 in the Seizures Priority Exemplar.

NurseThink® Time

✏️ Priority Assessments or Cues

1.

2.

3.

⚗️ Priority Laboratory Tests/Diagnostics

1.

2.

3.

⚠️ Priority Interventions or Actions

1.

2.

3.

🚩 Priority Potential & Actual Complications

1.

2.

3.

⚕️ Priority Nursing Implications

1.

2.

3.

💧 Priority Medications

1.

2.

3.

👤 Priority Education/Discharge Issues

1.

2.

3.

Seizures

Pathophysiology/Description

> Seizures are sudden, uncontrolled and excessive discharge of neurons within the brain. When seizure activity is chronic, meaning seizures occur frequently it is termed epilepsy

> Causes of seizures include brain injury, genetic factors, trauma, brain tumors, stroke, metabolic disorder and toxicity

> While most seizures are caused by conditions within the brain, disorders outside the brain, such as hypertension, septicemia, kidney disease and others, can also cause seizures

> Seizures are classified as generalized and focal. With general seizures, both sides of the brain are involved, and the client usually loses consciousness. Conversely, focal seizures involve one side of the brain and may stay to that side only. However, focal seizures can spread to involve other parts of the brain and eventually end in a generalized seizure

> There are several types of generalized seizures but tonic-clonic seizure is the most common of the generalized seizures. Patients usually lose consciousness and if standing, they fall to the ground

Priority Assessments or Cues

- Complete health history, to include seizure history
- Ask client about period just before seizure activity, as some clients experience an aura (a feeling that warns them a seizure is about to start)
- Seizure activity assessment
  - Type of seizure, generalized of focal
  - Onset, seizure activity, duration and client's status after the seizure
  - Factors that may have precipitated a seizure
  - Oral cavity after seizure to determine any damage, such as client biting tongue
  - Breathing during and after seizure, ensure no airway occlusion
  - Vital signs after a seizure
  - Incontinence, as some clients become incontinent of bladder and/or bowel during seizure
  - Client's behavior in the postictal phase
  - Status epilepticus, where seizure is prolonged

Priority Laboratory Tests/Diagnostics

- Electroencephalography (EEG), to examine the electrical activity of the brain
- Lumbar puncture to test cerebrospinal fluid (CSF)
- Complete blood cell count, liver and kidney function tests and blood chemistries to look for structural lesions causing seizures
- Computed tomography (CT) scan and Magnetic resonance imaging to determine structural lesions in seizure that is new

Priority Interventions or Actions

- Remove any unsafe objects from client's immediate environment during a seizure. Gently place client on floor if seizure starts while client is standing or sitting. Never leave client during seizure
  > In acute care setting, pad client's side rails. Do not restrain in active seizure
- Document details of seizure such as behavior before, onset, type of seizure, duration and postictal state
  > Refrain from placing objects in client's mouth in a seizure as it may cause more harm to the client and risk of injury to the nurse
  > Monitor client for loss of bowel and bladder continence
- Support client's airway, breathing and circulation. May need to open airway for suctioning after seizure. Administer oxygen if needed. Ongoing monitoring of level of consciousness, and oxygenation after seizure
  > Loosen clothing that is restrictive
  > If status epilepticus occurs, administer intravenous antiseizure medications

Priority Potential & Actual Complications

- Status epilepticus, which is continuous seizure activity with rapid spasms where the client does not experience consciousness between the seizures.
- Injury to self
- May be fatal
  > Mental issues, such as depression from ineffective coping

Priority Nursing Implications

- When clients do not benefit from prevention of seizures with medications, called medically refractory epilepsy, surgery is available where the epileptic focus in the brain is removed. This is not beneficial to all clients with seizures and an extensive evaluation must be done to determine candidacy

Priority Medications

> Several medications are used to treat seizures. Below are a few of the most commonly used ones

- phenytoin (extended-release capsules)
  - Anticonvulsant drug to manage seizures
  - Initial dose is 100 mg (1 capsule) orally 3 times daily
  - Maintenance dose is 100 mg (1 capsule) orally 3 to 4 times a day

- 💡 carbamazepine
  - An anticonvulsant that is also a mood stabilizer
  - Initial dose is 200 mg orally 2 times daily for the immediate and extended-release drug or 100 mg orally 4 times daily for the suspension
  - Maintenance dose is 800 to 1200 mg/day

- 💡 phenobarbital
  - Barbiturate used in acute seizures and maintenance therapy
  - Dose for acute seizures is 20 to 320 mg intramuscular or intravenous every 6 hours as necessary
  - Maintenance dose is 60 to 200 mg orally per day

- › clonazepam
  - Anticonvulsant drug to manage seizures
  - Dose is 1.5 mg orally divided into 3 doses daily
  - Maximum dose is 20 mg daily

- › lorazepam
  - benzodiazepine to manage status epilepticus
  - Dose is 4 mg intravenous given at a rate of 2 mg/min. Dosage is repeated 5 to 10 minutes, if needed
  - Maximum dose is 8 mg

👤 Priority Education/Discharge Issues

- 💡 Importance of taking life-long medications to prevent seizures, taking medications as ordered and reporting any side effects to health care provider. Instruct on wearing a MedicAlert bracelet
- › Teach client to identify events that trigger the seizures and how to avoid them
- › Teach avoidance of alcohol intake, poor sleep and excessive tiredness as they can trigger seizures
- › Assist client to locate resources, whether online or on ground to get additional information on seizures
- 💡 Teach client the importance of letting others in the immediate social circle know about their seizure disorder, in the event of an emergency
- 💡 Teach client that if seizure lasts more than 5 minutes, emergency medical care must be called
- › Provide client with a list of how others should manage the client during and after a seizure, so client might share it with family members

Go To Clinical Answers

Text designated by 💡 are the top answers for the Go To Clinical related to Seizures.

Stages of a Seizure

1 Aura Stage

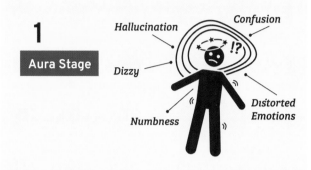

Hallucination · Confusion · Dizzy · !? · Distorted Emotions · Numbness

2 Tonic Stage

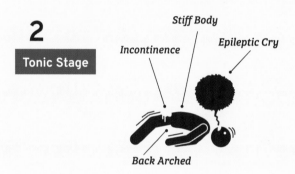

Stiff Body · Incontinence · Epileptic Cry · Back Arched

3 Clonic Stage

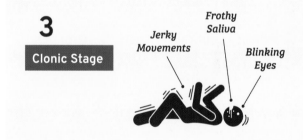

Jerky Movements · Frothy Saliva · Blinking Eyes

4 Postictal Stage

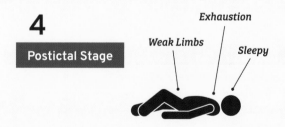

Exhaustion · Weak Limbs · Sleepy

Image 13-2: Create one note card for each stage of a seizure. On the front of the card DRAW the image representing that stage. On the back of the card, list 3 priority nursing concerns.

Osteoporosis

Pathophysiology/Description

> Osteoporosis is a progressive metabolic disease that is marked by breakdown of bone tissue and demineralization of bone resulting in fragile bones that are susceptible to fractures.

> Several risk factors for osteoporosis, among them are female gender, estrogen deficiency in women, low calcium diet, long-term use of corticosteroid drugs, older age (older than 65) and family history

> Diseases associated with osteoporosis: Kidney disease, hyperthyroidism, liver cirrhosis, rheumatoid arthritis, among others

Priority Assessments or Cues

> Back pain that is made worse when client bends or lifts and fractures, common with brittle bones

> Ask about pain to hips that is made worse when standing or walking. Assess for poor balance

> Determine height and compare with past adult height, reduction in height might be seen from vertebral compression

> Bent shape, called dowager's hump, manifested by a humped look to the thoracic spine

> Correct usage of assistive devices, such as walkers. Client's awareness of home mobility safety

Priority Laboratory Tests/Diagnostics

> Bone mineral densitometry evaluates mineral density of bones and compares to bone mineral density of a healthy adult. Serum calcium, vitamin D, phosphorus and alkaline phosphatase

> Dual-energy X-ray absorptiometry (DXA), the gold standard of bone mineral density tests, measures density of bones in hips, forearm and spine. A T-score of -2.5 or lower is indicative of osteoporosis

Priority Interventions or Actions

> Administer drug therapy as prescribed. Provide vitamin C, D, and calcium

> Provide diet high in protein to maintain muscle mass

> Instruct client in proper use of assistive devices. Encourage, and assist client with walking

> Provide range of motion exercises to client's tolerance to maintain functioning of joint

> Assist with application of orthotic device to protect areas of fracture

Priority Potential & Actual Complications

> Fractures, physical immobility and hunched-over posture

Priority Nursing Implications

> With zoledronic acid therapy, client must have serum calcium and renal function tests before administration

> Kyphoplasty and vertebroplasty are two surgeries used to repair vertebral fractures from osteoporosis. They are minimally invasive surgeries

Priority Medications

> There are several drugs used to treat osteoporosis. These are two of the most commonly used bisphosphonates

> alendronate
> - Dose is 10 mg orally once daily or 70 mg orally once weekly
> - Stay in sitting position for at least 30 minutes after taking. Take 30 minutes prior to taking other drugs or food

> ibandronate
> - Dose is 150 mg orally once monthly on the same day each month, or 3 mg by intravenous injection administered over 15 to 30 seconds every three months
> - Stay in sitting position for at least 30 minutes after taking. Take 30 minutes prior to taking other drugs or food

Priority Education/Discharge Issues

> Walking at least 30 minutes three times weekly to maintain bone mass

> Avoiding activities that place excessive stress on the bones, such as running

> Smoking cessation as nicotine exacerbates bone destruction

> Minimize alcohol intake as excessive alcohol consumption contributes to bone destruction

> Foods that contain calcium, vitamins C and D, and encourage intake of these foods

> Good body mechanics to avoid fractures. Good hydration to decrease formation of kidney stones

> Stress the importance for client to keep follow-up appointments

> Remove unsafe obstacles from home that might increase risk of falls, such as loose rugs

Osteoarthritis

Pathophysiology/Description

> A progressive disorder marked by destruction of articular cartilage of the joints

> With time and further degeneration of cartilage, bone rubs on bone causing pain

> Causes of OA: congenital disorders, repetitive use of joints, decreased estrogen, and damage to surrounding joint structures

Priority Assessments or Cues

> Joint pain that is worsened by activity and alleviated by rest (this is in early stage)

> Aggravating and relieving factors. Movement from sitting to standing position, difficult with OA

> Completion of daily activities. Joint pain prevents completion of activities of daily living

> Bony swelling to joints caused by osteophytes formation, called Heberden's nodes and cysts or bony outgrowths called Bouchard's nodes. Both cause redness and swelling

> Asymmetry of affected extremities. OA usually impacts one side of the body

> Stiffness of joints, usually occurs after client has been in one position for a long while

> Grating sound (called crepitation) in joint caused by cartilage particles in the cavity of the joint

> Arthritic process in knee which can manifest as bowlegged or knock-kneed

Priority Laboratory Tests/Diagnostics

> Computed tomography (CT) scan, magnetic resonance imaging (MRI) and bone scan are used to look for early arthritic chances to joint. X-rays used to stage the degree of damage to joints

> Synovial fluid analysis helps to differentiate OA from other types of arthritis. With OA, synovial fluid will be normal

Priority Interventions or Actions

> Administer drug therapy as prescribed. Assist with completion of activities of daily living

> Provide range of motion exercises. Initiate physical and occupational therapy consult as indicated

> Immobilize affected joint with brace or splint as prescribed, in acute phase of inflammation

> Use device such as a bed cradle to keep pressure from bed linens off client's affected feet

> Use moist heat to help with stiffness. Ensure client rests during acute flare-up

Priority Potential & Actual Complications

> Physical immobility, sleep disturbances, disability and social isolation

> Gout and bone death (called osteonecrosis)

Priority Nursing Implications

> Keep in mind that osteoarthritis can be quite debilitating in advanced stages impacting just about all functionality of a client's life. This must be considered in client teaching of the client with OA

Priority Medications

> Non-steroidal anti-inflammatory drugs (NSAIDs)
> - There are several NSAIDs that can be used. Ibuprofen is one that is commonly used
> - Low dose ibuprofen: 200 mg up to 4 times daily
> - Most significant adverse effect of NSAIDs is gastrointestinal bleeding

> capsaicin cream
> - Topical analgesic that blocks pain impulse
> - Apply to the affected site up to 4 times daily
> - Available by prescription and over-the-counter

> cortisone
> - Corticosteroids used to treat OA when joint is inflamed and swollen
> - Dose varies, administered into the joint
> - Further intervention is needed if after 4 injections the pain and swelling are not relieved

Priority Education/Discharge Issues

> Use heat to treat affected joints but use a cold compress with active inflammation

> Use of splints on affected joint as prescribed. Administration of drugs for pain

> Use of assistive device to assist with immobility, such as cane and walker

> Weight loss to minimize stress on the joints. End exercise and rest if pain starts in affected joint

> Teach importance of modifying the home environment to enhance safety

Fractures

Pathophysiology/Description

> A fracture is a break in the continuity of a bone that results from traumatic injuries or other disease processes

> There are many types of fractures classified in different ways

> Complete vs incomplete fractures: With incomplete fractures, the bone is still intact with the fracture only occurring across the shaft, while with a complete fracture, the bone is broken right through

> Open vs closed fracture: In an open fracture, bone is exposed through broken skin, while in a closed fracture, the skin is unbroken

> Displaced vs nondisplaced fracture: With displaced fractures, the bones are broken and separate, sometimes in fragments, while in nondisplaced fracture, the bone is broken but stays intact

Priority Assessments or Cues

> Assess for pain that is sudden and localized to the affected area

> Perform neurovascular assessment to include capillary refill, color, sensation, peripheral pulses, edema, and temperature

> Assess for tenderness at the injury site

> Assess client for guarding of the affected area

> Assess client's weight-bearing status. With a fracture bearing weigh causes pain

> Examine the affected site for swelling, redness and deformity

> Assess for type of fracture

> Complete history of injury occurrence

> Examine skin for bleeding and/or bone protrusion

> Assess for muscle spasms because of involuntary muscle reflex

> Listen for crunching of bone fragments, can occur with fragmented fracture

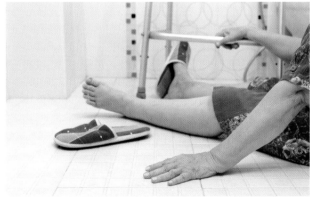

Image 13-3: The nurse finds a client in the bathroom on the floor. What are 3 priority assessments that are not related to orthopedics? Write down an anticipated finding for each assessment.

Priority Laboratory Tests/Diagnostics

> X-ray of the affected extremity will show the fracture

> Computed tomography (CT) scan and magnetic resonance imaging (MRI) will show fracture and any damage to surrounding structures

Priority Interventions or Actions

> Administer drug therapy as prescribed

> Immobilize the affected extremity to prevent movement that might cause further damage

> Cover open fracture wound with sterile dressing

> Interventions related to fixing fracture (traction, reduction, cast, fixation)
  - Inform client of the type of surgery and the device that will be used after surgery
  - Monitor neurovascular status of affected extremity
  - Provide proper alignment to promote comfort and prevent damage to fracture repair
  - Monitor drainage system used. Measure output
  - Monitor for bleeding and signs of infection on casts, dressings or at pin insertion sites
  - Plan client care with client's immobility status in mind
  - Provide adequate fluid to prevent constipation from immobility
  - Provide good skin care to prevent pressure ulcers as client is immobile
  - Check traction to ensure the weights are not touching any surfaces and are hanging freely
  - Manage internal fixation apparatus such as checking for intact screws, pins and plates
  - Monitor the traction ropes and pully mechanism to ensure no obstructions
  - Clean pin sites as prescribed
  - Provide measures to prevent a thromboembolism such as having client sit on side of bed and dangle feet, range of motion to unaffected extremity. Administer low dose anticoagulant as ordered
  - Have client perform deep breathing to prevent respiratory compromise
  - Monitor casted extremity to ensure cast is not too tight, causing circulatory compromise

Priority Potential & Actual Complications

> Infection
> Osteomyelitis
> Avascular necrosis
> Physical immobility
> Blood clots
> Compartment syndrome
> Fat embolism

Priority Nursing Implications

> A major and life-threatening complication of fractures is compartment syndrome, where the extremity gets swollen, increasing the pressure within the muscle compartment. Blood flow and nerves become compromised and capillary refill decreases drastically. Manifestations are pain in the limb that is not relieved by analgesics, loss of color, loss of sensation, loss of function, paleness, and inability to palpate pedal pulses. A surgical procedure(fasciotomy) is used to correct compartment syndrome and the wound is left open to decompress the tissue

Priority Medications

> There are several drugs used to treat osteoporosis. These are a few of the most commonly used ones

> carisoprodol
> • Muscle relaxant
> • Treat pain caused by muscle spasms
> • Dose is 250 to 350 mg orally 3 times daily for 2 to 3 weeks

> cyclobenzaprine
> • Muscle relaxant
> • Treat pain caused by muscle spasms
> • Immediate release initial dose is 5 mg orally 3 times daily. Extended-release dose is 15 mg orally once daily

> methocarbamol
> • Muscle relaxant
> • Treat pain caused by muscle spasms
> • Initial dose is 1500 mg four times daily for the first 48 to 72 hours. Maintenance dose is 4000 to 4500 mg/day in divided doses

Priority Education/Discharge Issues

> Teach client importance of walking at least 30 minutes three times weekly to maintain bone mass

> Teach to elevate extremity with cast above the heart level

> Educate on assessing extremity below cast and reporting any abnormalities, such as numbness and tingling, cool to touch, paleness

> Teach not to place objects under the cast as in trying to scratch the skin under the cast

> Instruct on reporting bad smell coming from under the cast

> Teach client and caregiver how to clean pin sites with an external fixator and assess for infection

> Teach client that if an internal fixator was used, frequent X-rays will be done to determine alignment and healing of the bone

> Stress the importance for client to keep follow-up appointments

> Teach client to remove unsafe obstacles from home that might increase risk of falls, such as loose rugs

> Alert client to the fact that when a cast is removed, the extremity may appear shrunken but with time it will start to appear normal again

> Teach importance of keeping physical and occupational therapy appointments

> Teach client that modifications may need to be made in the home to accommodate the impaired mobility

> Teach client to maintain the prescribed weight-bearing status

> Teach use of assistive devices

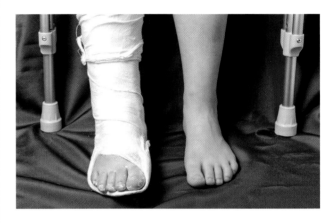

Image 13-4: Create one statement by this client that indicates discharge instructions were effective. Then create one statement by the client that indicates a need for further teaching. Next, find an online video you would recommend this client view at home to reinforce learning.

_____

_____

_____

_____

_____

_____

_____

_____

_____

Peripheral neuropathy

Pathophysiology/Description

> Peripheral neuropathy results when there is damage to peripheral nerves. The peripheral nervous system controls signals between the body and the central nervous system. Impairment in this system causes disruptions of signals and clinical manifestations in parts of the body, depending on the nerves that are affected

> Causes of peripheral neuropathy are multifactorial
> • Diabetes mellitus, infections, trauma, vascular problems and tumors
> • Excessive alcohol intake, inherited and autoimmune diseases

> The overarching symptoms of peripheral neuropathy are muscle atrophy, weakness, diminished reflexes, loss of sensation, numbness and tingling to extremities

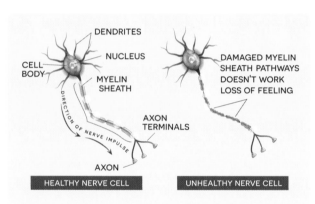

Image 13-5: Nerve damage in peripheral neuropathy.

Priority Assessments or Cues

> Clinical manifestations and assessment relate to the nerves that are affected in the body
> • Bowel and/or bladder incontinence. Decreased sensation
> • Extremities (primarily feet) for weakness, numbness, tingling and open wounds
> • Ask about heat intolerance. Burning or sticking pain in extremities
> • Decreased or heightened sensitivity to pain and pressure
> • Involuntary muscle twitching. Diminished reflexes
> • Assess for the main cause so it might be eliminated or controlled

Priority Laboratory Tests/Diagnostics

> Electromyography (EMG), and nerve conduction velocity tests assess the electrical activity of nerves and muscles

> Quantitative Sensory Testing (QST) is used to determine small and large nerve ending damages

> Autonomic Testing used to determine functioning of the autonomic nervous system

> Computed tomography (CT) scan and magnetic resonance imaging (MRI) will look for tumors or other conditions causing nerve impairment

> Nerve biopsy to look for nerve abnormalities

> Some of the many laboratory tests used for peripheral neuropathy
> • Thyroid panel for hypothyroidism and blood glucose to determine control of diabetes
> • Comprehensive metabolic panel to determine metabolic conditions
> • Vitamin B12 for vitamin deficiencies and antinuclear nuclear antibody for autoimmune conditions

Priority Interventions or Actions

> Clients are rarely seen in the acute setting for peripheral neuropathy but may be admitted for other illnesses and have peripheral neuropathy as a comorbidity. Interventions below are specific to managing the peripheral neuropathy
> • Administer pain medication as prescribed
> • Minimize client's risk for injury by removing obstacles in immediate environment
> • Apply any special extremity devices, such as hand splint or orthotic shoes, if prescribed
> • Assist with ambulation and use of assistive devices, like walker or cane to minimize risk of falls
> • Check bath water to ensure correct temperature to avoid burning skin
> • Use a bed cradle to protect feet from light touch, if client is hypersensitive to touch
> • Provide client with slippers or ask family members to bring slippers from home to avoid walking barefooted
> • Provide incontinent care or provide client with cleaning supplies, if client is incontinent
> • Perform range of motion to weakened muscles

Priority Potential & Actual Complications

> Trauma to skin, falls, infection and physical disability

Priority Nursing Implications

> A major implication for nurses is the fact that diabetes is a major cause of peripheral neuropathy and so when admitting clients with diabetes, it is crucial to remove socks and examine their feet. It is not uncommon to find wounds that they never realized were there because they had no sensation in their feet

> In the older client, it is challenging to diagnose peripheral neuropathy as many symptoms of the condition might be mistaken for the normal aging process

Priority Medications

> There are several drugs used to treat the neuropathic pain from peripheral neuropathy. These are a few of the most commonly used ones

> Non-steroidal anti-inflammatory drugs (NSAIDs)
  - There are several NSAIDs that can be used. Ibuprofen is one that is commonly used
  - Dose is 200 to 400 mg orally every 4 to 6 hours as needed
  - Most significant adverse effect of NSAIDs is gastrointestinal bleeding, from platelet aggregation

> gabapentin
  - Neuropathic pain agent
  - Treat nerve pain, causes drowsiness and dizziness
  - Dose varies but one dose is 600 mg orally once daily with food

> pregabalin
  - Neuropathic pain agent
  - Initial dose is 75 mg orally 2 times daily
  - Maintenance dose is 150 to 600 mg/day in divided doses

> capsaicin cream
  - Topical analgesic that blocks pain impulse
  - Apply to the affected site up to 4 times daily
  - Available by prescription and over-the-counter

> amitriptyline
  - Antidepressant that treats neuropathic pain by manipulating chemical processes in brain
  - Initial dose is 75 mg orally taken daily in divided doses
  - Maintenance dose is 40 to 100 mg orally taken daily

> nortriptyline
  - Antidepressant that treats neuropathic pain by manipulating chemical processes in brain
  - Dose is 25 mg orally 3 to 4 times daily
  - May cause crawling feeling and numbness

Priority Education/Discharge Issues

> Teach client who smokes about smoking cessation since smoking constricts blood vessels which causes poor circulation

> Encourage exercise to get more oxygen and blood flowing to nerves

> Teach good diabetes management, to include checking blood glucose, eating healthy and taking prescribed medications

> Instruct client to check feet daily for wounds. Demonstrate the use of a mirror to examine the plantar surface of feet

> Instruct client to wear shoes in and outside of the house to decrease risk of injury to feet

> Teach the importance of taking prescribed medications to manage conditions that cause peripheral neuropathy

> Teach that wearing splints and orthopedic shoes can help to take pressure off the nerves

> Educate on taking pain medication to relieve pain

> Provide instructions on use of a Transcutaneous electrical nerve stimulation (TENS) device, if prescribed

> Educate on importance of physical and/or occupational therapy to help improve function of impaired extremity

> Teach alcohol intake in moderation as excessive alcohol intake can worsen peripheral neuropathy

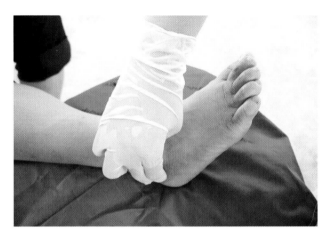

Image 13-6: List 6 important parts of diabetic foot care. Then watch an online video designed for a client. How did you do?

Trigeminal neuralgia

Pathophysiology/Description

> Trigeminal neuralgia (TN) is a form of chronic neuropathic pain that affects the 5th cranial nerve, the trigeminal nerve. It causes severe, sudden, stabbing, shock-like episodes of facial pain. This is type 1 TN which is classified as classic TN. There is also an atypical aspect to the condition called type 2 TN

> Type 2 TN is characterized by burning, aching and stabbing pain that is constant, but the severity may be less intense than type 1 TN. Clients with TN can experience both types

> Causes of TN are multiple sclerosis, tumor that causes nerve compression, vascular compression of the trigeminal nerve and shingles

> Medications are used to control TN, but clients can choose to have surgery to treat TN if medication therapy fails or if they cannot tolerate the medications

> Types of surgery
  - Microvascular decompression: removing/displacing blood vessels that compress the nerve
  - Brain stereotactic radiosurgery (Gamma knife): use of radiation to damage trigeminal nerve
  - Balloon compression: a hollow needle inserted through face, flexible catheter with balloon on end threaded through the needle. Pressure from the inflated balloon damages the nerve
  - Glycerol injections: needle inserted in face and guided to spinal fluid that surrounds the trigeminal nerve ganglion. Sterile glycerol is injected to damage the nerve
  - Radiofrequency rhizotomy: hollow needle inserted through face and electrode is inserted via the needle. Through alternating wakefulness and sedation, the part of the nerve associated with the pain is located and heat from the electrode damages the nerve fibers

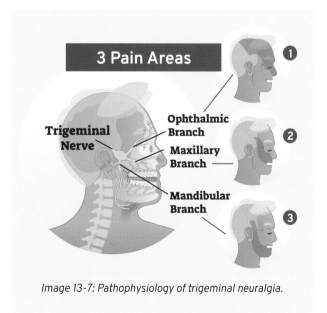

Image 13-7: Pathophysiology of trigeminal neuralgia.

Priority Assessments or Cues

> Ask client about onset of pain, usually described as sudden and abrupt

> Ask client to describe the pain, usually described as stabbing, burning, knife-like in type 1 TN or constant, aching and burning in type 2 TN

> Assess location of pain, usually pain is on the nose, lips, cheeks and gums

> Ask about triggers for the pain, clients usually state pain is triggered by touch, to a specific spot on the face, by actions such as yawning, washing the face, shaving, chewing, talking, wind exposure and applying makeup, among others

> Assess for severity of symptoms, which can be episodic in the beginning but with shorter pain free episodes as the condition progresses

> Assess sleep pattern as some clients will sleep excessively to avoid the pain

> Observe client to determine hygiene practices (especially facial, oral and hair care), as some clients may neglect hygiene care to avoid the pain

Priority Laboratory Tests/Diagnostics

> Magnetic resonance imaging (MRI) is done to see if there are other causes of the pain

> Complete neurologic examination

Priority Interventions or Actions

> Administer medications as prescribed

> Provide foods to client that are not at extremes of temperature

> Provide meals that are soft, where chewing is not needed

> Provide an environment that is not drafty/windy

> Provide hygiene care after client has been medicated to minimize pain

> Postoperative interventions
  - Monitor client's pain and compare with preoperative pain
  - Administer pain medication as prescribed
  - Monitor client's facial nerve, corneal reflex, hearing and extraocular muscles often to ensure no major damage
  - Apply cold compress/ice pack to face on the surgical side for 3 to 5 hours after a percutaneous radiofrequency rhizotomy
  - If surgery involved a small craniotomy, as with microvascular decompression procedure, monitor neurological status frequently, specifically intracranial cranial pressure and level of consciousness
  - Monitor surgery site for bleeding and signs of infection

Priority Potential & Actual Complications

> Facial paralysis

> Depression and social isolation

> Weight loss from fear of eating (due to pain triggered by chewing)

> Poor personal hygiene, especially oral and facial

Priority Nursing Implications

> The pain from trigeminal neuralgia can be so excruciating that clients with the condition avoid the triggers that cause the pain, such as mouth care, facial care (shaving) and eating. In addition, some clients withdraw from socialization because of fear of having attacks of pain in public

Priority Medications

> There are several antiseizure and tricyclic antidepressant drugs used to treat trigeminal neuralgia. These are a few of the most commonly used ones

> gabapentin
  - Neuropathic pain agent
  - Treat nerve pain, causes drowsiness and dizziness
  - Dose varies but one dose is 600 mg orally once daily with food

> amitriptyline
  - Antidepressant that treats trigeminal neuralgia by manipulating chemical processes in brain
  - Initial dose is 75 mg orally taken daily in divided doses
  - Maintenance dose is 40 to 100 mg orally taken daily

> carbamazepine
  - Antidepressant treats pain by blocking the firing of nerves
  - Initial dose is 100 mg orally of the immediate or extended-release tablets taken 2 times daily or, 50 mg orally of the suspension taken 4 times daily
  - Maintenance dose is 400 to 800 mg daily

> clonazepam
  - Antidepressant treats pain by blocking the firing of nerves
  - Dose is 1.5 mg orally administered daily in 3 divided doses
  - Drowsiness and dizziness are common side effects

Priority Education/Discharge Issues

> Teach client to chew foods on the side of the mouth that is not affected

> Instruct client to use a toothbrush that has soft bristles

> Teach client to protect face from temperature extremes such as strong winds

> Teach importance of proper hygiene and that medicating self before hygiene activities will reduce the pain

> Instruct client to avoid eating foods that are either too hot or too cold. Encourage lukewarm, soft foods that do not require much chewing

> Teach client to eat foods that have high caloric value and proteins

> Teach client having surgery that for percutaneous procedures, they will be awake

> Instruct client not to chew foods on the surgery side of the face until sensation returns to the face

> Teach client to assess surgery site for signs of infection

> If corneal damage occurred from surgery, instruct client to wear an eye shield. Reinforce importance of having regular eye exams

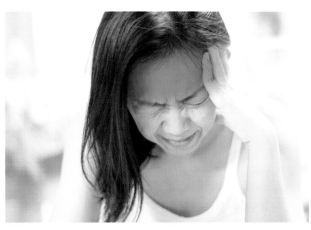

Image 13-8: This client is waiting for surgery. List 3 statements by her spouse on what they can do to help her manage the pain from the trigeminal neuralgia.

_____

_____

_____

_____

_____

_____

_____

_____

Carpal tunnel

Pathophysiology/Description

> Carpal tunnel syndrome (CTS) occurs when there is compression of the median nerve, the nerve that runs from the forearm into the palm of the hand via the carpal tunnel

> Persons who engage in occupations or hobbies that require repetitive wrist movement are at high-risk for getting CTS

> Additional contributing factors to CTS
  - Trauma to wrist
  - Hormonal involvement during pregnancy or menopause
  - Rheumatoid arthritis
  - Diabetes mellitus
  - Peripheral vascular disease

> For symptoms that persist longer than 6 months, carpal tunnel release surgery is recommended. This involves cutting a ligament around the wrist to take pressure off the median nerve. This is usually done in an outpatient setting

Priority Assessments or Cues

> Assess for weakness in affected arm

> Ask client about numbness, impaired sensation, itching and pain in affected hand and fingers

> Ask about onset of pain. Pain and numbness may cause client to awaken from sleep at nights

> Ask client to form a fist. This is sometimes difficult to do with CTS

> Assess use of client's thumb. With chronic CTS, the muscles at the base of the thumb may become dysfunctional

> Assess client's ability to perform fine hand movements. These are quite often impaired with CTS

> Assess for a positive Phalen's sign which manifests as tingling in the hands when the wrist is freely flexed for more than 60 seconds

> Assess for positive Tinel's sign, manifested as tingling in the hands when the medial nerve is tapped

Priority Laboratory Tests/Diagnostics

> X-rays of the arm and hand can show conditions that cause damage to the nerves, such as fractures

> Ultrasound will show abnormality in size of the median nerve

> Electromyography determines the severity of damage to the median nerve

> A nerve conduction study assesses the nerve's ability to send a signal along the nerve or to the muscle

Priority Interventions or Actions

> Administer medications as prescribed

> Immobilize the hand using a splint

> Postoperative interventions, if client opted for surgery
  - Monitor pain level and administer analgesics as prescribed
  - Monitor vital signs
  - Assess dressing for bleeding
  - Assess wound for signs of infection

  - Monitor neurovascular status of fingers
  - Referral to physical therapist

Priority Potential & Actual Complications

> Dysfunction of the affected hand, if no surgical intervention

> Complications related to surgery
  - Bleeding
  - Median nerve injury
  - Scar that is sensitive
  - Infection
  - Damage to blood vessels

Priority Nursing Implications

> Carpal tunnel release can take two approaches, open release surgery or endoscopic carpal tunnel release. When speaking with clients about both options, it is helpful to know that the endoscopic approach affords for quicker recovery time and has less discomfort postoperatively

Priority Medications

> Non-steroidal anti-inflammatory drugs (NSAIDs) is choice of pain medication for CTS
  - There are several NSAIDs that can be used. Ibuprofen is one that is commonly used
  - Dose is 200 mg up to 4 times daily
  - Most significant adverse effect of NSAIDs is gastrointestinal bleeding, from platelet aggregation

Priority Education/Discharge Issues

> Encourage the use of a hand splint at nights to decrease nighttime numbness and pain

> Instruct client to seek physical therapy care

> Teach client to be very careful when picking up objects that can slip from hand and cause damage, such as a cup with hot beverage

> Take frequent breaks from repetitive tasks

> Teach application of ice packs to wrist that becomes swollen and red

> Teaching following carpal tunnel release surgery
  - How to change dressing at the surgery site
  - How to assess for infection
  - How to don and doff splint
  - Full recovery is not instantaneous and may take a few months
  - Strength is decreased after surgery but will improve with time
  - Plan on modifying work for a few weeks, especially if it involves repetitive hand movements
  - Consider changing jobs, if possible
  - May develop nerve damage from surgery
  - Wear fingerless gloves at work to keep hands warm
  - Use a work desk that keeps hands in a neutral position while working

Amputation

Pathophysiology/Description

> Amputation is defined as removal of a body part, usually limb or part of a limb, due to trauma or by surgery

> Amputation is highest in older adults due to disease processes such as diabetes mellitus and peripheral vascular conditions. When younger individuals have amputations, it is quite often the result of trauma, such as land mines and motor vehicle accidents

Priority Assessments or Cues

> Assess client's and family's emotional state regarding amputation

> Assess client's knowledge of pre and postoperative care

> If amputation is from sudden traumatic event, assess for bleeding and hemodynamic instability of client, such as hypotension, tachycardia, hypovolemic shock and stabilize for surgery

Priority Laboratory Tests/Diagnostics

> Arteriogram, venogram and Doppler studies will show blood flow through the arteries and veins of the extremity, usually poor circulation is identified

> Complete blood cell count will show elevated white blood cell count if infection results from the amputation

Priority Interventions or Actions

> If traumatic amputation, stabilize the client to minimize hemorrhage and maintain hemodynamic status

> Preoperative interventions
  - Ensure client's questions regarding surgery are answered
  - Discuss what will occur in the postoperative phase of care
  - Provide instructions on use of incentive spirometry and deep breathing exercises that will be used after surgery
  - Discuss phantom limb pain that might be experienced when the limb is removed

> Postoperative interventions
  - Monitor for bleeding and signs of infection at surgery site
  - Ongoing monitoring of vital signs to determine hemodynamic stability
  - Administer pain medications as prescribed
  - Encourage client and family to discuss feelings about loss of limb. Monitor for posttraumatic stress disorder and provide appropriate consultations as needed
  - Ensure that a surgical tourniquet is available in the event of excessive bleeding
  - Prevent flexion contractures (common in hip joint). Assist client to lie on abdomen with hip extended a few times throughout the day
  - Maintain sterility in dressing changes to prevent infection
  - Ensure physical and occupational therapists are involved in client's care
  - Apply compression bandage as ordered to decrease swelling, promote healing, shrink residual limb and decrease pain
  - Assist client with ambulation

Priority Potential & Actual Complications

> Hemorrhage
> Phantom pain
> Physical disability
> Mental disorders such as depression

Priority Nursing Implications

> Amputations that occur in upper extremities are usually more devastating because they usually happen because of traumatic events, giving the client no time to prepare for the loss. The role of the nurse here is crucial when it comes to helping the client cope with the sudden loss

Priority Medications

> Pain medication is per the choice of the surgeon and the client's needs

Priority Education/Discharge Issues

> Teach client that phantom pain from missing limb usually subsides

> Teach client to use mirror therapy for phantom limb sensation and pain. Looking at the remaining limb in the mirror sends a signal to the brain that the other limb is not there

> Teach the importance of maintaining appointments for physical and/or occupational therapy

> Teach client not to hang or dangle the residual limb over the side of the bed as doing so may cause swelling

> Instruct client to clean residual limb nightly with bacteriostatic soap and warm water and do not use lotions or oils on the limb unless prescribed

> Instruct not to elevate residual limb on pillow

> Assist client with performing active range of motion exercises, when tolerable

> Educate client that when walking for the first time, the missing limb may distort their position in space, making them uncoordinated and increasing their risk of falling

> Teach the client crutch walking

> If client has a prosthesis, teach that full weight can be borne on the prosthesis about 90 days following amputation

> Teach how to change dressings and assess for infection

> Instruct client on complications that warrant a call to health care provider

> Instruct client to keep the prosthesis socket clean by washing with water and soap and rinsing well

> Teach the importance of properly maintaining the prosthesis and wearing shoes that are properly fitted

> Teach importance of modifying the home environment to enhance safety

Amyotrophic lateral sclerosis

Pathophysiology/Description

> Amyotrophic lateral sclerosis (ALS), known as Lou Gehrig's disease. A progressive, degenerative neuromuscular disorder that involves death of motor neurons in the brain and spinal cord

> More common in men than women and onset is usually somewhere between age 50 and 75

> Causes and risk factors
> • Genetic mutation and hereditary, dysfunctional immune response, and environmental toxins
> • Excess levels of glutamate in the brain and having served in the military

Priority Assessments or Cues

> Respiratory status to detect any early respiratory compromise. Energy level, ALS causes fatigue

> Client's speech may find speech is slurred. Skin for muscle wasting

> Ability to ambulate, may see that client trips while walking. Ask about falls at home

> Inquire whether client experiences muscle cramps and twitching, common with ALS

> Ask if client has been dropping things, common with ALS. Assess for spastic muscles

> Sleep pattern may have difficulty sleeping. Ask about bowel habits, constipation is common

> Observe when eating, may find difficulty swallowing and drooling

> Observe posture, may find that client has difficulty maintaining good posture

Priority Laboratory Tests/Diagnostics

> Electromyography determines the severity of damage to the median nerve. A nerve conduction study assesses the nerve's ability to send a signal along the nerve or to the muscle

> Magnetic resonance imaging (MRI) can show other conditions that may be causing the symptoms

Priority Interventions or Actions

> Administer medications as prescribed. Provide foods that are easy to swallow to prevent aspiration

> Assist with limb and trunk exercises to minimize spastic muscles. Maintain a safe environment

> Provide tracheostomy care if client has a tracheostomy

> Initiate physical, occupational, speech and psychological consults as prescribed

Priority Potential & Actual Complications

> Total dependence for all activities of daily living (ADLs), inability to speak

> Respiratory compromise from muscle paralysis, depression, and death

Priority Nursing Implications

> Riluzole causes liver function changes so monitor liver function while taking the drug

> Be empathetic as physical care is provided, understanding that client and family are likely very distressed with the diagnosis and the impending decline of client's status

Priority Medications

> riluzole
> • Works by decreasing the release of glutamate, thus minimizing damage to motor neurons
> • Dose is 50 mg orally every 12 hours
> • Must be taken at least an hour before, or two hours after, a meal

> edaravone
> • Slows decline in daily functioning
> • Initial treatment is 60 mg once a day as intravenous infusion given for 14 days then a 14-day drug-free period. Dosages and duration of future cycles are modified
> • May causes dizziness, tachycardia and skin rash

Priority Education/Discharge Issues

> The long-term trajectory of the disease. Advance directives and end-of-life care

> Exercises to reduce muscle spasticity. Foods that have high nutrition value and are easy to swallow

> Signs and symptoms of respiratory muscle decline and when emergency help is to be sought

> Safe home environment to minimize risk of falls. Speech, physical and occupational therapy

> Medication therapy, reinforcing that medications slow the progression but are not curative

> Other medications to treat symptoms of ALS such as constipation and sleep problems

> Psychosocial consult to manage the long-term emotional, social and financial implications of ALS

Guillain-Barré syndrome

📋 Pathophysiology/Description

> Guillain-Barré Syndrome (GBS) is an autoimmune, acute inflammation of peripheral and cranial nerves

> Myelin sheath is lost and the nerves that are affected become edematous and inflamed causing a slowing or inhibition of nerve impulses

> Guillain-Barré syndrome is usually seen after a person has had an infection of the respiratory or gastrointestinal tract

✏️ Priority Assessments or Cues

> Respiratory status to detect symptoms of respiratory failure, a major complication of GBS.

> Results of arterial blood gasses and need for ventilator support. Look for cardiac dysrhythmias

> Pain, worse during the night. Numbness and tingling of the extremities. Absent reflexes

> Muscle strength shows weakness and/or paralysis. Energy level may be decreased

> Hypertension, orthostatic hypotension and bradycardia.

> Paralytic ileus, drooling indicating inadequate gag reflex, and difficulty swallowing.

> Poor sleep pattern. Client may report less sleep because of pain at nights

> Assess bowel and bladder status, often see incontinence in both

🧪 Priority Laboratory Tests/Diagnostics

> Electromyography (EMG) shows cause of weakness. Lumbar puncture shows elevated protein level

> Nerve conduction tests response of the nerves and muscles to electrical impulses

⚠️ Priority Interventions or Actions

> Emergency equipment at bedside, cough and deep breathe, and monitor respiratory status.

> Monitor for progression of paralysis. Perform activities when muscle strength is optimal

> Turn and reposition every two hours or more frequently. Use pressure relieving devices

> Perform meticulous skin care if incontinent of bladder and bowel

> Provide foods that are easy to swallow to prevent aspiration

> Administer nutrition via enteral or parenteral route if unable to eat orally

> Prepare client for plasmapheresis or intravenous immunoglobulin as prescribed

> Ensure referrals to speech, occupational and physical therapists

🚩 Priority Potential & Actual Complications

> Respiratory infection, respiratory failure, paralysis and death

♻️ Priority Nursing Implications

> The symptoms in GBS can move very quickly and progress to a life-threatening stage in a few hours. Clients with early symptoms must be treated rapidly before more muscle groups, such as those in the chest and diaphragm are impacted, causing respiratory and cardiac failure

💧 Priority Medications

> immunoglobulin (IV Ig), given at a high dose

  • Best effect is seen when administered to client within 14 days of symptoms starting

  • Usual high dose is 400 mg/kg, given intravenous daily for 5 consecutive days

  • Blocks damaging antibodies. This is the preferred treatment over plasmapheresis

👤 Priority Education/Discharge Issues

> Recovery is slow, but most people usually recover fully

> Triggers that worsen the symptoms. Seek healthcare at the first sign of symptoms

> Signs and symptoms of an infection. Balance of rest and exercise

> Eating well-balanced nutritious meal that is easy to swallow

> Resources that may help client and family cope with the condition

Compare and Contrast		
	BOTULISM POISONING	**MYASTHENIA GRAVIS**
Reflexes		
Sensory		
Motor		
Autonomic		

Table 13-2: Compare and contrast helps you Save Time Studying. Complete this chart by searching online and textbook resources.

Multiple sclerosis

📋 Pathophysiology/Description

> Multiple sclerosis (MS) is a chronic, progressive condition in which demyelination of neurons in the central nervous system occurs

> The disease has been shown to have a genetic tendency, with genetic factors seen in families that have more than one person with the disease

> The disease usually has an onset between the second to the fifth decade of life with more women than men having the condition

> Factors that precipitate MS
> - Pregnancy
> - Emotional stress
> - Infection
> - Trauma
> - Fatigue
> - Climate change

✏️ Priority Assessments or Cues

> Assess respiratory status to detect any early symptoms of respiratory compromise

> Ask client about energy level, MS causes muscle weakness and fatigue

> Assess client's vision, may find double or blurred vision, or unilateral blindness

> Assess client's balance and coordination, may have poor balance and lack of coordination

> Assess client's speech, may find difficulty speaking

> Ask client about bladder incontinence or retention and constipation of bowels, common with MS

> Assess client's hearing as MS can cause hearing loss

> Assess for cognitive dysfunction such as processing of information, finding of words and memory which tend to present in late-stage MS

> Assess for emotional lability such as euphoria and anger, which sometimes manifest with MS

> Examine client's eyes, may find nystagmus

> Assess ambulation, may see that client trips while walking

> Ask client about falls at home, as falls are common with MS

> Inquire whether client experiences numbness and tingling to extremities, common with MS

> Assess client for spasticity to lower extremities

> Assess skin for pressure ulcers caused by immobility

🧪 Priority Laboratory Tests/Diagnostics

> Lumbar puncture to examine cerebrospinal fluid will indicate elevated gamma globulin level

> Evoked potential testing may show delayed response

> Computed tomography (CT) scan and magnetic resonance imaging (MRI) of brain and spinal cord can show tissue damage, inflammation and plaques

⚠️ Priority Interventions or Actions

> For client with diplopia, use an eye patch to cover the affected eye

> Provide proper skin care in acute exacerbation to prevent pressure ulcers

> Turn and reposition client who is dependent

> Encourage bladder training to minimize incontinence

> Encourage coughing and deep breathing exercises to prevent respiratory compromise

> Provide client with a meal that is well balanced and inclusive of fiber to help constipation

> Administer medications as prescribed

> Maintain client in a safe environment that is free of potential hazards for falling

> Provide foods that are easy to swallow to decrease risk of aspiration

> Initiate physical, occupational and speech consult as prescribed

> Assist client to make decisions about lifestyle modifications

> Encourage client and family to talk about the emotional aspect of the diagnosis. Provide psychological consult if needed

🚩 Priority Potential & Actual Complications

> Infections

> Respiratory conditions such as pneumonia

> Paralysis with total dependence for all activities of daily living (ADLs)

> Blindness

> Depression

⚕️ Priority Nursing Implications

> Sexual functioning is severely compromised in clients with MS. This is usually a sensitive topic to address but one that is worth discussing with the client so that alternate ways of intimacy with partner might be sought

> With interferon, it is important to alert client to the fact that protective clothing and sunscreen lotion must be worn while taking the drug and the site of injection administration must be rotated with each dose. It is normal to experience flu-like symptoms when the drug is first started

> Dalfampridine must not be used in clients with seizure disorder as it may precipitate seizures

> Prednisone should not be stopped abruptly as client will experience prednisone withdrawal symptoms, which include weakness, severe fatigue, and joint and body aches

💧 Priority Medications

> Drugs to treat MS are many and in various classes. Below are a few of the most common drugs used in each class

> Beta 1A interferon
  - Immunomodulator
  - Dose is 30 mcg intramuscular once weekly
  - Dose can be titrated to prevent side effect of flu-like symptoms

> mitoxantrone
  - Immunosuppressant
  - Dose is 12 mg/m^2 given as a 5 to 15-minute intravenous infusion every 3 months
  - Serious side effects of cardiotoxicity, infertility and leukemia

> alemtuzumab
  - Monoclonal antibody
  - First Treatment Course: 12 mg intravenous daily on 5 consecutive days
  - Second treatment course: 12 mg intravenous daily on 3 consecutive days administered 12 months after the first

> prednisone
  - Corticosteroid
  - Dose is 200 mg orally daily for 1 week, then 80 mg every other day for 1 month
  - Most beneficial when used to treat acute flare-ups

> dalfampridine
  - Enhances nerve conduction
  - Dose is 10 mg orally every 12 hours
  - Used to improve walking in MS

👤 Priority Education/Discharge Issues

> Educate client on the long-term trajectory of the disease and what the needs may be as the disease progresses

> Teach client to recognize triggers that worsen the symptoms of MS, such as heat and fatigue

> Teach client to avoid temperature extremes

> Teach client signs and symptoms of an infection and to seek care immediately

> Instruct on the importance of a good balance of rest and exercise

> Teach client to eat well-balanced nutritious meals

> Teach client to ensure fiber intake to help treat constipation

> Provide education measures to minimize injury due to sensory loss, such as decreasing water temperature

> Instruct on importance of seeking pharmacist or health care provider's opinion before taking over-the-counter medications

> Instruct on proper administration of medications, adhering to the cautions with each drug and observing for side effects

> Educate client on measures to make the home environment safe from hazards that may cause a fall, such as removing loose rugs and installing hand bars in showers

> Teach self-catheterization to the client who will need to empty the bladder via that method.

> Provide information on resources that may assist client with coping with the disease such as The National Multiple Sclerosis Society

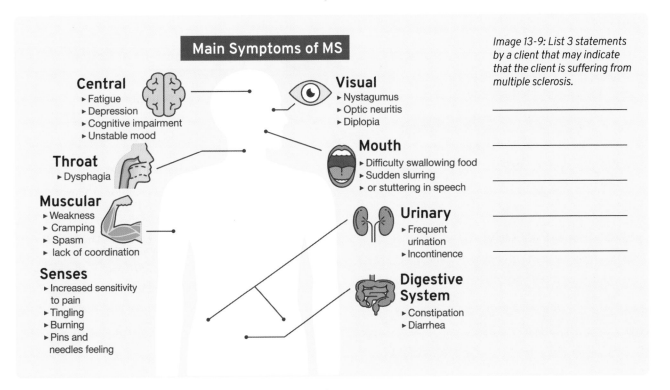

Image 13-9: List 3 statements by a client that may indicate that the client is suffering from multiple sclerosis.

_____

_____

_____

_____

Myasthenia gravis

Pathophysiology/Description

> Myasthenia gravis (MG) is an autoimmune, neuromuscular disease where significant weakness and fatigue of skeletal muscle groups occur

> The disease is characterized by an attack on acetylcholine by antibodies, resulting in decreased numbers of acetylcholine receptor sites at the neuromuscular junction

> Excessive secretion of cholinesterase, not enough secretion of acetylcholine, or muscle fibers that do not respond to acetylcholine are causes of MG

> Factors that precipitate MG
> • Pregnancy
> • Stress
> • Extremes of temperature
> • Certain drugs
> • Trauma
> • Menstruation

> The thymus gland, though small in adults, seems to foster the production of acetylcholine antibodies so clients can choose to have it removed in a procedure called a thymectomy

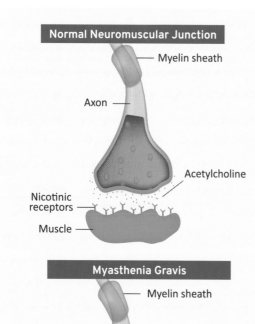

Normal Neuromuscular Junction

Myelin sheath

Axon

Acetylcholine

Nicotinic receptors

Muscle

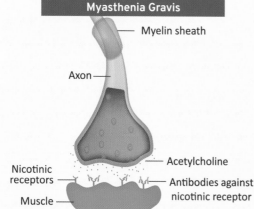

Myasthenia Gravis

Myelin sheath

Axon

Acetylcholine

Nicotinic receptors

Muscle

Antibodies against nicotinic receptor

Image 13-10: Pathophysiology of myasthenia gravis.

Priority Assessments or Cues

> Assess respiratory status to detect symptoms of respiratory compromise as MG can cause difficulty breathing and respiratory insufficiency

> Assess breath sounds as client is at risk for respiratory infection

> Ask client about energy level, MG causes muscle weakness and fatigue

> Assess client's vision, may find double vision. Observe eyes, may find ptosis

> Observe client eating, may see difficulty chewing and swallowing

> Assess client's speech, may find difficulty speaking and/ or client's voice fades away with continuous conversation, caused by progressive weakness to muscle. May hear hoarseness

> Assess client for infection as it can exacerbate MG, causing a myasthenic crisis

Priority Laboratory Tests/Diagnostics

> Edrophonium test (Tensilon test) elicits sudden improvement in muscle strength indicating MG

> Electromyography (EMG) examines electrical activity between client's brain and muscles, may find poor electrical activity

> Chest X-ray to look for respiratory involvement, like pneumonia

> Computed tomography (CT) scan to examine the thymus gland for tumors or other abnormalities in client already diagnosed with MG

> Acetylcholine receptor antibodies test will be positive for the antibodies

Priority Interventions or Actions

> Place emergency equipment at client's bedside in the event of a cholinergic or myasthenic crisis

> Monitor client's respiratory system. Ensure effective breathing. Encourage coughing and deep breathing. Monitor for respiratory failure

> Administer anticholinesterase drugs as prescribed and monitor for adverse effects

> Monitor for cholinergic crisis caused by excessive anticholinesterase drugs

> Monitor for myasthenic crisis caused by insufficient medication, infection, fatigue or progression of MG that was not identified

> Monitor muscles for improved strength, indicating therapeutic effect of drugs

> Ongoing monitoring of vital signs

> Encourage ambulation to prevent complications of immobility. Plan activities around times when client's muscle strength is optimal

- Balance activity and rest to prevent fatigue
- Provide foods that are easy to swallow to decrease risk of aspiration. Monitor for aspiration
- Prepare client for plasmapheresis if prescribed
- Prepare client for administration of intravenous immunoglobulin G, if prescribed

Priority Potential & Actual Complications

- Myasthenic crisis
- Cholinergic crisis
- Tumors of the thymus

Priority Nursing Implications

- Myasthenic crisis is an acute flare-up of weakness in the muscles that is triggered by certain illnesses, pregnancy, surgery or various other stressors. This crisis may cause respiratory insufficiency because of weakness to muscles that impact breathing and swallowing. Anticholinesterase medications must be increased to address this condition
- Cholinergic crisis occurs when too much anticholinesterase drug has been administered. The condition is manifested by nausea, vomiting, abdominal pain, increased bronchial secretions, blurred vision, sweating, pupillary miosis and hypotension. Stop anticholinesterase and administer atropine sulfate

Priority Medications

- pyridostigmine: anticholinesterase and a successful drug in treating MG
  - Oral dose for the immediate-release tablet and syrup is 60 mg 3 times daily
  - Oral dose for the sustained-release tablet is 180 to 540 mg orally once or twice daily
  - Parenteral dose is 2 to 5 mg intramuscular or slow intravenous administration every 2 to 3 hours
- neostigmine: anticholinesterase drug
  - Usual initial oral dose is 15 mg 3 times daily.
  - Usual intravenous, intramuscular and subcutaneous dose is 0.5 to 2.5 mg and the patient response dictates the appropriate dosing
  - Anticholinergic drug, such as atropine is given to prevent a cholinergic crisis
- atropine sulfate: Anticholinergic drug
  - Treat anticholinesterase toxicity
  - Usual dose is 0.4 mg to 0.6 mg, intravenous, intramuscular, or subcutaneous
  - Administer with or before giving neostigmine
- edrophonium
  - Used in tension test to diagnose myasthenia gravis

- Usual test dose is 2 mg administered intravenously
- Positive for MG if client's muscle strength improves within seconds after administration

- prednisone
  - Corticosteroid and most common drug in the class to treat MG
  - Dose is 5 to 60 mg orally per day
  - Used to suppress the immune response

Priority Education/Discharge Issues

- Educate client on the long-term trajectory of the disease and what the needs will be, living with the disease
- Teach client to recognize triggers that worsen the symptoms of MG
- Teach client signs and symptoms of an infection and to seek care immediately
- Instruct on the importance of a good balance of rest and exercise
- Teach client to eat a well-balanced nutritious meal that is semisolid and easy to swallow
- Teach client to schedule medications for maximal muscle strength effect at time of activity, such as eating
- Educate client on signs and symptoms of cholinergic and myasthenic crisis
- Educate client about other options of treatment for myasthenia gravis beyond medications, such as plasmapheresis or surgery
- Instruct on importance of seeking pharmacist or health care provider's opinion before taking over-the-counter medications
- Instruct on proper administration of medications, adhering to the cautions with each drug and observing for side effects
- Provide information on resources that may assist client with coping with the disease such as Myasthenia Gravis Foundation

Compare and Contrast		
	CHOLINERGIC	MYASTHENIC
Pulse		
Pupil		
Secretions		
Skin		
Muscles		

Table 13-3: Compare and contrast helps you Save Time Studying. Complete this chart by searching online and textbook resources.

Parkinson's disease

📋 Pathophysiology/Description

> Parkinson's disease (PD) is a chronic neurodegenerative disease that is characterized by lack of the chemical messenger, dopamine. Dopamine is needed for proper functioning of the extrapyramidal system so when dopamine is lacking, the extrapyramidal system malfunctions

> The main features of PD are gross slowness in starting and executing movement along with resting tremors and gait disturbance

> Parkinson's disease is seen mostly in men and diagnosis occurs as age increases. The disease slowly progresses, often ending in disability and total dependence for care needs

> Causes
> - Genetics
> - Environmental factors such as exposure to pesticides, well water, industrial chemicals
> - Residing in rural areas
> - Lewy bodies, which are clumps of protein found in brain of clients with PD

> Antiparkinsonian drugs are the mainstay of treating PD. However, surgical therapy is also available. These include ablation (destruction of affected part of brain), deep brain stimulation (using electrodes to decrease activity produced by depletion of dopamine) and transplantation of fetal neural tissue in the brain of person with PD. Transplantation research is continuing

✏️ Priority Assessments or Cues

> Assess client's gait, may observe shuffling gait, classic of later stage PD

> Assess movement, will see bradykinesia. Assess for purposeful movement, may find akinesia

> Examine client's stance, will find a stooped posture where trunk and head lean forward

> Ask client to write something and observe writing. Words may trail off the page and be smaller than when started, due to tremors

> Assess for tremors that increase at rest and decrease when hands are active

> Observe facial expression, may see a masklike expression (called deadpan expression)

> Observe client's posture, will see rigidity that can appear to have jerkiness (called cogwheel rigidity). Assess muscle strength, may find muscle weakness

> Assess client for postural instability by performing the pull test (stand behind client and tug client backward, eliciting a backward fall)

> Listen to client's speech, will hear slurred and monotone speech

> Assess for bowel and bladder incontinence which may manifest with PD

> Observe client eating, may see difficulty swallowing, as dysphagia is common as PD progresses. Assess for drooling

> Assess client for psychological complications of PD such as depression and apathy

🧪 Priority Laboratory Tests/Diagnostics

> Computed tomography (CT) scan and magnetic resonance (MRI) to rule out other conditions such as a brain tumor

> Response to antiparkinsonian drug test: improvement in symptoms when this drug is given, confirms the diagnosis of PD

⚠️ Priority Interventions or Actions

> Administer antiparkinsonian drugs

> Perform range of motion to client's tolerance to maintain mobility of joints and muscles. Initiate consult with physical therapy to prevent contractures and muscle wasting

> Turn and reposition client every two hours or more frequently, to prevent pressure ulcers. Use pressure relieving devices on bed

> Perform meticulous skin care for client who is incontinent of bladder and bowel

> Provide assistive device to help with ambulation

> Have client use strategies to minimize risk of falls, such as rocking from side to side, stepping over a line on the floor and lifting toes when stepping

> Plan activities around times when client's muscle strength is optimal

> Balance activity and rest to prevent fatigue

> Provide foods that are easy to chew and swallow to decrease risk of aspiration, because of dysphagia. Ensure food is cleared from mouth to prevent aspiration

> Provide foods that are high in calories

> Monitor constipation. Provide high fiber in diet and adequate fluids

> Administer nutrition via enteral or parenteral route if client is unable to eat orally

🚩 Priority Potential & Actual Complications

> Involuntary movements (dyskinesias)
> Psychiatric problems such as depression
> Dementia
> Dysphagia with resulting malnutrition
> Muscle weakness
> Injuries from falls

Priority Nursing Implications

> Parkinson's disease will become very debilitating for the client as the disease progresses and will take a toll on caregivers at some point in the trajectory of the disease. It is crucial that client and family teaching surround this fact so that caregivers will be fully knowledgeable about the expectations as the disease progresses and can better plan for care of the client

Priority Medications

> There are different classes of drugs used to treat PD. Below are a few of the most common drugs used in each class

> levodopa
> • Dopaminergic/Antiparkinsonian agent
> • Usual dose is 250 mg 2 to 4 times daily
> • Dose can be increased to reach desired effect

> levodopa/carbidopa
> • Dopaminergic/Antiparkinsonian agent
> • levodopa/carbidopa is a combination drug available in several dosage strengths. Choice of dosage is determined by the prescriber
> • May cause dyskinesia (involuntary and uncontrolled movement)

> ropinirole
> • Dopamine receptor agonist
> • Immediate release tablet: Initial dose is 0.25 mg orally three times daily. After the initial week, dosage may be titrated weekly for 3 weeks, to reach desired dosage
> • Extended-release tablet: Initial dose is 2 mg orally once daily for 1 to 2 weeks. Dose may be titrated up based on prescriber's judgment and therapeutic response

> benztropine
> • Anticholinergic drug. Works by balancing cholinergic and dopaminergic activities
> • Initial dose is 0.5 to 2 mg orally, intramuscularly or intravenously once daily
> • Usual dose: is 1 to 2 mg oral daily

> diphenhydramine
> • Antihistamine drug. Manages tremors in PD
> • Oral dose is 25 to 50 mg orally 3 to 4 times daily
> • Parenteral dose is 10 to 50 mg administered via deep intramuscular injection or intravenous, as needed

> selegiline
> • Monoamine Oxidase Inhibitor.
> • Dose is 5 mg orally twice a day
> • Used with levodopa/carbidopa to prolong the half-life of levodopa/carbidopa and enhance the levels of dopamine

Priority Education/Discharge Issues

> Discuss options with client and caregiver that will allow client to maintain independence

> Discuss use of adaptive devices and equipment, such as a wheelchair, long spoon, special mug, among others

> Teach ways to modify client's clothing and shoes to increase client's independence in manipulating them, such as using Velcro closure instead of buttons

> Educate client and family on the importance of making modifications in the home to facilitate client's independence and minimize risk for injuries. These include, removal of loose rugs, installing grab bars in shower, placing bench in shower, getting an elevated toilet set, among others

> Instruct caregivers to be patient and not rush the client when completing tasks, as task completion will be much slower than usual with PD

> Teach the importance of administering antiparkinsonian medications

> Educate client on foods that are high in pyridoxine (vitamin B6) as pyridoxine hinders the effect of antiparkinsonian drugs

> Educate on continued physical and occupational therapy for strengthening of muscles and use of adaptive strategies for activities of daily living

> Educate on eating foods that are easy to chew and swallow

> Encourage eating six small meals throughout the day instead of few large meals

> Provide information on resources that may help client and family cope with the condition, such as the American Parkinson Disease Association and referral to counseling

> Discuss the long-term burden of caring for someone with PD. Assist client and family with seeking alternate options for care outside of the home, such as a long-term care facility, if desired

> Have client use strategies to minimize risk of falls (mentioned in priority interventions)

Complete this MNEMONIC
Parkinson's Disease signs and symptoms

S _____

M _____

A _____

R _____

T _____

Table 13-4: Feel free to search the Internet or create your own.

Cataracts

Pathophysiology/Description

> Opacity of the lens that affects transparency, causing vision changes. Can occur in one or both eyes

> Causes include age related, eye trauma, congenital such as caused by maternal diseases, radiation and diabetes mellitus, among others

> Cataract surgery is usually done on one eye at a time. Most of the postoperative care is done by the client and/or caregiver at home

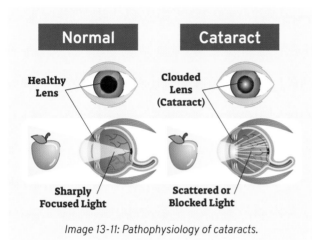

Image 13-11: Pathophysiology of cataracts.

Priority Assessments or Cues

> Decreased and/or blurred vision. Assess color perception, may be abnormal

> Glare from driving worsened by night driving. Double vision (diplopia)

> Redness and pain in eye, more prominent in age-related cataract

> Knowledge of surgical procedure. Ability to adhere to postoperative instructions

Priority Laboratory Tests/Diagnostics

> Visual acuity test shows vision impairment

> Slit lamp examination shows cataract on lens. Glare testing shows vision loss

> Pupil dilation test shows extent of cataract's impact on vision

Priority Interventions or Actions

> Preoperative interventions
  • Teaching on expectations of surgery and postoperative care. Administer eye medications
  • Decrease lighting to prevent photopia after administering mydriatic

> Postoperative interventions
  • Examine eye patch to ensure adequate coverage of eye. Elevate head of bed 30-40 degrees
  • Position off operative side. Administer analgesics if needed. Assist with ambulation
  • Prevent client actions that increase intraocular pressure, such as bending and coughing

Priority Potential & Actual Complications

> Infection, bleeding, vision loss and dislocation of implanted lens

Priority Nursing Implications

> Consider the impact of cataracts on older adults. Independence may be lost as poor vision allows them to be dependent on others to assist them with tasks such as driving. Be supportive and provide information on ways they might still maintain independence

Priority Medications

> tropicamide (one of many drugs used to dilate the eye)
  • Cycloplegic drug
  • Usual dose: instillation of 1 or 2 drops of 0.5% solution into eye 15 or 20 minutes prior to procedure
  • Produces both paralysis and dilation

> ketorolac ophthalmic solution (non-steroidal anti-inflammatory eye drops)
  • Used to reduce inflammation and decrease pain
  • Dose of 0.45% ophthalmic solution: Instill 1 drop in the affected eye twice daily beginning 1 day before cataract surgery, through the first 2 weeks after surgery
  • A 0.5% ophthalmic solution can also be used

Priority Education/Discharge Issues

> No actions that increase eye pressure. No lifting heavier than 5 pounds

> Wear sun shades to prevent photophobia. Expect eye discomfort for a few days

> No rubbing of eye, as it can result in an infection. Proper instilling of eye drops

> Notify health care provider of redness, unusual drainage, vision loss, floaters or light flashes

> Decreased depth perception while wearing the eye patch

> Visual acuity may not return to the operative eye until 1-2 weeks after surgery

> Importance of follow-up visits

Glaucoma

Pathophysiology/Description

> A group of eye disorders that damage the optic nerve due to increased ocular pressure

> Two types of glaucoma
> • Primary open-angle glaucoma (POAG): drainage path for aqueous humor is blocked so outflow is decreased in the trabecular network. This is the most common type of glaucoma
> • Primary angle-closure glaucoma (PACG): angle closure causes reduction in the outflow of aqueous humor. Some causes of angle closure might be pupil dilation or bulging lens

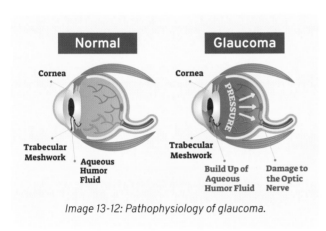

Image 13-12: Pathophysiology of glaucoma.

Priority Assessments or Cues

> Accommodation diminished with glaucoma. Sudden, severe eye pain with PACG

> Peripheral vision loss, indicative of POAG. Nausea and vomiting with PACG

> Blurred vision and visualization of colored halos with PACG

> Client's understanding of condition and ability to follow the long-term treatment regimen

Priority Laboratory Tests/Diagnostics

> Visual acuity test shows vision impairment. Perimetry shows impairment in visual fields

> Slit lamp examination shows fixed pupil and flat anterior chamber angle with PACG and normal angle with POAG. Tonometry shows elevated intraocular pressure

> Ophthalmoscopy shows a deeper and wider optic disc with POAG

Priority Interventions or Actions

> Eye medications to decrease intraocular pressure

> Preoperative interventions for PACG
> • Teaching regarding expectation of iridectomy surgery and postoperative care.
> • Administer intravenous or oral hyperosmotic drugs to decrease intraocular pressure

> Postoperative interventions
> • Examine eye patch to ensure adequate coverage of eye. Elevate head of bed 30-40 degrees
> • Position off operative side. Administer analgesics if needed. Assist with ambulation
> • Prevent client actions that increase intraocular pressure, such as bending and coughing

Priority Potential & Actual Complications

> Infection, bleeding, loss of vision and recurrence of glaucoma

Priority Nursing Implications

> Primary angle-closure glaucoma is an emergency that must be addressed immediately

Priority Medications

> There are several classes of drugs used to treat glaucoma. Below are two that are commonly used

> dipivefrin
> • a-Adrenergic agonist
> • Decreases production of aqueous humor
> • Usual dose is 1 drop every 12 hours

> carbachol
> • Cholinergic agent
> • Causes iris sphincter to contract and trabecular meshwork to open, allowing aqueous outflow
> • Dose is no more than 0.5 mL instilled into the anterior chamber of the eye

Priority Education/Discharge Issues

> No actions that increase eye pressure. No lifting heavier than 5 pounds

> Wear sun shades to prevent photophobia. Expect eye discomfort for a few days

> No rubbing of eye, as it can result in an infection. Proper instilling of eye drops

> Notify health care provider of redness, unusual drainage, vision loss, floaters or light flashes

> Decreased depth perception while wearing the eye patch

> Visual acuity may not return to the operative eye until 1-2 weeks after surgery

> Importance of follow-up visits. Regular eye exams. MedicAlert Identification

Conjunctivitis

Pathophysiology/Description

> Conjunctivitis is inflammation or infection of the conjunctiva. Conjunctivitis caused by bacteria is contagious and good handwashing must be done to prevent the spread

> Causes: bacteria, viruses, chemical irritants, trauma, foreign body in eye and chlamydia

> Most cases of conjunctivitis get better on their own

> Keratitis, infection or inflammation of the cornea, can also impact the conjunctiva resulting in a condition called keratoconjunctivitis

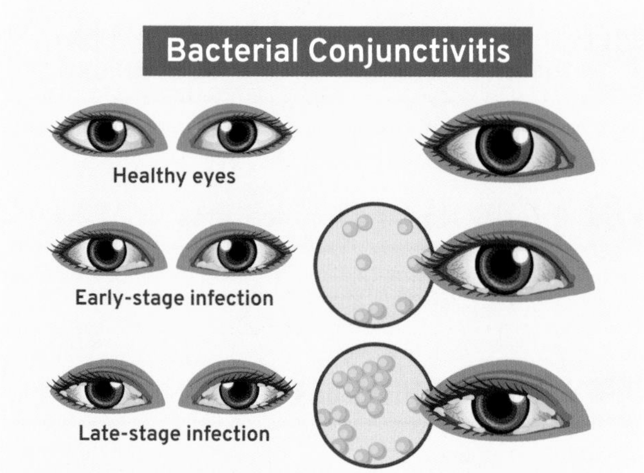

Bacterial Conjunctivitis

Healthy eyes

Early-stage infection

Late-stage infection

Image 13-13a: Pathophysiology of bacterial conjunctivitis.

Viral Conjunctivitis

Healthy eyes

Early-stage infection

Late-stage infection

Virus

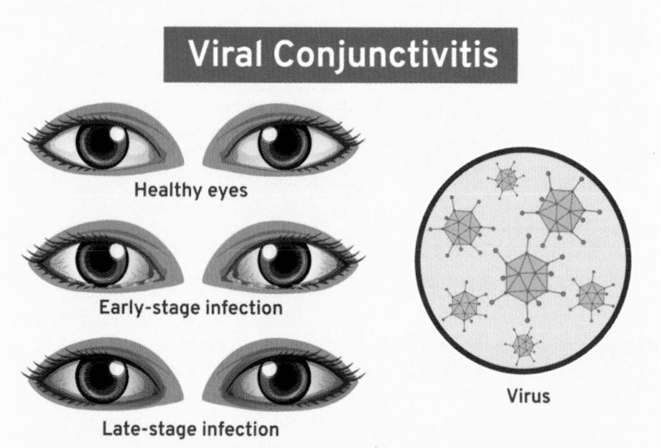

13-13b: Pathophysiology of viral conjunctivitis.

Priority Assessments or Cues

> Assess client for itchy, burning, teary and red eyes. Assess for swelling to the eyelids

> Examine eyes for drainage. Mucopurulent drainage usually indicates bacterial or chlamydial causes

> Ask client about tolerance to light as conjunctivitis may cause mild photophobia

> Ask client to describe feeling in the eyes, usually described as gritty or sandy feel to eyes

Priority Laboratory Tests/Diagnostics

> Visual acuity test to determine if conjunctivitis has affected vision

> Slit lamp examination is used to examine small sections of structures of the eye to detect small abnormalities. Conjunctivitis will be seen

> Eye culture to determine if cause of conjunctivitis is bacterial

Priority Interventions or Actions

> Administer eye drops as prescribed

> Maintain proper infection control practice

> Apply cold or warm compress

Priority Potential & Actual Complications

> Meningitis, if bacterial conjunctivitis is left untreated

> Keratitis

Priority Medications

> moxifloxacin (for bacterial conjunctivitis)
  - Quinolone antibiotic
  - Used to treat conjunctivitis caused by bacteria
  - Dose: Instillation of 1 drop in the affected eye(s) 3 times daily for 7 days

> ocular lubricant
  - Can be bought over-the-counter
  - Used to moisten the eye and alleviate dryness and irritation
  - Must not be used to treat a bacterial eye infection

Priority Education/Discharge Issues

> Instruct client on proper handwashing to prevent spread of the condition

> Instruct to not share make-up and to discard remaining make-up

> Instruct client to stop wearing contact lens until conjunctivitis is resolved and to discard current lens

> Teach client not to rub or scratch eyes

> Instruct client not to share towels and washcloths

> Instruct on proper administration of eye drops without touching eye

> Hold head back and pull lower eyelid down to form a pocket

> Dropper held above the eye without touching the eye

> Gaze up and look away from dropper. Squeeze drops into pocket of eye

> Finger pressed for 1 minute to the inside corner of eye, so fluid does not get into the tear duct

Macular degeneration

Pathophysiology/Description

> Macular degeneration (MD) occurs when the macula, which is the central part of the retina, deteriorates

> The vision loss from macular degeneration is irreversible. Though MD rarely causes complete blindness, the physical disability that limited vision causes can be life-altering

> The condition is seen as individuals age and so it is often referred to as age-related macular degeneration

> Risk factors
> - Genetics
> - Ethnicity: more common in Caucasians than other ethnic groups
> - Cardiovascular disease
> - Smoking or smoke exposure

> Types of macular degeneration
> - Dry MD: yellow deposits in the retinal pigment epithelium, called drusen, increase in numbers and size causing distorted vision. Dry MD is the most common type and is not curable
> - Wet MD: growth of abnormal blood vessels leaks fluid and blood into the retina causing scars to form. The scars result in distortion of vision

Priority Assessments or Cues

> Assess for blurred, darkened and distorted vision

> Asses for floaters or spots in field of vision, called scotomas. This is common in MD

> Assess for decreased central vision

> Ask about the need for brighter light when working, which is a consistent finding with MD

> Assess client's ability to read print, may find that words are blurred

Priority Laboratory Tests/Diagnostics

> Ophthalmoscopy shows drusen deposits and other changes consistent with MD

> Optical coherence tomography examines the anatomy of the retina and appearance of the macula

> Scanning laser ophthalmoscopy examines anatomy of the retina and appearance of the macula

> Amsler grid tests the integrity of the retina

> Fundus photography, indocyanine green dyes and intravenous angiography clarifies the extent of MD and whether it is wet or dry

Priority Interventions or Actions

> Assist with administration of intraocular injected medications to slow vision loss and monitor for side effects such as eye irritation, photosensitivity and eye pain

> If client had photodynamic therapy, ensure no part of their body is exposed before leaving to go home as sunlight on any part of the body can activate the drug used in the therapy, causing sunburn

Priority Potential & Actual Complications

> Progression from dry to wet macular degeneration

> Visual hallucinations

> Physical disability due to vision loss

Priority Nursing Implications

> Loss of central vision from macular degeneration can be very devastating for the client and family. It is important to understand the implications of this loss when it comes to caring for the client and interacting with the family. Help them to determine the best ways to cope with the vision loss and lifestyle changes that will need to be made

Priority Medications

> There are several selective inhibitors used to treat wet MD. Three commonly used drugs are below

> ranibizumab
> - selective inhibitors of endothelial growth factor
> - Slows vision loss in wet MD
> - Dose is 0.5 mg via intravitreal injection once monthly

> aflibercept
> - selective inhibitors of endothelial growth factor
> - Slows vision loss in wet MD
> - Dose is 2 mg (0.05 mL) administered by intravitreal injection every 4 weeks for the first 12 weeks, then 2 mg (0.05 mL) via intravitreal injection once every 8 weeks

> pegaptanib
> - selective inhibitors of endothelial growth factor
> - Slows vision loss in wet MD
> - Dose is 0.3 mg via intravitreal injection into the affected eye once every 6 weeks

Priority Education/Discharge Issues

> Teach the use of visual aids to maximize current vision, such as electronic hand-held magnifiers, E-readers, image zooming, among others

> Teach that taking high doses of vitamins and minerals can help to decrease the risk of vision loss

> Educate on the side effects of medications that are injected in the eye (mentioned in priority intervention above)

> Teach that injections are administered every 4 to 6 weeks

> Teach that the healthcare provider will determine response to medication therapy using the optic coherence tomography test

> If client had photodynamic therapy, teach to avoid intense light and sunlight for 5 days after the procedure as the drug used can be activated by light

> Teach that smoking cessation helps to slow vision loss

Hearing impairment

Pathophysiology/Description

> Hearing loss is the inability to hear sounds

> There are various factors that cause hearing loss. Impacted cerumen, foreign items in the ear, otitis media, damage to tympanic membrane, presbycusis and ototoxicity are just a few of the causes

> Types of hearing loss

- Sensorineural: occurs due to functional defect of inner ear, such as noise causing trauma over time. This type of hearing loss is usually permanent

- Conductive: transmission of sound waves to the inner ear is hindered because of conditions in the middle or outer ear such as impacted cerumen

- Mixed: hearing loss results from a combination of both sensorineural and conductive factors

- Central: the inability to interpret speech and sound due to problem occurring in the brain

- Functional: psychological factors seem to cause functional hearing loss. The person does not hear or respond even though there are no physical reasons for the hearing loss

Priority Assessments or Cues

> Determine onset of client's symptoms

> Determine history of ear infections or other ear injuries

> Ask about exposure to constant loud noise

> Engage client in speech to determine if client asks to repeat statements, as is common in hearing loss

> Assess to determine if client responds incorrectly to questions asked

> Observe if client turns head to one side to hear, as if favoring one ear

> Assess if client cannot respond when spoken to unless looking directly at the speaker's lips

> Assess client for ringing in the ear (tinnitus), among the first signs of hearing loss

> Assess client's tone of voice in conversation, shouting is usual

> Observe if the client increases the sound level on equipment, such as television or radio, when others in the room are hearing the sound perfectly

> Ask client about withdrawal from large or social gatherings. This is usually because of fear of being engaged in a conversation

> Assess the impact hearing loss has on client's quality of life

Priority Laboratory Tests/Diagnostics

> Tuning fork tests to determine hearing loss and the type (sensorineural vs conduction)

> Audiometer test determines degree of hearing loss and how best to treat it

> Whisper test determines if client is able to hear spoken words from a certain distance

Priority Interventions or Actions

> Get the client's full attention before speaking. Speak into the client's better ear

> Do not cover face or mouth with hand when speaking to client. Maintain eye contact

> Ensure there is no food in the mouth or chewing of gum when speaking

> Stand close to client and ensure speech is slow and words are properly formed

> Use written words if needed

> Ensure the room is quiet and there are no distractors, such as television on or other people speaking

> Decrease the decibel of the voice when speaking as shouting does not help the client

> Ensure the room is well lit

> Ensure non-verbal expression matches spoken words as client who lip reads relies on a match of words with non-verbal expressions

> Rephrase sentences if needed

Priority Potential & Actual Complications

> Complete hearing loss

> Social isolation

Priority Nursing Implications

> Some older adults with hearing loss due to presbycusis, may believe that their hearing loss results from the aging process and so they simply accept it as such and believe that nothing can be done to aid their hearing. As nurses, it is important to present all options for hearing assistive devices and techniques to older adults with hearing loss

Priority Education/Discharge Issues

> Teach client to face the person with whom a conversation is being had

> Instruct client to have conversations in good lighting so lip reading might be easier and ensure there is no background noise as distraction

> Teach client to ask others with whom a conversing is being held to speak clearly and into the unaffected ear

> Teach client to avoid high noise levels

> Provide information to client about types of hearing aids, listening devices and the cochlear implant procedure

> Provide information to client on the use of sign language (usually for clients who have severe hearing loss)

> Teach client to keep audiologist appointments

Scoliosis

Pathophysiology/Description

> Scoliosis is a deformity of the spine that is characterized by an S-shaped curvature of the lumbar and thoracic spine, occurring quite often during a child's growth spurts just before puberty (called idiopathic scoliosis), or seen at birth (called congenital scoliosis). The condition is seen mostly in girls than boys

> Some causes of scoliosis might be muscular dystrophy, cerebral palsy, defects from birth that affect spinal bone development and other factors such as infection or injuries to the spine

> The condition can be mild where there is no significant physical impairment or functioning, or so severe that it limits the child's physical functioning

> Scoliosis must be monitored as the child grows to determine any changes in spinal curvature

> Monitoring of scoliosis
> • With spinal curvature of 10-20 degrees (mild) the child must be evaluated every 3 months and X-rays done every 6 months, with prescribed exercises to increase muscle strength and improve posture
> • Spinal curvature 20-40 degrees (moderate), brace worn for 23 hours daily to prevent further curvature
> • Spinal curvature greater more than 40 degrees (severe), spinal fusion surgery with instrumentation is needed

Priority Assessments or Cues

> Have client bend over at the waist, will observe asymmetry of the trunk

> Inspect client from behind, uneven shoulders, scapula, hips and waist will be seen

> Ask caregiver about appearance of client's clothing. Caregiver may report uneven appearance in length of client's skirt

> Assess leg length when client is standing, will notice asymmetry

> Assess client and caregiver's understanding of various options for treatment depending on the degree of child's curvature

Priority Laboratory Tests/Diagnostics

> Scoliometer to measure symmetry of the trunk

> X-ray to confirm the diagnosis of scoliosis

> Magnetic resonance imaging (MRI) to detect underlying conditions that may be impacting scoliosis

Priority Interventions or Actions

> Prepare client for testing that will measure curvature and determine treatment protocol

> Explain course of treatment to client and caregiver

> Initiate exercises to treat client who has mild curvature

> Apply prescribed brace to client with moderate curvature

> Inspect skin under brace for signs of skin breakdown. Wash and dry skin before reapplying brace

> Instruct client in proper use of assistive devices. Prepare client for surgery, if severe scoliosis

> Postoperative interventions
> • Monitor dressing to surgical site for bleeding and infection. Administer analgesics
> • Perform log rolling when turning and repositioning client
> • Keep client's body in proper alignment. Do not twist or bend client's body
> • Prevent respiratory compromise by allowing client to cough and deep breathe. Have client use incentive spirometry
> • Use compression devices to minimize risk of blood clots. Assist with ambulation
> • Perform good skin care to prevent pressure ulcers. Place thoracolumbar sacral orthosis (TLSO) on client
> • Keep client nothing by mouth until able to eat oral foods, as prescribed
> • Monitor neurological and cardiac status

Priority Potential & Actual Complications

> Back problems such as pain. Cardiac and respiratory problems

> Physical appearance and physical disability

> Mental problems, such as depression and social isolation

Priority Nursing Implications

> As nurses, it is crucial that the emotional status of a client who must wear a brace for 23 of 24 hours in a day be considered as this is usually a child who might experience body image issues from socializing with peers

Priority Education/Discharge Issues

> Teach client how to don and doff the brace

> Educate that wearing of the brace will be discontinued after bones have stopped growing

> Teach to wear brace for 23 hours daily and importance of washing and drying skin under brace before reapplying. Instruct to wear t-shirt under brace for skin protection

> Teach to perform prescribed exercises daily to prevent further curvature

> Teach client how to log roll and get on and off the bed after surgery

> Teach not to bend or twist body. Teach to sit straight in chairs and not to slump

> Teach importance of maintaining restrictions on activity for up to 8 months after surgery as prescribed. Teach not to engage in sports that increase the risk of falls

> Teach that if a rod is placed in the spine, it will be lengthened every 6 months as the client grows

> Teach surgery site assessment for bleeding, signs of infection and when to contact health care provider

Labyrinthitis/Meniere's disease

Pathophysiology/Description

> Labyrinthitis and Meniere's disease are both disorders of the inner ear that cause dizziness and affect balance

> When one of the two vestibular nerves in the inner ear becomes inflamed, for various reasons, labyrinthitis occurs

> Meniere's disease has no known cause but with the disease, excessive amounts of endolymph is observed in the membranous labyrinth, causing the labyrinth to rupture. There is usually poor reabsorption or overproduction of the endolymph fluid. Meniere's disease is also known as endolymphatic hydrops

> Factors causing labyrinthitis: bacterial and viral infections of middle and inner ear, respiratory and gastrointestinal tract

> In some cases, viral and bacterial infections, head injury, allergic reactions, stress and biochemical issues may have an association with Meniere's disease

> Most people with these conditions do not require surgical intervention. However, when attacks from Meniere's disease becomes incapacitating, surgery is an option

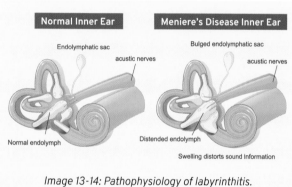

Image 13-14: Pathophysiology of labyrinthitis.

Priority Assessments or Cues

> Complete history and physical. Client may report symptoms that have lasted for hours or days

> Assess client for vertigo and dizziness. In Meniere's disease client may describe intense vertigo even when lying down. Assess for loss of balance

> Assess for headaches, that may be severe with Meniere's disease. Assess for nausea and vomiting

> Test client's hearing and may find hearing loss on affected side

> Examine client's eyes, may see nystagmus. Client may have difficulty focusing the eyes

> Assess client's stance, may see that client is unbalanced

> Ask client about ringing in the ear as this is common with labyrinthitis

> Ask client to describe feeling in ears, may say there is a feeling of fullness in the ear, with Meniere's

> Assess client's spatial awareness, may describe a feeling of spinning in space or being pulled to the ground, with Meniere's disease

Priority Laboratory Tests/Diagnostics

> Audiometer test determines if hearing loss is being experienced

> Electronystagmography (ENG) balance test. With Meniere's disease reduced balance response will be manifest in one ear

> Vestibular testing examines the inner ear to try and isolate the symptoms to a specific cause

> Glycerol test: the client is given an oral dose of glycerol and audiograms are performed. Diagnosis of Meniere's disease is supported if improvement in hearing and speech discrimination occurs

> Electroencephalogram, used to look at electrical activity in brain to rule out other causes of symptoms, in labyrinthitis

Priority Interventions or Actions

> In an acute attack, administer medications such as antihistamines, antivertigo, antiemetics and benzodiazepines. Diuretic may also be ordered for Meniere's disease

> Maintain a safe environment to prevent client from falls

> Allow client to stay in bed in a room that is dark, that has reduced stimulation

> Ensure client does not make sudden head movements or changes position suddenly as these actions will worsen vertigo

> Provide client with an emesis basin as vomiting is expected

> Keep the wheels of the bed locked, side rails up and the bed in a low position

> Instruct client to call for assistance before getting out of bed

> Ensure client gets diet low in sodium, helps to decrease fluid in the ear in Meniere's disease

> Surgical interventions (endolymphatic sac decompression and placement of a shunt, vestibular nerve section or labyrinthectomy)

- Monitor neurological system

- Assess dressing to affected ear. Assess packing for bleeding and signs of infection

- Administer medications for vertigo and nausea

- Place bedside commode in client's room and encourage client to use it rather than attempting to walk to the bathroom

- Ensure call bell is within client's reach and reinforce the importance of calling for assistance before getting up

- Do not allow client to ambulate alone, as dizziness may persist after surgery

- When conversing with client, speak on the nonoperative side

Priority Potential & Actual Complications

> Meningitis (with labyrinthitis)
> Hearing loss
> Loss of balance
> Social isolation

Priority Nursing Implications

> Prednisone should not be stopped abruptly as client will experience prednisone withdrawal symptoms, which include weakness, severe fatigue, and joint and body aches

Priority Medications

> There are several drugs used to treat both diseases in an acute attack. Below are some commonly used drugs
> diphenhydramine
  • Antihistamine used to decrease sensations in both conditions
  • Usual oral dose is 25 to 50 mg orally 3 to 4 times daily
  • Usual parenteral dose is 10 to 50 mg deep intramuscular or intravenous as needed
> lorazepam
  • Benzodiazepine used to decrease sensations in both conditions
  • Usual initial dose is 2 to 3 mg taken orally per day, given 2 to 3 times daily
  • Usual maintenance dose is 1 to 2 mg orally 2 to 3 times daily
> meclizine
  • Used to treat vertigo associated with both conditions
  • Usual dose is 25 to 100 mg taken oral, daily in divided doses
  • Exact dose depends on client's clinical response
> prednisone
  • Corticosteroid used to control swelling in labyrinthitis
  • Usual initial dose is 5 to 60 mg orally per day
  • Dosage to be tapered
> hydrochlorothiazide
  • Diuretic
  • Works by reducing fluid in inner ear
  • Usual dose is 25 mg daily
> prochlorperazine
  • Antiemetic used to treat nausea and vomiting in both conditions
  • Usual oral dose is 5 to 10 mg orally 3 to 4 times daily
  • Usual intramuscular dose is 5 to 10 mg intramuscular. The dose can be repeated every 3 to 4 hours as needed

Priority Education/Discharge Issues

> Teach client to take medications as prescribed and report adverse effects to health care provider
> Teach client to assess packing to ear for signs of bleeding or abnormal drainage and report to health care provider
> Instruct client to change positions slowly and avoid making jerking and quick motions with the head
> Teach client to maintain safety with attacks. Do not walk alone
> Teach removal of fall hazards from home, such as loose area rugs. Instruct on the use of nonslip mats in the shower
> Teach client about dietary factors that may help with Meniere's disease, such as limiting salt, monosodium glutamate (MSG), alcohol and caffeine
> Instruct client to rest and decrease environmental stimulation during an attack of Meniere's disease and labyrinthitis
> Teach client to stop smoking and avoid allergens as both are irritants that may worsen the conditions
> Teach importance of follow-up appointments

Otitis media/externa

Pathophysiology/Description

> Otitis media is an infection of middle ear that results in inflammation

> Otitis media is caused by a blockage of the eustachian tube because of swelling that occurs from allergies, colds or bacteria. An effusion can also occur with otitis media, which manifests as purulent or mucoid fluid, accumulating in the middle ear space following conditions such as trauma from pressure change and a sinus infection

> Children are particularly vulnerable to getting otitis media as they have shorter and flatter eustachian tubes than that of an adult's, making this condition a childhood disease

> Otitis media can become chronic with recurrent multiple attacks, causing cholesterol and epithelial cells to form in the middle ear leading to mastoiditis. These cholesterol formations must be surgically removed

> While otitis media is a middle ear infection, otitis externa (external otitis), also called swimmer's ear, is an inflammation or infection of the outer ear and ear canal. Swelling that occurs with otitis externa can lead to conductive hearing loss

> Otitis externa can be caused by several factors, such as swimming in contaminated water, trauma to the ear, fungi, bacteria or placing objects inside the ear to scratch the ear (such as a hairpin). Otitis externa is also more common in children than adults

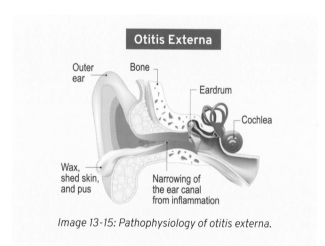

Image 13-15: Pathophysiology of otitis externa.

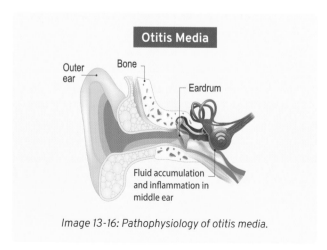

Image 13-16: Pathophysiology of otitis media.

Priority Assessments or Cues

> Assess vital signs, will likely find increased temperature as fever is common in otitis media and in otitis externa if the infection has spread to adjacent tissues

> Assess for ear pain as this is one of the first signs with both conditions

> Assess client for crying and fussiness because of the pain and discomfort. Client will be tugging and rubbing on the ear or placing finger in the ear

> Observe client's head movement, may see head moving from side to side

> Assess client for hearing loss or muffled hearing that can occur in both conditions

> Ask caregiver about client's eating, may find loss of appetite

> Examine ear for drainage, blood-tinged or purulent drainage may be seen in otitis externa. Purulent drainage in chronic otitis media

> Assess client's chewing, may find that chewing causes significant discomfort with otitis externa

> Assess for redness and edema, seen more with otitis externa

Priority Laboratory Tests/Diagnostics

> Otoscopic examination will reveal a bulging tympanic membrane with redness

> Tympanometry to measure the pressure in the ear and see if there is a ruptured eardrum

> X-ray, computed tomography (CT) scan and magnetic resonance imaging (MRI) of the mastoid, to look for bone involvement and a mass (with chronic otitis media)

> Culture and sensitivity of ear drainage to determine bacterial growth and best treatment course

Priority Interventions or Actions

> Apply moist heat for both conditions as prescribed

> Administer analgesics, antipyretics, antiemetics and antibiotics as prescribed

> Manipulate client's pinna gently when examining ear or instilling ear drops

> Monitor for therapeutic effect of medications

> Prepare client for surgery, if indicated

> Postoperative interventions for otitis media (myringotomy, tympanoplasty)

- Assess dressing to affected ear. Assess packing for bleeding and signs of infection

- Ensure use of proper infection control practices such as hand hygiene

- Prevent client from making quick, sudden movements of the head

- Encourage client not to cough or strain (as in having a bowel movement)
- Do not offer client a straw to use for drinking
- Clean hair by wiping with a clean washcloth to avoid wetting the head. Keep ear dry

🚩 Priority Potential & Actual Complications

> Facial paralysis from tympanoplasty surgery and hearing loss

☡ Priority Nursing Implications

> When caring for older adults with ear infections, be aware of malignant external otitis, which is an infection caused by a serious pathogen and usually afflicts older adults with diabetes. It can be potentially fatal if not treated because it can migrate from the external ear to the temporal bone causing osteomyelitis. Antibiotics must be administered to treat this infection

💧 Priority Medications

> Several antibiotics are used to treat otitis media and otitis externa and dosages vary based on the age and weight of the child. Below are some examples
> amoxicillin
  - Antibiotic to treat otitis media
  - Usual pediatric dose is immediate-release 80 to 90 mg/kg/day orally in 2 divided doses. Duration of therapy can vary based on provider's preference
  - Treat both otitis media and external otitis
> amoxicillin/clavulanate
  - Antibiotic
  - Usual adult dosage is 250 mg orally every 8 hours or 500 mg orally every 12 hours for 10 to 14 days
  - Pediatric dosage is based on the age and weight of the child
> ciprofloxacin and dexamethasone (combination drug)
  - Antibiotic and steroid ear medication
  - Usual adult and pediatric dosage 4 drops in the affected ear 2 times daily for 7 days
  - Treat otitis externa and otitis media in adults and children older than 6 months
> finafloxacin
  - Antibiotic otic suspension
  - Usual dosage for adults and children is 4 drops into the affected ear two times daily for 7 days.
  - Treat otitis externa in adults and children older than 12 months

👤 Priority Education/Discharge Issues

> Teach client/caregiver to take medications as prescribed and report adverse effects to health care provider
> Teach client to notify the health care provider if the tympanoplasty tubes fall out
> Instruct on the proper administration of ear drops
> Instruct client/caregiver to finish all prescribed antibiotics even if client starts to feel better
> Teach client/caregiver to assess packing to ear and dressing for signs of bleeding or abnormal drainage and report to health care provider
> Instruct client/caregiver on proper/safe cleaning of drainage
> Teach that while packing is in the ear, client may experience impaired hearing
> Instruct client/caregiver to change positions slowly and avoid making jerking and quick motions with the head
> Instruct to avoid forceful coughing and to not wash hair for 1 week
> Instruct not to travel by air in the weeks following surgery
> Teach not to blow the nose for about 1 week after surgery but if needed to blow, do so with 1 nostril at a time and with the mouth open
> Instruct on the use of earplugs when client returns to swimming or other water activities that involve water submergence
> Teach importance of follow-up appointments

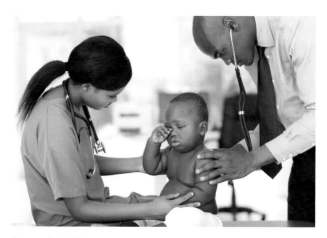

Image 13-17: The parent asks, "When should I take my child to the doctor for an ear infection?" What is the nurse's best response?

_____

_____

_____

Spina bifida

Pathophysiology/Description

> Neural tube forms in early pregnancy and usually closes around 4 weeks after conception. Spina bifida is a neural tube defect that occurs because the neural tube fails to close during development of the embryo

> Causes include maternal malnutrition, radiation, chemicals and a genetic mutation

> Risk factors include maternal obesity, low vitamin B12 and folate in pregnancy, and maternal diabetes, family history of neural tube defects, use of antiseizure medications in pregnancy

> The condition is seen more in females than males and among Caucasians and Hispanics than other ethnic groups

> There are two types of spina bifida, spina bifida cystica and spina bifida occulta

 • Spina bifida occulta: a mild form of the condition. There is no protrusion of meninges and only a small separation exists in the vertebrae. It usually goes undiagnosed as there are no neurologic deficits

 • Spina bifida cystica: spinal cord and meninges protrude and form a sac on the lumbar or sacral area. There are two types of spina bifida cystica, meningocele and myelomeningocele

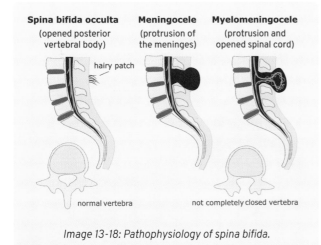

Image 13-18: Pathophysiology of spina bifida.

Priority Assessments or Cues

> Assess for flaccid paralysis of lower extremities

> Assess bowel and bladder status, may find incontinence of both

> Assess joints, may find deformities of joints primarily hip subluxation and dislocation

> Examine back, will see protruded sac in back. Assess sac for rupture, bleeding and signs of infection

> Examine posture, may see kyphosis and scoliosis

> Assess reflexes, may find missing deep tendon reflexes

> Assess for nuchal rigidity, somnolence and fussiness which may indicate meningitis

> Assess child's fontanels, bulging fontanel might indicate increased intracranial pressure

> Assess vital signs, elevated temperature may indicate an infection. Measure axillary temperature as a rectal thermometer might cause a rectal prolapse

Priority Laboratory Tests/Diagnostics

> Ultrasound scan of uterus, may show meningocele

> Maternal serum alpha-fetoprotein (MSAFP) test shows significantly high alpha-fetoprotein (AFP) levels

> Blood test to confirm the high AFP level, further evaluation is done if AFP is still high

> Amniocentesis, showing high levels of AFP

Priority Interventions or Actions

> Perform thorough neurological assessment

> Prevent meningocele from drying, cover with saline moistened sterile gauze. Change gauze dressing every 2-4 hours to prevent infection

> Measure child's head circumference as hydrocele can occur. Measure intracranial pressure

> Maintain aseptic technique when caring for meningocele

> Position child in prone position to take pressure off the meningocele

> Do not place diaper on child before surgery as it may cover the meningocele

> Measure intake and output

> Use measure to prevent stool from soiling the meningocele

> Provide gentle range of motion to prevent contractures and muscle wasting

> Prepare child for surgery. Initiate nothing by mouth

> Ensure caregivers' questions are answered preoperatively

> Postoperative interventions

 • Monitor surgery site for bleeding signs of infection and cerebrospinal fluid leak

 • Administer pain medication as prescribed

 • Place child in a prone or side-lying position as prescribed

 • Continue bowel and bladder care as preoperatively

 • Continue neurological assessments as preoperatively

 • Resume feedings as prescribed when child is awake and alert from anesthesia

 • Involve caregivers in child's care

Priority Potential & Actual Complications

> Immobility

> Bowel and bladder incontinence

> Meningitis

> Orthopedic issues

> Sleep disorders

> Hydrocephalus

> Restricted or tethered spinal cord (spinal nerves become bound to the scar where surgery occurred)

Priority Nursing Implications

> In most cases of spina bifida, surgery occurs after the infant is born. However, when spina bifida is detected in pregnancy, prenatal surgery can be done to repair the spinal cord. Surgery must occur before week 26 of pregnancy

Priority Education/Discharge Issues

> Teach caregiver how to perform dressing changes and assess surgical site for infection

> Educate on proper positioning of child, prone or side-lying as prescribed

> Teach caregiver to perform proper skin care and to avoid stools getting to the surgery site

> Teach caregiver to perform intermittent urinary catheterization, if prescribed

> Teach to perform gentle range of motion on child joints to prevent contractures

> Teach signs of complications and who to call if complications occur

> Educate on importance of feeding child a diet that has high fiber and fluids to prevent constipation

> Educate caregiver that child may have latex allergy because of repeated exposure to latex in the acute care setting

> Educate caregiver how to use mobility aids for child, as prescribed

> Educate caregiver on the trajectory of spina bifida and the long-term needs of the child

> Educate caregiver that child may need ongoing care from several professionals such as neurology, orthopedics, urology, physical/occupational/speech therapy and special education professionals

> Assist caregiver with resources for support groups, if needed. Provide information for the Spina Bifida Association of America

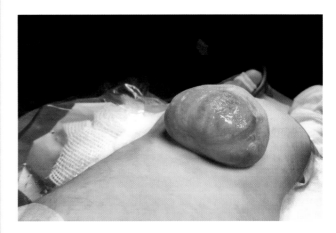

Image 13-19: The client's parent is very overwhelmed after their infant's spina bifida surgery. List 5 statements by the parent that indicates that post operative teaching was effective.

1. _____

_____

2. _____

_____

3. _____

_____

4. _____

_____

5. _____

_____

_____

_____

_____

_____

Spinal cord injury

Pathophysiology/Description

> Spinal cord injury (SCI) is caused by damage to the spinal cord, usually from a traumatic event, which causes temporary or permanent changes in function

> Classified as primary vs secondary injury. Primary refers to the initial injury caused by a specific event, such as a gunshot. Secondary refers to the ongoing damage that continues after the initial injury has occurred. There are many factors that can impact secondary injury, among them are cellular necrosis and vascular changes.

> Characterized by the level of injury, degree of injury and mechanism of injury

> Level of injury

  • Tetraplegia (used to be called quadriplegia): trunk, arms, hands, pelvic organ and legs all impacted by the spinal cord injury

  • Paraplegia: all or part of the trunk, legs and pelvic organs are affected

> Degree of injury

  • Complete injury: sensory and motor function are lost below the level of injury

> Incomplete injury: there is some motor or sensory function below the level of injury.

> Mechanism of injury: Hyperflexion, flexion, extension-rotation, flexion-rotation and compression

Priority Assessments or Cues

> Respiratory issues, likely with cervical injuries, especially above C4

> Vital signs and oxygen saturation. Ensure saturation is greater than 90%

> Cause of trauma, open wounds and signs of internal injuries

> Neurologic system, using the American Spinal Injury Association (ASIA) Impairment Scale

> Cardiovascular system, hypotension and bradycardia due to deficit in sympathetic nervous system

> Absence of reflexes and other deficits below the injury

> Neurogenic bladder and bowel, common in SCI. Treat as prescribed

> Paralysis in all four extremities or in lower extremities only

> Nutritional status. Client will have significant nutritional needs

> Neuropathic pain, often described as tingling, burning, or shooting

> Catheter-associated urinary tract infection because of the extended usage of urinary catheters

Priority Laboratory Tests/Diagnostics

> Computerized tomography (CT) scan showing degree and location of injury. X-ray, viewing spinal column

> Magnetic resonance imaging (MRI) showing neurological changes and any soft tissue damages

Priority Interventions or Actions

> Immobilize client and maintain a patent airway. Ensure oxygen saturation greater 90%

> Initiate placement of endotracheal tube as needed. Monitor arterial blood gasses and determine need for client to be placed on a mechanical ventilator

> Initiate intravenous lines and start fluids as prescribed. Place nasogastric tube to suction

> Ensure client receives nutrition via alternate routes in the initial days of the injury

> Head in neutral position. Do not place in sitting position. Move with log roll technique

> Maintain normal body temperature. Monitor for signs of respiratory infection

> Perform ongoing monitoring of all systems. Provide prophylaxis for stress ulcers as prescribed

> Compression devices to prevent venous thromboembolism. Low-dose heparin as prescribed

> Pressure ulcer prevention protocol, ensuring meticulous skin care

> Monitor for signs indicating spinal shock and/or autonomic dysreflexia/hyperreflexia

> Consultations for speech, occupational and physical therapists

> If autonomic hyperreflexia occurs: raise head of bed, loosen tight clothing, assess for cause and relieve the cause. Most often it occurs because of a full bladder or bowel. Perform urinary catheterization and bowel evacuation if needed. Administer antihypertensive and monitor blood pressure every 15 minutes

> Postoperative interventions (skeletal traction for cervical or upper thoracic injuries)

  • Weights to the traction. Check to ensure weights hang freely without touching

  • Client's body in good alignment. Maintain use of Stryker frame or other types of special bed

  • Monitor proper fit of the halo jacket. Ensure 1 finger fits under the jacket

  • Place foam or fleece at pressure points under halo vest to prevent pressure ulcers

  • Clean pin sites on halo and skull tongs daily and monitor for signs of infection

- High-protein, calcium-rich diet to promote bone healing and prevent muscle wasting
- Wrench at the bedside that can open the halo in an emergency if needed

> Postoperative interventions (laminectomy or spinal fusion for thoracic, lumbar and sacral injuries)

- Monitor circulation and motor function in lower extremities. Monitor respiratory function
- Monitor surgery site for bleeding and infection. Provide cast care for full-body casts
- Client flat and in good alignment. Turn and reposition every 2 hours using log rolling.
- Encourage incentive spirometry and coughing and deep breathing
- Nothing by mouth until bowel sounds return. Monitor intake and output

🚩 Priority Potential & Actual Complications

> Autonomic dysreflexia/hyperreflexia, spinal shock, neurogenic shock

> Complete or partial paralysis, total dependence, depression and social isolation

℧ Priority Nursing Implications

> During the first 2 days of a spinal cord injury, edema may cause severe respiratory dysfunction, placing client at risk for respiratory failure. Respiratory problems are the main cause of death in persons who sustain a spinal cord injury

> When reflexes for a client with thoracic spinal injury at T6 or higher has returned after a spinal shock, autonomic hyperreflexia can occur. This is manifested as significantly high blood pressure, severe headache, bradycardia, flushing and sweating above the injury, blurred vision and nausea. Autonomic hyperreflexia is a medical emergency to avoid a stroke

🩸 Priority Medications

> Several drugs are used for various aspects of spinal cord injury. Below are some examples

> enoxaparin
- Low molecular weight heparin
- Usual dose is 40 mg subcutaneously once daily
- Used to prevent venous thromboembolism

> phenylephrine
- Vasopressor drug

- Usual intramuscular or subcutaneous dose is 2 to 5 mg every 1 to 2 hours as needed
- Used to maintain mean arterial pressure at a level that improves perfusion to spinal cord

> oxybutynin
- Anticholinergic drug used to treat neurogenic bladder
- Recommended immediate-release dose is 5 mg orally 2 to 3 times daily
- Recommended extended-release dose is 5 to 10 mg once a day at approximately the same time each day

> nifedipine
- Calcium channel blocker: one of many used to treat autonomic dysreflexia
- Usual Initial dose is 30 to 60 mg orally once daily
- Usual maintenance dose is 30 to 90 mg orally once daily

👤 Priority Education/Discharge Issues

> Teaching regarding nutritional intake and bowel management
- Eat 3 well-balanced meals daily that consist of high protein, and 20-30 grams of daily fiber to prevent constipation. Drink adequate fluids. Exercise as able
- Determine schedule for bowel movements and manual rectal stimulation

> Teaching regarding care of halo vest
- Clean pin sites as prescribed and apply antibiotic ointment. Report signs of infection
- Open vest one side at time while lying down, clean, inspect, dry skin and replace brace
- Dry vest with hair dryer if wet
- Do not twist body. Always keep wrench close. Wear sheepskin pad under vest

> Teaching regarding autonomic hyperreflexia
- Signs of autonomic hyperreflexia (aforementioned) and report immediately
- Raise head of bed, check for bowel impaction or full bladder and relieve cause

> Teaching regarding skin care
- Change position in bed every 2 hours, at least. Shift position in wheelchair every 15 minutes. Use pressure relief mattress and chair cushion
- Cut fingernails short. Examine skin daily for skin breakdown

> Trajectory of spinal cord injury and the long-term care needs

> Need for ongoing care from several professionals. Resources for support groups

1. A client returns to the orthopedic unit after surgery for a traumatic amputation of the left foot in a farming accident. What statement or query by the client requires immediate follow-up by the nurse?
   1. "It feels like the tractor is still crushing my foot!"
   2. "Should I feel tingling in my toes?"
   3. "Thank God I didn't lose my whole leg!"
   4. "My father had a similar accident years ago."

2. The nurse is doing discharge teaching for a client in day surgery who had carpal tunnel release of the dominant hand. Which question by the client indicates additional teaching is needed?
   1. "If I see blood soaking through the dressing, I need to call or come back immediately."
   2. "I am to take the pain medication as it is prescribed as needed."
   3. "I can only lift 10 pounds with that hand, so my infant is OK to lift."
   4. "I should be able to return to work on limitations until the dressing is removed."

3. The clinic nurse is planning to teach a group in the community center about prevention and risks of osteoporosis. Which statement by the nurse would be important to include in the teaching plan?
   1. "Everyone, especially those at risk, should include adequate calcium in their diets."
   2. "Genetics have no role in development of osteoporosis."
   3. "Osteoporosis is totally preventable for those over 65, with screenings."
   4. "People who are less active are at less risk for fractures from osteoporosis."

4. A client presents to the clinic looking extremely tired and complains that movements of the legs have prevented sleep for several nights. What statement by the nurse would be most appropriate?
   1. "I can't imagine living with my legs moving about all night. I wouldn't be able to sleep either."
   2. "Losing sleep like that can be very exhausting. Let's do a complete assessment to help find the cause(s)."
   3. "My husband has restless legs syndrome and tosses about all night. That would be that's what's going on with you."
   4. "Oh, my! You look so tired like you could just drop. Sit down and rest a bit."

5. The clinic nurse is evaluating a client with Parkinson's disease who was ordered levodopa/carbidopa. What assessment by the nurse would be highest priority?
   1. "Are you having any side effects of the medication?"
   2. "Do you experience fewer freezing motion episodes?"
   3. "Have you had any difficulty with urination?"
   4. "Do you experience a bit less shaking of your hands?"

6. The clinic nurse is teaching a client about improving quality of life while living with osteoarthritis. Which statement by the client demonstrates that more teaching is needed?
   1. "I can alternate heat and cold to alleviate my pain and tenderness in my knee."
   2. "I will call the outpatient therapy unit for appointments when you send the order."
   3. "So, which over-the-counter medications will help with pain after the injection into my knee?"
   4. "This is just part of aging since nothing can be done to decrease my pain or disability."

7. A female client who sustained a cervical spinal cord injury with quadriplegia states she has a headache. Which is the first nursing action?
   1. Conduct a comprehensive pain assessment.
   2. Palpate and bladder scan the client's lower abdomen.
   3. Turn the client to the side and reposition extremities.
   4. Assess the client's body temperature.

8. The nurse is caring for a client with a medical diagnosis of amyotrophic lateral sclerosis (ALS) and pneumonia. The client's spouse calls the nurses station reporting the client coughing and choking. What would be the priority nursing action?
   1. Give the client a drink of water with a straw.
   2. Medicate the client for the cough as needed.
   3. Place prescribed oxygen on per nasal canula and suction after assessing lung sounds.
   4. Talk gently to the client in a calm voice while assessing the severity of the symptoms.

9. The nurse is implementing discharge teaching with an athlete that sustained a closed fracture of the femur after an injury at a track meet. The healthcare provider placed a long-leg soft cast until swelling diminishes. What statement by the client demonstrates a need for clarification?
   1. "I can put light weight on the leg since the provider put a heel on the cast."
   2. "I can go to school after two days at home."
   3. "I will use the crutches like this (and demonstrates)."
   4. "I won't take pain medicine unless I begin to feel like I need it."

10. The home health nurse is visiting a client with multiple sclerosis who is complaining of urinary leakage. What information should the nurse gather first?
    1. "Do you feel full in the lower abdomen?"
    2. "Have you been using pads or briefs? Do I need to bring you more?"
    3. "Are you leaking stool also?"
    4. "Let me call the provider and get an in-and-out catheter order."

11. The nurse is caring for a client admitted with a possible diagnosis of Guillain-Barré syndrome (GBS). What statement by the client requires immediate follow-up?
    1. "I had the flu about a month ago and thought I was over it."
    2. "I'm having difficulty breathing and feel like I can't catch my breath."
    3. "I am having trouble doing my routine activities."
    4. "My hands and feet are numb and feel very heavy."

12. The nurse is working with young adults with cerebral palsy (CP). Which client should be assessed first for a risk for injury?
    1. A client who is non-ambulatory and has weakness of the extremities and inability to move voluntarily.
    2. A client in a wheelchair that does not appear to fit correctly and causes mal-alignment of the spine.
    3. A client with difficulty with articulation and communicating, causing the client frustration.
    4. An ambulatory client with uncontrolled muscle movements, spasticity, and a wide gait.

13. A client who has had Myasthenia Gravis for five years is admitted to the hospital for an unrelated problem. What nursing interventions would be most effective in avoiding triggering a myasthenic crisis?
    1. Assess the client's ability to maintain a usual lifestyle and role responsibilities.
    2. Help client plan around activities in the hospital to minimize stress and fatigue.
    3. Monitor for side effects of the myasthenia drugs.
    4. Well-balanced diet with fresh fruits and vegetables.

14. The nurse is caring for a client with diabetic peripheral neuropathy. The client reports that sometimes there's an inability to determine the position of his feet when standing from a sitting position. What would be the priority nursing actions? Select all that apply.
    1. Be sure the client's feet are securely planted on the floor before helping the client to stand.
    2. Help the client sit on side of bed with the feet on a stool.
    3. Place client on fall precaution and caution the other staff.
    4. When making the bed, be sure to give the client's toes room under the sheet and blanket.
    5. Ensure that the client understands the need for assistance with standing and ambulation.

15. A nurse is conducting screening for scoliosis of middle school children Which assessment would warrant referral for further evaluation for this condition? Select all that apply.
    1. Back pain with significant twisting.
    2. Decreased lateral range of motion.
    3. Scapular hump with forward bending.
    4. Uneven shoulder height when standing.
    5. Palpable lesions on the vertebrae.
    6. Uneven appearance of bra straps.

16. The nurse is caring for an adult client with paraplegia secondary to spina bifida admitted for treatment of a Stage 3 pressure ulcer on the coccyx. Several methods have been discussed with the client and caregiver to treat the pressure ulcer. What should the priority focus be in treating the pressure ulcer?
    1. Change the wet-to-dry dressings twice daily.
    2. Eat a diet with many fruits, vegetables, and high protein.
    3. Keep off the coccyx by changing positions frequently and using a pressure reduction pillow or gel pad.
    4. Take a vitamin supplement with Vitamin C, B, iron, and others to promote healing.

17. The school nurse is caring for a child in third grade with spastic cerebral palsy, demonstrating hypertonia, tense muscles, hip flexion, toe walking, and scissor gait. What strategies does the nurse communicate to the classroom teacher to address safety of the child?
    1. Ensure the child is academically similar to the other children in the classroom.
    2. Explain to the other students that the child walks with difficulty because of a birth injury.
    3. Get an adapted table and chair for the child to use for ease of sitting to work.
    4. Treat the child as any other child in the classroom to prevent self-esteem issues.

18. A client presents to the clinic with sudden onset of pain when brushing his teeth and shaving. The pain continued ranging from a dull ache to severe pain. The clinic healthcare provider diagnoses trigeminal neuralgia and decides to try medical management of episodes. What action should the nurse take first?
    1. Administer pain medication.
    2. Do a thorough assessment of the nature and onset of the attacks.
    3. Prepare the client for a future surgery to relieve the symptoms.
    4. Refer the client to a psychologist in the clinic.

19. The nurse in the ophthalmology clinic has completed teaching for a client with macular degeneration. What statement by the client indicates additional teaching is needed?
    1. "I guess I will have to give up my needlepoint."
    2. "I hope my vision will improve with the medications."
    3. "I may have to quit driving when my vision decreases."
    4. "I will use a scanning technique with my peripheral vision to read."

20. A client in the post-op recovery unit after mastoidectomy with tympanoplasty, after suffering with chronic otitis media for many years. Intravenous orders include ceftazidime 4 grams in 24 hours in divided doses every 12 hours, diluted in 250 mL normal saline. The nurse begins the initial dose of _____ mg in 250 mL normal saline.

21. A home health nurse is caring for a client with severe arthritis in both knees. The client shares that he doesn't move around a lot because he is afraid of falling. What would the nurse ask first to assess the client's needs?
    1. "Are you able to attend church and other social functions?"
    2. "Can you get your groceries delivered by the market you shop?"
    3. "Why don't you ask your family to drive you for groceries and appointments?"
    4. "Will you show me any assistive devices you use to get around home or out?"

22. The nurse is preparing to care for a client newly diagnosed with Meniere's disease. What should be included in the nursing actions? Select all that apply.
    1. Keep an emesis basin at the bedside.
    2. Keep side rails up to minimize chance of falls.
    3. Leave the television on for the client for distraction.
    4. Tell the client to avoid sudden head movements.
    5. Turn off the lights and darken the blinds in the client's room during an attack.

23. A nurse is assessing a client who reports having been diagnosed with cataracts in the right eye last year. What information would be appropriate for the nurse to ask to gather further data? Select all that apply.
    1. "Do you attend social functions?"
    2. "Does closing one eye help you to see better?"
    3. "Are you able to drive at night?"
    4. "Do you often read for pleasure?"
    5. "Do you wear protective shades when outside?"

24. A client presents to the clinic with complaints of continued pain and paresthesia on the face and neck after a shingles infection (herpes zoster). What nursing actions should be taken next? Select all that apply.
    1. Assess the nature, quality/intensity, and location of the pain.
    2. Determine what exacerbates or alleviates the pain.
    3. Gently massage the painful area to see if that will alleviate it.
    4. Administer the prescribed antiviral agent.
    5. Tell the client that the infection is healed so the pain should be gone.

25. The client is diagnosed with bacterial conjunctivitis in the left eye. What factors should the nurse evaluate to prevent the spread of the infection to the other eye or others? Select all that apply.
    1. Allergies to pollens.
    2. Children in the home.
    3. Contact with other infected individuals.
    4. Practice frequent handwashing.
    5. Tearing, drainage.

26. The client with chronic open angle glaucoma is being sent home from the clinic with cholinergic agent carbachol eye drops—2 drops 3% solution TID. How much of the medication is the client receiving daily?

_____

27. A client with a fracture of the left hand is casted and the nurse is providing discharge teaching. What statements/questions from the client demonstrate a good understanding of discharge teaching? Select all that apply.
    1. "I can still play ball again in this weekend's game. I'm the best catcher they have."
    2. "I can shower as long as I cover the cast with plastic."
    3. "I have a follow-up appointment in two weeks."
    4. "I won't put anything in the cast to scratch any itches."
    5. "Throbbing pain is expected as my broken bones heal."

28. A client comes to the clinic with complaints of an earache from chronic otitis media. After consultation with the clinic provider, the nurse prepares to administer an antibiotic and pain medication. In what order would the nurse perform these actions? Rank order the responses.
    1. Administer the medications.
    2. Ask the client about any drug allergies.
    3. Complete the physical assessment.
    4. Give the client prescriptions from provider to be filled.
    5. Have the client sit or lie down quietly for at least 30 minutes for observation.

29. The nurse in the clinic is assessing a new client, when the nurse suspects the client has a hearing loss. In what order would the nurse perform these actions? Rank order the responses.
    1. Enunciate words clearly to the client.
    2. Get a bit closer and face the client when speaking in a normal voice.
    3. Repeat each question louder to the client.
    4. Turn off the radio and close the door.
    5. Write what is being asked of the client on a pad.

30. The nurse is planning care for a client with a new diagnosis of generalized seizure disorder. Which nursing strategy from the following exhibit would be deemed most important for the nurse to address?

Nursing Care of the Client with Generalized Seizures
NURSING EXPECTED OUTCOME
1. Client will maintain open airway during seizures.
2. Client will have satisfactory psychosocial functioning while maintaining compliance with treatment regimen.
3. Client will have optimal mental and physical functioning while taking antiseizure drugs.
4. Client will be free from injury during a seizure.

1. A client returns to the orthopedic unit after surgery for a traumatic amputation of the left foot in a farming accident. What statement or query by the client requires immediate follow-up by the nurse?
   1. 🔑 "It feels like the tractor is still crushing my foot!"
   2. "Should I feel tingling in my toes?" *This is a common response from the nerve endings in the stump.*
   3. "Thank God I didn't lose my whole leg!" *This does not require an immediate follow-up.*
   4. "My father had a similar accident years ago" *Although the nurse would need to respond to this question, the severe pain issue would be a higher priority.*

   Rationale: By the client's description that it feels like the tractor is still crushing the foot, it's apparent that acute pain is a high priority. The nurse should use the 1-10 pain scale to determine how much pain is experienced, check vital signs and surgical dressing, check the post-op prescriptions for what the client can have, and administer it.

   THIN Thinking: Help Quick – *Pain management is a priority for immediate nursing care.* **NCLEX®:** Basic Care and Comfort **QSEN:** Patient-centered Care

2. The nurse is doing discharge teaching for a client in day surgery who had carpal tunnel release of the dominant hand. Which question by the client indicates additional teaching is needed?
   1. "If I see blood soaking through the dressing, I need to call or come back immediately." *Bleeding through the dressing is excessive and needs follow-up – this statement demonstrates understanding.*
   2. "I am to take the pain medication as it is prescribed as needed." *Pain medicine is taken as needed and as prescribed.*
   3. 🔑 "I can only lift 10 pounds with that hand, so my infant is OK to lift."
   4. "I should be able to return to work on limitations until the dressing is removed." *Accurate statement.*

   Rationale: Carpal tunnel release is often recommended if symptoms last more than six months. In most cases, it is done on an out-client/day-stay basis. Although symptoms may be relieved immediately after surgery, full recovery may take months. Instruct the client about wound care and appropriate assessments to perform at home. Clients usually return to work on limitations after a few days, and daily activities are curtailed so as not to re-injure the hand, including lifting and repetitive motions, to prevent further injury.

   THIN Thinking: Identify Risk to Safety – *Lifting more than the prescribed weight could cause damage to the surgical area. An infant can be up to 1 year and weight > 10 pounds.* **NCLEX®:** Safety and Infection Control **QSEN:** Safety

3. The clinic nurse is planning to teach a group in the community center about prevention and risks of osteoporosis. Which statement by the nurse would be important to include in the teaching plan?
   1. 🔑 "Everyone, especially those at risk, should include adequate calcium in their diets."
   2. "Genetics have no role in development of osteoporosis." *Inaccurate statement, osteoporosis is genetic.*
   3. "Osteoporosis is totally preventable for those over 65, with screenings." *Inaccurate statement.*
   4. "People who are less active are at less risk for fractures from osteoporosis." *Inaccurate statement.*

   Rationale: Prevention and treatment of osteoporosis focus on adequate calcium intake. Foods high in calcium include dairy products, yogurt, some green leafy vegetables (broccoli, kale, turnip greens, spinach), sardines, and seafood. The amount of elemental calcium varies in different calcium preparations. Calcium is difficult to absorb in doses greater than 500 mg, so the client should be taught to take the supplements in divided doses for better absorption.

   THIN Thinking: Nursing Process – *Providing accurate information/teaching should include the risks of osteoporosis.* **NCLEX®:** Health Promotion and Maintenance **QSEN:** Patient-centered Care

4. A client presents to the clinic looking extremely tired and complains that movements of the legs have prevented sleep for several nights. What statement by the nurse would be most appropriate?
   1. "I can't imagine living with my legs moving about all night. I wouldn't be able to sleep either." *Statement does not help client.*
   2. 🔑 "Losing sleep like that can be very exhausting. Let's do a complete assessment to help find the cause(s)."
   3. "My husband has restless legs syndrome and tosses about all night. That would be that's what's going on with you." *Not the nurse's role to diagnosis.*
   4. "Oh, my! You look so tired like you could just drop. Sit down and rest a bit." *Does not help client.*

   Rationale: The nurse should complete a thorough assessment prior to implementing a plan of care. The goals of management of restless leg syndrome (RLS) are to reduce client discomfort and distress and to improve sleep quality.

   THIN Thinking: Nursing Process – *Assessment should be completed before planning the client's care.* **NCLEX®:** Basic Care and Comfort **QSEN:** Patient-centered Care

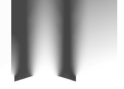

5. The clinic nurse is evaluating a client with Parkinson's disease who was ordered levodopa/carbidopa. What assessment by the nurse would be highest priority?
   1. "Are you having any side effects of the medication?" *This question is too general to be helpful.*
   2. "Do you experience fewer freezing motion episodes?" *Assessing effectiveness of medication is not as important as assessing for serious side effects.*
   3. 🔘 "Have you had any difficulty with urination?"
   4. "Do you experience a bit less shaking of your hands?" *Assessing effectiveness of medication is not as important as assessing for serious side effects.*

   Rationale: For clients with Parkinson's disease, drug therapy is designed to control the symptoms. Levodopa/carbidopa does have side effects, including urinary retention which can be serious.

   THIN Thinking: Identify Risk to Safety – *Understanding the side effects for medications can prevent injury for clients.* **NCLEX**®: Phrenological and Parenteral Therapies **QSEN:** Patient-centered Care

6. The clinic nurse is teaching a client about improving quality of life while living with osteoarthritis. Which statement by the client demonstrates that more teaching is needed?
   1. "I can alternate heat and cold to alleviate my pain and tenderness in my knee." *The use of heat and cold may relieve pain.*
   2. "I will call the outpatient therapy unit for appointments when you send the order." *Outpatient therapy can build strength and movement.*
   3. "So, which over-the-counter medications will help with pain after the injection into my knee?" *Over-the-counter medications including NSAIDs can help with pain.*
   4. 🔘 "This is just part of aging since nothing can be done to decrease my pain or disability."

   Rationale: The individual will most often complain of pain, stiffness, and limitation of function, as well as daily frustration in coping with limitations. Determine what makes the pain better or worse, and how the pain affects the ability to perform ADL's. Ask about pain management practices, and success of each treatment. Adjust home management goals to meet the client's needs, including family or caregivers. Assess safety, accessibility, and self-care abilities in the client's environment, and help address any deficits noted.

   THIN Thinking: Nursing Process – *During a teaching session, it is important for the nurse to evaluate an inaccurate statement in order to address areas where additional teaching is needed.* **NCLEX**®: Health Promotion and Maintenance **QSEN:** Patient-centered Care

7. A female client who sustained a cervical spinal cord injury with quadriplegia states she has a headache. Which is the first nursing action?
   1. Conduct a comprehensive pain assessment. *Although important, the first action would be to check for the most likely cause of the headache for this client- autonomic dysreflexia.*
   2. 🔘 Palpate and bladder scan the client's lower abdomen.
   3. Turn the client to the side and reposition extremities. *This would not address client's complaint.*
   4. Assess the client's body temperature. *This would not address client's complaint.*

   Rationale: The headache could be a sign of autonomic dysreflexia which may occur with high level spinal cord injuries. Bladder distension is usually the cause of this condition and is relieved by slowly emptying the bladder. Other causes include bowel impaction, pressure ulcers, tight clothing, menses, trauma, or deep vein thromboses. If unmanaged, it could lead to encephalopathy and shock.

   THIN Thinking: Help Quick – *A headache in a client with quadriplegia may be a result of autonomic dysreflexia, a medical emergency and needs to be address quickly.* **NCLEX**®: Physiological Adaptation **QSEN:** Safety

8. The nurse is caring for a client with a medical diagnosis of amyotrophic lateral sclerosis (ALS) and pneumonia. The client's spouse calls the nurses station reporting the client coughing and choking. What would be the priority nursing action?
   1. Give the client a drink of water with a straw. *This would worsen the client's condition and increase the risk of aspiration.*
   2. Medicate the client for the cough as needed. *Cough indicate airway clearance issue and shouldn't be suppressed.*
   3. 🔘 Place prescribed oxygen on per nasal canula and suction after assessing lung sounds.
   4. Talk gently to the client in a calm voice while assessing the severity of the symptoms. *The priority action would be to address the problem by suctioning and applying oxygen.*

   Rationale: Nursing interventions for ALS include: 1) facilitating communication, 2) reducing risk of aspiration, 3) facilitating early identification of respiratory insufficiency, 4) decreasing risk of injury related to falls, 6) provide diversional activities such as reading and companionship, 7) support the client's cognitive and emotional functions, 8) help the client and family manage the disease process, including grieving over loss of motor function or death.

   THIN Thinking: Help Quick – *With ALS, there is a risk for aspiration. It is important to provide oxygen and clear the airways as quickly as possible.* **NCLEX**®: Physiological Adaptation **QSEN:** Safety

9. The nurse is implementing discharge teaching with an athlete that sustained a closed fracture of the femur after an injury at a track meet. The healthcare provider placed a long-leg soft cast until swelling diminishes. What statement by the client demonstrates a need for clarification?

1. 🔵 "I can put light weight on the leg since the provider put a heel on the cast."
2. "I can go to school after two days at home." *In most cases, this is acceptable.*
3. "I will use the crutches like this (and demonstrates)." *Accurate response.*
4. "I won't take pain medicine unless I begin to feel like I need it." *Accurate response.*

Rationale: Soft casting is be used after reduction to maintain alignment and immobilize the injured part during the initial phase when the extremity is swollen. Under no circumstances should any weight bearing occur until the provider applies the permanent cast and gives the go ahead to do so.

THIN Thinking: Top Three – *Prevention of further injury is the priority. Placing weight on the leg can worsen the injury until it is more effectively immobilized.* **NCLEX®:** Reduction of Risk Potential **QSEN:** Patient-centered Care

10. The home health nurse is visiting a client with multiple sclerosis who is complaining of urinary leakage. What information should the nurse gather first?

1. 🔵 "Do you feel full in the lower abdomen?"
2. "Have you been using pads or briefs? Do I need to bring you more?" *Does not address cause of new problem.*
3. "Are you leaking stool also?" *Does not assist with urinary leakage.*
4. "Let me call the provider and get an in-and-out catheter order." *More information is needed before using a catheter.*

Rationale: The client with multiple sclerosis (MS) may have bladder control and bowel problems (especially constipation), and measures to deal with those are taught. A full bowel or bladder may cause pressure and leakage.

THIN Thinking: Nursing Process – Further assessment is needed before intervention. **NCLEX®:** Basic Care and Comfort **QSEN:** Patient-centered Care

11. The nurse is caring for a client admitted with a possible diagnosis of Guillain-Barré syndrome (GBS). What statement by the client requires immediate follow-up?

1. "I had the flu about a month ago and thought I was over it." *This may be related to the cause of GB but does not require immediate follow-up.*
2. 🔵 "I'm having difficulty breathing and feel like I can't catch my breath."
3. "I am having trouble doing my routine activities." *Completion of activities is important related to GB but does not require immediate follow-up.*
4. "My hands and feet are numb and feel very heavy." *Although important to note, this does not require immediate follow-up as it doesn't involve client's breathing.*

Rationale: In the management of GBS the primary concern is compromised respiratory ability and ventilatory support as the ascending paralysis progresses. Some clients progress into respiratory failure and require artificial ventilation for a period, as the syndrome is characterized by an autoimmune process that occurs a few days or weeks following a viral or bacterial infection.

THIN Thinking: Identify Risk to Safety – *Since GBS can impair the ability to breathe, shortness of breath is an urgent finding.* **NCLEX®:** Physiological Adaptation **QSEN:** Safety

12. The nurse is working with young adults with cerebral palsy (CP). Which client should be assessed first for a risk for injury?

1. A client who is non-ambulatory and has weakness of the extremities and inability to move voluntarily - *This client is not in immediate risk of a safety issue.*
2. A client in a wheelchair that does not appear to fit correctly and causes mal-alignment of the spine. *Not as important as risk for injury.*
3. A client with difficulty with articulation and communicating, causing the client frustration. *Not as important as risk for injury.*
4. 🔵 An ambulatory client with uncontrolled muscle movements, spasticity, and a wide gait.

Rationale: The ambulatory client is at risk for falls due to uncontrolled muscle movements, spasticity, and a wide gait. The nurse should assess the environment in and around the client's room. Then work with the client and family on safety principles in the unfamiliar hospital environment, as well as at home, work, and social settings, to reduce the risk for injury—clearing items out of the path for mobility, about the room and hall and to/from the bathroom, as well as any assistive devices.

THIN Thinking: Identify Risk to Safety- *This client is at risk for falls and requires surveillance to avoid injury.* **NCLEX®:** Health Promotion and Maintenance **QSEN:** Safety

13. **A client who has had Myasthenia Gravis for five years is admitted to the hospital for an unrelated problem. What nursing interventions would be most effective in avoiding triggering a myasthenic crisis?**
    1. Assess the client's ability to maintain a usual lifestyle and role responsibilities. *Important, but the goal is to prevent crisis (eliminating triggers).*
    2. 💡 Help client plan around activities in the hospital to minimize stress and fatigue.
    3. Monitor for side effects of the myasthenia drugs. *Important but the goal is to prevent crisis (eliminating triggers).*
    4. Well-balanced diet with fresh fruits and vegetables. *Identifying triggers would be more important.*

    Rationale: The primary feature of MG is fluctuating weakness of the skeletal muscles used to move the eyes/eyelids, chew, swallow, speak, and breathe; fatigue occurs after repeating actions. Myasthenic crisis is an acute event and marked exaggeration of symptoms may be triggered by respiratory infections, emotional distress, fatigue and stress, pregnancy, and beginning treatment with drugs that interfere with the MG drugs or steroids.

    THIN Thinking: Identify Risk to Safety – *Prevention of MG crisis is the priority to protect the client from injury.* **NCLEX®:** Physiological Adaptation **QSEN:** Safety

14. **The nurse is caring for a client with diabetic peripheral neuropathy. The client reports that sometimes there's an inability to determine the position of his feet when standing from a sitting position. What would be the priority nursing actions? Select all that apply.**
    1. 💡 Be sure the client's feet are securely planted on the floor before helping the client to stand.
    2. Help the client sit on side of bed with the feet on a stool. *This would not be helpful for ambulation.*
    3. 💡 Place client on fall precaution and caution the other staff.
    4. When making the bed, be sure to give the client's toes room under the sheet and blanket. *This would help decrease friction on toes, but not keep client safe when trying to ambulate.*
    5. Ensuring that the client understands the need for assistance with standing and ambulation.

    Rationale: Individuals with diabetic peripheral neuropathy often complain of burning, intermittent, shock-like pain, as well as numbness, changes in reflexes, and decreased motor strength. All are results of nerve damage that occurs because of metabolic derangements associated with diabetes mellitus. Foot injuries, falls, and ulcers can occur without the client being aware of pain, so client safety is paramount.

    THIN Thinking: Identify Risk to Safety – *The client statement indicates a risk for injury. The nurse must determine actions for prevention.* **NCLEX®:** Safety and Infection Control **QSEN:** Safety

15. **A nurse is conducting screening for scoliosis of middle school children Which assessment would warrant referral for further evaluation for this condition? Select all that apply.**
    1. Back pain with significant twisting. *Unrelated to scoliosis.*
    2. Decreased lateral range of motion. *Not a symptom of scoliosis.*
    3. 💡 Scapular hump with forward bending.
    4. 💡 Uneven shoulder height when standing.
    5. Palpable lesions on the vertebrae. *Not a sign of scoliosis.*
    6. 💡 Uneven appearance of bra straps.

    Rationale: Screening all preadolescents is somewhat controversial but is recommended for girls ages 10-12 years and boys 13 to 14 years. Findings requiring referral include the scapular hump deformity when bending forward, uneven shoulders, and changes in the spine which cause bra straps to appear uneven. Definitive diagnosis is done through X-ray.

    THIN Thinking: Nursing Process – *The nurse should understand the assessment changes that indicate scoliosis.* **NCLEX®:** Reduction of Risk Potential **QSEN:** Evidence-based Practice

16. **The nurse is caring for an adult client with paraplegia secondary to spina bifida admitted for treatment of a Stage 3 pressure ulcer on the coccyx. Several methods have been discussed with the client and caregiver to treat the pressure ulcer. What should the priority focus be in treating the pressure ulcer?**
    1. Change the wet-to-dry dressings twice daily. *Helpful but more important to remove pressure from injured area.*
    2. Eat a diet with many fruits, vegetables, and high protein. *Will help with healing, but more important to remove pressure from injured area.*
    3. 💡 Keep off the coccyx by changing positions frequently and using a pressure reduction pillow or gel pad.
    4. Take a vitamin supplement with Vitamin C, B, iron, and others to promote healing. *It is more important to remove pressure from injured area.*

    Rationale: Although all of these measures will help with the healing of a pressure ulcer, taking the pressure off it will be the priority. The overall goals are that the client with a pressure ulcer will 1) have no deterioration of the ulcer, 2) reduce or eliminate the factors that lead to pressure ulcers, 3) not develop new pressure ulcers or infection in the ulcer, and 4) have healing of the ulcer.

    THIN Thinking: Nursing Process – *Interventions for a pressure ulcer include the reduction of pressure on the bony areas of the skin.* **NCLEX®:** Reduction of Risk Potential **QSEN:** Evidence-base practice

17. **The school nurse is caring for a child in third grade with spastic cerebral palsy, demonstrating hypertonia, tense muscles, hip flexion, toe walking, and scissor gait. What strategies does the nurse communicate to the classroom teacher to address safety of the child?**

    1. Ensure the child is academically similar to the other children in the classroom. *This is not accurate and would not help to keep child safe.*
    2. Explain to the other students that the child walks with difficulty because of a birth injury. *This would not help to keep the child safe.*
    3. 🔵 Get an adapted table and chair for the child to use for ease of sitting to work.
    4. Treat the child as any other child in the classroom to prevent self-esteem issues. *Child will require some adaptive equipment to maintain safety.*

    Rationale: Spastic CP is the most common type, and is characterized by increase deep tendon reflexes, hypertonia, and sometime contractures, as with this child's toe walking and scissor gait. Assess the environment in and around the classroom for any potential safety issues that could cause injury. Assess the need for physical and learning adaptations in the school setting. Consider the use of assistive devices, depending on severity of symptoms. At the same time, it is important that the other children understand why the other child has different abilities and not to bully or make fun of the child.

    THIN Thinking: Identify Risk to Safety – *The nurse needs to recognize the physical accommodations that need to be made to keep this child safe.* **NCLEX®:** Reduction of Risk Potential **QSEN:** Safety

18. **A client presents to the clinic with sudden onset of pain when brushing his teeth and shaving. The pain continued ranging from a dull ache to severe pain. The clinic healthcare provider diagnoses trigeminal neuralgia and decides to try medical management of episodes. What action should the nurse take first?**

    1. Administer pain medication. *Assess before treatment.*
    2. 🔵 Do a thorough assessment of the nature and onset of the attacks.
    3. Prepare the client for a future surgery to relieve the symptoms. *Treatment plan is to use medical interventions rather than surgical.*
    4. Refer the client to a psychologist in the clinic. *This is a medical issue, not a psychological one.*

    Rationale: Once diagnosis is made the goal of treatment is relief of pain either medically or surgically. Various medical and surgical therapies are available, including drugs like antiseizure drugs, tricyclic antidepressants, analgesics, and local nerve blocks. The nurse should assess the attacks in detail, including triggers, characteristics, frequency, and pain management techniques, as well as the client's nutritional status, oral hygiene, and behavior. Evaluate the effects of the pain on the client's lifestyle, drug use, emotional state, and suicidal tendencies.

    THIN Thinking: Nursing Process – *Assessment should occur before planning interventions.* **NCLEX®:** Basic Care and Comfort **QSEN:** Patient-centered Care

19. **The nurse in the ophthalmology clinic has completed teaching for a client with macular degeneration. What statement by the client indicates additional teaching is needed?**

    1. 🔵 "I guess I will have to give up my needlepoint."
    2. "I hope my vision will improve with the medications." *Accurate statement, medication can improve vision.*
    3. "I may have to quit driving when my vision decreases." *Decreased vision will lead to loss of driver's license.*
    4. "I will use a scanning technique with my peripheral vision to read." *Accurate statement.*

    Rationale: Macular degeneration a progressive eye disease with gradual loss of central vision. There are new drugs and therapies used to improve or at least arrest the progress of the disease. Individuals with macular degeneration adapt and learn to use their peripheral vision and continue with their normal lives if they can--reading, sewing, using computers, driving—until their vision impedes their doing so.

    THIN Thinking: Nursing Process – *Understanding the progression of the illness will also assist the nurse to evaluate a client's understanding.* **NCLEX®:** Health Promotion and Maintenance **QSEN:** Patient-centered Care

20. **A client in the post-op recovery unit after mastoidectomy with tympanoplasty, after suffering with chronic otitis media for many years. Intravenous orders include ceftazidime 4 grams in 24 hours in divided doses every 12 hours, diluted in 250 mL normal saline. The nurse begins the initial dose of _____ mg in 250 mL normal saline.**

    Answer: 2000 mg.

Rationale: Since chronic otitis media sometimes results in mastoiditis (infection in the mastoid bone, often with purulent drainage from the ear), a mastoidectomy is performed with tympanoplasty to remove infected portions of the mastoid bone. The surgical repair can be negatively impacted by conditions such as a sudden change in pressure or infections that develop after surgery. Therefore, the IV medication would be given over a longer period (90 min) to prevent sudden pressure changes. Third generation cephalosporins such as ceftazidime are sometimes given in chronic conditions that have been treated with other antibiotics over time, to which individuals may have developed resistance or allergy. 4 grams divided by 2 = 2000 mg.

THIN Thinking: Identify Risk to Safety- *Medication calculations need to be 100% accurate in order to provide safe care.* **NCLEX®:** Pharmacological and Parental Therapies **QSEN:** Safety

21. **A home health nurse is caring for a client with severe arthritis in both knees. The client shares that he doesn't move around a lot because he is afraid of falling. What would the nurse ask first to assess the client's needs?**
    1. "Are you able to attend church and other social functions?" *This would not be the first question to ask.*
    2. "Can you get your groceries delivered by the market you shop?" *This may be a strategy to help client but would not be the first question.*
    3. "Why don't you ask your family to drive you for groceries and appointments?" *Probing question that does not provide helpful information.*
    4. 🔘 "Will you show me any assistive devices you use to get around home or out?"

Rationale: The individual will most often complain of pain, stiffness, and limitation of function, as well as daily frustration in coping with limitations. Determine what makes the pain better or worse, and how the pain affects the ability to perform ADL's. Ask about pain management practices, and success of each treatment. Adjust home management goals to meet the client's needs, including family or caregivers. Assess safety, accessibility, and self-care abilities in the client's environment, and help address any deficits noted.

THIN Thinking: Identify Risk to Safety – *Further assessment is needed to determine the risk for falls.* **NCLEX®:** Safety and Infection Control **QSEN:** Safety

22. **The nurse is preparing to care for a client newly diagnosed with Meniere's disease. What should be included in the nursing actions? Select all that apply.**
    1. 🔘 Keep an emesis basin at the bedside.
    2. 🔘 Keep side rails up to minimize chance of falls.
    3. Leave the television on for the client for distraction. *Client should avoid TV, which may worsen symptoms.*
    4. 🔘 Tell the client to avoid sudden head movements.
    5. 🔘 Turn off the lights and darken the blinds in the client's room during an attack.

Rationale: Plan nursing interventions to minimize vertigo and provide for client safety. Teach the techniques to the client for control of symptoms at home. During an acute attack keep the client in a quiet, dark room in a comfortable position. Teach the client to avoid sudden head movements or position changes. Avoid flickering fluorescent lights and televisions. Make an emesis basis available as vomiting is common. Keep the side rails up and bed in low position to minimize falls and instruct the client to call for assistance to get up. Monitor intake and output.

THIN Thinking: Nursing Progress – *Understanding the best interventions to prevent worsening of the symptoms and protect from injury.* **NCLEX®:** Physiological Adaption **QSEN:** Patient-centered Care

23. **A nurse is assessing a client who reports having been diagnosed with cataracts in the right eye last year. What information would be appropriate for the nurse to ask to gather further data? Select all that apply.**
    1. "Do you attend social functions?" *Question would not give pertinent data.*
    2. "Does closing one eye help you to see better?" *Question would not give pertinent data.*
    3. 🔘 "Are you able to drive at night?"
    4. 🔘 "Do you often read for pleasure?"
    5. 🔘 "Do you wear protective shades when outside?"

Rationale: Cataracts are an opacity in the lens and may occur in one or both eyes. The client may complain of a decrease in vision (with frequent change in glasses prescription), abnormal color perception, and glare with flaring of lights. This is magnified significantly at night when the pupil dilates, causing many to quit driving at night. Since most cataracts occur in older clients, they may experience loss of independence, lack of control over life, and significant change in self-perception. Asking about attending social functions and closing one eye are not helpful assessments.

THIN Thinking: Identify Risk to Safety – *Recognition of times when vision is reduced will allow the nurse to create a plan for safety.* **NCLEX®:** Safety and Infection Control **QSEN:** Safety

24. A client presents to the clinic with complaints of continued pain and paresthesia on the face and neck after a shingles infection (herpes zoster). What nursing actions should be taken next? Select all that apply.
    1. 💡 Assess the nature, quality/intensity, and location of the pain.
    2. 💡 Determine what exacerbates or alleviates the pain.
    3. Gently massage the painful area to see if that will alleviate it. *Massage would worsen pain.*
    4. 💡 Administer the prescribed antiviral agent.
    5. Tell the client that the infection is healed so the pain should be gone. *Pain may be present even if there are no longer open areas.*

    Rationale: Individuals with peripheral neuropathy from various causes often complain of burning, intermittent, shock-like pain, as well as numbness, changes in reflexes, and decreased motor strength. All are results of nerve damage that occurs because of metabolic derangements or injury and may be felt along the distribution of one or more peripheral nerves, as with that of shingles, and may occur during the prodrome or long after the obvious infection heals. As clients experience peripheral neuropathies and live with them, they may cope differently and may or may not be willing to try different strategies to manage it. Massage does not ease neuropathic pain.

    THIN Thinking: Nursing Process – *The nurse needs to understand the focused assessment and plan for peripheral neuropathy in order to teach appropriately.* **NCLEX®:** Basic Care and Comfort **QSEN:** Patient-centered Care

25. The client is diagnosed with bacterial conjunctivitis in the left eye. What factors should the nurse evaluate to prevent the spread of the infection to the other eye or others? Select all that apply.
    1. Allergies to pollens. *This is unrelated to spread of infection.*
    2. 💡 Children in the home.
    3. 💡 Contact with other infected individuals.
    4. 💡 Practice frequent handwashing.
    5. 💡 Tearing, drainage.

    Rationale: Conjunctivitis is an infection or inflammation of the conjunctivae, and may be caused by bacteria or viruses, as well as from exposure to allergens or chemical irritants. It may occur at any age, but bacterial conjunctivitis (pinkeye) is most common in children, with epidemics occurring. Thorough assessment, treatment, and measures to prevent spread of the infection are important, including that of good handwashing technique.

    THIN Thinking: Identify Risk to Safety – *Since conjunctivitis is highly contagious by touch the nurse needs to identify the risk associated with the spread of infection.* **NCLEX®:** Safety and Infection Control **QSEN:** Safety

26. The client with chronic open angle glaucoma is being sent home from the clinic with cholinergic agent carbachol eye drops—2 drops 3% solution TID. How much of the medication is the client receiving daily?

    Answer: 6 gtts

    Rationale: Carbachol is used to used to foster contraction of the sphincter in the iris of the eyes. It promotes fluid outflow by opening up the trabecular meshwork. Carbachol is in a class of drugs called cholinergic agents. 2 gtts X 3 time/day= 6 gtts.

    THIN Thinking: Identify Risk to Safety- *Medication calculations need to be 100% accurate in order to provide safe care.* **NCLEX®:** Pharmacological and Parental Therapies **QSEN:** Safety

27. A client with a fracture of the left hand is casted and the nurse is providing discharge teaching. What statements/questions from the client demonstrate a good understanding of discharge teaching? Select all that apply.
    1. "I can still play ball again in this weekend's game. I'm the best catcher they have." *The client would not be able to play ball this weekend as it may injure the affected arm or displace the fracture.*
    2. 💡 "I can shower as long as I cover the cast with plastic."
    3. 💡 "I have a follow-up appointment in two weeks."
    4. 💡 "I won't put anything in the cast to scratch any itches."
    5. "Throbbing pain is expected as my broken bones heal." *If the extremity starts throbbing, it may indicate that the cast is too tight or swelling has increased, warranting further inspection.*

    Rationale: In the case of a fracture that's not misaligned, there may be no need for realignment or it may be done in the Emergency Department. Casting is used to immobilize the injured part. The individual will most likely be sent home with cast care and activity instructions. This may include showering instructions, correct cast care (including not putting anything down into the cast), activity restrictions, and symptoms that require healthcare provider follow-up.

    THIN Thinking: Identify Risk to Safety – *It is important for the client to fully understand the care of the cast and the prevention of circulatory impairment that can result from them.* **NCLEX®:** Safety and Infection Control **QSEN:** Safety

28. A client comes to the clinic with complaints of an earache from chronic otitis media. After consultation with the clinic provider, the nurse prepares to administer an antibiotic and pain medication. In what order would the nurse perform these actions? Rank order the responses.
   1. Complete the physical assessment.
   2. Ask the client about any drug allergies.
   3. Administer the medications.
   4. Have the client sit or lie down quietly for at least 30 minutes for observation.
   5. Give the client prescriptions from provider to be filled.

Rationale: Acute otitis media is an inflammation of the tympanum, ossicles, and space of the middle ear and can be the result of infection or allergies. Pressure from the inflammation causes the tympanic membrane to bulge and become red and painful. Other symptoms accompanying OM can be fever, malaise, headache/earache, or reduced hearing. If effusion is present, a feeling of fullness or "popping" may be complaints. Antibiotics are used if infection is present. Repeated attacks of OM may lead to chronic OM, especially in adults who have history of OM as a child. This is the correct order of these steps.

THIN Thinking: Nursing Process – *Assessment is first for the collection of baseline information should there be a problem. Allergy review needs to take place before the medication administration.* **NCLEX®:** Physiological Adaption **QSEN:** Safety

29. The nurse in the clinic is assessing a new client, when the nurse suspects the client has a hearing loss. In what order would the nurse perform these actions? Rank order the responses.
   1. Turn off the radio and close the door.
   2. Get a bit closer and face the client when speaking in a normal voice.
   3. Enunciate words clearly to the client.
   4. Repeat each question louder to the client.
   5. Write what is being asked of the client on a pad.

Rationale: Hearing disorders are a common cause of disability in the U.S. With the aging of the population, the incidence is growing. There are several signs that indicate a client has hearing loss. These include always asking speakers to repeat themselves, not answering when spoken to, asking for others to speak louder, and placing the hand over the ear in a cupping motion. It is also common for the client with a hearing impairment to become frustrated with others and act

irritable. Standing close to a speaker and attempting to read the speaker's lips and increased sensitivity to slight increases in noise level or ambient noise, are also indicative of hearing loss. Interference in communication and interaction with others can be the source of problems for the client and caregiver.

THIN Thinking: Nursing Process – *Prioritizing actions is important to obtain the best results.* **NCLEX®:** Basic Care and Comfort **QSEN:** Patient-centered Care

30. The nurse is planning care for a client with a new diagnosis of generalized seizure disorder. Which nursing strategy from the following exhibit would be deemed most important for the nurse to address?

Nursing Care of the Client with Generalized Seizures
NURSING EXPECTED OUTCOME
1. Client will maintain open airway during seizures.   2. Client will have satisfactory psychosocial functioning while maintaining compliance with treatment regimen.   3. Client will have optimal mental and physical functioning while taking antiseizure drugs.   4. Client will be free from injury during a seizure.

Answer: 1

Rationale: Generalized seizures are characterized by tonic-clonic movements, loss of consciousness, falling to the ground or slumping in a chair, cyanosis, incontinence, and a post-ictal stage (soreness, fatigue, sleepy). Although prevention of injury is of utmost importance, following A-B-C's of care, airway is priority during a seizure. One should assess airway patency and position the client to maintain airway during and after the seizure. Preemptively in hospital, the nurse should remove potentially harmful objects from the bedside and pad the side rails to protect the client from injury.

THIN Thinking: Nursing Process – *Prioritization with ABCs when setting care goals.* **NCLEX®:** Management of Care **QSEN:** Patient-centered Care

Comfort

Pain / Pressure / Fatigue

This chapter discusses a variety of Priority Exemplars addressing alterations in comfort. Pain and pain management, dealing with skin disorders (including burns), and addressing sleep issues with clients may be very challenging. We learned that the skin is the key protective barrier to infection, that pain is the fifth vital sign, and we will sleep about one-quarter of our lives. These validate the importance of this chapter in studying for NCLEX®!

Priority Exemplars:

> Pressure ulcers
> Burns
> Acute pain
> Chronic pain
> Contact dermatitis/ impetigo
> Fatigue
> Sleep disorders

Next Gen Clinical Judgment

Consider the number of clients you have cared for who presented with acute or chronic pain. How were the assessment findings different? How were they the same? Compare and contrast the nursing care for clients dealing with acute and chronic pain.

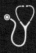
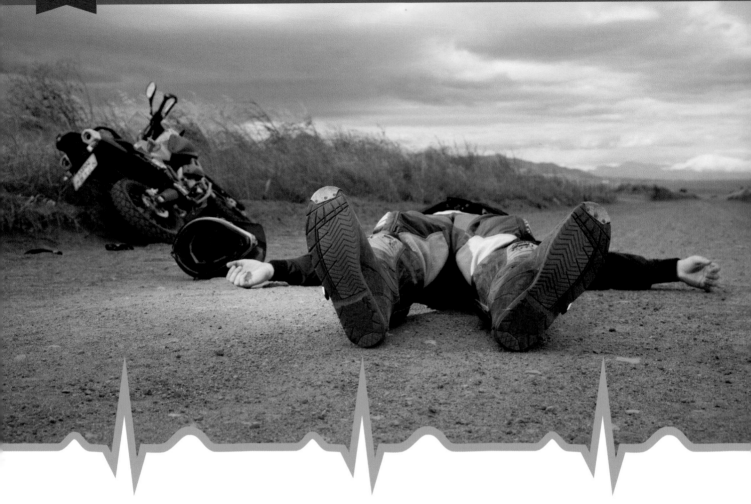

Go To Clinical Case 1

A 38-year-old man sustains a C-5 spinal cord injury subsequent to a motorcycle accident. The client was stabilized at an acute care facility. The client has quadriplegia, has a tracheostomy, is dependent on ventilatory support, and is sustained by gastrostomy tube feedings. The client is about to be transferred to a rehabilitation center for the developing a bowel and bladder programs, attempting to be weaned off the ventilator, resuming oral feedings, and discharge teaching.

The admission nurse at the rehabilitation center notes a 2 cm by 1 cm red, maroon pressure area on the sacral area. The nurse notes that this area does not blanch with pressure and is darker than the skin around it. There is no drainage from the area. The client's vital signs are 98.9°F—88-16-132/86.

NurseThink® Time

Using the NurseThink® system, complete priorities. Check your answers designated by 💡 in the Pressure ulcers Priority Exemplar.

NurseThink® Time

✏️ Priority Assessments or Cues

1.

2.

3.

🧪 Priority Laboratory Tests/Diagnostics

1.

2.

3.

⚠️ Priority Interventions or Actions

1.

2.

3.

🚩 Priority Potential & Actual Complications

1.

2.

3.

⚕️ Priority Nursing Implications

1.

2.

3.

💧 Priority Medications

1.

2.

3.

👤 Priority Education/Discharge Issues

1.

2.

3.

Pressure ulcers

Pathophysiology/Description

> The local injury to tissue created by pressure or a combination of shearing forces (friction of tissue pulling against a surface) and pressure. Most commonly found on bony prominences where pressure is exerted by chairs, beds, or equipment. May also be impacted by the presence of moisture

> Severity of pressure ulcer is associated with amount of pressure (client weight, location of pressure point), length of time area is exposed to pressure, and client tissue characteristics

> The heels and sacrum are the most common sites for pressure ulcers

> Protruding tissues or those prone to being a pressure point may also be at risk, including ears, shoulders, hips, ankles, chin, elbows, and sides of knees

Priority Assessments or Cues

○ Assess for risk factors associated with pressure ulcers/poor perfusion including increased age, immobility/bedrest, poor wound healing, diabetes mellitus, conditions causing poor perfusion, incontinence, confusion/disorientation, neurological compromise, spinal cord injury/paralysis, anemia, pain, poor nutrition, obesity, contractures, long surgical procedures, and hyperthermia

○ Assess for characteristics of pressure ulcers associated with each stage

  • Suspected deep tissue injury described as a local area, purple or maroon in color, skin may blister or be intact, be painful, warm or cool, firm or mushy,

  • **Stage I** described as intact skin with non-blanching redness, darker areas at location of injury, may be different from peripheral coloring of skin

  • **Stage II** described as a fluid-filled blister with a red-pink wound bed or open shallow ulcer, partial loss of dermis

  • **Stage III** described as a full thickness tissue erosion, may see subcutaneous fatty layer, may show beginnings of undermining and tunneling

  • **Stage IV** described as full thickness tissue loss with exposure of bone, tendons, or muscle tissue. May include eschar and necrotic tissue, undermining and tunneling present

> Assess for signs of pressure ulcer infection including fever, redness, swelling, and drainage

○ Wounds are described in detail, measured by width and depth of the wound, and this information is carefully documented in the medical record to assess severity and response to treatment. Ulcers are described by stage, size, location, type of wound, drainage, and presence of signs of infection or pain

Priority Laboratory Tests/Diagnostics

○ Wound cultures should be done. Wounds may be contaminated or colonized with bacteria but chronicity of wound or client immunosuppression may mask the signs of infection

Priority Interventions or Actions

○ Address health status and conditions increasing risk for pressure ulcers

○ Ensure adequate nutrition for healing. Oral, enteral or parenteral feedings, with supplementary proteins and vitamins, are often needed

> Assess and manage pain

> Ensure adequate hygiene and cleanliness of tissues

○ Wound care includes debridement and removal of dead tissue, wound cleaning via gentle irrigation with non-cytotoxic solutions, application of moist dressings (wet to dry dressing should not be used as they may disrupt healing tissue), and ensuring area is not experiencing pressure

> Wounds may require advanced healing mechanisms, wound vacuums, skin grafting, skin flaps, or surgical repair

Priority Potential & Actual Complications

○ Cellulitis and chronic infection

○ Sepsis

○ May be fatal

Priority Nursing Implications

○ Clients should be assessed on admission for risk for skin breakdown. The Braden scale is a validated tool often used for this purpose. A full head to toe assessment of the skin is warranted

> Nurses should be aware of the challenges in assessing variations in skin colors for changes and pressure areas

○ Significant emphasis may be on prevention through basic processes such as turning/repositioning, not pulling clients along sheets to avoid shearing forces, positioning, splints, position changes when seated, providing supports/cushions/specially designed pads, and encouraging activity/ambulation when appropriate

○ Clients most at risk for pressure ulcers may benefit from special beds which provide varying exposure to pressure/air movement mattresses, facilitate turning and movement, and relieve pressure areas. Wheelchair cushions, padded toilet seats, foam mattresses, overbed lifts, and lift sheets may be indicated; never position on the pressure ulcer

- Pressure ulcers commonly recur in the same or similar areas, warranting vigilant assessments and nursing care. Admission assessments should note locations and timing of previous pressure ulcers

- Serial pictures or images of pressure ulcers are often helpful in comparing the wound to previous time periods and assessing response to treatment

- Massage of pressure ulcers is contraindicated to prevent further skin breakdown

- Although most eschar (dry, necrotic tissue) must be removed (debrided), the dry tissue on the heels should remain to protect those areas

- Referral to a wound care specialist is often indicated

Priority Medications

- Pain medications as indicated

Priority Education/Discharge Issues

- Ensure that the client, family, and caregivers are aware of the risk factors and means to prevent pressure ulcers, along with locations of bony prominences. Teach caregivers positioning strategies and the use of pads, pillows, and equipment to periodically move the client. Use strategies such as timers and turning logs to ensure frequent turning

- Encourage client, family, and caregivers to be aware of assistive devices for lifting, moving, and positioning clients

- Teach client, family, and caregivers the importance of hygiene, cleanliness, hydration, and adequate nutrition

- Encourage the use of community resources and respite services to relieve caregiver role strain

- Teach caregivers the signs and symptoms of pressure ulcers and infection such that they may be detected early

Complete these MNEMONICS

SKIN

S _____

K _____

I _____

N _____

NO ULCER

N _____

O _____

U _____

L _____

C _____

E _____

R _____

Table 14-1: Pressure ulcer prevention. Feel free to search the Internet or create your own.

Go To Clinical Answers

Text designated by 💡 are the top answers for the Go To Clinical related to Pressure ulcers.

Stages of Pressure Sores

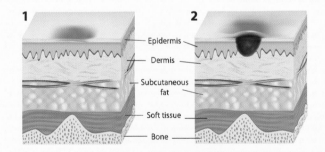
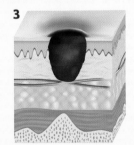
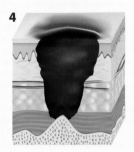

Image 14-1: Can you stage pressure ulcers? Using this chart, search for pressure ulcer images on the internet and stage them. Compare with a friend.

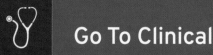

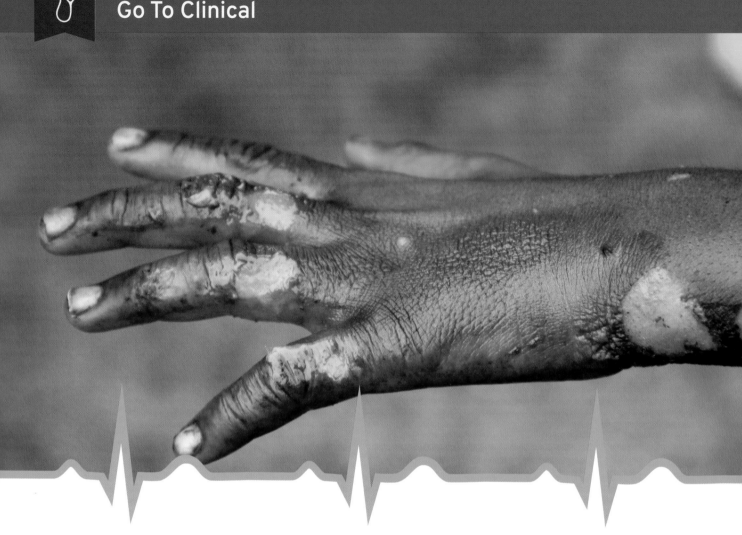

Go To Clinical Case 2

The emergency department receives notification of an incoming client. It is a 12-year-old boy who was "experimenting" with a lighter and gasoline while attempting to prepare a charcoal grill for a family meal. The fire flashed back and burned his hands, almost all of his right arm, front of his chest, abdomen, and the anterior portion of his left thigh. Only a small area on his chin was burned. The paramedic estimates mostly superficial and partial thickness burns, with a small 3 inch in diameter circle on his chest of full thickness from his shirt catching on fire.

The family indicates that the client is otherwise healthy, on no medications, and has no allergies.

The client is receiving 100% oxygen via mask, has an intravenous line in each antecubital space, one capped and one with normal saline infusing.

The client is shivering and is wrapped in damp gauze dressings. The client vomited once on route to the hospital. The client's vital signs are: 97°F–140-32-82/42.

NurseThink® Time

Using the NurseThink® system, complete priorities. Check your answers designated by 💡 in the Burns Priority Exemplar.

✎ Priority Assessments or Cues

1.

2.

3.

⚗ Priority Laboratory Tests/Diagnostics

1.

2.

3.

⚠ Priority Interventions or Actions

1.

2.

3.

⚑ Priority Potential & Actual Complications

1.

2.

3.

℞ Priority Nursing Implications

1.

2.

3.

◆ Priority Medications

1.

2.

3.

👤 Priority Education/Discharge Issues

1.

2.

3.

Burns

📋 Pathophysiology/Description

> One of the leading causes of morbidity and mortality due to trauma

> Defined as injury to body caused by heat/fire (thermal/ smoke inhalation), chemicals, electricity, or radiation

> Impact of burn dependent on client characteristics, burning agent, length of exposure, and temperature of the burning agent

✏️ Priority Assessments or Cues

💡 Assess impact on airway/breathing circulation; assess vital signs

> Assess impact of burn in clients with selected co-morbidities (very young, older adults, poor nutrition, those with chronic illness, those with other injuries)

💡 Assess the severity of burn as dictated by depth, extent, and location

• Depth including superficial partial thickness (epidermis), partial thickness (dermis), and full thickness (into the layers of fat, muscle, and bone)

• Extent guided by the Rule of Nines or Lund Browder formula

• Location of the burn, including burns in areas that may impact breathing (face, neck, head, around chest), impair self-care (eyes, hands, feet, joints), or increase risk for infection (nose, ears, and perineum)

💡 Assess response to treatment (work of breathing, urine output, heart rate, blood pressure, mean arterial pressure (> 65 mmHg)

> Monitor body temperature frequently to assess for hypothermia or infection

🧪 Priority Laboratory Tests/Diagnostics

💡 Hemoglobin and hematocrit including elevated hematocrit with hemoconcentration during emergent and acute phases

💡 Electrolytes including serum sodium (decreased serum sodium in emergent; increased sodium in acute phase due to high sodium fluids/enteral feedings); hyperkalemia in emergent phases due to cellular destruction or hypokalemia in acute phase due to loss from wounds

> Bronchoscopy to monitor airway for damage or edema

💡 ABGs to assess oxygenation and ventilation

> Assess kidney function/potential for acute tubular necrosis

⚠️ Priority Interventions or Actions

> Prehospital

• Maintain patent airway/provide oxygen as indicated

• Remove from source/remove clothing

• Smaller burns may be covered with tap-water dampened soaks, larger burns should be covered for shorter periods to avoid hypothermia

• For chemical burn, remove the agent and flush with water

• Check for other injuries and transport as needed

> Emergent (up to 72 hours after the burn)

💡 Continued airway management/intubate and ventilate as indicated, monitor for airway edema and progressing respiratory distress

💡 Fluid shifts from blood vessels into interstitial and other/ third spaces due to increased capillary permeability/ protein levels require fluid resuscitation

- Establish 2 intravenous sites

- Use the Parkland formula (4 mL lactated ringers X weight in Kg. X % of total body surface area); ½ the first fluids in first 8 hours, ¼ in second 8 hours, ¼ in third 8 hours

💡 Ensure pain management via intravenous route dependent upon the severity of pain, the extent of the burn, and client perceptions of pain

• Provide wound care including showering, dressing changes, debridement/enzymatic debridement, escharotomies/fasciotomies, grafting (allografting, artificial skin, cultured epithelial autografts)

• Prevent contractures, prevent deficits to/maintain functioning including splinting/positioning, physical/ occupational therapies, turning, range-of-motion exercises, and encourage participation in self-care

• Assess readiness for and toleration of feedings (bowel sounds, abdominal tenderness/distension/firmness, bowel function, vomiting/nausea)

> Rehabilitation (weeks to months after the burn)

• Continue measures to prevent contractures and skin breakdown

• Evaluate wound healing and subsequent treatments (reconstructive surgeries, use of water-based moisturizers, antihistamines for itching skin)

• Provide encouragement during slow healing process

> Assess psychosocial responses to trauma, pain, body image changes, treatments, and recovery

Go To Clinical Answers

Text designated by 💡 are the top answers for the Go To Clinical related to Burns.

Priority Potential & Actual Complications

- Upper/lower airway burns with or without smoke inhalation
- Hypovolemic shock
- Infection/sepsis
- Metabolic asphyxiation (carbon monoxide/hydrogen cyanide)
- Reduction of circulation to affected extremities
- Curling's ulcers
- Hyperglycemia with insulin resistance
- Heart failure/pulmonary edema
- Pneumonia
- Delirium
- Venous thromboembolism
- Acute tubular necrosis

Priority Nursing Implications

- Nurses have a significant role in the prevention of burns, providing education, and monitoring safety
- Burns are very painful and cause anxiety, nurses are active in managing pain, fear, anxiety, and the physiological status
- Implement venous thromboembolism prophylaxis procedures as prescribed
- Because burns create a hypermetabolic/hypercatabolic state, nutrition is key to promote wound healing and health. Early initiation of oral or enteral feedings is now recommended to ensure adequate nutrition and positive nitrogen balance. Nurses need to ensure safe enteral feedings to avoid aspiration

Priority Medications

- enoxaparin
  - Venous thromboembolism prophylaxis
  - Assess for perfusion to subcutaneous tissues during fluid shifts
- ranitidine
  - Intravenous or oral
  - Prevent Curling's and stress ulcers
  - Assess for occult blood in stools and other signs of ulceration
- morphine
  - Management of severe pain
  - Intravenous (IM poorly absorbed with fluid shifts)
  - Assess for respiratory depression and constipation
- tetanus toxoid
  - Given to all burn victims to prevent tetanus
  - If the client has not had an immunization in 10 years, administer tetanus immunoglobulin

- silver sulfadiazine
  - Silver containing topical ointment to decrease microbial growth
  - More effective than systemic antibiotics in early stages when perfusion is poor
  - Assess for allergy to sulfur

Priority Education/Discharge Issues

- Ensure that client and family have the support and resources to cope with a potentially long, painful, and difficult healing period
- Provide emotional support related to changes in body appearance and function, including sexuality, self-esteem, and perceptions of self-worth
- Encourage use of support systems and community resources to aid in rehabilitation
- Teach client and family about wound care, physical/occupational therapies, diet, medications, signs of infection, pain management, and follow-up
- Teach client about potential for itching, sensitivity, pigmentation changes, contractures, scarring, and hypersensitivity of burn sites
- Ensure that burn prevention information is available to the client and family

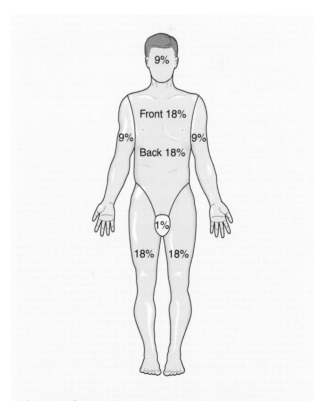

Image 14-2: Using the rule of 9's, what body surface area is covered by burns for the boy in Case 2? Remember for pediatric patients, the head is a slightly larger percentage and the legs is a smaller percentage.

Acute pain

Pathophysiology/Description

> Pain is one of the most prominent healthcare issues today, with subjective and objective interpretations, current management controversies, and debilitating consequences

> Pain was described by Margot McCaffery as "whatever the person experiencing the pain says it is, existing whenever the person says it does." Other definitions discuss unpleasant sensory and emotional experiences related to actual or potential tissue damage

> Two types of pain (these may be acute or chronic)

• Nociceptive pain

- May be superficial somatic (skin/mucous membranes), deep somatic (muscles/bones/tendons), or visceral (deep organs/GI tract/bladder)

- Pain perception is impacted by physiologic, affective, cognitive, behavioral, and sociocultural dimensions

- Nociception processing of pain includes transmitting message from site of tissue damage to central nervous system and is made up of 4 processes including transduction (release of chemicals in response to tissue damage), transmission (message transferred from periphery to spinal cord/dorsal root to thalamus and cortex), perception (personal interpretation of message), and modulation (descending messages that inhibit or facilitate effects of pain transmission)

- Causes include trauma, surgery, injury, burns, disease, or necrosis

- Usually responsive to opioid and non-opioid drugs

- Nociceptive pain may be described as sharp, aching, dull, or cramping

• Neuropathic pain

- Including central pain (lesion in CNS), peripheral neuropathies (related to diabetes/alcoholism), deafferentation pain (loss of afferent transmission as in phantom pain), and sympathetically maintained pain (complex regional pain syndrome)

- Causes include trauma, infection, metabolic disease, infection, alcoholism, tumors, toxins, or neurologic diseases

- Treatment usually requires adjuvant drugs

- Neuropathic pain may be described as burning, shooting, itching, or stabbing

> Acute pain is defined as lasting less than three months, may be mild to severe levels, pain is generally associated with a specific event decreases over time and generally goes away. Acute pain may signal tissue damage and allow for adaptation. Unremitting acute pain may become chronic in nature but goal of management of acute pain is relief of pain. Relief may not be total, but pain is reduced to a tolerable level

Priority Assessments or Cues

> Screen all clients for pain (pain is the fifth vital sign)

> Use standardized pain assessment tools

> Assess risk factors for acute pain experiences including injury/trauma, surgery, pathophysiological changes in the body (necrosis of myocardial tissue, ischemia to peripheral extremities, acute degeneration of bone/muscle, vascular changes of cerebral vessels), labor/delivery, or infection

> Assess client's personal interpretation of the meaning of pain

> Assess self-report of pain (as client is able), including:

• Onset (clients with acute pain may recall event or injury)

• Pattern (may increase with activity or change based on medication dosing/duration of medication effects)

• Duration

• Location/radiation (more often specific rather than generalized)

• Intensity

• Quality (nature and characteristics)

• Associated factors (pain may increase or decrease with activity, increases or decreases during sleep)

• Previous and current management strategies/healthcare seeking/utilization/previous experiences

• Impact on social and occupational functioning

• Impact on sleep, activity, function, emotions, sexual libido/performance, and relationships with others

> Assess objective signs of acute pain including how they hold their body/positioning, sitting very still or restless, pallor, elevated heart rate/respiratory rate/blood pressure, fatigue, anxiety, agitation, diaphoresis, confusion, facial expressions/gestures, moaning, or urinary retention

> Assess for breakthrough pain, procedural/incident pain, or end-of-dose failure

Priority Laboratory Tests/Diagnostics

> Diagnostic tests to detect underlying causes

Priority Interventions or Actions

> Ensure accurate documentation of assessments and treatments

> Treat underlying cause (antibiotics for infections, splint postoperative surgical site, cast fractured limb, manage cardiovascular function)

> Non-pharmacologic methods should accompany pharmacologic methods, including application of heat/cold, acupuncture, relaxation strategies, distraction, imagery, hypnosis, transcutaneous electrical nerve stimulation, massage, and use of complementary/alternative strategies

> Frequently reassess pain levels and evaluate effectiveness of management strategies

> Acute pain management may be facilitated by implantable pain pumps, client-controlled analgesia, and alternative administrations routes, including transmucosal, buccal, intranasal, and rectal routes

Priority Potential & Actual Complications

> Untreated pain is associated with prolonged healing, immunosuppression, emotional/physical discomfort/dysfunction, depression, and sleep disorders

> Physiological complications may include weight loss, hypertension, hyperglycemia/glucose intolerance, atelectasis/pneumonia, paralytic ileus/constipation, immobility/deep vein thromboses, weakness/fatigue, infections, confusion/poor decision-making, fluid and electrolyte imbalance, social withdrawal, and isolation

Priority Nursing Implications

> Nurses may use standardized pain assessment tools, body maps to pinpoint pain location and radiation, and scales/analogs/FACES/ranking tools to assess pain intensity. These tools are valuable with clients with developmental/cognitive/communication barriers

> Self-report and description (rating) is critical, but often nurses must use other methods to assess pain for those who are unable to participate (clients who are non-verbal, unconscious, or who have communication disorders)

> Clients in acute pain often benefit from around-the-clock analgesia, rather PRN scheduling. This prevents pain from getting to a level too high/difficult to manage

> Multimodal analgesia dictates that two or more agents are used together to manage pain, thereby increasing pain medication effectiveness, increasing client perceptions of pain management, and decreasing potential side effects of each medication (opioid-sparing effect of acetaminophen when delivered with hydrocodone)

> Nurses need to vigilantly assess for respiratory depression in clients receiving opioid agents and carefully monitor during first doses, when dose is increased, or when multiple agents are used to manage pain

Priority Medications

> acetaminophen
  - May be PO, PR, IV/sustained-release available in oral forms
  - For mild to moderate pain and is an antipyretic, no antiplatelet or anti-inflammatory effects
  - Long-term use or high doses may impair liver function, cause liver toxicity

> ibuprofen
  - PO
  - May cause GI side effects (bleeding, perforation, or ulceration, especially in older adults)
  - May increase hypertension, myocardial infarction, and stroke

> ketorolac
  - For < 5 days
  - Ensure hydration to avoid kidney dysfunction

> celecoxib
  - Inhibits COX-2, not COX-1, and creates less GI side effects (risk still exists)
  - May be associated with cardiovascular thrombosis, MIs, and CVAs (increased risk with long-term use or CV risk factors)

> codeine with acetaminophen
  - Associated with high incidence of nausea and constipation
  - Oral agent for moderate pain relief, acetaminophen has opioid-sparing effects
  - 5-10% of European Americans lack the enzymes needed to metabolize codeine to endogenous morphine

> hydrocodone with acetaminophen
  - Oral combination of opioid with co-analgesics
  - Used for moderate to severe pain
  - Short-term management of acute pain

> morphine
  - PO, PR, IV, subcutaneous, epidural, intrathecal, sublingual
  - For moderate to severe pain

> lidocaine
  - Topical local anesthetic
  - Used for painful procedures (venipuncture, lumbar puncture, bone marrow aspiration)
  - Takes about 30 minutes to achieve effect, lasts about 60 minutes

> naloxone
  - Reverses effects of opioids
  - IV, Subq, nasal spray
  - If opioids used for pain management for several days, client may experience severe pain and/or withdrawal symptoms when naloxone administered

Priority Education/Discharge Issues

> Teaching is incorporated into all components of assessment and management of pain

> Emphasis should be placed on education about the side effects of medications, including constipation, sedation, nausea, itchiness, and respiratory depression associated with opioids, dose or agent limiting side effects, adverse reactions, and scheduling. Side effects are major causes of poor pain control and non-adherence in cases of acute and chronic pain

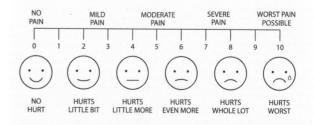

Image 14-3: Think of three clients. For whom would this pain scale not work? Conduct an internet search for 'cultural variation in pain assessment.'

Chronic pain

📋 Pathophysiology/Description

> Chronic pain is defined as mild to severe pain lasting more than three months, may appear gradually or suddenly, onset may not be traced to a stimulating event, cause may or may not be known, continues past the anticipated time of relief, usually not adaptive in nature, does not go away, and may increase and decrease throughout the day despite analgesia. May or may not be eliminated but interventions are focused on reduction of disability and resumption of function

> The financial and personal costs of all pain in general, but most markedly with chronic pain, are significant

> There are concerns that chronic pain is often undertreated, especially associated with cancer and end-of-life care. Conversely, chronic pain management is often associated with the current opioid crisis, calling into question some current practices

> Pain is one of the most prominent healthcare issues today, with subjective and objective interpretations, current management controversies, and debilitating consequences

> Pain was described by Margot McCaffery as "whatever the person experiencing the pain says it is, existing whenever the person says it does." Other definitions discuss unpleasant sensory and emotional experiences related to actual or potential tissue damage

> Two types of pain (these may be acute or chronic)
  - Nociceptive pain
    - May be superficial somatic (skin/mucous membranes), deep somatic (muscles/bones/tendons), or visceral (deep organs/GI tract/bladder)
    - Pain perception is impacted by physiologic, affective, cognitive, behavioral, and sociocultural dimensions
    - Nociception processing of pain includes transmitting message from site of tissue damage to central nervous system and is made up of 4 processes including transduction (release of chemicals in response to tissue damage), transmission (message transferred from periphery to spinal cord/dorsal root to thalamus and cortex), perception (personal interpretation of message), and modulation (descending messages that inhibit or facilitate effects of pain transmission)
    - Causes include trauma, surgery, injury, burns, disease, or necrosis
    - Usually responsive to opioid and non-opioid drugs
    - Nociceptive pain may be described as sharp, aching, dull, or cramping
  - Neuropathic pain
    - Including central pain (lesion in CNS), peripheral neuropathies (related to diabetes/alcoholism), deafferentation pain (loss of afferent transmission as in phantom pain), and sympathetically maintained pain (complex regional pain syndrome)
    - Causes include trauma, infection, metabolic disease, infection, alcoholism, tumors, toxins, or neurologic diseases
    - Treatment usually requires adjuvant drugs
    - Neuropathic pain may be described as burning, shooting, itching, or stabbing

> Chronic pain may cause significant and long-term suffering, perceptions of lack of self-control, anxiety, depression, and insecurity

✏️ Priority Assessments or Cues

> Screen all clients for pain (pain is the fifth vital sign)

> Use standardized pain assessment tools

> Assess risk factors for chronic pain experiences including pathophysiological changes in the body (joint and musculoskeletal changes leading to arthritis and back pain, vascular changes related to chronic migraine headaches, muscle aches due to fibromyalgia), or age/physiological deterioration

> Assess client's personal interpretation of the meaning of pain

> Assess self-report of pain (as client is able), including onset (clients with chronic pain may not know exact initiation of pain), pattern (chronic pain may increase or decrease over time, may increase or decrease with sleep cycles or during times of activity), duration (may be less specific than acute pain), location/radiation (may be specific or more generalized), intensity, quality (nature and characteristics, may be less able to describe with chronic pain), associated factors (chronic pain may be associated with depression/emotional factors that increase pain perception, pain may increase or decrease with activity), previous and current management strategies/healthcare seeking/utilization/previous experiences, impact on social and occupational functioning, and impact on sleep, activity, function, emotions, sexual libido/performance, and relationships with others (more significant impacts with chronic pain)

> Assess objective signs of chronic pain which may be similar to and/or different from those with acute pain; client may state pain is severe without objective signs due to the body's adaptation to the pain state (may not reflect sympathetic nervous system stimulation). Additional classic symptoms include flat affect, depression, irritability, reduced level of activity and social interaction, and fatigue

> Assess for breakthrough pain, procedural/incident pain, or end-of-dose failure. Clients with chronic pain may struggle to cope with the additional pain associated with procedures, lack of management, or experiences associated with fear or apprehension

🧪 Priority Laboratory Tests/Diagnostics

> Diagnostic tests to detect underlying causes

⚠️ Priority Interventions or Actions

> Ensure accurate documentation of assessments and treatments and compare with previous assessments at each healthcare encounter

- Treat underlying cause (back pain may indicate need for physical therapy, exercises and stretching, or surgical repair, chronic migraines may benefit from identification and elimination of triggers)
- Non-pharmacologic methods should accompany pharmacologic methods, including application of heat/cold, acupuncture, relaxation strategies, distraction, imagery, hypnosis, transcutaneous electrical nerve stimulation, massage, and use of complementary/alternative strategies
- Frequently reassess pain levels and evaluate effectiveness of management strategies
- New chronic pain interventions include therapeutic nerve blocks, neuroablative procedures, neuroaugmentation, and surgical intervention

⚑ Priority Potential & Actual Complications

- Untreated pain is associated with prolonged healing, immunosuppression, emotional/physical discomfort/ dysfunction, depression, and sleep disorders
- Physiological complications may include weight loss, hypertension, hyperglycemia/glucose intolerance, atelectasis/pneumonia, paralytic ileus/constipation, immobility/deep vein thromboses, weakness/fatigue, infections, confusion/poor decision-making, fluid and electrolyte imbalance, social withdrawal, and isolation
- Chronic pain may lead to significant decreases in social, self-care, and occupational functioning

℧ Priority Nursing Implications

- Nurses may use standardized pain assessment tools, body maps to pinpoint pain location and radiation, and scales/ analogs/FACES/ranking tools to assess pain intensity. These tools are valuable with clients with developmental/ cognitive/communication barriers
- Multimodal analgesia dictates that two or more agents are used together to manage pain, thereby increasing pain medication effectiveness, increasing client perceptions of pain management, and decreasing potential side effects of each medication (opioid-sparing effect of acetaminophen when delivered with hydrocodone)
- Nurses need to vigilantly assess for respiratory depression in clients receiving opioid agents and carefully monitor during first doses, when dose is increased, or when multiple agents are used to manage pain
- Nurses need to be aware of opioid-induced hyperalgesia wherein clients appear to be more sensitive to pain following pharmacological pain management strategies
- Clients with chronic pain often find relief in use of the cannabinoids. These medications, whether smoked or in oral/pill form, provide pain relief, decrease nausea, increase appetite, are opioid-sparing, and reduce the impact of opioid withdrawal. Their use in pain management continues to be researched and current legislation demonstrates the value of these medications for some clients

- Chronic pain management is often made more complex by tolerance, physical dependence, pseudoaddiction, and addiction
- Providing pain management for clients with opioid and other addictions may be complex, but these clients deserve respectful and high-quality pain assessment and management

◌ Priority Medications

- See medications in Acute pain Priority Exemplar
- Clients with chronic pain may receive adjuvant medications to support pain management, including corticosteroids, antiseizure medications, antidepressants, adrenergic agonists, GABA receptor agonists, or local anesthetics
- fentanyl
  - Very potent analgesic
  - Transdermal route indicated for chronic pain
  - Assess for symptoms of overdose, including decreased respirations, excessive sleepiness, confusion, or lethargy
- tapentadol
  - For moderate to severe chronic pain, available in sustained-release formula
  - Less nausea and constipation than other opioids
- clonidine
  - Alpha-adrenergic agonist
  - Used for chronic headaches or neuropathic pain
- mexiletine
  - Oral/systemic anesthetic for neuropathic pain
  - Watch for nausea, dizziness, paresthesias, tremoring, and seizures
  - Avoid with clients with cardiac disorders
- trolamine salicylate
  - Topical, locally absorbed aspirin-containing cream
  - Used for muscle and joint pain
  - Avoids GI irritation
- dronabinol
  - Cannabinoid medication approved for medical use
  - May be smoked or in a prepared oral form
  - Enhance endogenous opioid system, alleviates nausea, and increases appetite
  - May be effective in decreasing the impact of withdrawal

👤 Priority Education/Discharge Issues

- Teaching is incorporated into all components of assessment and management of pain
- Emphasis should be placed on education about the side effects of medications, including constipation, sedation, nausea, itchiness, and respiratory depression associated with opioids, dose or agent limiting side effects, adverse reactions, and scheduling. Side effects are major causes of poor pain control and non-adherence in cases of acute and chronic pain

Contact dermatitis/ impetigo

Pathophysiology/Description

> Atopic dermatitis is an inflammatory response to environmental allergens, may be chronic and recurrent, may occur with asthma and nasal congestion

> Allergic contact dermatitis is a delayed hypersensitivity reaction of the skin after a chemical has penetrated the skin and becomes antigenic. After 7-10 days, memory cells form an antibody response. Subsequent exposures yield skin lesions within 48 hours. Often related to exposure to metal, rubber, oils associated with plants, and some cosmetics or dyes

> Latex allergies yield a contact dermatitis related to the chemical processes of making gloves

> Impetigo is a bacterial infection of the skin, often associated with Group A Beta-hemolytic streptococcus or Staphylococcus. May be a primary or secondary infection

Priority Assessments or Cues

> Assess the characteristics of atopic dermatitis including acute phase (erythema, seeping vesicles, and pruritis). During subacute phase, lesions may become scaly with red/brown plaques. Chronically, skin may become thickened, hyperpigmented, dry, and scaled

> Assess for allergic contact dermatitis including red papules or vesicles, may be pruritic, burn or cause pain. If rash is extended over a period of time, the skin may become thick and scaly

> Assess for response to latex which may be 6-48 hours after exposure including symptoms of drying, mild swelling, fissuring, and cracking of the skin. May progress to redness, marked swelling, and crusting. May lead to scaling and hyperpigmentation

> Impetigo may be associated with poor hygiene. Assess client's hygiene practices. With children, assess for open lesions and potential for contamination with scratching, lack of hygiene, and exposure to infectious agents (stools, urine, etc.)

> Other risk factors to be assessed that are associated with impetigo include obesity, diabetes mellitus, moist skin folds, history of atopic dermatitis, and treatment with corticosteroids, immunosuppressants, or antibiotics

> Assess for appearance of impetigo, including vesicular-papular rash with yellow-brown drainage. Redness noted around the edges and are often pruritic

Priority Laboratory Tests/Diagnostics

> Skin cultures if drainage is accessible

> Other diagnostic procedures for associated risk factors/illnesses

> In severe cases, allergy testing to determine hypersensitivities

Priority Interventions or Actions

> Use moisturizers on dry skin areas

> Topical immunomodulators and corticosteroids

> Phototherapy sometimes used to dry skin and allow for healing

> Identify and limit exposure to allergic or latex stimulators of skin change

> Impetigo is often treated with systemic antibiotics

> Topical care of impetigo includes warm saline compresses followed by gentle washing to remove exudate and crusting. Areas are left open to air to dry and heal. May be treated with topical antiinfectives

Priority Potential & Actual Complications

> Secondary bacterial infections (impetigo) may occur with untreated skin irritations that are exposed to infectious agents

> Untreated impetigo may lead to bacterial acute glomerulonephritis

Priority Nursing Implications

> Nurses need to be cognizant of their personal risk for contact dermatitis, especially latex, related to extensive and long-term exposure. Many agencies have latex exposure policies or latex free practices

Priority Medications

> pimecrolimus
  - Immunosuppressant/suppresses the inflammatory response
  - Used to treat atopic and contact dermatitis
> mupirocin
  - Topical antibiotic
  - Used to treat impetigo
> penicillin
  - Oral medication administered for impetigo
  - Provides systemic treatment to reduce severity and spread of impetigo

Priority Education/Discharge Issues

> Teach clients to avoid agents that cause allergic contact dermatitis

> Emotional stress may exacerbate skin reactions

> Instruct clients that those who are prone to contact and allergic dermatitis may experience hypersensitivity reactions, allergic reactions, and drug intolerances/allergies

> Teach the importance of hygiene and effective handwashing

> Impetigo may be contagious, ensure that clients and family are aware of means to prevent spread of infection

Fatigue

Pathophysiology/Description

> Described as the ongoing, persistent feeling of tiredness; lasting more than a few days or weeks

> Subjective description of lack of energy that hampers functioning in the social, personal, and occupational areas

> May be a symptom of an underlying healthcare issue (such as cancer) or may be unexplained

> May indicate a sleep deficit or may be associated with the increased energy required in the healing process or the body's response to disease

> Fatigue may be associated with end-of-life, may be an early sign of other illnesses, such as heart failure or chronic obstructive pulmonary disease, or may be the most significant side effect of treatment and last for a long period after treatments for cancer

> Chronic fatigue syndrome is described as debilitating fatigue along with other symptoms. Although cause is unknown, may be triggered by stress/stressful event and illnesses with flu-like symptoms, or triggered by organisms such as Epstein-Barr virus, cytomegalovirus, and others

> Fibromyalgia is described as a chronic disorder associated with fatigue, pain, morning stiffness, depression, difficulty coping with stress, anxiety, inflammatory bowel syndrome, and non-restful sleep; thought to be associated with neurotransmitter dysregulation

Priority Assessments or Cues

> Assess for risk factors associated with fatigue, including depression, anxiety, dehydration, hypothyroidism, insomnia, infection, or concurrent or chronic disease or disorders (diabetes, heart failure, respiratory illnesses)

> Assess for reversible causes of fatigue (poor sleep, dehydration, illness)

> Assess client's tolerance to activities and determine those activities/interests in which the client most wants to participate

> Fatigue is a subjective symptom. To assess, ask the client to describe fatigue, use numeric scales to quantify level of fatigue, or administer standardized fatigue scales

> Assess for pallor, adequacy of perfusion, oxygenation, and ventilation

> Determine if client takes medications that may cause or increase fatigue

> Administer standardized depression or anxiety scales, if indicated

> Assess for risk factors for chronic fatigue syndrome including significant stress, trauma, or illness

> Assess for symptoms of chronic fatigue syndrome including fatigue not associated with exertion and not relieved by rest, changes in memory function and ability to concentrate, sore throat, muscle and joint pain, headache, and malaise

> Assess for risk factors associated with fibromyalgia including familial history of this and other sleeping disorders, or a recent trauma or illness that may trigger the illness

> Assess for symptoms of fibromyalgia including fatigue, malaise, burning pain, facial/head/neck pain, joint tenderness/point tenderness at 11 of the 18 identified and specific body points associated with fibromyalgia, cognitive changes and changes in level of consciousness, and diarrhea, constipation, bloating, and pain associated with irritable bowel syndrome

Priority Laboratory Tests/Diagnostics

> Complete blood count-assess for anemia, a potential causal factor of fatigue and elevations in white blood cells may indicate infection

> With fibromyalgia, ANA levels (antinuclear antibodies) may be low

> Muscle biopsies with fibromyalgia may demonstrate muscle atrophy

Priority Interventions or Actions

> Determine and manage underlying cause for fatigue; if cause is unknown, treatment is often symptomatic

> Balance time for activity with time for rest, discuss favorite activities with client and create a plan to create time for each, determine and maximize activities during the time of day when the client feels most energetic. Ensure adequate rest prior to periods of activity

> Ensure client is awake and active, as able, during the day to optimize nighttime sleep

> Ensure adequate hydration. Many believe dehydration is a root cause of fatigue in otherwise healthy individuals

> Encourage optimal nutrition, including foods high in protein, iron, and whole fiber, some recommend limiting sugar, caffeine, and alcohol which may disrupt sleep and irritate muscles

> Develop progressive exercise programs, as able, to increase time and intensity of exercise

> In hospitalized clients, reduce disruption during nighttime sleep and group activities to allow for uninterrupted rest

> Implement strategies to reduce stress, including coping strategies, biofeedback, cognitive behavioral therapy, psychotherapy, massage, yoga, progressive relaxation, Tai Chi, walking and low-impact exercise programs, use of hot and cold therapies, mindfulness strategies, and sleep hygiene practices

Priority Potential & Actual Complications

> Social withdrawal/social isolation/depression/anxiety

> Immobility/disuse syndrome

Priority Nursing Implications

> Many clients experience fatigue and pain. Make sure pain is managed and analgesics are used to ensure adequate pain relief. Once pain is managed, then consider hypnotic agents and other sleep-inducing strategies

> For hospitalized clients, nurses may advocate for rest times so clients have uninterrupted times of restful sleep. In intensive care and other environments, dim lights at night, limit nighttime activities, group interventions, provide comfort measures, and establish quiet hours to assist in attaining restful sleep and quiet rest periods

> Chronic fatigue syndrome and fibromyalgia may be extremely frustrating for clients and families; clients may not be "believed" or their symptoms and limitations may not be deemed as credible by others in their social or occupational circles

Priority Medications

> oral NSAIDS
  • Manage mild to moderate pain levels
  • These may allow for restful sleep by addressing the pain that disturbs sleep

> ferrous sulfate
  • Oral forms of iron should be enteric coated or sustained-release to ensure absorption in the duodenum for optimal absorption
  • Liquid oral-forms of iron will stain the teeth so a straw and diluting the solution is recommended

> zolpidem
  • Short-term hypnotic; long-term use should be closely monitored
  • May be used with severe sleep problems (including to fibromyalgia and chronic fatigue syndrome)

> clonazepam
  • Anticonvulsant agent
  • Effective with stimulating sleep and reducing anxiety

> duloxetine
  • Antidepressant
  • Administer early in the day to avoid insomnia
  • Used with fibromyalgia

> pregabalin
  • Used to treat the pain associated with fibromyalgia

> cyclobenzaprine
  • Muscle relaxant with sedative effects
  • May increase productive sleep

Priority Education/Discharge Issues

> For home care, instruct clients on sleep hygiene practices including going to bed only when sleepy, getting out of bed if haven't fallen asleep in 20 minutes, limiting liquids at night, quiet reading (not screen time) prior to sleep, warm baths or showers just prior to sleep, limiting exercise before bedtime (at least 6 hours prior to) but getting adequate exercise during the day, liming caffeine/stimulants/nicotine/alcohol before bed, having a small protein snack/warm milk prior to sleep to avoid hunger, reducing light and noise if sleeping time is not at night, keeping bed for sleeping and only sleeping activities, staying out of bed during the day, set a regular sleep and wake up time, limiting day-time naps, limiting use of hypnotics, and stress reducing strategies to avoid anxiety at sleep time

> Instruct clients about the importance of a balance of sleep, rest, and activity in their lives

> Teach about short-term use of hypnotic agents to attain restful sleep, consider melatonin or lavender oil via diffuser

> Fibromyalgia and chronic fatigue syndrome may interfere with working, attaining health insurance, and receiving needed healthcare. Encourage clients to use available resources to meet basic and healthcare needs

> Fatigue disorders have an unknown course, some resulting in a long recovery period or a lack of full recovery. Teaching is essential to deal with the anger, frustration, and sadness felt by clients and the skepticism or negative reactions of those in the client's world.

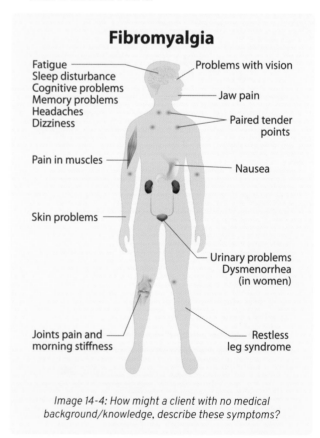

Fibromyalgia

Fatigue
Sleep disturbance
Cognitive problems
Memory problems
Headaches
Dizziness

Problems with vision

Jaw pain

Paired tender points

Pain in muscles

Nausea

Skin problems

Urinary problems
Dysmenorrhea
(in women)

Joints pain and morning stiffness

Restless leg syndrome

Image 14-4: How might a client with no medical background/knowledge, describe these symptoms?

Sleep disorders

📋 Pathophysiology/Description

> Defined as a group of disorders associated with sleep or times of rest, conditions may lead to poor quality sleep

> Sleep deprivation may lead to moodiness, cognitive impairment, obesity, depressed immune response, hypertension, GERD, and increased insulin resistance/type 2 diabetes

> About 87% of American society claims to have some sleep disorder

> Insomnia is the difficulty falling asleep, waking during sleep and having difficulty falling back asleep, or waking early. May be acute or chronic; may be primary or secondary

> Restless leg syndrome is the unpleasant sensory/motor activity of one or both legs. May be primary or secondary. May be associated with diabetes, hypertension, anemia, pregnancy, renal failure, or rheumatoid arthritis

> Narcolepsy is the disordered sleep pattern in a client which causes uncontrolled, spontaneous sleep during waking hours, may occur during activities, clients may pass immediately into rapid eye movement sleep from the awake state. Clients with narcolepsy are protected by the Americans with Disabilities Act. May be triggered by a head trauma, change in sleep patterns, or an infection

> Obstructive sleep apnea (OSA) is the partial or complete obstruction of the airway during sleep

✏️ Priority Assessments or Cues

> Assess for symptoms of sleeplessness including sleep patterns, fatigue level, and impact of sleep issues on social, personal, and occupational functioning

> Assess for chronic disorders that disturb sleep (COPD, heart failure)

> Assess for difficulties falling asleep, waking during sleep and having difficulty falling back asleep, or waking early

> Use standardized measures to assess sleep

> Determine if client takes medications that may cause or increase sleep disorders

> Assess for symptoms of restless leg syndrome including the uncontrollable urge to move/involuntary movement of legs, paresthesias, creeping/crawling sensations in the legs, numbness/tingling, restlessness, or pain at rest

> Assess for symptoms of narcolepsy including witnessed or experienced periods of sudden sleep states, sleep paralysis, hallucinations, or cataplexy (falling during sudden sleep episodes)

> Assess clients at risk for OSA including clients older than 65 years, or with a BMI > 28 kg/m² , neck circumference > 17 inches, acromegaly, history of smoking, craniofacial abnormalities, and COPD

> Assess for signs/symptoms of OSA including insomnia, audible snoring, startling during sleep, daytime sleepiness, morning headaches, and irritability

🧪 Priority Laboratory Tests/Diagnostics

> Complete blood count to assess for anemia

> Serum ferritin levels

> Renal function (BUN, creatinine)

> Actigraphy to monitor sleep, rest, and activity levels

> Polysomnography (PSG) assesses muscle tone (EMG), eye movements (EOG), and brain activity (EEG) to assess for narcolepsy and other sleep disorders. May include chest/abdominal movement sensors and oral/nasal airflow measurements to diagnose OSA

> Multiple sleep latency tests/sleep studies for narcolepsy

> Overnight oxygen saturation measurement for OSA

⚠️ Priority Interventions or Actions

> Treat underlying cause of sleep disorder

> Institute sleep hygiene measures (see below)

> Consider cognitive behavioral therapy or other counseling to deal with stressors

> Restless leg syndrome may be relieved by activity (walking, stretching, kicking, rocking)

> Narcolepsy is most successfully treated with a combination of medications and behavioral therapies

> OSA
  - If mild, client is instructed to sleep on side or elevate head of bed/use pillows
  - Avoid alcohol or sedatives 3-4 hours before sleep
  - Weight loss
  - Use an oral appliance to maintain an open airway
  - If these measures unsuccessful, clients are recommended to use continuous positive airway pressure (CPAP) or bilevel positive airway pressure (BiPAP) via mask to open airways. Clients are encouraged to select a mask most comfortable for them. Adherence to nightly CPAP or BiPAP is often poor due to the mask, noise, the interference with partner sleep, and that fact that the machine needs to be transported with the client for overnight stays. Client may complain of nasal stuffiness after use
  - Surgical repair or radiofrequency ablation may be effective for clients with refractory OSA

🚩 Priority Potential & Actual Complications

> Social, personal, and occupational dysfunction from sleep disorders/disturbed sleep

> Social withdrawal/isolation/depression

> Motor vehicle and work-related injuries related to lack of attentiveness/sleepiness/falling asleep

> Untreated sleep apnea may lead to hypertension, heart failure, dysrhythmias, and impotence

Sleep disorders

Priority Nursing Implications

> Prolonged sleep deprivation in hospitalized clients may lead to delirium and prolonged recoveries. Nurses need to employ measures to foster sleep in clients, including rest times so clients have uninterrupted times of restful sleep. In intensive care and other environments, dim lights at night, limit nighttime activities, group interventions, provide comfort measures, and establish quiet hours may assist in attaining restful sleep and quiet rest periods

> Many sleep disorders go untreated, nurses have an important role in detecting and assisting clients to manage sleep disorders

> Support groups are often helpful for clients with sleep disorders

> For clients with OSA, nurses need to use caution when administering central nervous system depressants or opioids to avoid respiratory depression

Priority Medications

> melatonin
  - Available over-the-counter as a sleep aid/supplement
  - Relieves insomnia associated with jet lag and shift work
  - May lower blood pressure and interact with warfarin and CNS depressants

> zolpidem
  - First line agents for insomnia
  - May be safely used for one year under close medical surveillance
  - Available as oral pills, dissolvable oral tablets, and sublingual tablets

> carbidopa/levodopa
  - Antiparkinsonian medication to increase dopamine
  - May relieve restless leg syndrome

> enacarbil
  - Anticonvulsant
  - May relieve the sensory symptoms of restless leg syndrome

> modafinil
  - First line agent for narcolepsy
  - Non-amphetamine wake-promotion drug

Priority Education/Discharge Issues

> For home care, instruct clients on sleep hygiene practices including going to bed only when sleepy, getting out of bed if haven't fallen asleep in 20 minutes, limiting liquids at night, quiet reading (not screen time) prior to sleep, warm baths or showers just prior to sleep, limiting exercise before bedtime (at least 6 hours prior to) but getting adequate exercise during the day, limiting caffeine/stimulants/nicotine/alcohol before bed, having a small protein snack/warm milk prior to sleep to avoid hunger, reducing light and noise if sleeping time is not at night, keeping bed for sleeping and only sleeping activities, staying out of bed during the day, set a regular sleep and wake up time, limiting day-time naps, limiting use of hypnotics, and stress reducing strategies to avoid anxiety at sleep time

> Encourage clients to keep a sleep diary to maintain an accurate account of sleep, encourage sleep partners to participate in recording sleep activity

Complete this MNEMONIC
INSOMNIA
I _____
N _____
S _____
O _____
M _____
N _____
I _____
A _____

Table 14-2: Insomnia causes and symptoms. Feel free to search the Internet or create your own.

1. A client who has Alzheimer's Disease is in an intensive care unit following major abdominal surgery. The nurse is getting ready to transfer the client to a general surgical unit. During handoff report, which assessment data are important for the nurse to provide regarding the client's pain?
   1. The nurse's beliefs on how severe the client's pain is.
   2. The client's most recent vital signs.
   3. A description of the client's facial expressions and changes in mental status.
   4. The nurse cannot provide information about the client's pain because the client has dementia.

2. The nurse is caring for an older adult client who is experiencing chronic back pain and is receiving an opioid analgesic. The nurse plans care for this client knowing that the client is at a high-risk for experiencing which health concern?
   1. Renal failure.
   2. Falls.
   3. Liver failure.
   4. Alterations in hearing.

3. The nurse is planning to teach a 16-year-old client with contact dermatitis. What teaching strategy does the nurse plan to use during the educational session?
   1. Provide education to the client's mother.
   2. Use a formal lecture style when delivering the information.
   3. Assess the client's motivation and ability to learn.
   4. Provide printed information written at the high school reading level.

4. A nurse is caring for a client who has third-degree burns on the right hand from a kitchen fire. The client is scheduled to go for a skin graft procedure tomorrow. Physical therapy is coming within the hour. The client is sitting in the room with the lights out and is staring out the window. What action does the nurse take first?
   1. Provide client education about the upcoming skin graft and sign the informed consent for surgery.
   2. Assess the status of the dressing on the client's hand.
   3. Say to the client, "People with burns experience a lot of emotions and frustrations. Tell me what you are feeling right now."
   4. Help the client put on shoes and get ready for the physical therapy visit.

5. A client with a pressure ulcer is receiving negative-pressure wound therapy. What finding indicates the need for follow-up by the nurse?
   1. The negative-pressure wound therapy unit is hanging on the side of the bed.
   2. The diameter of the wound has not changed since a week ago.
   3. There is a small amount of clear, odorless drainage from the wound.
   4. The client rates pain as a 3 on a 0-10 pain scale.

6. The nurse is caring for a client who fell off a ladder and broke his arm. The client is receiving naproxen 500 mg BID orally PRN for pain associated with the injury. What statement made by the client requires immediate follow-up by the nurse?
   1. "My pain is worse when I move my arm."
   2. "I had a stomach ulcer last year."
   3. "I need to take the medication around the clock to relieve my pain."
   4. "I wonder if I can switch to acetaminophen to control my pain when I go home."

7. The nurse is caring for a young adult who reports fatigue due to chronic insomnia. What instructions does the nurse give first?
   1. Work towards having a consistent time you go to sleep and wake up.
   2. Exercising 1-2 hours before bedtime will help you feel more tired and fall asleep.
   3. Put a night light in the room to help you get to the bathroom safely during the night.
   4. Make sure the room is warm and you cover yourself with a blanket when you go to bed.

8. A nurse is caring for a client who is obese. Which statement made by the client requires further assessment by the nurse?
   1. "I walk about 15 minutes twice a day; when I get up and right after dinner."
   2. "I usually fall asleep within 20 – 30 minutes of laying down."
   3. "I sleep 6-7 hours every night."
   4. "My wife says I wake her up a couple of times from snoring every night."

9. A charge nurse is making assignments for the nursing staff on a medical-surgical care unit that includes registered nurses and licensed practical/vocational nurses. Which client is it most appropriate to assign to a registered nurse?
    1. A client who had a total hysterectomy yesterday and is requesting a fan.
    2. A client who had a thoracotomy yesterday and is receiving morphine by IV push (IVP).
    3. A client with cholecystitis who is experiencing abdominal pain and is having surgery tomorrow.
    4. A client with arthritis who had a total knee replacement 2 days ago and is taking hydrocodone for pain.

10. The nurse is caring for a client who reports falling asleep while stopped at a red light in the car. The nurse suspects the client has obstructive sleep apnea. What assessment finding is consistent with this diagnosis?
    1. Body mass index (BMI) 25.3 kg/m².
    2. Neck circumference of 16 inches (40.6 cm).
    3. Client states has difficulty falling asleep.
    4. Client startles during sleep.

11. A nurse is caring for a client who states, "I wake up at night sometimes with a feeling of panic. My heart races, I breathe really hard and fast and I'm usually really sweaty." The nurse plans care knowing this client is probably experiencing which health problem?
    1. Parasomnias.
    2. Narcolepsy.
    3. Insomnia.
    4. Obstructive sleep apnea.

12. A nurse is teaching a client about the use of home bilevel positive airway pressure (BiPAP) due to a diagnosis of obstructive sleep apnea. What nursing action is essential to improve the client's adherence to this therapy?
    1. Tell the client to take diphenhydramine 25 mg by mouth every night to help the client fall asleep at night.
    2. Suggest the client evaluate surgical options to treat sleep apnea to make an informed decision.
    3. Make sure the mask fits well and makes a tight seal.
    4. Include the client in the selection of the mask and device before starting the therapy.

13. A male client sustains burns and is brought to the emergency department for care. The client is estimated to weigh 160 pounds. The client is estimated to have 25% of his body burned. Using the Parkland formula, how much lactated ringers should be administered in the first eight hours of his care?

14. The nurse is caring for a client who was in a house fire and has full-thickness burns on the back of both arms and the back of the head. The client's face has superficial burns on the face. The client weighs 60 kg. Using the Rule of Nines and the Parkland formula with 4 mL lactated Ringers IV, how much IV fluid does the client need in the first 24 hours following the burns?
    1. 1620 mL.
    2. 3240 mL.
    3. 4320 mL.
    4. 8640 mL.

15. The nurse is administering IV fluids to a client who sustained full-thickness burns on the front of both legs and the feet. The client weighs 55 kg. What finding by the nurse indicates the effectiveness of fluid resuscitation?
    1. Mean arterial pressure (MAP) 40 mmHg.
    2. Systolic blood pressure of 82 mmHg.
    3. Urine output 30 mL in the last hour.
    4. Heart rate 130 beats per minute.

16. While assessing a client's skin, the nurse finds a reddened spot on the sacral area that remains red when pressing on it. The skin in this area is warm, swollen, and painful. The nurse plans care knowing this client has which classification of pressure ulcer?
    1. Category/Stage I.
    2. Category/Stage II.
    3. Category/Stage III.
    4. Category/Stage IV.

17. A nurse is planning care for a client with chronic low back pain. What is the priority outcome of care for this client?
    1. The client is able to dress self.
    2. The client will not experience pain.
    3. The client will state three ways to cope with anxiety.
    4. The client's discomfort will not interfere with sleep.

18. A nurse is caring for a client who is experiencing pain following abdominal surgery. The client has a prescription for morphine IV push. What is the nurse's first action when administering the medication?
    1. Explain the procedure to the client.
    2. Identify the client using 2 identifiers.
    3. Flush the IV line.
    4. Clean injection port with alcohol swab.

19. A client has prescription for fentanyl citrate 75 mcg slow IV Bolus on call to surgery. The label on the vial states 100 mcg/2 mL. How much fentanyl (in mL.) does the nurse need to prepare in the syringe, rounding to the nearest tenth mL.?

20. A nurse completed discharge teaching for a client who had back surgery three days ago and is going home with a prescription for naproxen 500 mg twice a day for pain. What statement by the client indicates additional follow-up by the nurse is needed?
    1. "If my pain is not controlled well on this medication, I should call my doctor."
    2. "I am glad my doctor didn't send me home on aspirin, because I'm allergic to it."
    3. "I should take this medication with food."
    4. "I need to stop taking this medication as soon as I can."

21. What should a nurse do to assess the behavioral aspects of a client's pain?
    1. Ask the client to rate pain on a scale of 0 – 10.
    2. Watch the client walk down the hall observing impaired mobility related to pain.
    3. Assess what the client does to relieve the pain.
    4. Determine if the client avoids participating in conversations with visitors.

22. The nurse is caring for a client who is experiencing fatigue from iron-deficiency anemia. The client has an iron supplement ordered. What action does the nurse implement at this time? Select all that apply.
    1. Ask the client to rate fatigue on a scale of 0 – 10.
    2. Teach the client to eat eggs, nuts, and whole-grain rice.
    3. Explain the normal values of hemoglobin and hematocrit.
    4. Teach the client ways to prevent constipation.
    5. Tell the client to report black stools immediately.

23. A nurse is determining a client's pressure ulcer risk using the Braden Scale. What is important for the nurse to assess? Select all that apply.
    1. The client's ability to sense pain or discomfort in the extremities.
    2. If the client has any risk factors for melanoma.
    3. How well the client moves in the bed and chair.
    4. If the client experiences pain while turning onto the side.
    5. The client's 3-day food diary.

24. A nurse is inserting an intermittent catheter in a female client who sustained full and partial thickness burns to the chest and abdomen. In what order would the nurse perform these actions?
    1. Open packet of lubricant and lubricate catheter.
    2. Clean labia and urinary meatus.
    3. Place sterile drape on bed between client's thighs.
    4. Insert catheter into urethral meatus.
    5. Apply sterile gloves.
    6. Perform hand hygiene.

25. The nurse is caring for a client who sustained a spinal cord injury four days ago and now has quadriplegia. What assessments are a priority of the nurse in preventing pressure ulcers? Select all that apply.
    1. Assess the client for constipation and urinary retention.
    2. Visualize and touch the client's skin over the sacrum, ischial tuberosity, hips, and heels.
    3. Auscultate the client's heart and breath sounds.
    4. Assess the client's total protein, albumin, and prealbumin levels.
    5. Monitor the client's blood pressure.

26. A nurse is providing teaching to a client who has contact dermatitis. Which statements made by the client indicate an understanding of the information? Select all that apply.
    1. "Contact dermatitis happens when my skin touches something I am allergic to."
    2. "I should probably wear gloves when I work in my garden."
    3. "Because of my contact dermatitis, I am at an increased risk for having blood transfusion reactions."
    4. "Skin testing may help us figure out what is causing my skin to become red, swollen, and itchy."
    5. "Contact dermatitis is usually caused by a viral or bacterial infection in the skin."

27. A client comes to the emergency department after sustaining burns from a house fire. The client has 27% total body surface area that is affected by the burns. What are the priority nursing actions? Select all that apply.
    1. Immerse the client in cool water.
    2. Remove as much of the client's clothing as possible.
    3. Administer opioid analgesics as prescribed.
    4. Flush the client's eyes with tap water.
    5. Initiate two intravenous lines.
    6. Insert an indwelling urinary catheter.

28. A nurse is assessing an adult client with chronic pain. Which of the nurse's actions or statements could lead to an inaccurate pain assessment? Select all that apply.
    1. The nurse uses the FACES/Oucher® Scale to assess the client's pain.
    2. "Tell me about the onset, duration, and pattern of your pain."
    3. "I'm sure your pain is preventing you from getting a good night's sleep."
    4. "How does your pain interfere with your sexual health?"
    5. The nurse assesses the client's pain systematically.

29. A client was admitted to a post-surgical unit following an abdominal hysterectomy. Based on the orders in the chart below, what care can the nurse delegate to the nursing assistant?

Diagnosis: Total Abdominal Hysterectomy	Allergies: None
Order Date	**Client Orders**
10/17	1. Admit to post-surgical unit 2. Start PCA with morphine; give 5 mg loading dose; PCA dose/interval: 1.5 mg every 15 minutes with 1-hour limit of 10 mg 3. Apply compression stockings to legs bilaterally 4. Clear liquid diet, advance as tolerated 5. Walk 200 – 300 feet in hallway QID Dr. S. Thompson

1. Walk the client down the hallway for the first time.
2. Ask the client if she would like to advance her diet when delivering lunch.
3. Explain to the client why she needs to wear the compression stockings.
4. Notify the nurse if the client has signs of over sedation.

30. A home health nurse is caring for a client who has a prescription for fentanyl citrate patch. Place an x on the client's medical record below on the data that indicates the client is experiencing an adverse effect of the medication that requires follow-up by the nurse.

ID# 467325	DOB: 4/7/1971	Allergies: Latex, Penicillin					
Date	Height (inches)	Weight (Pounds)	Temp	B/P	Pulse	Resp	Pain Level	Last Bowel Movement
1/31	62 in	131	99°F	115/77	75	16	5	1/27
2/7	61 in	125	98.6°F	110/70	64	18	4	2/3
2/14	61.5 in	123	98.4°F	108/62	62	16	3	2/10
2/21	61 in	120	98.6°F	102/60	60	14	1	2/15

1. A client who has Alzheimer's Disease is in an intensive care unit following major abdominal surgery. The nurse is getting ready to transfer the client to a general surgical unit. During handoff report, which assessment data are important for the nurse to provide regarding the client's pain?
   1. The nurse's beliefs on how severe the client's pain is. *The nurse should not guess about the client's pain level.*
   2. The client's most recent vital signs. *Client's with chronic pain may not have any vital sign changes.*
   3. ⚲ A description of the client's facial expressions and changes in mental status.
   4. The nurse cannot provide information about the client's pain because the client has dementia. *Even if the client can't verbalize pain level, there are objective scales the nurse can use to assess pain.*

   Rationale: Clients with dementia experience pain. Nurses use client behaviors, such as facial expressions and changes in mental status, to assess pain, especially if clients are not able to describe their pain. Using the nurse's beliefs leads to an inaccurate pain assessment. Vital signs are not sensitive or specific indicators of pain.

   THIN Thinking: Nursing Process – *An accurate assessment of pain should be factual with subjective and objective observations only.* **NCLEX®:** Basic Care and Comfort **QSEN:** Patient-centered Care

2. The nurse is caring for an older adult client who is experiencing chronic back pain and is receiving an opioid analgesic. The nurse plans care for this client knowing that the client is at a high-risk for experiencing which health concern?
   1. Renal failure. *Opioids generally do not have an effect on kidney function.*
   2. ⚲ Falls.
   3. Liver failure. *Opioids generally do not cause liver failure.*
   4. Alterations in hearing. *Opioids generally do not cause issues with hearing.*

   Rationale: Older adults require special attention when receiving pain medications because they can have increased drug sensitivity and side effects. Opioids most commonly place the elderly at increased risk for falls and other injuries. Liver and renal failure may impair the metabolism and excretion of medications. Opioids can cause visual disturbances but do not cause alterations in hearing.

   THIN Thinking: Identify Risk to Safety – *Risks for safety include age, pain, and medication. The nurse should recognize this and institute safety measures.* **NCLEX®:** Safety and Infection Control **QSEN:** Safety

3. The nurse is planning to teach a 16-year-old client with contact dermatitis. What teaching strategy does the nurse plan to use during the educational session?
   1. Provide education to the client's mother. *A 16-year-old should be able to understand teaching and be involved in self-care.*
   2. Use a formal lecture style when delivering the information. *The nurse needs to determine the clients best learning preference before instituting.*
   3. ⚲ Assess the client's motivation and ability to learn.
   4. Provide printed information written at the high school reading level. *For ease of readability, most educational handouts should be written at a 5th grade level.*

   Rationale: It is important to provide effective health promotion for clients who experience contact dermatitis. Nurses need to assess a client's motivation and ability to learn when planning client education. This information helps the nurse determine if the client is ready to learn. Teaching the client's mother and providing a formal lecture does not encourage the client to engage in learning. Printed information should be written at a fifth-grade reading level and not any higher if possible.

   THIN Thinking: *Nursing* Process – *Assessment of motivation and learning style should be included with the readiness to learn. Once this is determined the focused plan can be put into place.* **NCLEX®:** Health Promotion and Maintenance **QSEN:** Patient-centered Care

4. A nurse is caring for a client who has third-degree burns on the right hand from a kitchen fire. The client is scheduled to go for a skin graft procedure tomorrow. Physical therapy is coming within the hour. The client is sitting in the room with the lights out and is staring out the window. What action does the nurse take first?
   1. Provide client education about the upcoming skin graft and sign the informed consent for surgery. *This does not address client's emotional status, which is a higher priority.*
   2. Assess the status of the dressing on the client's hand. *This does not address client's emotional status which is a higher priority.*
   3. ⚲ Say to the client, "People with burns experience a lot of emotions and frustrations. Tell me what you are feeling right now."
   4. Help the client put on shoes and get ready for the physical therapy visit. *This does not address client's emotional status.*

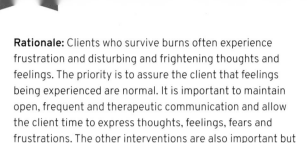

Rationale: Clients who survive burns often experience frustration and disturbing and frightening thoughts and feelings. The priority is to assure the client that feelings being experienced are normal. It is important to maintain open, frequent and therapeutic communication and allow the client time to express thoughts, feelings, fears and frustrations. The other interventions are also important but are not the priority. They can all be performed later.

THIN Thinking: Nursing Process – *The nurse must assess the emotions of a client and adjust the plan of care accordingly.* **NCLEX®:** Psychosocial Integrity **QSEN:** Patient-centered Care

5. **A client with a pressure ulcer is receiving negative-pressure wound therapy. What finding indicates the need for follow-up by the nurse?**
   1. ⦿ The negative-pressure wound therapy unit is hanging on the side of the bed.
   2. The diameter of the wound has not changed since a week ago. *Pressure ulcers heal very slowly.*
   3. There is a small amount of clear, odorless drainage from the wound. *This is an expected finding.*
   4. The client rates pain as a 3 on a 0-10 pain scale. *This may be expected.*

Rationale: When using negative-pressure wound therapy, the unit needs to hang freely from the foot of the bed or sit on a level surface. The other assessment findings in this question are expected and do not require follow-up by the nurse.

THIN Thinking: Help Quick – *Quick identification and intervention of the placement of the wound therapy will prevent problems.* **NCLEX®:** Physiological Adaptation **QSEN:** Safety

6. **The nurse is caring for a client who fell off a ladder and broke his arm. The client is receiving naproxen 500 mg BID orally PRN for pain associated with the injury. What statement made by the client requires immediate follow-up by the nurse?**
   1. "My pain is worse when I move my arm." *This would be expected.*
   2. ⦿ "I had a stomach ulcer last year."
   3. "I need to take the medication around the clock to relieve my pain." *Taking medications round the clock can provide better pain control.*
   4. "I wonder if I can switch to acetaminophen to control my pain when I go home." *This would be a reasonable request but doesn't require immediate attention.*

Rationale: Naproxen is a non-steroidal anti-inflammatory drug (NSAID). Gastrointestinal (GI) bleeding is a common side effect of NSAIDs; the risk increases in clients with a history of peptic ulcer disease. The nurse needs to follow-up and ensure the client also has a prescription for a medication such as a proton pump inhibitor to reduce the risk of GI bleeding. Pain associated with arm movement is expected. Administering pain medications as ordered around the clock, especially in acute pain, helps control the client's pain. Determining if the client can switch pain medications at discharge to acetaminophen will require follow-up but this does not need to be addressed immediately.

THIN Thinking: Identify Risk for Safety – *It is important for the nurse to recognize the side effects of medication and how they may conflict with the client's health history.* **NCLEX®:** Pharmacological Integrity **QSEN:** Safety

7. **The nurse is caring for a young adult who reports fatigue due to chronic insomnia. What instructions does the nurse give first?**
   1. ⦿ Work towards having a consistent time you go to sleep and wake up.
   2. Exercising 1-2 hours before bedtime will help you feel more tired and fall asleep. *Exercise early in the day can help with sleep, but not shortly before bedtime.*
   3. Put a night light in the room to help you get to the bathroom safely during the night. *This does not address problem of insomnia.*
   4. Make sure the room is warm and you cover yourself with a blanket when you go to bed. *People sleep better in a cool environment.*

Rationale: Having a consistent bedtime routine and avoiding exercise in the evening within 2 hours of bedtime promotes sleep. Sleep is enhanced through controlling the environment, which includes ensuring a comfortable temperature and minimizing distractions, such as light and noise. A warm environment is not conducive to sleep.

THIN Thinking: Nursing Process – *Instruction should include common interventions that promote sleep.* **NCLEX®:** Basic Care and Comfort **QSEN:** Patient-centered Care

8. **A nurse is caring for a client who is obese. Which statement made by the client requires further assessment by the nurse?**
   1. "I walk about 15 minutes twice a day; when I get up and right after dinner." *Exercise would be helpful for weight loss.*
   2. "I usually fall asleep within 20 – 30 minutes of laying down." *This is typical and not a cause for alarm.*
   3. "I sleep 6-7 hours every night." *This is common.*
   4. 🔎 "My wife says I wake her up a couple of times from snoring every night."

Rationale: This client is reporting possible signs of sleep apnea. Common signs and symptoms include reports from the client's bed partner of wakening due to the client snoring or not breathing. A risk factor for sleep apnea is obesity. Sleep apnea greatly affects a client's health. Thus, the nurse needs to further assess this client and report findings to the client's health care provider. The other statements made by this client are expected findings.

THIN Thinking: Nursing Process – *The nurse must recognize the assessment findings for sleep disturbance including awakening from snoring.* **NCLEX®:** Reduction of Risk Potential **QSEN:** Patient-centered Care

9. **A charge nurse is making assignments for the nursing staff on a medical-surgical care unit that includes registered nurses and licensed practical/vocational nurses. Which client is it most appropriate to assign to a registered nurse?**
   1. A client who had a total hysterectomy yesterday and is requesting a fan. *This is a routine surgery and so could be assigned to a licensed practical nurse; nothing in the question indicates that the client is unstable.*
   2. 🔎 A client who had a thoracotomy yesterday and is receiving morphine by IV push (IVP).
   3. A client with cholecystitis who is experiencing abdominal pain and is having surgery tomorrow. *- Client has expected abdominal pain and does not require a registered nurse.*
   4. A client with arthritis who had a total knee replacement 2 days ago and is taking hydrocodone for pain. *Client is stable does not require a registered nurse.*

Rationale: All these clients are experiencing or will likely experience pain, which can be managed by registered nurses and licensed practical/vocational nurses. The charge nurse needs to assign clients with the highest complexity to the registered nurse. In this situation, the client with the thoracotomy who is receiving morphine IVP is the most complex.

THIN Thinking: Identify Risk to Safety – *A client who is unstable or requires care outside the licensed practical/ vocational nurse's scope of practice would be the best to assign to the registered nurse.* **NCLEX®:** Management of Care **QSEN:** Teamwork and Collaboration

10. **The nurse is caring for a client who reports falling asleep while stopped at a red light in the car. The nurse suspects the client has obstructive sleep apnea. What assessment finding is consistent with this diagnosis?**
    1. Body mass index (BMI) 25.3 kg/m². *Risk factor when BMI is > 30 kg/m².*
    2. Neck circumference of 16 inches (40.6 cm). *Risk factor when neck circumference is > 17.*
    3. Client states has difficulty falling asleep. *Not a usual problem for clients with sleep apnea.*
    4. 🔎 Client startles during sleep.

Rationale: Clients with obstructive sleep apnea frequently arouse at night due to a generalized startle response. Risk factors for sleep apnea include a BMI greater than 30 kg/m² and a neck circumference greater than 17 inches (43 cm). Difficulty falling asleep is an assessment finding consistent with insomnia.

THIN Thinking: Nursing Process – *The nurse needs to identify the risks and assessment findings for developing sleep apnea so that further testing can be suggested.* **NCLEX®:** Safety and Infection Control **QSEN:** Safety

11. **A nurse is caring for a client who states, "I wake up at night sometimes with a feeling of panic. My heart races, I breathe really hard and fast and I'm usually really sweaty." The nurse plans care knowing this client is probably experiencing which health problem?**
    1. 🔎 Parasomnias.
    2. Narcolepsy. *This disorder is falling asleep while doing activities.*
    3. Insomnia. *This is difficulty falling asleep.*
    4. Obstructive sleep apnea. *This is a physical condition where client has periods of apnea.*

Rationale: This client is experiencing signs and symptoms of parasomnias, which include sudden awakening, signs of panic, tachycardia, increased respirations and diaphoresis. Narcolepsy, insomnia, and sleep apnea are also sleep disorders, but they have different signs and symptoms.

THIN Thinking: Nursing Process – *Understanding the symptoms will help the nurse identify the sleep disturbance.* **NCLEX®:** Health Promotion and Maintenance **QSEN:** Safety

12. A nurse is teaching a client about the use of home bilevel positive airway pressure (BiPAP) due to a diagnosis of obstructive sleep apnea. What nursing action is essential to improve the client's adherence to this therapy?
 1. Tell the client to take diphenhydramine 25 mg by mouth every night to help the client fall asleep at night. *This is unnecessary.*
 2. Suggest the client evaluate surgical options to treat sleep apnea to make an informed decision. *Less invasive treatment measures should be tried first.*
 3. Make sure the mask fits well and makes a tight seal. *Client needs to be involved in decision making to ensure compliance.*
 4. Include the client in the selection of the mask and device before starting the therapy.

Rationale: BiPap is often better tolerated than CPAP (continuous positive airway pressure) in clients with sleep apnea because it delivers a higher inspiration pressure and a lower pressure when the client exhales. Many clients have difficulty adhering to using BiPap daily. To improve adherence, the nurse needs to include the client in selecting the mask and blower device at the beginning of therapy. Clients do not need to take diphenhydramine or consider surgical options when therapy starts. Ensuring the mask fits well promotes effectiveness of BiPap therapy but does not enhance adherence.

THIN Thinking: Nursing Process – *When planning care, it is important to include the client in the decision-making process to improve compliance.* **NCLEX®:** Psychosocial Integrity **QSEN:** Patient-centered Care

13. A male client sustains burns and is brought to the emergency department for care. The client is estimated to weigh 160 pounds. The client is estimated to have 25% of his body burned. Using the Parkland formula, how much lactated ringers should be administered in the first eight hours of his care?

 Answer: 3635 mL.

 Rationale: 160 pounds equals 72.7 kg.

 The Parkland formula dictates that 4 mL lactated ringers X weight in Kg. X % of total body surface area); ½ the first fluids in first 8 hours, ¼ in second 8 hours, ¼ in third 8 hours.

 4 X 72.7 X 25 = 7270; ½ of 7270 = 3635 mL.

 THIN Thinking: Identify Risk to Safety – *The nurse must consistently perform accurate medication calculations for safety.* **NCLEX®:** Pharmacological and Parenteral Therapies **QSEN:** Teamwork and Collaboration

14. The nurse is caring for a client who was in a house fire and has full-thickness burns on the back of both arms and the back of the head. The client's face has superficial burns on the face. The client weighs 60 kg. Using the Rule of Nines and the Parkland formula with 4 mL lactated Ringers IV, how much IV fluid does the client need in the first 24 hours following the burns?
 1. 1620 mL.
 2. 3240 mL.
 3. 4320 mL.
 4. 8640 mL.

Rationale: Using the Rule of Nines, the nurse calculates the total body surface affected (TBSA) by full-thickness burns. The back of the head is 4.5% and the back of both arms is 9%. The nurse does not include the face in this calculation because it has superficial partial-thickness burns. Thus, the TBSA is 13.5%. For a client who weighs 60 kg, the nurse uses the Parkland formula to determine the amount of fluid needed in the first 24 hours:
4 mL x 60 kg x 13.5 (%TBSA burned) = 3240 mL in 24 hours.

THIN Thinking: Identify Risk to Safety – *Safe fluid calculation is critical to the client's recovery.* **NCLEX®:** Physiological Adaptation **QSEN:** Safety

15. The nurse is administering IV fluids to a client who sustained full-thickness burns on the front of both legs and the feet. The client weighs 55 kg. What finding by the nurse indicates the effectiveness of fluid resuscitation?
 1. Mean arterial pressure (MAP) 40 mmHg. *MAP should be >65 mmHg.*
 2. Systolic blood pressure of 82 mmHg. *Systolic should be greater than 90.*
 3. Urine output 30 mL in the last hour.
 4. Heart rate 130 beats per minute. *HR should be <120.*

Rationale: Clients who sustain full-thickness burns require IV fluid resuscitation titrated on the client's response to therapy. Indicators of effective fluid therapy include urine output of 0.5 – 1 mL/kg/hour, MAP greater than 65 mmHg, systolic B/P greater than 90 mmHg, and heart rate less than 120 beats per minute.

THIN Thinking: Top Three – *Identification of adequate perfusion from fluid resuscitation would include sufficient blood pressure, mean arterial pressure, level of consciousness, and urine output.* **NCLEX®:** Pharmacological and Parenteral Therapies **QSEN:** Safety

16. While assessing a client's skin, the nurse finds a reddened spot on the sacral area that remains red when pressing on it. The skin in this area is warm, swollen, and painful. The nurse plans care knowing this client has which classification of pressure ulcer?

1. 💡 Category/Stage I.
2. Category/Stage II. *Stage II involves open area on skin.*
3. Category/Stage III. *Stage III involves skin and fatty tissue.*
4. Category/Stage IV. *Stage IV involves skin, fatty tissue and muscle layers.*

Rationale: Category/Stage I pressure ulcers have nonblanchable redness. They are in a localized area and are usually over a bony prominence. The skin can be discolored, warm, painful, hard, and swollen.

THIN Thinking: Nursing Process – *Assessment of Stage 1 pressure ulcers can prevent further skin breakdown when identified early and implementing an aggressive plan of care.* **NCLEX®:** Reduction of Risk Potential **QSEN:** Patient-centered Care

17. **A nurse is planning care for a client with chronic low back pain. What is the priority outcome of care for this client?**
    1. The client is able to dress self. *Although important, this would not be the priority outcome.*
    2. The client will not experience pain. *This likely is unrealistic.*
    3. The client will state three ways to cope with anxiety. *No evidence client has anxiety.*
    4. 💡 The client's discomfort will not interfere with sleep.

Rationale: Chronic pain often interferes with a client's sleep. If chronic pain is controlled, it should not interfere with sleep. The first and third outcomes address areas which may be affected by pain but as stated, they do not directly address the client's pain. It is unrealistic for this client to never experience pain. Thus, the second outcome is not appropriate.

THIN Thinking: Nursing Process – *The plan of care should be directed in managing the pain so it does not interfere with rest, sleep, and activities of daily living as best as possible.* **NCLEX®:** Basic Care and Comfort **QSEN:** Patient-centered Care

18. **A nurse is caring for a client who is experiencing pain following abdominal surgery. The client has a prescription for morphine IV push. What is the nurse's first action when administering the medication?**
    1. Explain the procedure to the client. *First step is to ID client.*
    2. 💡 Identify the client using 2 identifiers.
    3. Flush the IV line. *First step is to ID client.*
    4. Clean injection port with alcohol swab. *First step is to ID client.*

Rationale: Before administering a medication, it is essential to identify the client using at least 2 identifiers, such as asking the client's name and birthday. Once the nurse identifies the client, the nurse explains the procedure to the client, cleans the injection port with an alcohol swab and flushes the IV line.

THIN Thinking: Identify Risk for Safety – *Proper identification is always a high priority in medication administration.* **NCLEX®:** Safety and Infection Control **QSEN:** Safety

19. **A client has prescription for fentanyl citrate 75 mcg slow IV Bolus on call to surgery. The label on the vial states 100 mcg/2 mL. How much fentanyl (in mL.) does the nurse need to prepare in the syringe, rounding to the nearest tenth mL.?**

Answer: 1.5 mL

Rationale: Use the medication calculation method that works best for you to minimize errors. Using the formula method, the answer is calculated as follows:

Dose ordered x Amount on hand = Amount to administer.

Dose on hand:
$\frac{75 \text{ mcg} \times 2 \text{ mL}}{100 \text{ mcg}} = 0.75 \times 2 \text{ mL} = 1.5 \text{ mL}$

THIN Thinking: Identify Risk to Safety – *The nurse must consistently perform accurate medication calculations for safety.* **NCLEX®:** Pharmacological and Parenteral Therapies **QSEN:** Safety

20. **A nurse completed discharge teaching for a client who had back surgery three days ago and is going home with a prescription for naproxen 500 mg twice a day for pain. What statement by the client indicates additional follow-up by the nurse is needed?**
    1. "If my pain is not controlled well on this medication, I should call my doctor." *This is appropriate.*
    2. 💡 "I am glad my doctor didn't send me home on aspirin, because I'm allergic to it."
    3. "I should take this medication with food." *This is appropriate.*
    4. "I need to stop taking this medication as soon as I can." *The client shouldn't take the medication any longer than necessary.*

Rationale: Clients who have an allergy to aspirin may also be allergic to other NSAIDs. Thus, the nurse needs to follow-up and explore other medications that might be safer for the client to take with the physician. Clients should notify their doctor if their pain is unrelieved. Taking NSAIDs with food helps reduce GI effects. Naproxen should only be taken at the lowest possible dose for the least amount of time.

THIN Thinking: Identify Risk to Safety – *The nurse needs to quickly identify potential allergic reactions with medication to prevent injury.* **NCLEX®:** Safety and Infection Control **QSEN:** Safety

21. **What should a nurse do to assess the behavioral aspects of a client's pain?**
    1. Ask the client to rate pain on a scale of 0 – 10. *This is providing subjective information.*
    2. Watch the client walk down the hall observing impaired mobility related to pain. *This supports objective data collection.*
    3. Assess what the client does to relieve the pain. *-Does not focus on behavioral aspects.*
    4. ⊚ Determine if the client avoids participating in conversations with visitors.

    Rationale: Pain affects many aspects of a client's life. Behavioral aspects of a client's pain include changes in social interaction (e.g., avoiding conversation, reduced attention span), facial expressions (e.g., grimacing wrinkled forehead), and unexpected body movements (e.g., restlessness, muscle tension). The first three options also are important factors to assess but do not focus on the behavioral aspects of the client's pain.

    THIN Thinking: Nursing Process – *Pain assessment can be completed using subjective, objective, and behavioral assessments.* **NCLEX®:** Basic Care and Comfort **QSEN:** Patient-centered Care

22. **The nurse is caring for a client who is experiencing fatigue from iron-deficiency anemia. The client has an iron supplement ordered. What action does the nurse implement at this time? Select all that apply.**
    1. ⊚ Ask the client to rate fatigue on a scale of 0 – 10.
    2. ⊚ Teach the client to eat eggs, nuts, and whole-grain rice.
    3. ⊚ Explain the normal values of hemoglobin and hematocrit.
    4. ⊚ Teach the client ways to prevent constipation.
    5. Tell the client to report black stools immediately. *Black stool would be expected with the intake of iron supplement.*

    Rationale: Ranking fatigue on a scale of 0 – 10 is an assessment measure. Clients who have iron-deficiency anemia need to eat foods that stimulate erythropoiesis such as eggs, nuts, and whole grains. They need to understand lab values related to their anemia. Iron supplements usually cause constipation and black stools. Thus, it is important to teach ways to prevent constipation and to expect a change in the appearance of their stools.

    THIN Thinking: Nursing Process – *Implementations and teaching are important with iron ingestions and fatigue monitoring.* **NCLEX®:** Pharmacology and Parenteral Therapies **QSEN:** Patient-centered Care

23. **A nurse is determining a client's pressure ulcer risk using the Braden Scale. What is important for the nurse to assess? Select all that apply.**
    1. ⊚ The client's ability to sense pain or discomfort in the extremities.
    2. If the client has any risk factors for melanoma. *This not a concern, Braden does not measure melanoma risk.*
    3. ⊚ How well the client moves in the bed and chair.
    4. If the client experiences pain while turning onto the side. *-Although significant, this doesn't affect pressure ulcer risk.*
    5. ⊚ The client's 3-day food diary.

    Rationale: When using the Braden Scale, the nurse assesses the client's sensory perception, nutrition, mobility, and friction and shear. The nurse also assesses the amount of moisture the skin is exposed to. Risk factors for melanoma and pain when turning onto the side are not a part of the Braden Scale.

    THIN Thinking: Nursing Process – *Use of the Braden Scale will determine the client's risk for developing skin breakdown and is a priority assessment for those at risk.* **NCLEX®:** Basic Care and Comfort **QSEN:** Evidence-based Practice

24. **A nurse is inserting an intermittent catheter in a female client who sustained full and partial thickness burns to the chest and abdomen. In what order would the nurse perform these actions?**
    1. Perform hand hygiene.
    2. Apply sterile gloves.
    3. Place sterile drape on bed between client's thighs.
    4. Open packet of lubricant and lubricate catheter.
    5. Clean labia and urinary meatus.
    6. Insert catheter into urethral meatus.

    Rationale: This is the order of the steps involved in the beginning of inserting a straight catheter into a female client. It is important for the nurse to maintain the sterile field as well as the client's privacy during the procedure.

    THIN Thinking: Identify Risk to Safety – *Performing a sterile skill in the correct sequential order will prevent the risk of infection.* **NCLEX®:** Safety and Infection Control **QSEN:** Safety

25. **The nurse is caring for a client who sustained a spinal cord injury four days ago and now has quadriplegia. What assessments are a priority of the nurse in preventing pressure ulcers? Select all that apply.**
    1. Assess the client for constipation and urinary retention. *Although important, these assessments wouldn't affect pressure ulcer risk.*
    2. ⊚ Visualize and touch the client's skin over the sacrum, ischial tuberosity, hips, and heels.
    3. Auscultate the client's heart and breath sounds. *These assessments wouldn't affect pressure ulcer risk.*
    4. ⊚ Assess the client's total protein, albumin, and prealbumin levels.

5. Monitor the client's blood pressure. *This assessment wouldn't affect pressure ulcer risk.*

Rationale: Clients with spinal cord injuries have multiple needs. Assessing the skin by visualizing and touching it, especially over bony prominences, and assessing the client's nutritional status focus on the client's skin. Assessing for elimination alterations, heart and breath sounds, and blood pressure are not part of the focused assessment for a client's risk for pressure ulcers.

THIN Thinking: Nursing Process – *Assessment for pressure ulcers in important for early identification, intervention, and prevention.* **NCLEX®:** Reduction of Risk Potential **QSEN:** Safety

26. **A nurse is providing teaching to a client who has contact dermatitis. Which statements made by the client indicate an understanding of the information? Select all that apply.**
    1. 🔘 "Contact dermatitis happens when my skin touches something I am allergic to."
    2. 🔘 "I should probably wear gloves when I work in my garden."
    3. "Because of my contact dermatitis, I am at an increased risk for having blood transfusion reactions." *This is not true.*
    4. 🔘 "Skin testing may help us figure out what is causing my skin to become red, swollen, and itchy."
    5. "Contact dermatitis is usually caused by a viral or bacterial infection in the skin." *This is not true.*

Rationale: Contact dermatitis is a delayed hypersensitivity reaction that involves the skin. It usually occurs when a client's skin touches an allergen; it is not caused by a bacteria or virus. Common allergens include poison ivy, oak and sumac, so wearing gloves while gardening may prevent the client from getting contact dermatitis. Skin testing can be done to determine the client's allergen. Contact dermatitis does not increase the risk of developing blood transfusion reactions.

THIN Thinking: Nursing Process – *Understanding the risks and causes of contact dermatitis will allow the nurse to perform proper assessment and teaching for prevention.* **NCLEX®:** Safety and Infection Control **QSEN:** Safety

27. **A client comes to the emergency department after sustaining burns from a house fire. The client has 27% total body surface area that is affected by the burns. What are the priority nursing actions? Select all that apply.**
    1. Immerse the client in cool water. *May cause hypothermia.*
    2. 🔘 Remove as much of the client's clothing as possible.
    3. 🔘 Administer opioid analgesics as prescribed.
    4. Flush the client's eyes with tap water. *-Not indicated for thermal burns.*
    5. 🔘 Initiate two intravenous lines.
    6. 🔘 Insert an indwelling urinary catheter.

Rationale: Emergent care of the client with burns occurs during the first 72 hours and focuses on controlling pain and restoring fluid and electrolyte balance. Thus, it is important to establish multiple IVs and give pain medications as prescribed. An indwelling urinary catheter is inserted to evaluate the effectiveness of IV fluid replacement. It is also important in the emergent phase to remove as much of the client's clothing as possible. Do not immerse the client's burns in cool water because it can cause hypothermia. Flushing the eyes with tap water is indicated for chemical burns, not thermal burns.

THIN Thinking: Help Quick – *Quick intervention can prevent worsening of the burns, infection, and hypovolemic shock.* **NCLEX®:** Physiological Adaptation **QSEN:** Safety

28. **A nurse is assessing an adult client with chronic pain. Which of the nurse's actions or statements could lead to an inaccurate pain assessment? Select all that apply.**
    1. 🔘 The nurse uses the FACES/Oucher® Scale to assess the client's pain.
    2. 🔘 "Tell me about the onset, duration, and pattern of your pain."
    3. 🔘 "I'm sure your pain is preventing you from getting a good night's sleep."
    4. "How does your pain interfere with your sexual health?" *Appropriate question for an adult will tell the impact of pain on activities of daily living.*
    5. The nurse assesses the client's pain systematically. *Appropriate way to assess pain.*

Rationale: Sources of inaccurate pain assessment include using an assessment tool that is not supported by research. The FACES/Oucher® Scale has been tested for use with children; it is not tested or recommended to be used with adults. Using medical terms during the assessment that the client cannot understand lead to bias in assessment. Use terms a client can understand instead of using words such as, "onset, duration, and pattern," when assessing pain. Option number 3 shows the nurse is assuming that pain is interfering with the client's sleep. Allowing the nurse's biases and preconceived ideas affect the accuracy of pain assessment. The last two options lead to accurate pain assessment.

THIN Thinking: Nursing Process – *Age appropriate pain assessment is important so that the nurse has a good understanding as to how to best treat the pain.* **NCLEX®:** Basic Care and Comfort **QSEN:** Evidence-based Practice

29. A client was admitted to a post-surgical unit following an abdominal hysterectomy. Based on the orders in the chart below, what care can the nurse delegate to the nursing assistant?

Diagnosis: Total Abdominal Hysterectomy	Allergies: None
Order Date	**Client Orders**
10/17	1. Admit to post-surgical unit 2. Start PCA with morphine; give 5 mg loading dose; PCA dose/interval: 1.5 mg every 15 minutes with 1-hour limit of 10 mg 3. Apply compression stockings to legs bilaterally 4. Clear liquid diet, advance as tolerated 5. Walk 200 – 300 feet in hallway QID Dr. S. Thompson

1. Walk the client down the hallway for the first time. *It is unknown how the client will tolerate ambulating the first time, must be done with a registered nurse.*
2. Ask the client if she would like to advance her diet when delivering lunch. *-This requires a registered nurse's evaluation.*
3. Explain to the client why she needs to wear the compression stockings. *-This requires teaching which the registered nurse should do.*
4. ⊙ Notify the nurse if the client has signs of over sedation.

Rationale: The nurse should ask the nursing assistant to notify the nurse if the client is over sedated. Nurses are responsible for assessing and teaching their clients. The nurse should walk with the client the first time she gets up from surgery. This allows the nurse to assess the client's tolerance to activity and intervene in case the client experiences complications the first time she is up and walking.

THIN Thinking: Help Quick – *Over sedation should be reported to the nurse quickly so the registered nurse can perform an appropriate assessment and interventions.* **NCLEX®:** Safety and Infection Control **QSEN:** Teamwork and Collaboration

30. A home health nurse is caring for a client who has a prescription for fentanyl citrate patch. Place an x on the client's medical record below on the data that indicates the client is experiencing an adverse effect of the medication that requires follow-up by the nurse.

ID# 467325		DOB: 4/7/1971		Allergies: Latex, Penicillin				
Date	**Height (inches)**	**Weight (Pounds)**	**Temp**	**B/P**	**Pulse**	**Resp**	**Pain Level**	**Last Bowel Movement**
1/31	62 in	131	99°F	115/77	75	16	5	1/27
2/7	61 in	125	98.6°F	110/70	64	18	4	2/3
2/14	61.5 in	123	98.4°F	108/62	62	16	3	2/10
2/21	61 in	120	98.6°F	102/60	60	14	1	X

Answer: The X should be on the date of the client's last bowel movement (2/15)

Rationale: Fentanyl is an opioid analgesic. Common side effects of opioid analgesics include constipation, nausea and vomiting, sedation, respiratory depression and pruritis. With continued use, many side effects diminish. However, constipation does not. The frequency of the client's bowel movements has consistently decreased over time. The nurse needs to follow-up with the client's health care provider and provide teaching on ways to reduce constipation.

THIN Thinking: Nursing Process – Assessment of regular bowel movements is important for the client on an opioid analgesic. **NCLEX®:** Pharmacological and Parenteral Therapies **QSEN:** Safety

Adaptation

Stress / Violence / Coping / Addiction

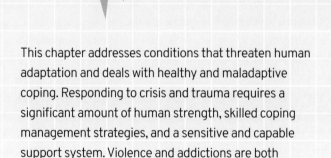

This chapter addresses conditions that threaten human adaptation and deals with healthy and maladaptive coping. Responding to crisis and trauma requires a significant amount of human strength, skilled coping management strategies, and a sensitive and capable support system. Violence and addictions are both stressors and may be perceived as coping mechanisms.

Nurses have a significant role in assisting clients to cope with stressors, recover from trauma, and deal with the ramifications and recovery from addiction. The challenge for the new nurse is that Adaptation-related issues and concerns can arise at anytime. The nurse must be ready to address these concerns by performing Priority Assessments and implementing Priority Interventions. As you care for the clients on the following pages, think about clients you have cared for and where you saw Adaptation-related nursing concerns in actual client care.

Next Gen Clinical Judgment

As you are reviewing these Priority Exemplars, consider how SAFETY plays into each one. Think about the client's threat to safety to self or others. Remember that NCLEX-RN® is an exam about Safety!

Priority Exemplars:

> Eating disorders
> Post-traumatic stress disorder (PTSD)
> Trauma: Abuse, rape, and sexual assault
> Crisis intervention
> Obsessive-compulsive disorder
> Substance abuse

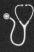
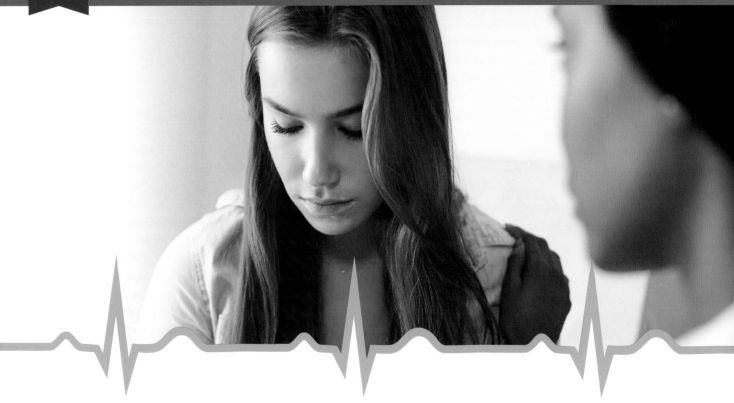

Go To Clinical Case 1

B.C. is a 16-year-old female who enters the emergency department (ED) with her mother. B.C. is pale and looks anxious, with tears in her eyes. Her mother is angry and yells at the triage nurse, stating that her daughter needs to see a doctor immediately. As the triage nurse begins to assess B.C., the mother becomes more agitated and paces the floor. B.C. begins to cry and is unable to answer the triage nurse's questions.

The Charge Nurse escorts the mother to the visitor lounge and tries to console her while the triage nurse calms B.C. and begins the interview. B.C. shared that this is her third visit to the ED in six months. Each time her mother has brought her because B.C. will not eat as much as her mother wants her to and they argue, leading to today's visit to the ED. B.C. says "I am just not hungry, I am fine. I do well in school, I am on the track team, and my grades are good. I just don't need to eat a lot and I need to keep my weight down to do well in track." Each previous ED visit resulted in discharge from the ED and a referral to an eating disorders clinic. B.C. then "talked her mother out of going" and bargained that she would "be better."

Today, B.C. fainted in school during physical education class and the school nurse expressed her concerns to B.C.'s mother. The school nurse noted that B.C. is extremely underweight, appears dehydrated, and that B.C. does not appear to realize the dangers of not eating. B.C.'s mother left work to pick her up and drove immediately to the ED.

B.C.'s initial assessment finds her vital signs: 97.8°F—66-11-88/58. She is 5 feet 3 inches and weighs 97 lbs/44 kg. She is pale and has few tears, her mucous membranes are pale and dry. Her skin is cool and the nurse notes fine lanugo on her shoulders and upper arms. B.C. states she has not had her period in four months which "is fine with me since I run track," and she is chronically constipated. B.C. states she fainted because "I skipped lunch to work on a project."

B.C. is to be admitted to the adolescent unit.

NurseThink® Time

Using the NurseThink® system, complete priorities. Check your answers designated by 💡 in the Eating disorders Priority Exemplar.

✎ Priority Assessments or Cues

1.

2.

3.

⚗ Priority Laboratory Tests/Diagnostics

1.

2.

3.

⚠ Priority Interventions or Actions

1.

2.

3.

⚑ Priority Potential & Actual Complications

1.

2.

3.

℞ Priority Nursing Implications

1.

2.

3.

◌ Priority Medications

1.

2.

3.

👤 Priority Education/Discharge Issues

1.

2.

3.

Eating disorders

Pathophysiology/Description

> Anorexia nervosa
- Fear of obesity with a distortion of body image, preoccupation with food, and refusal to eat
- Perception of being overweight despite being emaciated
- May or may not be accompanied by a loss of appetite
- Reduced food intake/fasting, extensive exercising, and self-induced vomiting/use of laxatives or diuretics
- Increased incidence in western cultures, societal and cultural pressures on appearance and weight
- Primarily in women ages 12-30 years, male rate may be underestimated
- May be restricting (weight loss achieved through not eating and increased exercise) or binge-eating/purging

> Bulimia nervosa
- Episodic, uncontrolled, rapid, and compulsive eating of large quantities of food over a short period of time followed by attempts to rid the body of calories (vomiting, laxatives, diuretics, exercise, fasting)
- Report of lack of control during eating episodes
- Most common in women during late adolescence/early adulthood

> Binge eating disorder
- Recurrent eating of large amounts of food
- Usually eat alone and may feel guilty and depressed after episode
- Does not include purging
- More common in women than men
- May be related to obesity
- May increase risk for type 2 diabetes, hypertension, and cancer
- Most common in adults ages 46-55
- Binge eaters have high rates of impulsivity and are more likely to abuse drugs and alcohol

> Co-morbidities of eating disorders with substance use and mood/anxiety disorders (bulimia with anorexia nervosa; binge eating with depression)

> Conditions associated with physiological, environmental, familial, psychodynamic, and individual characteristics

Priority Assessments or Cues

- Assess vital signs. Client may be bradycardic, hypotensive, and hypothermic. May have marked hypotension with position changes

- Weigh client. With anorexia, may be less than 85% of normal weight, may be normal or fluctuating weight with bulimia, binge eating may lead to substantial weight gain and obesity

- Ask about eating patterns including lack of eating with anorexia, binging with bulimia and binge eating (often sweet, high-calorie, soft foods - rapid eating without chewing)

> Assess purging methods including diuretics, laxatives, exercise, self-induced vomiting, fasting

> Ask about what stops food binges including abdominal distension and discomfort, self-induced vomiting, self-blame/disgust, or other activities

> Physical assessments:
- Assess for lanugo (downy-like body hair) with anorexia, peripheral edema from low serum protein levels
- With self-induced vomiting, assess client for erosion of tooth enamel, calluses on fingers (Russell's sign), history of esophagitis, mouth ulcers, parotid enlargement, dental caries
- Assess hydration status

> History may include menstrual irregularities or amenorrhea, orthostatic hypotension, obsession with food and preparation, compulsive hand-washing

> Assess for depression, anxiety, guilt, self-blame, preoccupation with appearance, boredom, stressors, low self-esteem

> Assess client's perceptions of their body and appearance

> Assess using standardized screening tests including the Eating Disorders Inventory, Body Attitude Test, Eating Attitudes Test, or Diagnostic Survey for Eating Disorders

Priority Laboratory Tests/Diagnostics

- Serum electrolytes (purging, dehydration)
- Obtain ECG for ST segment and T wave changes associated with electrolyte changes
- CBC: Elevated hematocrit (dehydration)
> Urine specific gravity for dehydration
> Serum protein levels

Priority Interventions or Actions

- Hospitalization indicated in cases of
- Malnutrition
- Dehydration with electrolyte disturbances
- Bradycardia and cardiac dysrhythmias, hypotension, hypothermia
- Suicidal ideations

> To address nutritional needs

- If refusing PO, may require nasogastric feedings (may also be required if condition deteriorates)

- If taking PO, work with dietitian to slowly increase calories

- Small, frequent feedings

- Encourage a high fiber diet low in sodium and caffeine

- Focus on weight gained, not food eaten—weigh daily and establish weight gain goals—use behavior modification strategies (privileges and consequences)

- Assess intake and output

- Contract for a set time period for meals and stay with client during and after meals, look for stashed or discarded food

> To address emotional needs

- Explore feelings of inadequacy, coping mechanisms, and fears that lead to eating disorder, family issues/feelings of control or lack of control

- Discuss body image and credibility of distorted perceptions

- Examine areas of personal self-worth other than appearance

- Refer for group, family, or individual therapy

> To address overeating

- Establish a food diary

- Discuss feelings and thoughts related to overeating

- Create an eating and exercise plan that allows for reasonable weight loss

Priority Potential & Actual Complications

- Malnutrition/emaciation
- Electrolyte disturbance/cardiac dysrhythmias
> Heart disease and other consequences of obesity
> Obesity (binge eating)
> Renal failure
- May be fatal

Priority Nursing Implications

- Nurses may be instrumental in building relationship with client, ensuring that manipulative behaviors are limited
- Focus on healthy eating to meet body needs and the consequences of over or under-eating
- Nurses may play a key role in assessing and assisting clients and families to address issues such as control, coping, stress, and healthy communication

Priority Medications

- lorcaserin
  - Appetite suppressant
  - Collaborate with healthcare provider
  - Along with nutritional and exercise plan
- fluoxetine
  - SSRI antidepressant
  - Assist with depression, bulimia (may decrease craving for carbohydrates) and anorexia
  - May take 1-2 weeks to take effect
  - May increase risk of suicide
  - In conjunction with counseling/therapy

Priority Education/Discharge Issues

- Provide client and family with education about the nature of the illness, the management of the illness, and potential support services
- Refer to community organizations for all forms of eating disorders
- Support clients and families as they address the chronic nature of eating disorders and the complexity of the emotional and physical issues

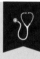

Go To Clinical Answers

Text designated by 💡 are the top answers for the Go To Clinical related to Eating disorders.

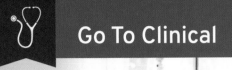
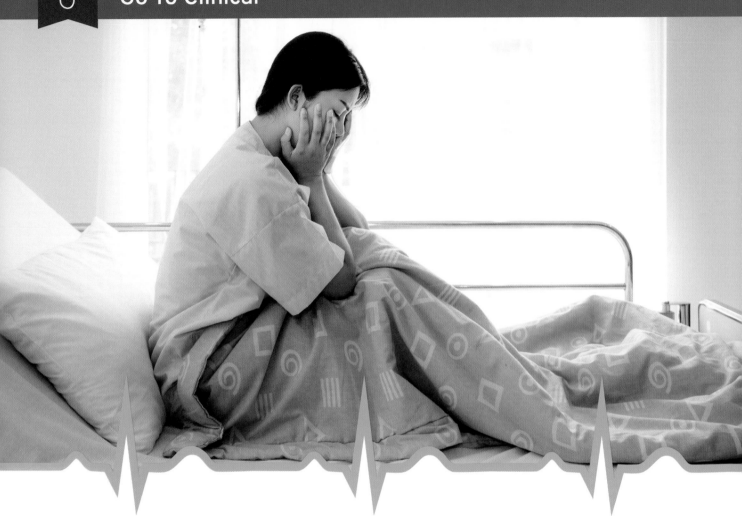

Go To Clinical Case 2

A 26-year-old female veteran is brought to the drop-in clinic of a mental health facility by her spouse. The client, L.N., is visibly upset, shaking, pale, and unable to make eye contact. The nurse asks the client to have a seat and calmly asks some questions. L.N. is restless and stands up and paces during the interview. The spouse explains that L.N. returned home from combat duty four months ago. At first, L.N. was happy to be home and settling into her routine. One month ago, L.N. lost her temper while working at her job as a sales clerk at an appliance store. L.N. walked off the job and came home saying "I hate that place, I never want to go back there."

Her employer was understanding and allowed L.N. to come back but had shared with L.N. that she seemed distracted and unable to "connect" with the customers. The spouse relayed that L.N. has been having trouble sleeping, is very restless, and frequently "zones out" of conversations.

L.N. continues to pace and becomes more agitated. She states "I just can't do it anymore. I am not sure I can ever handle being home. My life has changed forever. I keep thinking about what I saw and did over there. I don't deserve a happy life."

The nurse assesses L.N.'s vital signs: 98.7°F—96-18-124/86. L.N. reports decreased appetite, lack of sleep, and a low level of energy.

L.N. is admitted for evaluation to the short-term unit.

NurseThink® Time

Using the NurseThink® system, complete priorities. Check your answers designated by 💡 in the Post-traumatic stress disorder Priority Exemplar.

✎ Priority Assessments or Cues

1.

2.

3.

🏺 Priority Laboratory Tests/Diagnostics

1.

2.

3.

⚠ Priority Interventions or Actions

1.

2.

3.

🚩 Priority Potential & Actual Complications

1.

2.

3.

☊ Priority Nursing Implications

1.

2.

3.

💧 Priority Medications

1.

2.

3.

👤 Priority Education/Discharge Issues

1.

2.

3.

Post-traumatic stress disorder (PTSD)

Pathophysiology/Description

> Trauma—an extremely stressful and distressing experience that leads to emotional shock and incurs significant and long-lasting psychological effects

> Classified as:

- Post-traumatic stress disorder (stress response to an event outside the usual human experience and of significant magnitude such as rape, war, disasters)
  - Diagnosis with PTSD is based on severity of symptoms, persistence of more than a month, and significant impact on social or occupational functioning
- Acute stress disorder (symptoms are similar to PTSD, but resolution occurs within one month)
- Adjustment disorder (stress reactions from routine daily events, such as failure, rejection, or divorce, disorder usually resolved within six months of stressor)
  - May occur with or without anxiety or depressed mood
  - May occur with or without conduct disturbance

> Based on client history (or family observations), client may exhibit a pattern of difficulty accepting change or ineffective coping skills

> Symptoms may occur immediately post-trauma or may be delayed

> Adjustment disorders, as well as PTSD, may occur across the lifespan

> Emotional reactions may include guilt, anger, aggression

> Individual response to a trauma/disaster: Influenced by the severity and scope of the event and the individual's ego-strength, coping resources, temperament, previous experiences with stress

> Coping may be influenced by individual perception of the event

Complete this MNEMONIC
TRAUMA = PTSD
T _____
R _____
A _____
U _____
M _____
A _____

Table 15-1: Feel free to search the Internet or create your own.

Priority Assessments or Cues

> General

- Use standardized tools to assess levels of depression and anxiety
- Assess client's risk for harm to self or others
- Elicit client history from family and others as needed
- Assess for substance use and abuse

> Post-traumatic stress disorder

- Assess the impact of the trauma on client's abilities for self-care, socialization, work, engagement in activities
- Determine the event causing symptoms, the client's role in the event, and current factors related to the event
- Assess for intrusive memories, dissociative reactions (flashbacks) or dreams/nightmares
- Determine if client experiences high level of anxiety or arousal
- Assess about support systems and other coping mechanisms
- Ask about avoidance behaviors of experiences or stimuli (noises, reminders of event)
- Explore psychotic behaviors, distorted thoughts, and self-blame
- Ask about sleep and sleep disturbances

> Acute stress disorder

- Ask about recurrent memories, distressing dreams, dissociative reactions, and intense reactions
- Assess for depression, dissociative symptoms, and avoidance behaviors
- Assess for hypervigilance or hyperarousal

> Adjustment disorder

- Assess ability to work, engage in social activities
- Assess mood level, tearfulness, feelings of hopelessness, nervousness, worry, and restlessness
- Ask about history of conduct disorders, including truancy, vandalism, reckless driving, fighting

Priority Laboratory Tests/Diagnostics

- Determine serum alcohol levels or drug toxicology screens

Priority Interventions or Actions

- Encourage safety-related behaviors and provide precautions as needed

> Create a non-threatening environment with consistent caregivers

- Ensure a therapeutic, trusting relationship

- Stay with client during flashbacks, nightmares, and intrusive memories
- 💡 Encourage client communication about experiences and emotions at client's pace
- Explore coping mechanisms and support systems, discuss with client the coping mechanisms that were effective before the trauma
- Address client's feelings of guilt or self-blame
- Promote healthy grieving (see Bereavement Priority Exemplar)
- Allow for expression of pent-up anger, guilt, and frustration including physical exercise, walking, work, crafts, routes of expression (artwork, poetry)
- Use role-play to act out stressful situations and potential responses
- Refer client for therapy, including cognitive therapy, prolonged exposure therapy (like flooding or implosion therapy), group and family therapy, self-help groups, crisis intervention, eye movement desensitization and reprocessing (allows client to understand traumatic events as they are explored during rapid eye movement initiated by watching therapist's finger)

🚩 Priority Potential & Actual Complications

- 💡 Suicide or harm of others
- 💡 Debilitating social and/or occupational dysfunction

☋ Priority Nursing Implications

- 💡 Nurses' roles implementing trauma-informed care: *Realize* the increased prevalence of trauma-related incidents, *Recognize* signs/symptoms in clients, families, and others, *Respond* in practice, and avoid *Retraumatization*
- 💡 Current attention is focused on the impact of war and sexual assault on victims and the need for increased awareness and resources in the community. Nurses have a key role in advocating for clients with these experiences as they work through their trauma.
- 💡 Nurses may encounter clients who experienced a variety of traumas in their lives and nurses should employ sensitive and astute assessments to ensure clients receive the help they need to cope with physical, emotional, and sexual traumatic events

💧 Priority Medications

- 💡 paroxetine
  - SSRI
  - Found to be effective with PTSD
  - May take 1-4 weeks to be effective

- 💡 amitriptyline
  - Tri-cyclic antidepressant
  - Effective with PTSD
- 💡 carbamazepine
  - Anticonvulsant
  - Reduces intrusive thoughts and flashbacks
- cannabinoids
  - May be helpful in calming client and controlling symptoms
  - Clients with PTSD have low endogenous cannabinoid levels
- prazosin
  - Antihypertensive
  - Used to manage recurrent nightmares

👤 Priority Education/Discharge Issues

- 💡 Educate family on the nature of the traumatic response, the methods of intervention, and supports
- 💡 Consider community resources to provide support, self-help groups, peer counseling, education, protective respite care, and other resources
- Reinforce past coping mechanisms that have proven effective
- 💡 Provide teaching about relaxation techniques and anxiety-reducing strategies

Go To Clinical Answers

Text designated by 💡 are the top answers for the Go To Clinical related to PTSD.

_____

_____

_____

_____

_____

_____

_____

_____

Trauma: Abuse, rape, and sexual assault

Pathophysiology/Description

> Abuse is the maltreatment of a person by another

> Etiologies of violence/abusive behaviors have biological, psychological, and sociocultural dimensions. Organic brain syndromes, mental health disorders, role modeling of violent behaviors, poverty, and other conditions may predispose an individual to violence perpetration

> May involve intimate partner violence (violence between intimate partners, domestic violence, battering), child abuse and neglect, elder abuse, and sexual violence, including sexual trafficking

> Battering is a pattern of physical, emotional, and sexual violence to exert coercive control over an intimate partner

  • Victims of battering often have a low self-esteem, guilt/self-blaming for the violence, socially isolated, may have experienced violence in childhood, wish to protect children and keep family intact, may be financially dependent, fear retaliation, fear losing custody of children, lack a support network, or ascribe to social/cultural beliefs about marriage, role of women/men, and power

  • Perpetrators of battering are often jealous, maintain two demeanors (outside world, in home as abuser), highly stressed with limited coping, often emotionally degrading and controlling, withhold opportunities, money, and transportation to keep the victim under control

  • Cycle of battering includes tension/building phase, Acute battering incident, Honeymoon phase (calm, apologetic, loving)

> Child abuse is maltreatment that may include physically, emotionally, or sexually violent acts imposed on a child by a caregiver, may result in physical injury and emotional consequences

> Elder abuse is physical, sexual, or emotional violence against elder adults, may include neglect or economic exploitation, older adults may be vulnerable due to illness, dependency, immobility, or altered mental status

> Neglect may be physical (denying physical needs, such as food, shelter, health care, or supervision) or emotional (failure to meet individual's needs for love and support)

> Sexual exploitation is when a child or dependent individual is induced or coerced to engage in sexual conduct to promote a business, performance, or adult's sexual pleasure

> Sexual violence may include rape (use of power and violence over a sexual partner), sexual assault (sexual act in which the individual is coerced or forced), sexual coercion, unwanted sexual contact, acquaintance/date rape, statutory rape (between a person above the age of consent and a person less than the age of consent), marital rape (spousal rape if against the partner's will)

Priority Assessments or Cues

> Assess client's safety

> Assess vital signs and client's physiological level of stability

> Signs of physical abuse

  • Unexplained bruises, marks, black eyes, burns, or broken bones

  • Inconsistent or conflicting recounting of experiences

  • Changes in behavior including aggressiveness, excessive fears, hyperactivity, apathy, withdrawal

  • Marks or bruises at various stages of healing

  • Marked reactions to abuser including fear, withdrawal, or ignoring

  • Caregiver/perpetrator reports conflict with victims, describe victim as bad or deserving, harsh discipline, perpetrators may have history of abuse in their life

> Signs of emotional abuse

  • Emotional lability

  • Emotional developmental delay

  • Lack of attachment to caregiver

  • Suicidal ideations or attempts

  • Caregiver belittles/berates individual, rejects the person

> Signs of neglect

  • Absence from school/work, lack of home involvement in school/work

  • Lack of health care and hygiene, not meeting nutritional and shelter needs

  • Caregiver may be a substance abuser, may be depressed or indifferent

> Signs of sexual abuse

  • Difficulty walking, sitting, or increased reaction to touching by others

  • Reports of regressive behaviors, including bed wetting, and refuses to change in front of others

  • Torn or stained clothes/underwear

  • Unusual sexual knowledge or behaviors

  • May become pregnant, contract an STI, or demonstrate unusual behaviors

  • Perpetrator may be over-protective, isolative, or controlling

> Signs of elder abuse

  • Similar to those above

  • Assess for financial abuse or medication overdose

Priority Laboratory Tests/Diagnostics

> Tests to assess physical status based on abuse and symptoms

> Pregnancy test

> Sexually transmitted infection testing

Priority Interventions or Actions

> Maintain safety of client/victim

> Convey comfort, safety, and acceptance of victim

> Explain all assessments and treatments explicitly

> Photograph all injuries if permitted by the client

> Do not bathe or change clothes until after examination to preserve evidence

> Engage a sexual assault nurse examiner as indicated

> Ensure privacy during history and physical

> Allow client to pace their discussion of the assault

> Ensure client has support and refer, as indicated, to community resources

Priority Potential & Actual Complications

> Violent behaviors may breed additional violence and subsequent generations of abusers

> Serious physical and emotional sequelae from rape, abuse, and assault

> Violence may be extreme causing morbidity and mortality

> Rape trauma syndrome-see PTSD Priority Exemplar

Priority Nursing Implications

> Nurses must focus on the safety of the client/victim

> Current attention is devoted to the need for explicit consent prior to participation in sexual activity. Consent can only be received when an individual is sober, conscious, at age of consent and aware of the circumstance/consequences. Nurses are involved in educating and reinforcing positive relationship skills and about the concept of consent

> Nurses are often a front-line, sensitive intervener with victims. Providing support, caring, and thoughtful communication are critical to gain client's trust and ensure atraumatic care

> State laws differ about an abused victim's ability to report and press charges against a perpetrator. Maltreatment of children (< 18 years) and elders are, in most states, subject to mandatory reporting laws. Victims not covered by these parameters have the choice to disclose abuse. Nurses need to be aware of local and national laws related to abuse

> Play, art, games, and creative therapies may be used to elicit information from children about abuse episodes

> Nurses should be sensitive to ensuring a safe environment when interviewing a client for potential abuse. For example, away from partner/spouse if intimate partner violence is suspected

> Nurses may need to collaborate with law enforcement to obtain evidence (photographs, specimens)

Priority Education/Discharge Issues

> Educate victims about community resources including self-help groups, crisis hotlines, shelters, support groups, the civil/criminal justice system, and counseling services

> Prevention of child abuse may include teaching parents/caregivers about the realistic abilities of children, providing resources and information on healthy parenting, ensuring methods to relieve stress, and encourage seeking services for mental health issues

> Teach that rape is a crime of violence, not of passion. Teach about bystander advocacy and methods to promote stress management, reduction in alcohol and substance abuse, and gender equity to promote primary prevention of rape and sexual abuse.

> Assist families to find alternative residences for older adults who are victims and respite services to reduce stress levels when caregiving

Next Gen Clinical Judgment

Remember a time when you were faced with a significant challenge:

1. What coping mechanisms did you use to adapt to this challenge?

2. What actions or statements by others were especially helpful and not helpful during that time?

3. What assisted you through that difficult time?

4. How can these thoughts and memories inform your actions as a professional nurse?

_____

_____

_____

_____

_____

Crisis intervention

📋 Pathophysiology/Description

- Crisis is a sudden event that impacts the individual and current coping mechanisms prove inadequate to address issues and problem solving
- Hospitalization may be indicated if client expresses potential to harm self or others
- Characteristics
  - All people, at some time, experience a crisis
  - Crises are connected to a precipitating event
  - Crises are interpreted and perceived by the individual (a crisis for one person may not be for another)
  - Crises are, by definition, resolved in a short period of time (1-3 months)
  - Crises provide the opportunity for personal growth or may erode at individual's coping for subsequent problems and crises
- Human responses to crisis include feeling powerless, overwhelmed, and anxious. May perceive coping strategies are inadequate and may become obsessive, solely directed on addressing crisis. May experience physical manifestations of anxiety
- Crisis response is based on individual's perception of the event, availability of supports, and availability of coping strategies
- Phases of crisis
  - Phase 1 Exposure to the stressor
  - Phase 2 Current coping mechanisms fail, anxiety increases
  - Phase 3 Client seeks assistance and/or uses all coping and resources to resolve conflict/crisis
  - Phase 4 If unresolved, leads to psychological distress, panic, and disordered thinking
- Types of crises
  - Dispositional: acute response to an external stressor
  - Anticipated life transitions: lack of coping to normal times of transition
  - Crisis from traumatic stress: response to an external stressor over which the client has no control
  - Maturational/developmental: response to lack of coping with normal developmental stressors
  - Psychiatric emergencies: severe impairments secondary to the stressor. These may include overdose, suicide attempts, anger episodes, or intoxication

✏️ Priority Assessments or Cues

- Assess the client's capacity for harming self or others/ Assess if client has a plan
- Have client share about the precipitating event and describe the event and when it occurred
- Ask client about personal capacity to cope with this and previous crises / determine pre-crisis functioning
- Complete a brief assessment of the client's physical and emotional status / assess for pre-existing psychiatric issues
- Determine previous experiences with this crisis/coping mechanisms employed
- Ask about current coping mechanisms and their effectiveness
- Assess existence and adequacy of support systems
- Assess for use of substances

⚠️ Priority Interventions or Actions

- Management is focused on short-term identification and mobilization of resources
- Focus of management is problem-solving and productive change to restore functioning and achieve personal growth
- Establish a therapeutic relationship based on acceptance and active listening
- Set limits on aggressive, hostile, impulsive, or violent behavior
- Clarify the current crisis/problem, explore causes, and compare nurse's perceptions with the client's
- Discuss feelings of anger, resentment, guilt, or disappointment
- Discuss potential changes and coping mechanisms/ alternative strategies to deal with the crisis. Deliberate the pros and cons of different coping options / assist client to select coping strategies
- Clarify those components of the crisis that cannot be changed and feelings those evoke
- Identify and refer to resources and support systems

🧪 Priority Laboratory Tests/Diagnostics

- Serum blood alcohol levels and drug/toxicology screens

🚩 Priority Potential & Actual Complications

- Unresolved crisis may lead to anxiety, depression, and post-traumatic stress disorder
- May harm self or others

🖑 Priority Nursing Implications

- Nurses may work with peer-support teams including those with personal experience in dealing with crisis
- Crisis intervention skills may be used by nurses to help individuals after a disaster, diagnosis with a life-threatening illness, or any significant life change
- As clients learn to cope with current crisis, nurses may be instrumental in fostering new coping mechanisms and ways to deal with future crises

👤 Priority Education/Discharge Issues

- Ensure that clients and family members are aware of crisis hotlines, crisis centers, and hospital/agency resources focused on crisis intervention

In each of the following scenarios, you are being asked to create 3 PRIORITY assessment questions that you would ask a client who you suspect is in crisis. This is an important skill to have as you prepare for NCLEX® and more importantly, for professional nursing. Being able to perform a quick focused assessment with priority questions is vital in crisis intervention.

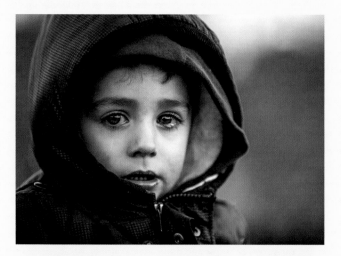

Image 15-1:

Three priority questions you must ask in this situation.

1. _____

_____

2. _____

_____

3. _____

_____

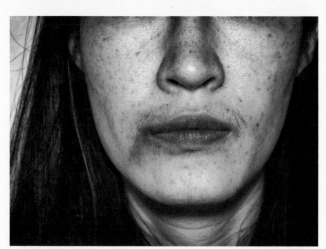

Image 15-2:

Three priority questions you must ask in this situation.

1. _____

_____

2. _____

_____

3. _____

_____

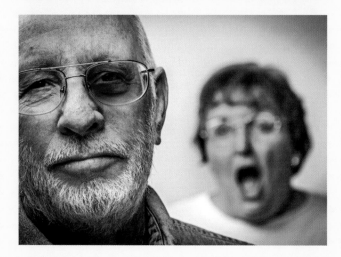

Image 15-3:

Three priority questions you must ask in this situation.

1. _____

_____

2. _____

_____

3. _____

_____

Substance abuse

Pathophysiology/Description

> A complex set of issues and disorders characterized by legal or illegal substance use, addiction, intoxication, and withdrawal

- Addiction is a chronic disease of usage of a substance that stimulates the reward and motivation regions of the brain, leading to pathological seeking of more substance. Characterized by tolerance where greater amounts of substance are needed and may impair social and occupational functioning
- Substance use disorder is when use of a substance impairs social and occupational function
- Intoxication is a state of euphoria, exhilaration, lethargy, or stupor as a result of substance ingestion, may have physical and emotional dimensions
- Withdrawal is physical and emotional readjustment after addictive substances are discontinued abruptly

> The breadth of symptoms depends upon the substance used, amount of substance used, and the duration for usage

> Substance use disorder and addiction have physical, genetic, environmental, and cultural etiological factors

> Alcohol and substances have significant impacts on the body, including the nervous, hepatic, cardiac, and renal systems

Priority Assessments or Cues

> Client's safety status, potential for injury to self and others

> Vital signs during withdrawal include tachycardia, hypertension

> Vital signs with sedative/opioid use/overdose include hypotension, respiratory depression, and poor perfusion

> Assess substance and substance-specific effects
- Alcohol—socially and culturally approved substance, potential for misuse
- Caffeine—readily available and used stimulant
- Cannabis—marijuana
- Opioids—prescription drug misuse
- Sedatives, hypnotics, anxiolytics—benzodiazepine, prescription drug misuse, illegally obtained substances
- Stimulants—cocaine, crack cocaine
- Others—Hallucinogens, inhalants, tobacco

> Standardized tools for substance use
- Clinical Institute Withdrawal Assessment of Alcohol Scale
- Michigan Alcoholism Screening Test
- CAGE (Ever felt you need to Cut down drinking? People Annoyed you by criticizing your drinking? Ever felt Guilty about your drinking? Ever had an Eye-opener in the morning?)(May be modified for other substances)
- Drug Abuse Screening Test (DAST)
- Clinical Opiate Withdrawal Scale (COWS)

> Determine potential for dual diagnosis in all mental health clients

> Determine patterns of usage

> Observe for symptoms of withdrawal including diaphoresis, tremor of eyelids, hands, or tongue, nausea and vomiting, irritability or depressed mood, weakness, anxiety, hallucinations, headache, insomnia, illusions (dependent on substance)

Priority Laboratory Tests/Diagnostics

> Blood alcohol level in which intoxication occurs between 100 to 200 mg/dL

> Breathalyzer for alcohol in most states, 0.08% legal intoxication

> Serum toxicology levels for substances

Priority Interventions or Actions

> Care during withdrawal
- Monitor vital signs and neurological status, re-orient client as needed
- Remove objects from and minimize stimulation in the environment
- Provide one-on-one supervision as appropriate
- Institute seizure precautions, determine the need for restraints, security devices
- Administer medications to control symptoms
- Maintain client hygiene

> Addressing addiction/misuse
- Develop nurse-client relationship
- Convey an attitude of acceptance, discouraging manipulation, rationalization, denial, and projection
- Address misconceptions about substance use with objective facts
- Teach client about the impact of substances on the body
- Encourage group participation
- Use motivational interviewing to allow client to set goals for personal recovery, identify assets of goal attainment, assess personal strength to facilitate change, determine obstacles to change, and develop strategies for goal attainment
- Provide referrals to self-help, crisis intervention, and counseling services

> Provide nutritional support and consult a dietician, limit protein with liver impairment, decrease dietary sodium to prevent fluid overload, provide small, frequent meals of non-irritating food if gastritis or esophagitis exists, thiamine supplements as indicated

> Individual counseling and group therapy

Priority Potential & Actual Complications

- Peripheral neuropathy, alcoholic myopathy, alcoholic cardiomyopathy, esophagitis, gastritis, pancreatitis, alcoholic hepatitis, cirrhosis, leukopenia, thrombocytopenia, sexual dysfunction
- Wernicke's encephalopathy/ Korsakoff's psychosis (thiamine deficiency-confusion, memory loss, lethargy, stupor)
- In pregnant women, fetal alcohol syndrome (craniofacial abnormalities, developmental delays, learning disabilities, organ dysfunction)
- Alcohol withdrawal delirium (see Delirium Priority Exemplar)
- Sedatives/hypnotics/opioids-respiratory depression/cough suppression
- May be fatal
- Stimulants-myocardial infarction, cardiac dysrhythmias

Priority Nursing Implications

- No safe alcohol use has been determined during pregnancy, therefore nurses need to instruct pregnant women to abstain during pregnancy
- During withdrawal from sedatives/opioids-clients may experience rapid eye movement (REM) rebound with insomnia and dreaming
- Nurses should be aware of potential drug diversion in the workplace and chemically-impaired co-workers
- Nurses may assess clients who enter clinical agency for other diagnoses/procedures who demonstrate signs of withdrawal
- With older adults, the use of alcohol, drug interactions, or polypharmacy may impact functional ability, sleep patterns, urinary continence, and cognitive function, including increased risk for falls

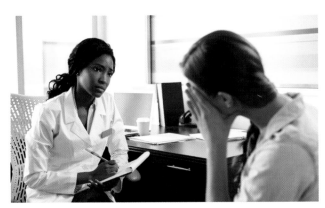

Image 15-4: The urgent care nurse is assessing a client for headaches. What would be some signs or symptoms that would indicate that the client is struggling with substance abuse?

Priority Medications

- naloxone
  - Antagonist to narcotic agents
  - Given nasally
  - May stimulate withdrawal
- disulfiram
  - Alcohol deterrent
  - Generates symptoms if alcohol is ingested
  - Range of symptoms from nausea/vomiting to death based on amount of alcohol ingested and individual sensitivity
  - Should not be started until 12 hours after alcohol abstinence
  - Instruct client about alcohol in selected over-the-counter medications and substances
- naltrexone
  - Opiate antagonist
  - To treat alcohol and heroin addiction
- lorazepam
  - Benzodiazepine-anti-anxiety agent
  - To reduce withdrawal symptoms
  - High doses provided routinely, with bolus doses for breakthrough symptoms
- vitamin supplementation
  - Folic acid, multivitamins, thiamine
  - With long-term alcohol use
- flumazenil
  - Antidote
  - Benzodiazepine overdose
- methadone
  - Prevents withdrawal in clients addicted to opioids
  - Part of a comprehensive cessation program

Priority Education/Discharge Issues

- Teach client alternative coping strategies to using substances: Reading, hobbies, exercise, meditation, music, relaxation techniques, and physical activity
- Ensure that client and family understand the need for abstinence, the impacts of substance use, their role in enabling substance use, management of substance use, and community resources to support recovery (Alcoholics Anonymous, etc.)
- Employ motivational interviewing to enhance client engagement in behavior change

Obsessive-compulsive disorder (OCD)

Pathophysiology/Description

> Characterized as one of the anxiety disorders

> Obsessions are intrusive thoughts that are recurrent and stressful, may be recognized as irrational, but are so powerful and repetitive that cannot be ignored, may try to repress/ignore them, but "giving" into the obsession allows for stress relief

> Compulsions are repetitive and ritualistic behaviors or mental acts that individuals feel driven or forced to perform, are completed in order to reduce the associated anxiety that is generated by obsession, significant dread of a negative event exists if the compulsions cannot be carried out

> Obsessive-compulsive disorder (OCD)includes either obsessions, compulsions, or both and is so significant that is causes social and/or occupational dysfunction and the behaviors take up more than one hour per day

> Engaging in obsessive-compulsive behaviors is stress-relieving for the client

> Common compulsions include handwashing, checking, ordering, praying, counting, and repeating words silently

> Equally common in men and women

> May be associated with hoarding disorder

> Usually begins in adolescence or early adulthood, but may begin earlier

> Usually a chronic illness, may be made more complex by substance use or episodes of depression

> Causes-changes in the anatomy and physiology of the brain, along with changes in brain biochemistry, are associated with OCD

Priority Assessments or Cues

> Assess client's level of anxiety using standardized scales

> Assess client's and family's reports of ritualistic behavior, obsessive thoughts, inability to meet basic needs, inability to meet responsibilities, or levels of anxiety

> Assess level of anxiety when client is unable to engage in OCD behaviors

> Determine client's ability to engage in alternative coping strategies to replace ritualistic behaviors

> Assess risk for suicide

Priority Interventions or Actions

> Establish a trusting environment, reassure client that they are safe and use open-ended questions

> Stay with client when in a panic or highly anxious

> Use brief messages—stay calm and describe agency routines

> Manage hyperventilation—take several breaths in a paper bag, then slow deep abdominal breaths, repeat as needed

> Decrease environmental stimuli

> Use sedation as needed

> Explore sources of anxiety once "attack" has subsided

> Assist client to identify triggers or early onset of anxiety and how to deal with these including deep breathing, imagery, prayer, meditation, or exercise

> For specific OCD behaviors consider use of controlled systematic desensitization (gradual exposure to stimuli) or implosion therapy (flooding with stimuli)

> Explore coping strategies and anxiety-management methods to replace ritualistic behavior

Priority Potential & Actual Complications

> Substance use/abuse as self-medication

> Generalized anxiety disorder

> Major depressive disorder

Priority Nursing Implications

> Times of stress, such as illness or trauma, may cause client to revert to OCD behaviors and require the nurse to assist with coping mechanisms or refer as indicated for a psychiatric consultation or counseling

> Methods to deal with stress that may be explored include progressive muscle relaxation, yoga, exercise, music, meditation, imagery, prayer, or affirmations

Priority Medications

> fluoxetine, paroxetine, sertraline
  - SSRIs
  - May require higher doses than those with depression
  - Side effects: Sleep disturbance, headache, and restlessness

> clomipramine
  - Tricyclic antidepressant
  - Side effects: Orthostatic hypotension, sedation, sexual side effects
  - May lower seizure threshold

Priority Education/Discharge Issues

> Assist client to recognize and avert rising anxiety levels that cause client to resort to OCD behaviors

> Reinforce healthy coping mechanisms to replace ritualistic behavior

> Teach client and family about the nature of the illness, the management of the illness, and community support services/potential for ongoing counseling

1. The nurse is assessing a client being admitted following a suspected incident of intimate partner abuse. What statement by the client requires immediate follow-up by the nurse?
   1. "Will I be safe here if my partner comes to visit?"
   2. "This is really nothing to worry about I will be fine."
   3. "My partner always comes around and apologizes."
   4. "What happens if I decide not to press charges?"

2. The nurse is instructing an unlicensed assistive personnel (UAP) prior to delegating care of a client diagnosed with an obsessive-compulsive disorder. What statement by the UAP indicates that additional teaching is needed?
   1. "I should encourage the client to participate in deciding what order we will organize his daily cares."
   2. "I need to encourage the client to stay on schedule regardless of the repetitive behaviors that are distracting."
   3. "The client does his ritualistic behaviors for a reason, so I need to let him do them as part of his normal day."
   4. "I need to communicate with the client in a calm, matter of fact manner even if I get frustrated with his behavior."

3. The nurse is planning care for a client diagnosed with post-traumatic stress disorder. What is the priority nursing intervention?
   1. Teach the client coping strategies.
   2. Establish a routine to help decrease anxiety.
   3. Administer anti-anxiety medications as prescribed.
   4. Develop a therapeutic nurse-client relationship.

4. The client who has recently experienced a sexual assault states "I am going to be afraid to go out by myself again especially at night." What is the most appropriate response by the nurse?
   1. "You need to resume your normal activities as soon as possible."
   2. "Tell me more about being afraid to go out at night."
   3. "Do you have friends that you can do things with at night?"
   4. "I am sure with time you will be able to go out alone again."

5. The nurse has completed teaching for a client recently diagnosed with anorexia. What statement by the client indicates additional teaching is needed?
   1. "I need to start eating three meals a day even if they are small."
   2. "Weighing myself every day is probably not a good idea."
   3. "If I gain 5 pounds this month my clothes will still fit."
   4. "The prom is coming up and I don't want to be fat again."

6. The nurse is caring for a client brought into the emergency room with suspected opioid intoxication. What assessment findings would the nurse expect to see?
   1. Slurred speech, bradycardia and hypotension.
   2. Muscle spasms, irritability and delusions.
   3. Hypertension, rapid speed, and paranoia.
   4. Sweating, hypersensitivity to noise and nausea.

7. The nurse is caring for a postoperative client with a history of heavy alcohol use. What assessment will the nurse want to add to the plan of care being implemented?
   1. Nutritional assessment.
   2. Musculoskeletal assessment.
   3. Cognitive assessment.
   4. Gastrointestinal assessment.

8. A client with a diagnosis of obsessive-compulsive disorder reports "I have been trying to stop worrying about my rituals but I just feel like I am ready to explode." What assessment would be a priority?
   1. Identify what alternate coping skills the client has tried to decrease the anxiety.
   2. Assess the need to administer a PRN dose of an antianxiety medication.
   3. Assess the potential for any self-harm due to increased anxiety.
   4. Ask the client to tell you more about the rituals that they are trying to avoid.

9. The nurse has delegated the care of a client with an anxiety disorder who has a pattern of needing crisis management to a new graduate nurse. What statement by the new graduate nurse indicates an understanding of the care of this client?
   1. "If the client's anxiety level seems to be increasing, I will check to see what prescriptions are available on the client's chart."
   2. "I need to be alert to the client's potential to act out if approached while experiencing an increase in anxiety."
   3. "When the client gets anxious, I will reassure the client that everything will be okay and there is no need to worry."
   4. "I will encourage the client the client to take some deep breaths and then we can explore some coping strategies."

10. The home care nurse is assessing an elderly client who was recently discharged from a rehabilitation setting. The client states "I wish I could go back to the rehab place, I felt so much safer there." What assessment question by the nurse would be the priority?
    1. "Tell me what made you feel safer at the rehab place."
    2. "Oh my gosh, this is a beautiful home, why don't you feel safe here?"
    3. "Your family seems to be taking good care of you, is this a safe neighborhood?"
    4. "Are you getting your needs met here by your family?"

11. When evaluating assessment data collected regarding an adolescent with a diagnosis of anorexia, what would be the priority for planning care for the client?
    1. Nutritional status.
    2. Coping skills.
    3. Family support.
    4. Risk for injury.

12. The nurse is planning care for a child who may have been abused prior to admission. What is a priority goal for the plan of care?
 1. Identify the potential source of the abuse.
 2. Develop a trusting relationship with the child.
 3. Do not allow the parents to visit the child alone.
 4. Encourage the child to identify coping skills.

13. The nurse is orienting a new nurse who will be caring for a client with a diagnosis of bulimia. What statement by the new nurse would be of immediate concern?
 1. "I certainly can identify with this client because I was bulimic as a teenager."
 2. "It must really be hard for this client to cope with life."
 3. "I don't understand why people do this to themselves, it must be very difficult."
 4. "I will need to be sure that I pay close attention to the client's behavior."

14. The nurse has completed discharge teaching for a client with a diagnosis of obsessive-compulsive disorder and a prescription for fluoxetine. What statement by the client indicates that additional teaching is needed?
 1. "I understand that I cannot drink alcohol while I am taking this medication."
 2. "I can continue to drink caffeinated soft drinks without any problems."
 3. "Carpooling instead of driving myself to school really limits my control."
 4. "To avoid any stomach issues I should take my fluoxetine with meals."

15. The emergency department nurse is admitting a client who reportedly was raped earlier that evening. What assessment would be a priority?
 1. Support systems.
 2. Coping skills.
 3. Physical trauma.
 4. Level of anxiety.

16. The nurse manager has called a meeting of the staff to debrief following a critical incident on the unit. Why is the debriefing an important process for crisis management?
 1. Identify who was responsible for the incident.
 2. Understand the incident to prevent future incidents.
 3. Evaluate staff that were present at the time of the incident.
 4. Teach the staff the correct procedure to avoid future incidents.

17. The clinic nurse noted that the same client has been in repeatedly over a short period of time for a renewal of the opioid prescription for pain. What would be the priority goal when planning care for this client?
 1. Identify alternate strategies to cope with pain.
 2. Recognize that addiction is a concern.
 3. Replace the opioid with another drug.
 4. Seek a second opinion regarding pain levels.

18. The clinic nurse is assessing a 40-year-old client who has come in for a routine physical examination. The nurse notes multiple older bruises on the client's back and legs. What is the nurse's role in reporting these findings?
 1. Mandated to report suspected abuse.
 2. Responsible for documenting observations.
 3. Nothing if the client denies abuse.
 4. Bruises are old and not significant.

19. The home care nurse is visiting an elderly client who lives with his son and family. What observation could be indicative of elder abuse?
 1. Medications are all out of date.
 2. The environment is disorganized.
 3. No one else is at home at the time of the visit.
 4. The client is more confused than last visit.

20. The nurse is assessing a client with a diagnosis of suspected post-traumatic stress disorder. What assessment finding would support this diagnosis?
 1. Able to block feelings about the event.
 2. Actively involved unit activities.
 3. Re-lives the traumatic event.
 4. Able to cope with anxiety.

21. The nurse is providing teaching for a client with a diagnosis of anorexia. What behaviors should the client continue to do at home? Select all that apply.
 1. Weigh daily for the first week.
 2. Continue with prescribed supplements.
 3. Avoid looking in the mirror.
 4. Avoid stress prior to meals.
 5. Eat several small meals each day.

22. What assessment data should be collected prior to planning care of a client with post-traumatic stress disorder? Select all that apply.
 1. Family and social support available.
 2. Level of distress and anxiety.
 3. Sleep patterns.
 4. Social interactions.
 5. Life before the traumatic event.

23. The nurse is caring for a client on the medical unit with a long history of alcohol abuse. While implementing care for the primary diagnosis, what symptoms will the nurse want to be alert to indicating alcohol withdrawal? Select all that apply.
    1. Lethargy.
    2. Tremors.
    3. Change in orientation.
    4. Anorexia.
    5. Irritability.
    6. Restlessness.

24. The nurse is providing teaching for a client who has had a long-term prescription for opioids for chronic pain. The client's dosage has been decreased and the goal is to shift to a non-opioid prescription for pain. What symptoms of potential withdrawal does the nurse want to include in the teaching? Select all that apply.
    1. Tachycardia.
    2. Hypothermia.
    3. Diaphoresis.
    4. Lethargy.
    5. Hypotension.

25. The nurse is implementing a plan of care for a child who was admitted with multiple traumatic injuries that were the result of suspected child abuse. What nursing actions would be included on the plan of care? Select all that apply.
    1. Develop a trusting relationship with the child.
    2. Encourage the parents to spend time with the child.
    3. Reassure the child that everything will be fine.
    4. Listen to the child in a non-judgmental manner.
    5. Focus on the injuries and not the suspected abuse.

26. The nurse is implementing care for a client with a diagnosis of bulimia. Prioritize the nursing actions on the plan of care. Rank order the responses.
    1. Observe the client's eating patterns.
    2. Listen empathetically to the client.
    3. Review dietary plans with the client.
    4. Develop a therapeutic relationship.
    5. Monitor the client's lab values.

27. The nurse is teaching a group of adolescents about the risks of addiction. Which topics would the nurse prioritize topics to include? Select all that apply.
    1. Family history of addiction.
    2. Using a substance to cope with stress.
    3. Experimenting with alcohol or another substance.
    4. Long-term use of a substance for pain.
    5. Experiencing chronic stresses such as socioeconomic factors.

28. The nurse is planning a crisis intervention for a client with acute anxiety. What should be the priority goals for crisis management? Select all that apply.
    1. Administration of prescribed medications.
    2. Identify the root cause of the anxiety.
    3. Safety of the client.
    4. Teach alternate coping strategies.
    5. Strategies to reduce the client anxiety.

29. The nurse is caring for a client in acute alcohol withdrawal. The prescription reads "administer diazepam 10 mg. IV immediately and 5-10 mg. after 4 hours if needed." The available vial is labeled 5 mg/mL. How much will the nurse draw up to administer the initial dose?

    _____

30. The nurse is observing a new nurse prepare the medications for a client diagnosed with obsessive-compulsive disorder. The prescription reads "paroxetine 20 mg PO daily for one week, then increase by 10 mg weekly until reaches 40 mg daily." The client has been on the medication for 10 days, what dose should the nurse be administering?

    _____

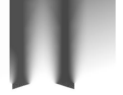

1. The nurse is assessing a client being admitted following a suspected incident of intimate partner abuse. What statement by the client requires immediate follow-up by the nurse?
   1. 💡 "Will I be safe here if my partner comes to visit?"
   2. "This is really nothing to worry about I will be fine." *Statement does not demonstrate immediate safety concern and may indicate reality or denial.*
   3. "My partner always comes around and apologizes." *Statement does not demonstrate immediate safety concern.*
   4. "What happens if I decide not to press charges?" *Statement does not demonstrate immediate safety concern.*

   Rationale: If the client is asking about their safety that should be an immediate concern for everyone. The nurse's role should be to provide a safe environment for the client.

   THIN Thinking: Identify Risk to Safety – *The nurse needs to quickly identify statements that could indicate that the client is afraid or at risk for injury.* **NCLEX**®: Psychosocial Integrity **QSEN:** Safety

2. The nurse is instructing an unlicensed assistive personnel (UAP) prior to delegating care of a client diagnosed with an obsessive-compulsive disorder. What statement by the UAP indicates that additional teaching is needed?
   1. "I should encourage the client to participate in deciding what order we will organize his daily cares." *This allows patient some control.*
   2. 💡 "I need to encourage the client to stay on schedule regardless of the repetitive behaviors that are distracting."
   3. "The client does his ritualistic behaviors for a reason, so I need to let him do them as part of his normal day." *Correct statement and indicates understanding of the disorder.*
   4. "I need to communicate with the client in a calm, matter of fact manner even if I get frustrated with his behavior." *Correct statement, these behaviors may be frustrating.*

   Rationale: Allowing the client to complete ritualistic behavior is a coping mechanism to decrease anxiety. Changing these behaviors is a very slow process. The rituals of obsessive-compulsive behaviors may lead to frustration experienced by the caregiver because it disrupts schedules.

   THIN Thinking: Top 3 – *The goal of care is to allow the client to continue their ritualistic behavior to prevent anxiety.* **NCLEX**®: Psychosocial Integrity **QSEN:** Patient-centered Care

3. The nurse is planning care for a client diagnosed with post-traumatic stress disorder. What is the priority nursing intervention?
   1. Teach the client coping strategies. *This would occur after developing a relationship and after the acute phase.*
   2. Establish a routine to help decrease anxiety. *This would occur after developing a relationship and may occur because of a therapeutic relationship.*
   3. Administer anti-anxiety medications as prescribed. *The priority would be to develop a therapeutic relationship.*
   4. 💡 Develop a therapeutic nurse-client relationship.

   Rationale: The primary consideration when caring for a client with post-traumatic stress disorder is to develop a therapeutic relationship. Once the nurse has developed the trusting relationship then the client will be more accepting of other nursing actions.

   THIN Thinking: Top 3 – *the first step in creating a relationship is to develop a therapeutic nurse-client relationship.* **NCLEX**®: Psychosocial Integrity **QSEN:** Evidence-based Practice

4. The client who has recently experienced a sexual assault states "I am going to be afraid to go out by myself again especially at night." What is the most appropriate response by the nurse?
   1. "You need to resume your normal activities as soon as possible." *This response does not demonstrate compassion or understanding.*
   2. 💡 "Tell me more about being afraid to go out at night."
   3. "Do you have friends that you can do things with at night?" *This statement does not allow client to explain her fears.*
   4. "I am sure with time you will be able to go out alone again." *False reassurance.*

   Rationale: The priority is to encourage the client to talk about their concerns in order to work through their fears. Providing unconditional acceptance of the client as a person to help them realize there are still valued.

   THIN Thinking: Nursing Process – *the nurse needs to further assess and get additional clarification when hearing a statement of safety concern.* **NCLEX**®: Psychosocial Integrity **QSEN:** Patient-centered Care

5. The nurse has completed teaching for a client recently diagnosed with anorexia. What statement by the client indicates additional teaching is needed?
   1. "I need to start eating three meals a day even if they are small." *Accurate response and demonstrates understanding the need for food.*
   2. "Weighing myself every day is probably not a good idea." *Accurate response and demonstrates that one can't obsess about weight.*
   3. "If I gain 5 pounds this month my clothes will still fit." *Accurate response and demonstrates acceptance of modest gains in weight.*
   4. 💡 "The prom is coming up and I don't want to be fat again."

Rationale: The client's perceived body image is a concern that the nurse needs to help the client deal with to recover from any eating disorder. The client needs to eat three meals per day and not weighing daily may help decrease anxiety associated with any weight gain.

THIN Thinking: Top Three – *Recognition of statements that will derail treatment plans is important.* **NCLEX®:** Psychosocial Integrity **QSEN:** Patient-centered Care

6. **The nurse is caring for a client brought into the emergency room with suspected opioid intoxication. What assessment findings would the nurse expect to see?**
   1. 🔹 Slurred speech, bradycardia and hypotension.
   2. Muscle spasms, irritability and delusions. *These are signs and symptoms of withdrawal.*
   3. Hypertension, rapid speed, and paranoia. *These are signs and symptoms of withdrawal.*
   4. Sweating, hypersensitivity to noise and nausea. *These are signs and symptoms of withdrawal.*

Rationale: Signs and symptoms of opioid intoxication include slurred speech, bradycardia, hypotension, hypothermia, sedation, pinpoint pupils, and calmness. Opioid withdrawal is also characterized by tachycardia, hypertension, hyperthermia, insomnia, muscle spasms, and runny nose.

THIN Thinking: Nursing Process – *Assessment of the signs of intoxication differ from the assessment findings of withdrawal.* **NCLEX®:** Pharmacological and Parenteral Therapies **QSEN:** Safety

7. **The nurse is caring for a postoperative client with a history of heavy alcohol use. What assessment will the nurse want to add to the plan of care being implemented?**
   1. Nutritional assessment. *This is part of routine post-op assessment, not specific to this client.*
   2. 🔹 Musculoskeletal assessment.
   3. Cognitive assessment. *This is part of routine post-op assessment, not specific to this client.*
   4. Gastrointestinal assessment. *This is part of routine post-op assessment, not specific to this client.*

Rationale: The early signs of alcohol withdrawal include tremors and restlessness. Most postoperative plans of care would include assessing levels of consciousness due to the anesthesia, gastrointestinal and nutritional assessments would also be included in routine postoperative assessments.

THIN Thinking: Identify Risk to Safety – *Alcohol withdrawal is dangerous and the nurse should identify risk factors and intervene appropriately.* **NCLEX®:** Basic Care and Comfort **QSEN:** Safety

8. **A client with a diagnosis of obsessive-compulsive disorder reports "I have been trying to stop worrying about my rituals but I just feel like I am ready to explode." What assessment would be a priority?**
   1. Identify what alternate coping skills the client has tried to decrease the anxiety. *Important, but the priority is to determine safety risk.*
   2. Assess the need to administer a PRN dose of an antianxiety medication. *The priority is to determine safety risk.*
   3. 🔹 Assess the potential for any self-harm due to increased anxiety.
   4. Ask the client to tell you more about the rituals that they are trying to avoid. *Important, but does not give the nurse more information regarding client's immediate safety risk.*

Rationale: The priority is to assess for the potential for self-harm or suicide as a means of decreasing anxiety. Once the client's safety is assessed, then the nurse could move on to exploring alternate coping skills or the possible need to administer an antianxiety prescription.

THIN Thinking: Identify Risk to Safety – *The nurse should prioritize statements that show escalation of anxiety.* **NCLEX®:** Reduction of Risk Potential **QSEN:** Safety

9. **The nurse has delegated the care of a client with an anxiety disorder who has a pattern of needing crisis management to a new graduate nurse. What statement by the new graduate nurse indicates an understanding of the care of this client?**
   1. "If the client's anxiety level seems to be increasing, I will check to see what prescriptions are available on the client's chart." *A non-pharmacological option should be tried first.*
   2. "I need to be alert to the client's potential to act out if approached while experiencing an increase in anxiety." *This statement is false.*
   3. "When the client gets anxious, I will reassure the client that everything will be okay and there is no need to worry." *False reassurance is not helpful in reducing anxiety.*
   4. 🔹 "I will encourage the client the client to take some deep breaths and then we can explore some coping strategies."

Rationale: Providing support and instructing the client regarding some immediate coping strategies such as deep breathing would be the first steps in crisis management. Once the client begins to regain control it is time to start exploring coping skills that could be used for anxiety reduction. Typically clients who are anxious are at risk of self-harm not striking out at others.

THIN Thinking: Top Three – *When prioritizing care for someone with anxiety disorder the nurse should focus care on identification of early symptoms and initiating relaxation techniques.* **NCLEX®:** Psychosocial Integrity **QSEN:** Patient-centered Care

10. The home care nurse is assessing an elderly client who was recently discharged from a rehabilitation setting. The client states "I wish I could go back to the rehab place, I felt so much safer there." What assessment question by the nurse would be the priority?
    1. 💡 "Tell me what made you feel safer at the rehab place."
    2. "Oh my gosh, this is a beautiful home, why don't you feel safe here?" *This question would make a client feel defensive.*
    3. "Your family seems to be taking good care of you, is this a safe neighborhood?" *This is the nurse's opinion.*
    4. "Are you getting your needs met here by your family?" *This question does not address client's concern of being less safe than when at the rehab center.*

    Rationale: It is important for the nurse to remain non-judgmental and collect more information. Allowing the client to tell his/her story does not influence the client's perceptions and/or place any blame on caretakers.

    THIN Thinking: Identify Risk to Safety – *Subtle signs and statements can cue to concern. The nurse needs to seek clarification from the client and not jump to conclusions.* **NCLEX®**: Safety and Infection Control **QSEN:** Safety

11. When evaluating assessment data collected regarding an adolescent with a diagnosis of anorexia, what would be the priority for planning care for the client?
    1. Nutritional status. *Although important, this is less important than determining potential self-injury risk.*
    2. Coping skills. *Although important, this is less important than determining potential self-injury risk.*
    3. Family support. *Although important, this is less important than determining potential self-injury risk.*
    4. 💡 Risk for injury.

    Rationale: Clients with anorexia frequently have self-esteem issues and limited coping skills. Therefore, assess the risk for self-injury or suicide is the highest priority. Nutritional status and the potential for electrolyte imbalances would be the next priority area needing to be addressed.

    THIN Thinking: Identify Risk to Safety – *Safety is the priority when caring for someone with anorexia.* **NCLEX®**: Health Promotion and Maintenance **QSEN:** Safety

12. The nurse is planning care for a child who may have been abused prior to admission. What is a priority goal for the plan of care?
    1. Identify the potential source of the abuse. *The nurse would need to develop a trusting relationship before asking questions about the potential abuse.*
    2. 💡 Develop a trusting relationship with the child.
    3. Do not allow the parents to visit the child alone. *At this point, the abuse is not validated and the abuser is unknown.*
    4. Encourage the child to identify coping skills. *This would be something to work on after the nurse/child have developed a trusting relationship.*

    Rationale: The nurse needs to develop a trusting relationship with the child before trying to explore the situation or alternatives. Children who have experienced abuse tend to be suspicious of adults.

    THIN Thinking: Top Three – *A child of abuse is often untrusting of adults. The nurse needs to develop trust in order form a relationship.* **NCLEX®**: Psychosocial Integrity **QSEN:** Evidence-based Practice

13. The nurse is orienting a new nurse who will be caring for a client with a diagnosis of bulimia. What statement by the new nurse would be of immediate concern?
    1. 💡 "I certainly can identify with this client because I was bulimic as a teenager."
    2. "It must really be hard for this client to cope with life." *Appropriate statement.*
    3. "I don't understand why people do this to themselves, it must be very difficult." *This statement would be concerning and require follow-up, but does not need to be addressed immediately.*
    4. "I will need to be sure that I pay close attention to the client's behavior." *Appropriate statement.*

    Rationale: It is important to develop a therapeutic relationship that includes being empathetic and open to understanding the client's perceptions. Identification with the client can be problematic because it could move the focus to the nurse and away from the client's unique experiences.

    THIN Thinking: Help Quick – *The nurse should recognize that with a history of the illness, the new nurse may focus the care on personal experiences which is not therapeutic for the client.* **NCLEX®**: Psychosocial Integrity **QSEN:** Patient-centered Care

14. **The nurse has completed discharge teaching for a client with a diagnosis of obsessive-compulsive disorder and a prescription for fluoxetine. What statement by the client indicates that additional teaching is needed?**
    1. "I understand that I cannot drink alcohol while I am taking this medication." *Accurate statement.*
    2. 🔘 "I can continue to drink caffeinated soft drinks without any problems."
    3. "Carpooling instead of driving myself to school really limits my control." *Statement is not of concern.*
    4. "To avoid any stomach issues I should take my fluoxetine with meals." *Accurate statement.*

    Rationale: While taking prescribed antianxiety medications the client not only needs to avoid alcohol but also caffeinated beverages. Most clients can drive while taking fluoxetine. Taking the medication with meals or a snack can decrease any GI discomfort.

    THIN Thinking: Top Three – *Understanding that alcohol and caffeine should be avoided is a teaching priority.* **NCLEX®:** Pharmacological and Parenteral Therapies **QSEN:** Evidence-based Practice

15. **The emergency department nurse is admitting a client who reportedly was raped earlier that evening. What assessment would be a priority?**
    1. Support systems. *Important, but not the immediate priority.*
    2. Coping skills. *Important, but not the immediate priority.*
    3. 🔘 Physical trauma.
    4. Level of anxiety. *Important, but not the immediate priority.*

    Rationale: Assessing the client's physical status is the initial priority to determine what immediate care is needed. Assessing the client's support systems, coping skills and level of anxiety will be important for care planning.

    THIN Thinking: Top Three – *Prioritization is to meet physical needs first.* **NCLEX®:** Basic Care and Comfort **QSEN:** Patient-centered Care

16. **The nurse manager has called a meeting of the staff to debrief following a critical incident on the unit. Why is the debriefing an important process for crisis management?**
    1. Identify who was responsible for the incident. *The goal of debriefing is to identify the cause of incident to prevent future incidents.*
    2. 🔘 Understand the incident to prevent future incidents.
    3. Evaluate staff that were present at the time of the incident. *The goal of debriefing is to identify the cause of incident to prevent future incidents.*
    4. Teach the staff the correct procedure to avoid future incidents. *The goal of debriefing is to identify the cause of incident to prevent future incidents.*

    Rationale: A critical incident on a health care unit is a crisis that needs to be addressed and managed. The goal of debriefing is to identify the root cause of the incident to prevent future incidents. The goal is not to place blame or accuse anyone.

    THIN Thinking: Identify Risk to Safety – *The first step for debriefing for crisis management is to fully understand the incident in order to prevent future incidents.* **NCLEX®:** Reduction of Risk Potential **QSEN:** Safety

17. **The clinic nurse noted that the same client has been in repeatedly over a short period of time for a renewal of the opioid prescription for pain. What would be the priority goal when planning care for this client?**
    1. 🔘 Identify alternate strategies to cope with pain.
    2. Recognize that addiction is a concern. *This option doesn't address client's pain issues.*
    3. Replace the opioid with another drug. *This option doesn't provide client with options in managing pain.*
    4. Seek a second opinion regarding pain levels. *No indication that this would be necessary.*

    Rationale: Encouraging the client to look for alternate strategies to cope with pain and/or discomfort could decrease the client's psychological dependency on the opioid medications. Initial client teaching should have included the potential for addiction but may not be heard by the client. Replacing the opioid with another drug does not address the concern but rather transfers it to something else.

    THIN Thinking: Top Three – *Understanding the opioids can lead to addiction, it is important for the nurse to help establish and practice alternative strategies for pain management.* **NCLEX®:** Management of Care **QSEN:** Patient-centered Care

18. **The clinic nurse is assessing a 40-year-old client who has come in for a routine physical examination. The nurse notes multiple older bruises on the client's back and legs. What is the nurse's role in reporting these findings?**
    1. Mandated to report suspected abuse. *Client is not a child or vulnerable adult, so reporting is not mandated.*
    2. 🔘 Responsible for documenting observations.
    3. Nothing if the client denies abuse. *Skin assessment should still be documented.*
    4. Bruises are old and not significant. *Bruises still need to be documented. They could be indicative of abuse, or of a bleeding issue.*

    Rationale: The nurse is responsible for documenting assessment findings even if the client denies abuse. The nurse is legally mandated to report suspected or actual cases of child and vulnerable adult abuse.

THIN Thinking: Nursing Process – *Further assessment could include asking where the bruising came from but the priority is documentation.* **NCLEX®:** Safety and Infection Control **QSEN:** Safety

19. **The home care nurse is visiting an elderly client who lives with his son and family. What observation could be indicative of elder abuse?**
    1. 🔘 Medications are all out of date.
    2. The environment is disorganized. *Disorganization is a subjective observation and does not indicate that the client is being abused.*
    3. No one else is at home at the time of the visit. *The client may be safe alone for periods of time.*
    4. The client is more confused than last visit. *Increased confusion may be due to natural cognitive decline or a physiological issue like an infection.*

    Rationale: Factors that could be assessed during a home visit that might indicate elder abuse include medications mismanaged, poor hygiene, lack of assistive devices and unsafe housing.

    THIN Thinking: Top Three – *Abuse includes medication mismanagement that could lead to injury, such as with outdated medications.* **NCLEX®:** Health Promotion and Maintenance **QSEN:** Safety

20. **The nurse is assessing a client with a diagnosis of suspected post-traumatic stress disorder. What assessment finding would support this diagnosis?**
    1. Able to block feelings about the event. *Incorrect, clients are unable to block or control feelings related to the event.*
    2. Actively involved unit activities. *Incorrect, clients may withdraw.*
    3. 🔘 Re-lives the traumatic event.
    4. Able to cope with anxiety. *Incorrect, clients may be unable to deal with anxiety.*

    Rationale: Post-traumatic stress disorder (PTSD) is characterized by persistent re-experiencing the traumatic event.

    THIN Thinking: Nursing Process – *The nurse should understand the assessments related to PTSD when caring for the client.* **NCLEX®:** Psychosocial Integrity **QSEN:** Evidence-based Practice

21. **The nurse is providing teaching for a client with a diagnosis of anorexia. What behaviors should the client continue to do at home? Select all that apply.**
    1. 🔘 Weigh daily for the first week.
    2. 🔘 Continue with prescribed supplements.
    3. Avoid looking in the mirror. *This would be an unrealistic expectation.*
    4. 🔘 Avoid stress prior to meals.
    5. 🔘 Eat several small meals each day.

    Rationale: The client with anorexia needs to develop a pattern of eating small meals on a frequent basis. Weight gain of about 2 pounds per week is the goal and weighing self daily for the first week demonstrates that there is not a huge weight gain by eating regularly. Stress around meals may re-introduce past behaviors. Prescribed food or fluid supplements help to prevent electrolyte imbalances.

    THIN Thinking: Nursing Process – *The nurse should plan appropriate interventions upon discharge for the client with anorexia.* **NCLEX®:** Physiological Adaptation **QSEN:** Evidence-based Practice

22. **What assessment data should be collected prior to planning care of a client with post-traumatic stress disorder? Select all that apply.**
    1. 🔘 Family and social support available.
    2. 🔘 Level of distress and anxiety.
    3. 🔘 Sleep patterns.
    4. 🔘 Social interactions.
    5. Life before the traumatic event. *This data would not be necessary to plan care for this client.*

    Rationale: Assessment should include the client's level of distress and/or anxiety and how they cope with it. Identifying social and/or family support available can provide data for care planning. Sleep disturbances are frequently related to PTSD as well as social isolation so these factors need to be assessed.

    THIN Thinking: Nursing Process – *The nurse should identify the appropriate assessments for someone with PTSD.* **NCLEX®:** Safety and Infection Control **QSEN:** Safety

23. The nurse is caring for a client on the medical unit with a long history of alcohol abuse. While implementing care for the primary diagnosis, what symptoms will the nurse want to be alert to indicating alcohol withdrawal? Select all that apply.
    1. Lethargy. *This is not a sign of alcohol withdrawal.*
    2. 💡 Tremors.
    3. 💡 Change in orientation.
    4. 💡 Anorexia.
    5. 💡 Irritability.
    6. 💡 Restlessness.

    Rationale: Even though the client is admitted for an unrelated diagnosis, the nurse needs to be alert for possible withdrawal based on the client's history. In addition, uncomplicated mild to moderate alcohol withdrawal symptoms include restlessness, irritability, anorexia, tremors, insomnia, impaired cognitive functions and mild perceptual changes.

    THIN Thinking: Nursing Process – *The nurse should be able to recognize the signs of alcohol withdrawal.* **NCLEX®**: *Psychosocial Integrity* **QSEN**: Patient-centered Care

24. The nurse is providing teaching for a client who has had a long-term prescription for opioids for chronic pain. The client's dosage has been decreased and the goal is to shift to a non-opioid prescription for pain. What symptoms of potential withdrawal does the nurse want to include in the teaching? Select all that apply.
    1. 💡 Tachycardia.
    2. Hypothermia. *This is not a sign of withdrawal.*
    3. 💡 Diaphoresis.
    4. Lethargy. *This is not a sign of withdrawal.*
    5. Hypotension. *This is not a sign of withdrawal.*

    Rationale: Clients need to be taught the potential symptoms of opioid withdrawal as a means of health promotion and risk prevention. Symptoms of opioid withdrawal include tachycardia, diaphoresis, hyperthermia, insomnia, hypertension, piloerection, rhinorrhea, muscle spasms, abdominal cramps, bone and muscle pain and anxiety.

    THIN Thinking: Nursing Process – *The nurse needs to recognize the assessment changes that occur in withdrawal.* **NCLEX®**: Reduction of Risk Potential **QSEN**: Patient-centered Care

25. The nurse is implementing a plan of care for a child who was admitted with multiple traumatic injuries that were the result of suspected child abuse. What nursing actions would be included on the plan of care? Select all that apply.
    1. 💡 Develop a trusting relationship with the child.
    2. Encourage the parents to spend time with the child. *If parents are suspected abusers, time with child should be supervised.*
    3. Reassure the child that everything will be fine. *False reassurance.*
    4. 💡 Listen to the child in a non-judgmental manner.
    5. Focus on the injuries and not the suspected abuse. *This measure will not help protect child from further abuse.*

    Rationale: Children that have been potentially abused tend to be suspicious of other adults. Therefore, developing a trusting relationship is the first step in helping the child feel safe in their environment. Listening to the child empathetically and without judgment may allow the child to tell their story. If the parent is the suspected abuser, their time with the child should be limited and supervised. Do not provide unrealistic reassurances or false hope.

    THIN Thinking: Top Three – *The nurse needs to first develop a trusting relationship with a child while preventing them from danger or anxiety.* **NCLEX®**: Safety and Infection Control **QSEN**: Patient-centered Care

26. The nurse is implementing care for a client with a diagnosis of bulimia. Prioritize the nursing actions on the plan of care. Rank order the responses.
    1. Develop a therapeutic relationship.
    2. Monitor the client's lab values.
    3. Listen empathetically to the client.
    4. Review dietary plans with the client.
    5. Observe the client's eating patterns.

    Rationale: Developing a therapeutic relationship is the foundation of any care for a client diagnosed with bulimia. Monitoring the client's lab values is a safety concern with bulimia and therefore a high priority. Listening to the client to understand their perspective and experience needs to be a precursor to client teaching such as reviewing the dietary plans and finally observing eating patterns is a strategy to evaluate the plan of care.

    THIN Thinking: Top Three – *Determine the priority of care is important to the best outcomes.* **NCLEX®**: Physiological Adaptation **QSEN**: Patient-centered Care

27. **The nurse is teaching a group of adolescents about the risks of addiction. Which topics would the nurse prioritize topics to include? Select all that apply.**
    1. 🔍 Family history of addiction.
    2. 🔍 Using a substance to cope with stress.
    3. 🔍 Experimenting with alcohol or another substance.
    4. 🔍 Long-term use of a substance for pain.
    5. 🔍 Experiencing chronic stresses such as socioeconomic factors.

    Rationale: Multiple factors can lead to the risk of addiction. An uncontrollable risk factor is family history or genetics. Using a substance to cope with stress or pain for an ongoing period of time can increase the risk of addiction.

    THIN Thinking: Nursing Process – *The nurse needs to recognize factors that lead to addiction.* **NCLEX**®: Basic Care and Comfort **QSEN**: Evidence-based Practice

28. **The nurse is planning a crisis intervention for a client with acute anxiety. What should be the priority goals for crisis management? Select all that apply.**
    1. 🔍 Administration of prescribed medications.
    2. Identify the root cause of the anxiety. *This would not be a priority when the client is in crisis.*
    3. 🔍 Safety of the client.
    4. Teach alternate coping strategies. *This would not be a priority when the client is in crisis.*
    5. 🔍 Strategies to reduce the client anxiety.

    Rationale: The focus of crisis intervention is on the present problem and should focus on client safety, the prescribed treatment, and reduction of anxiety. When the client's anxiety level is at crisis level is not the time for teaching or seeking to identify the root cause.

    THIN Thinking Top Three – *The nurse needs to recognize the priorities of care for crisis management.* **NCLEX**®: Psychosocial Integrity **QSEN**: Evidence-based Practice

29. **The nurse is caring for a client in acute alcohol withdrawal. The prescription reads "administer diazepam 10 mg. IV immediately and 5-10 mg. after 4 hours if needed." The available vial is labeled 5 mg/mL. How much will the nurse draw up to administer the initial dose? Fill in the blank.**

    Answer: 2 mL

    Rationale: If there are 5 mg/mL then 10 mg would be double that amount = 2 mL. For acute alcohol withdrawal the recommended prescription for diazepam is 10 mg IM or IV initially and then 5 – 10 mg in 3 – 4 hours as needed.

    THIN Thinking: Identify the Risk to Safety – *The nurse must safely perform calculations to deliver medications.* **NCLEX**®: Pharmacological and Parenteral Therapies **QSEN**: Safety

30. **The nurse is observing a new nurse prepare the medications for a client diagnosed with obsessive-compulsive disorder. The prescription reads "paroxetine 20 mg PO daily for one week, then increase by 10 mg weekly until reaches 40 mg daily." The client has been on the medication for 10 days, what dose should the nurse be administering?**

    Answer: 30 mg

    Rationale: The initial dose of 20 mgs will be increased after day 7 to 30 mg until day 14. For obsessive-compulsive disorders the recommended dosage is 20 mg per day initially and increase at weekly intervals up to 40 mg daily.

    THIN Thinking: Identify Risk to Safety– *The nurse must safely perform calculations when delivering care.* **NCLEX**®: Pharmacological and Parenteral Therapies **QSEN**: Safety

Emotion

Mood / Anxiety / Grief

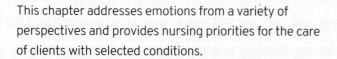

This chapter addresses emotions from a variety of perspectives and provides nursing priorities for the care of clients with selected conditions.

At no time in history has humankind realized the impact, scope, and complexity of emotions, mental health, and context. This chapter has us review several conditions across the continuum of mental health to illness.

Study Hint: Psychosocial or mental health nursing and science sometimes uses terms that are different from other specialties. When studying for NCLEX-RN®, make sure you are familiar with this unique set of terms. Such areas as defense mechanisms, symptoms of specific mental health disorders, and psychotropic medications, all may demand your understanding of these specialty-specific languages.

Priority Exemplars:

> Anxiety disorders
> Schizophrenia
> Depression
> Postpartum depression (PPD)
> Bipolar disorders
> Death and dying
> Bereavement

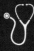
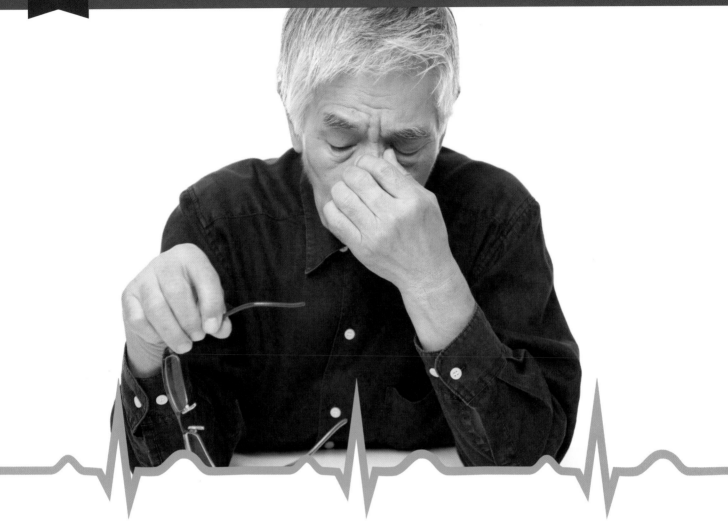

Go To Clinical Case 1

J.C. is a 61-year-old man who is brought to the crisis intervention clinic by his partner. Three weeks ago J.C. is laid off from the company for which he has worked for 43 years. They tell him he can retire and he "should be happy and enjoy life." J.C. has a history of anxiety which may be exacerbated by situational crises. J.C. shared with the nurse that he feels like nothing is going well and "something really bad is going to happen."

He denies the desire or plan to hurt himself or others. He presents to the clinic pacing constantly, is trembling, and is ruminating over money. He says his chest hurts and his heart is beating "out of his chest."

He becomes irritable when the nurse takes his vital signs. They are 98.9°F—120-36-162/98. His baseline blood pressure was 140/80. He claims to feel totally out of control and begins breathing deeply and rapidly when the nurse asks him about his worries. The client is admitted to the short-stay unit for observation.

NurseThink® Time

Using the NurseThink® system, complete the priorities. Check your answers designated by 💡 in the Anxiety disorders Priority Exemplar.

✎ Priority Assessments or Cues

1.

2.

3.

🧪 Priority Laboratory Tests/Diagnostics

1.

2.

3.

⚠ Priority Interventions or Actions

1.

2.

3.

🚩 Priority Potential & Actual Complications

1.

2.

3.

⚕ Priority Nursing Implications

1.

2.

3.

💧 Priority Medications

1.

2.

3.

👤 Priority Education/Discharge Issues

1.

2.

3.

Anxiety disorders

📋 Pathophysiology/Description

> Anxiety is the subjective response to stress

> Feelings of dread, impending doom, apprehension, fear, or discomfort which may or may not be associated with real stressors, may be out of proportion with stressor, and impairs functioning in social and work contexts

> Fear is the cognitive response to a threat, anxiety is emotional

> Most common of all psychiatric illnesses

> Twice as common in women than men; prevalence of 18% in adults; 25% in children

> Often exist with co-morbidities of depression, substance abuse, or other anxieties

> Attributed to biological, genetic, cognitive, and psychological causative factors

> Types
- Panic disorder
  - Sudden feelings of doom and physical symptoms
  - Are not triggered by a specific stressor or situation
  - Onset in early 20s
  - Variable frequency and severity
- Generalized anxiety disorder
  - Unrealistic, persistent, and excessive worry and anxiety
  - Occur more days than not for duration of at least 6 months
  - Impair social and occupational functioning
  - Onset may occur in childhood or adolescence, but also in the 20s
- Phobias
  - Persistent, exaggerated, irrational, and intense fear of a situation, object, or activity
  - Agoraphobia is the fear of open spaces causing confinement to home environment
  - Social anxiety disorder is the fear that one might do something embarrassing or be negatively evaluated by others. May be specific to public speaking or performance or more vague and non-specific.
  - Other phobias include fear of heights, snakes, dogs, strangers, homosexuals
  - Onset in the 20s and 30s
- Obsessive-compulsive disorder (see Priority Exemplar)
- Body dysmorphic disorder-exaggerated belief that the body is deformed
- Trichotillomania is a hair pulling disorder
- Hoarding disorder is the difficulty discarding or excessive acquisition of objects, regardless of value

> Client may hyperventilate and become lightheaded, short of breath, tachycardic, faint, or numbness/tingling of hands and feet

✏️ Priority Assessments or Cues

> Consider use of standardized anxiety assessments scales

> Assess for symptoms/signs of panic disorder including palpitations, tachycardia, diaphoresis, anxious expression, trembling, chest pain or pressure, nausea or vomiting, dizziness, chills, hot flashes, feelings of choking, shortness of breath, abdominal pain, feeling unsteady, paresthesias, depersonalization, feeling of losing control, or fear of dying

> Assess for signs and symptoms of generalized anxiety disorder including muscle tension, restlessness, "feeling on edge," avoiding social events or activities, procrastination, or excessive worry. Manifestations may or may not have a trigger event or stressor

> Assess for symptoms/signs of phobias including anxious response to a stressful object, activity, or situations including panic symptoms, sweating, tachycardia, and dyspnea

> Ask client about feelings of powerlessness such as feeling lack of control, expressions of doubt about personal capacity, withdrawal from decision-making or anxiety-producing situations, ritualistic behavior, preoccupation with feared object

⚠️ Priority Interventions or Actions

> Support client in therapies: Individual, cognitive, behavioral along with medications

> To address chronic anxiety
- Explore client's perceptions of threat
- Assist client to examine those factors that can and cannot be changed
- Explore selected coping and stress-management strategies
- Encourage independence and decision-making as able
- Provided structured activity and distractions
- Discuss replacing behaviors and thoughts with constructive thoughts and coping mechanisms
- With phobias and specific anxieties--Consider use of controlled systematic desensitization (gradual exposure to stimuli) or implosion therapy (flooding with stimuli)
- Allow for exploration, discussion, and reflection on thoughts and feelings

> During acute episode
- Stay with client—do not leave alone when in a panic or highly anxious
- Maintain a calm demeanor
- Use brief messages—stay calm and describe agency routines
- Manage hyperventilation, ask the client to take several breaths in a paper bag, then take slow deep abdominal breaths, repeat as needed
- Decrease environmental stimuli

- Use sedation as needed
- Once "attack" has subsided, explore sources of anxiety
- Assist client to identify triggers or early onset of anxiety and how to deal with these using deep breathing, imagery, prayer, meditation, or exercise

Priority Potential & Actual Complications

- Lack of social and occupational functioning
- Total social withdrawal
- Inability to meet personal daily needs

Priority Nursing Implications

- Anxiety is contagious. Nurses have a role to maintain calm when clients are escalating
- Deceleration techniques may be effective in addressing rising anxiety

Priority Medications

- buspirone
  - Anti-anxiety agent
  - Takes 10-14 days to be effective (not for PRN use)
  - Does not cause dependence or tolerance
  - Interacts with alcohol
- lorazepam
  - Benzodiazepine, calming agent
  - Client may become physically dependent and tolerant
  - Withdrawal if abruptly withdrawn
- alprazolam
  - Benzodiazepine, calming agent
  - Client may become physically dependent and tolerant
  - Withdrawal if abruptly withdrawn
- › imipramine
  - Tricyclic antidepressant
  - Higher doses needed to address panic with increased side effects

Priority Education/Discharge Issues

- Reassure client that healing is a long process and there may be times of regression
- Encourage clients to maintain therapy and medication regimen
- Counsel clients that most anti-anxiety agents cause sedation and orthostatic hypotension

Go To Clinical Answers

Text designated by 💡 are the top answers for the Go To Clinical related to Anxiety disorders.

Next Gen Clinical Judgment

Consider the impact personal hygiene, self-care, and ability to do activities of daily living have on the assessment and evaluation of clients with mental health issues:

1. How can a nurse use assessment of these parameters to judge the severity of symptoms?

2. How can a nurse use evaluation of these parameters to assess progress?

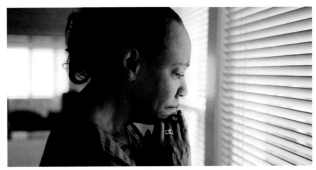

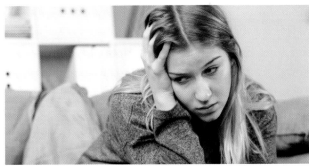

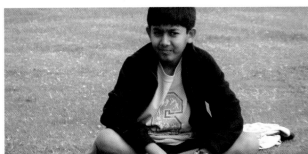

Image 16-1a / 16-1b / 16-1c: Anxiety can show up in any patient at anytime for many different reasons. Understanding the basics of priority assessment and intervention is vital. Using your clinical imagination, where might a nurse encounter these 3 patients above?

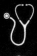

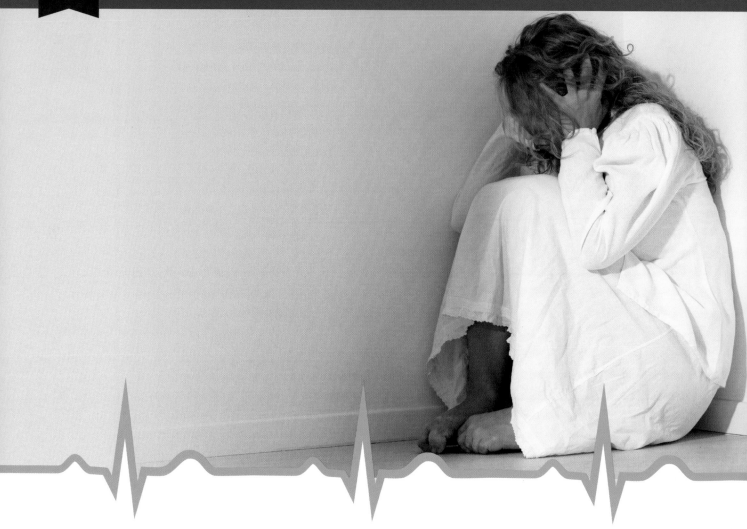

Go To Clinical Case 2

R.B. is 36 and was diagnosed with schizophrenia at 26 years of age. She is brought to the psychiatric triage center by her parents. R.B. is saying that she is being told the world is coming to an end and she needs to get ready by packing up food and supplies. Her parents found her this morning emptying cabinets and pacing the floor.

She becomes extremely agitated and starts yelling and throwing things. She grabs a pen on the counter and threatens to stab herself saying "I don't want to be here at the end of the world, I am going to kill myself...stab myself...you all are going to die when the end of the world comes."

R.B. has been able to control her symptoms in the past both with psychotropic medications, including risperidone and clozapine, and weekly therapy sessions. At home, R.B. is responsible for taking her own medications. She reports that she "stopped taking the medications because the voices told her they were 'poison'."

NurseThink® Time

Using the NurseThink® system, complete the priorities. Check your answers designated by 💡 in the Schizophrenia Priority Exemplar.

Priority Assessments or Cues

1.

2.

3.

Priority Laboratory Tests/Diagnostics

1.

2.

3.

Priority Interventions or Actions

1.

2.

3.

Priority Potential & Actual Complications

1.

2.

3.

Priority Nursing Implications

1.

2.

3.

Priority Medications

1.

2.

3.

Priority Education/Discharge Issues

1.

2.

3.

Schizophrenia

Pathophysiology/Description

> Known as a spectrum of disorders with a variety of etiological factors (biological, psychological, and environmental) and a wide variety of treatments that must be tailored to the individual and their symptoms

> Suicide is highly prevalent—1/3rd of clients have suicidal ideations, 10% die from suicide

> Effects about 1% of the Population

> Early onset begins in childhood, but generally begins late adolescent and early adulthood

> Progressive disease with exacerbations and chronic course

> Phases of Schizophrenia

- Premorbid

- Prodromal

- Active Psychotic/Acute schizophrenic episode

- Residual

> Other psychotic disorders

- Delusional disorders-clients have delusions without bizarre behaviors

  - Erotomaniac type-believes high status people are in love with them

  - Grandiose type—delusions of grand status, personal worth, and talents

  - Jealous type-perseverating that sexual partner is unfaithful

  - Persecutory-belief that one is being treated badly

  - Somatic type-false fixed beliefs about a medical condition

- Brief psychotic disorder

  - Sudden onset of psychotic symptoms, including catatonia

- Substance/medication-induced psychotic disorder

- Psychotic disorders due to medical condition

- Catatonic disorders due to a medical condition

- Schizophreniform disorder-psychotic behaviors of short duration

- Schizoaffective disorder-schizophrenic behaviors along with signs of depression and/or mania

Priority Assessments or Cues

○ Assess risk of suicide

> Assess for symptoms of schizophrenia:

- Positive symptoms

  - Delusions (false, fixed beliefs)

  - ○ Hallucinations (distorted sensory perceptions),

  - Disorganized speech-echolalia (echoing previous word), incoherence, neologisms (new language), loose associations (speech or topics do not make sense)

  - Disorganized behavior-hyperactivity, hostility, agitation, hostility

- Negative symptoms

  - Lack of speech/lack of intonation of speech/lack of gesturing

  - Withdrawal

  - Lack of ability to move or initiate activity

  - Blunted affect

  - Poor hygiene and lack of ADLs

○ Assess history from client, family, and others in the client's world to determine progression of symptoms

> Observe for: Waxy flexibility (body is not moved after positioning), posturing, pacing and rocking, regression, eye movement abnormalities

⚠ Priority Interventions or Actions

> General

  ○ Pharmacotherapy with psychotherapy

- Strategies that foster social skills, activities of daily living, and rehabilitation

- Individual psychotherapy, group therapy, family, assertive community therapy (team creates community experiences to regain skills), and behavioral therapy

○ Suicide prevention strategies/Dealing with aggression

- Observation of client at frequent, irregular intervals

- Maintain a low-stimulus environment

- Support client during agitated periods with additional staff and restraint as necessary

- Initiate suicide precautions

  - Provide one-on-one supervision

  - No harmful objects/tell visitors no harmful objects

  - Assess for ideations of plan

  - Develop a no-suicide contract

○ During hallucinations

- Listen attentively and observe for hallucination behaviors

- Avoid touch but convey an attitude of acceptance

- Do not reinforce the client's perceptions-state you do not see, hear, and use words "the voices" to decrease credibility, etc.

- Try to distract, listen to music/television, and engage in activities

- Use "reasonable doubt" technique to relay lack of belief in hallucinations

- Assist client to see association between stress and hallucinations (I know you believe you see/hear them, but I do not)

- Teach clients to use voice dismissal where they verbally tell the voice to go away
> Enhance relationships
  - Promote trust and avoid physical contact
  - Avoid talking or laughing around clients if they suspect it is about them
  - Maintain an assertive, matter-of-fact means of dealing with the client
  - Encourage consistent caregivers
  - Orient client to surroundings
  - Use concrete communication techniques
> Physical priorities
  - Attempt to meet client needs if they are non-verbal and unable to do on own
  - Assist client with self-care needs and encourage hygiene
  - Develop a toileting schedule, as needed
  - Encourage independence and decision-making as able
  - Provide canned, packaged, or home foods if the client is suspicious of foods (client may also suspect foods from home)

🚩 Priority Potential & Actual Complications

> Total withdrawal from/lack of participation in society
> Suicide

⚕ Priority Nursing Implications

💡 Nurses need to be vigilant for clients who may be suicidal or at risk for self-harm

💡 Nurses need to know that schizophrenia is associated with longer hospitalizations, higher costs, and greatest disruptions to family and personal life than any other mental health condition

💡 Evaluate and treat for extrapyramidal symptoms

💡 Treatment may include changing the psychotropic medication, reducing the dose, or adding an anticholinergic agent (benztropine, diphenhydramine)

💧 Priority Medications

💡 chlorpromazine
  - Phenothiazine antipsychotic
  - Leading antipsychotic medication
  - Watch for extrapyramidal symptoms
  - Assess for gynecomastia and sedation
  - Watch for anticholinergic effects

💡 risperidone
  - Atypical antipsychotic
  - Determine client's history—decreases seizure threshold
  - Encourage water or hard candy to alleviate dry mouth
  - May cause nausea and vomiting

💡 clozapine
  - Atypical antipsychotic
  - Need to have weekly blood levels monitored
  - Check allergic reaction
  - May lead to weight gain

> benztropine/diphenhydramine
  - anticholinergics
  - Decrease extrapyramidal symptoms (EPS)
  - Increased anticholinergic effects-sedation, dry mouth, orthostatic hypotension, constipation, urinary retention

👤 Priority Education/Discharge Issues

💡 Tell clients to refrain from smoking due to increased metabolism of antipsychotic medications—or adjust dosage accordingly

💡 Instruct clients to be careful with activities and operating equipment due to orthostatic hypotension and sedation

💡 Teach client about photosensitivity and need to use sunscreen

Go To Clinical Answers

Text designated by 💡 are the top answers for the Go To Clinical related to Schizophrenia.

_____

_____

_____

_____

_____

_____

Depression

Pathophysiology/Description

> Depression is an alteration in mood manifested by sadness, despair, and pessimism

> Characterized as a chronic mood disorder

> Mood is defined as a significant and sustained emotion that impacts a person's perception of the world.

> Lifetime prevalence of depression is 17% which is a common psychiatric disorder

> Increasing incidence among adolescents and young adults, especially girls; twice as common in women than men

> May be linked to socioeconomic well-being

> May have seasonal links (research continues)

> Types
  - Major depressive disorder (MDD)
  - Symptomatic for at least two weeks
  - No mania associated
  - Not attributed to substances or medical condition
    - Single episode or recurrent
    - Transient, mild, moderate, or severe symptoms
    - May include anxiety and suicidality
    - May have psychotic or catatonic symptoms with lack of contact with reality
  - Persistent depressive disorder (dysthymia)
    - Less severe than MDD
    - No psychotic symptoms
    - Chronic mood depression and irritability
    - May be early onset (< 21 years) or late onset (> 21 years)
  - Premenstrual dysphoric disorder
    - Depressed mood, anxiety, mood swings and disinterest in activities one week prior to menstruation
    - Decreases/eliminated after menstrual cycle
  - Substance/medication-induced depressive disorder
    - Related to effects of a medication
    - Associated with intoxication/withdrawal
  - Depressive disorder due to another medical condition
  - Postpartum depression
    - Depressed mood after delivery-more significant than minor sadness
    - May have psychotic features

> Causality related to genetic, biochemical, and psychosocial influences

Priority Assessments or Cues

> Assess for depressed mood using standardized depression assessments, assess for anger, hopelessness, self-negating comments, pessimism, lack of control

> Assess for suicidality including ideations, plan, energy level

> Assess client's self-esteem/feelings of hopelessness

> Assess for lack of interest in usual activities, changes in appetite (weight loss or gain), sleep patterns (insomnia or hypersomnia), and cognition (inability to concentrate, confusion, thoughts of death)

> Assess client's ability or lack of ability to feel pleasure (anhedonia is the lack of ability to feel pleasure)

> Assess level of activity—client may be active or inactive

> Assess fatigue level—client may have decreased energy levels

> Assess hygiene and self-care because depression may decrease attention to self

> Assessment of depression in children
  - Infants/toddlers-feeding problems, lack of play, delays in speech/motor development
  - Preschool children-phobias, aggressiveness, auditory hallucinations
  - School age-vague physical complaints, poor social skills, aggressiveness, worry, poor self-esteem, lack of play
  - Adolescence-anger, aggressiveness, high-risk behaviors, apathy, social withdrawal, sexual acting out, restlessness, substance use

> Assessment of depression in older adults
  - Bereavement overload
  - Memory loss, confusion, or apathy may be manifested as pseudodementia

Priority Laboratory Tests/Diagnostics

> Serum toxicology to determine substance use

> Labs based on physiological needs (hydration/nutrition)

Priority Interventions or Actions

> Individualized psychotherapy, group therapy, family therapy

> Cognitive therapy
  - Designed to assist client to replace negative with positive automatic thoughts
  - Consider realistic potential complications
  - Focus on learning new methods to conceptualize and perceive life tasks

> Electroconvulsive therapy

> Transcranial magnetic stimulation-stimulates nerve cells in the brain

> Light therapy

> Medications

> Care for clients at risk for suicide
  - Create a safe environment—observe closely and stay with client as needed
  - Ensure room and surroundings are cleaned of any objects that may be used for self-harm. Constant observation is warranted

- Assess for risk/lethality/ideations of suicide
- Portray unconditional acceptance
- Allow for expression of feelings such as anger and guilt
> With depression
  - Develop a trusting relationship with an accepting attitude
  - Allow for ventilation of feelings such as anger
  - Provide education on mood and grief
  - Promote feeling of positive self-worth
  - Reassure that crying is healthy and acceptable
  - Provide distraction, physical activity, and outlets for anger and tension
  - Encourage group attendance
  - Teach assertiveness and positive communication
  - Promote realistic goal-setting and decision-making and means for goal attainment

Priority Potential & Actual Complications

> Catatonia, stupor
> Physiological impact of lack of meeting nutritional, sleep, and activity needs

Priority Nursing Implications

> Nurses should be aware of the "black box warning" wherein some antidepressants are associated with increased rates of suicide in young people when first starting medications

> Nurses need to ensure clients' safety when suicide is a concern. Nurses may need to ensure taking of medications (so they are not "stockpiled" for overdose) by making frequent rounds at irregular times and observe clients closely

Priority Medications

> amitriptyline
  - Tricyclic antidepressant
  - Takes 1-3 weeks to take effect
  - Avoid smoking—increases metabolism
> fluoxetine
  - Selective serotonin reuptake inhibitor (SSRI)-antidepressant
  - May take 2-3 weeks to work
  - Take in morning to avoid insomnia
> phenelzine
  - Monoamine oxidase inhibitor (MAOI), antidepressant
  - Large number of food interactions which could lead to hypertensive crisis
  - Later agent to be used-if depression refractory to other treatments

> bupropion
  - Atypical antidepressant
  - May decrease seizure threshold
  - Should not "double-up" doses if a dose is missed
  - Also used for smoking cessation
> duloxetine
  - Serotonin-norepinephrine reuptake inhibitor, antidepressant
  - May cause orthostatic hypotension
  - May cause sweating and constipation

Priority Education/Discharge Issues

> Provide referral as needed to community resources including support groups, mental health clinics, crisis intervention
> Encourage adherence to medication regimens
> Ensure family education and support
> Ensure that family and others are aware of client's risk for suicide, potential signs of suicidality, means to keep client safe, and emergency procedures

Complete this MNEMONIC
SIG E CAPS for Depression
S _____
I _____
G _____
E _____
C _____
A _____
P _____
S _____

Table 16-1: Feel free to search the Internet or create your own.

_____

_____

_____

Postpartum depression (PPD)

📋 Pathophysiology/Description

> Postpartum depression affects up to 20% of women who give birth.

> Changes in levels of hormones in the body after childbirth place some women at risk for postpartum depression

> There are many other factors that place women at risk for postpartum depression. Among them are marital disunity, history of major depression, substance abuse, low self-esteem, severe psychological stressors, lack of social support and having a sick neonate, among others

> Treatment for postpartum depression includes psychotherapy, drugs or a combination of both

✏️ Priority Assessments or Cues

> Unprovoked irritability and rage

> Intense feeling of dread and fear

> Inability to sleep, or oversleeping

> Sadness and crying without a cause

> Feeling of guilt

> Indifference to the newborn

> Obsessions, including thoughts of injuring the newborn or self

> Avoiding friends and family

> Binging on food or eating too little

⚗️ Priority Laboratory Tests/Diagnostics

> There are no lab tests that diagnosis postpartum depression. Interview with the mother and completion of depression scales help to make the diagnosis
  - Postpartum Depression Screening Scale
  - Edinburg Postnatal Depression Scale

⚠️ Priority Interventions or Actions

> Hypervigilance to detect behaviors that clue into the mother's postpartum depression

> Probing questions to determine mother's state of mind and relationship with infant

> Empathetic discussion with mother and partner regarding feelings

> Initiate process for prescribed psychotherapy sessions

> Initiate antidepressant therapy

🚩 Priority Potential & Actual Complications

> Poor child/maternal bonding

> Developmental delays in baby

> Dysfunctional family relationship

> Major depression

> Suicide or homicide (of baby)

☞ Priority Nursing Implications

> Nurses must be aware that even though postpartum depression impacts women primarily, a small percentage of men also experience the condition. The implication is that when both parents are experiencing postpartum depression, measures to ensure proper care of the infant must become a priority. Therefore, nurses must be very observant and watchful for signs of depression in mothers, as well as fathers.

🩸 Priority Medications

> The class of antidepressants used to treat postpartum depression is the selective serotonin reuptake inhibitors (SSRIs). There are many drugs in this class. Four of the most commonly used ones are below

> fluoxetine
  - Usual initial dose of the immediate-release preparations is 20 mg orally, given daily
  - Usual maintenance dose is 20 – 60 mg orally, given daily
  - Usual initial dose of delayed-release capsule is 90 mg orally, given once weekly. This is started 7 days after ending a dose of the immediate-release preparation

> paroxetine
  - Usual initial dose of the immediate-release preparations is 20 mg orally, given daily
  - Usual maintenance dose of immediate-release tablet is 20-50 mg orally, given daily
  - Usual initial dose of controlled-release tablet is 25 mg orally, given daily; usual maintenance dose is 25 mg – 62.5 mg orally, given orally

> escitalopram
  - Usual initial dose is 10 mg given by mouth daily
  - Usual maintenance dose is 10 – 20 mg given by mouth daily
  - Common side effects are dizziness and irregular heartbeat

> sertraline
  - Usual initial dose is 50 mg given by mouth daily
  - Usual maintenance dose is 50 – 200 mg given by mouth daily
  - May cause drowsiness so to take at bedtime

Priority Education/Discharge Issues

> Importance of maintaining scheduled psychotherapy sessions

> Importance of taking antidepressants as prescribed

> Recognizing and reporting adverse effects of medications

> Who to contact if a crisis occurs at home that impacts safety of self or the baby

> Provide information about postpartum support groups

> Benefit of getting uninterrupted sleep for several days

> Exercise and time for daily relaxation

> Importance of keeping all follow-up medical appointments

> Allowing friends and family to help with care of newborn

> That antidepressant medications may not be effective immediately but might take a few weeks to start working

> Benefit of other non-pharmacological treatment such as acupuncture, herbs and light therapy, among others

> Importance of partner offering ongoing affection and care

Clinical Hint

Postpartum depression can occur in a new mother, or one who has had children previously. Mothers should be screened before they are discharged. Experts also recommend screening for maternal depression when the mother brings the baby for the 1, 2, and 4-month visits, since postpartum depression frequently occurs at about 4 weeks after the woman gives birth.

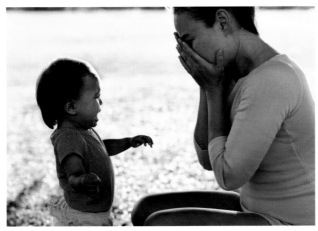

Image 16-2

Bipolar disorders

Pathophysiology/Description

> Characterized as a chronic mood disorder. Mood is defined as a significant and sustained emotion that impacts a person's perception of the world

> Affect is the external appearance of the emotional experience

> Bipolar disorders are manifested with cycles of depression and mania (elation in mood including exaggerated and risk-laden behaviors)

> Impacts about 2.6% of the US population. 83% are profoundly impacted. Impacts men and women equally, average onset is at 25 years

> Often misdiagnosed or undiagnosed

> Types
  • Bipolar I (major depression with mania)
  • Bipolar II (major depression with hypomania)
  • Cyclothymic disorder (mood cycling including less severe levels of depression and elevated mood not quite as significant as hypomania)
  • Substance/medication-induced bipolar disorder (directly caused by drugs during intoxication or withdrawal; or reaction to other medications such as steroids)
  • Bipolar disorder due to medical condition (electrolyte imbalance, brain tumor)
  • Disruptive mood dysregulation disorder is mainly a syndrome associated with childhood, manifested by irritability, temper tantrums, and mood swings

> Causation attributed to hereditary, genetic, and physiological (neurotransmitter/neuroanatomical) elements along with stress/trauma factors in the client's life or environment

> May occur in children and adults

> Comorbidity with attention-deficit/hyperactivity disorder(ADHD) in children (see ADHD Priority Exemplar)

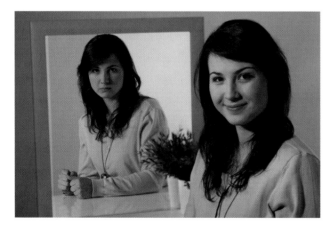

Image 16-3: Search for internet videos that say "I have bipolar disorder." As you study the following Priority Assessments, think about the people in the videos.

Priority Assessments or Cues

> Assess for signs and symptoms of depression (see Depression Priority Exemplar)

> Assess symptoms of mania including elation, inflated self-esteem, grandiosity, hyperactivity, agitation, racing thoughts/flight of ideas, distractibility, accelerated/forced speech, engagement in high-risk behaviors (substance use, promiscuity/exaggerated sexual behaviors, excessive shopping, gambling, investing), irritability, frenzied motor activity, decreased need for sleep, rapid mood swings, lack of hygiene/self-care

> Assess for impact on social and work life, to be considered mania it must have a significant impact on life functioning

> Observe for hypomania-behaviors similar to those above but not so severe as to cause significant social or work dysfunction, may begin as cheerful but devolve to irritability and volatility, may experience weight loss, engage in inappropriate and high-risk behaviors

> Assess for delusions (false fixed beliefs) and hallucinations (distorted sensory experiences)

> Assess for substance use

Priority Laboratory Tests/Diagnostics

> Electrolyte levels

> Drug and toxicology screens

Priority Interventions or Actions

> Medications including monotherapy with mood stabilizers

> Second-generation antipsychotics

> Psychoeducational focused family therapy concerning early warning signs and management

> Individual or group therapy (self-help or support groups) and cognitive therapy

> Electroconvulsive therapy

> Client management during acute episodes
  • Decrease external stimuli such as lights, noise
  • Remove dangerous objects
  • Check on client frequently/stay with client during increased agitation
  • Provide activities and distraction when feasible
  • Intervene as mood becomes anxious or agitated
  • Maintain calm attitude/set limits on manipulation and reinforce non-manipulative behaviors
  • Use a team approach to calm client including deceleration, medications, mechanical restraints
  • Implement gradual removal of client restraints as situation warrants

⚑ Priority Potential & Actual Complications

> Negative events related to poor decision-making/high-risk behaviors

> Physical exhaustion and life-threatening malnutrition

> Delirious mania may lead to intensified symptoms that threaten safe of self and others, confused thinking, and stupor

⚕ Priority Nursing Implications

> Nurses need to work with dietician to ensure adequate calories such as use finger foods, high calorie shakes during acute episodes—maintain I & O, calorie counts

> During manic periods clients often feel powerful and capable, leading them to decide to not take medications, leading to exacerbations

> Nurses may need to assist in facilitating restful sleep

⬤ Priority Medications

> lithium carbonate
  - Mood stabilizer
  - Effective in about 1/3 of clients
  - Ensure adequate sodium and water intake
  - Cautious use of diuretics
  - Monitor serum levels (0.6-1.2 mEq/L)

> valproic acid
  - Anticonvulsant used to stabilize moods
  - May cause sedation
  - Cannot be discontinued abruptly
  - Avoid alcohol
  - May increase suicidal thoughts and behaviors

⬤ Priority Education/Discharge Issues

> Instruct client to avoid caffeine in diet to foster sleep

> Reinforce the need for strict adherence with medication schedule

> Remind about need for regular blood draws to monitor serum levels

> Reinforce the need for therapy, in addition to medications, to manage chronic and acute elements of disorder

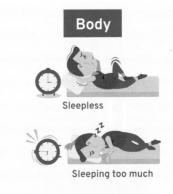

Body

Sleepless

Sleeping too much

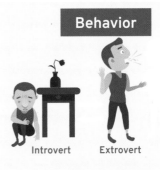

Behavior

Introvert   Extrovert

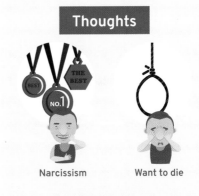

Thoughts

Narcissism   Want to die

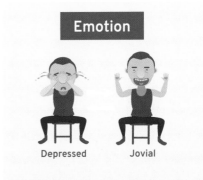

Emotion

Depressed   Jovial

Image 16-4: Make a note card for each of the 4 areas of concerns for people with bipolar disorder.

Death and dying

Pathophysiology/Description

> There is specific care revolving around the death and dying process

> Also known as end-of-life care

Priority Assessments or Cues

> Assess client's religious and spiritual preferences

> Assess client's end-of-life wishes including advanced directive

> Assess for other legal and ethical issues, including withdrawal of treatment, organ and tissue donation, legal documentation, cardiopulmonary resuscitation

> Assess the physiological status of the client near death
  - Slowing of metabolism until organ function ceases
  - Decreases in sensory function such as changes in vision, taste, smell, pain, touch, loss of blinking/staring (hearing preserved until late in the process)
  - Respirations become shallow and irregular, with tachypnea or bradypnea, may develop audible crackles or wet sounds ("death rattle") or Cheyne-Stokes breathing (alternating deep and rapid breathing)
  - Skin may become cool and waxy, extremities become cool, pale, mottled, and cyanotic
  - Urine output decreases and client may be incontinent
  - Peristalsis slows leading to constipation and distention, client may be incontinent
  - Client moves less with depressed gag and swallow reflexes
  - Death occurs as organs fail, cardiac/respiratory arrest
  - Brain death occurs when the cerebral cortex ceases function/damage is irreparable

> Assess clients frequently for status and need for comfort measures

Priority Interventions or Actions

> Encourage clients to have an advanced directive, including a living will and durable power of attorney

> Referral to hospice
  - Provides palliative and supportive care where focus is on comfort, rather than cure
  - Ensure the optimum pain management
  - Multidisciplinary team of nurses, physicians, chaplains, social workers, and others ensure to comfort and symptom control
  - Provides holistic care to allow client to be as active and involved as able
  - May be in the home, part of a hospital, or at a specific hospice center
  - Provides services to family members, respite care, and emotional support

> Provide physical care
  - Provide pain management
  - Elevate the head of the bed, suction as needed, and provide oxygen
  - Provide oral and other hygiene measures as tolerated
  - Keep perineal area clean and change pads frequently
  - Provide rest as needed
  - Allow or restrict visitors to meet the needs of the client
  - Provide anti-emetics as needed
  - Offer small quantities of favorite foods or beverages

> Provide emotional care
  - Allow for privacy of client and family
  - Provide support and advocacy
  - Encourage family to communicate with client as able, using verbalizations and touch to relate with client
  - Encourage client and family to discuss fears at end-of-life, including pain, loneliness, and remorse

> Postmortem procedures
  - Close client's eyes, replace dentures (as needed), remove IV tubing, catheters, and dressings (check hospital policy if autopsy is to be performed)
  - Wash client and redress (check policy and if autopsy is to be performed)
  - Place pads under client, place a pillow under head, and position client for family viewing
  - When transporting to the morgue, follow agency policy and ensure client identification, cover or use special bed for transport

Priority Nursing Implications

> Ensure that the client's dignity is preserved and family is respected

> Consider cultural practices, laws, and hospital policy when rendering postmortem care

> Provide privacy for family to spend time with the client after death

> Consider the nurse's own need for support when caring for dying clients

Priority Medications

> morphine
  - Analgesic
  - End-of-life pain management
  - May slow respirations
  - May be given intravenously or orally

> fentanyl
  - For severe, ongoing pain
  - Dose titrated to ensure safe pain relief
  - Patch provides sustained-release pain management
  - May be given via buccal, nasal, and sublingual membranes

> Oral lubricant solution or spray
  - Available over-the-counter
  - Relieves dry mouth

Bereavement

Pathophysiology/Description

> Bereavement is the human response characterized by grief and/or sadness in response to a loss

> Characterized by loss (when something of value is taken away) and grief (emotional grief subsequent to a loss)

> The real or perceived loss may be a person, pet, occupation, partner, health status or function, developmental milestone or crisis, or possession

> Anticipatory grief
  • Feeling grief before the loss
  • May lead to detachment prior to the loss

> Stages of grief
  • Kubler Ross
    - Denial
    - Anger
    - Bargaining
    - Depression
    - Acceptance
  • Worden
    - Accepting the reality of the loss
    - Processing the pain of grief
    - Adjusting to the world without the lost entity
    - Finding an enduring connection with the lost entity while resuming or finding a new life
  • Bowlby
    - Numbness/protest
    - Disequilibrium
    - Disorganization and despair
    - Reorganization

> Length of grief
  • Varies with the individual
  • Acute grief period-6-8 weeks

Priority Assessments or Cues

> Assess client's developmental level. Grief responses vary based on developmental age and capacity of the client

> Assess for financial or personal implications of the loss, coping skills, history of mental illness or substance abuse, history of trauma, number of previous losses, role of individual in the client's life

> Assess for cultural and spiritual variables impacting the bereavement experience

> Assess client's stage of grief and risk factors

Priority Interventions or Actions

> Develop trust and show empathy

> Encourage discussion about the loss when appropriate—allow client to ventilate

> Help client identify emotions such as guilt, anger, anxiety, helplessness, bitterness

> Provide support and encouragement as appropriate

> Reassure the client and reinforce positive coping and periods of grief

> Examine previous coping or spiritual strategies used in the past to cope with loss

> Contact a spiritual leader as requested

Priority Potential & Actual Complications

> Delayed or inhibited grief
> Distorted or exaggerated grief
> Chronic or prolonged grief
> Maladaptive grieving/loss of self-esteem
> Clinical depression characterized by disturbed self-esteem, anhedonia, hopelessness, guilt, and dysphoria
> Suicidal ideations

Priority Nursing Implications

> Nurses may provide the role of listener and support person in the bereavement process

> Hospice services may provide support for the bereaved in addition to the dying. The interdisciplinary team focuses on client and family physical and emotional needs, especially pain and symptom management

> Stages of grief provide the nurse and client some structure and comfort as this process proceeds

> Nurses need to be aware of the individual, cultural, and spiritual dimensions of bereavement, along with the developmental factors impacting the grief response

Priority Education/Discharge Issues

> Encourage clients to have an advanced directive, including a living will and durable power of attorney

> Ensure supports are available in the family, community, and healthcare setting for those responding with maladaptive grief

1. The nurse is assessing a client recently admitted to hospice care. When trying to determine the needs of the client, which assessment is a priority?
   1. Exploring the relationships and communication patterns within the family.
   2. Identifying the client's religious preferences and name of their spiritual counselor.
   3. Reviewing the prescribed medications with the client to see if they understand them.
   4. Determining whether the client's insurance will pay for hospice care.

2. The spouse of a client nearing death states "she has been my whole life, I don't think I can go on without her." What is the appropriate response by the nurse?
   1. "You are a strong person and you will be able to carry on."
   2. "Tell me more about your concern that you cannot go on without her."
   3. "Losing someone is always difficult, but it will get easier with time."
   4. "Tell me more about those many years you have shared with her."

3. The interprofessional team is planning end-of-life care for a client with terminal cancer. The client's young children recently climbed into bed to snuggle their mom which is an infection control concern. What suggestion by the nurse would be appropriate?
   1. "We may need to limit the time the client's young children visit."
   2. "The kids need to touch their mother, maybe we could encourage holding hands."
   3. "If the kids wash their hands before snuggling, short periods should be fine."
   4. "We could encourage the client's spouse to snuggle with the kids at home."

4. The nurse is delegating the care of a client with bipolar disorder to an unlicensed assistive personnel (UAP). What instruction is critical to a successful plan of care?
   1. "Allow the client to maintain as much control as possible."
   2. "Do not argue with the client if they don't want to eat lunch."
   3. "Be sure to consistently implement the limits set for the client."
   4. "Encourage the client to play card games to keep them busy."

5. The hospice nurse is visiting a client who is terminally ill. What assessment is the priority when caring for a client on hospice care?
   1. Level of consciousness.
   2. Pain management.
   3. Intake and output.
   4. Respiratory rate.

6. The client with a diagnosis of major depression states "I have been on these antidepressant medications for a week now and I don't feel any better." What statement by the nurse would appropriate?
   1. "It took you a long time to get this depressed, don't expect an immediate turnaround."
   2. "Oh, I see improvements in your mood every day since you started the prescription."
   3. "Sometimes the antidepressant medications take up to 3 weeks before you see a change."
   4. "I will check with your healthcare provider, maybe we need to change medications."

7. While the nurse is caring for a client with a diagnosis of schizophrenia, the client states "I keep hearing those voices telling me to run away." What response by the nurse is appropriate?
   1. "Those voices are just in your head and the medication will help in a few days."
   2. "Can you tell me who the voice sounds like and what you think you need to do?"
   3. "Sometimes those voices tell you things that don't make any sense just ignore them."
   4. "Try to listen to me and the others around you that you can see."

8. While walking through the dining room the nurse overhears a client with a diagnosis of paranoid schizophrenia whisper to another client "they are all out to get us and probably poisoned the food too." What would be the priority nursing action?
   1. "Don't worry you are safe here. Watch I will take a bite of the food to prove it."
   2. "This is a safe place and no one is going to poison your food here."
   3. "Can I sit down and join you while you eat? What are you having for lunch?"
   4. "Don't be silly all of the food here is safe. The staff have the same meals."

9. The nurse is planning care for client with a history of anxiety disorder who is admitted for pneumonia. What would be the priority goal for the care plan?
   1. Client will participate in care planning.
   2. Anxiety levels will be managed.
   3. Client will be compliant with treatment plan.
   4. Anti-anxiety medications will be administered as needed.

10. The nurse has completed the admission assessment of a client with a diagnosis of acute bipolar disorder. Based on the assessment, what is the priority focus for the nursing plan of care?
    1. Control the client's hyperactivity.
    2. Monitor relevant lab values.
    3. Hydration and nutrition.
    4. Client teaching.

11. The nurse is meeting with the interdisciplinary team to discuss the care plan for a client with a diagnosis of depression. What statement by the nurse indicates that the care needs to be re-evaluated?
    1. "We have been letting the client make decisions about activities of daily living."
    2. "The client has lost another 2 pounds and reports being constipated."
    3. "The family says that the client is more talkative when they come to visit."
    4. "Antidepressant medications were started 10 days ago but no apparent effect."

12. The nurse is instructing an unlicensed assistive personnel (UAP) who will be caring for a client with a diagnosis of schizophrenia. The UAP has asked how to deal with the client who reports hearing voices. What is the appropriate response by the nurse?
    1. "Just ignore the client's report of hearing voices."
    2. "Tell the client that the voices are just in his head."
    3. "Distract the client by changing the subject."
    4. "Ask the client what the voices are saying."

13. The nurse is preparing a presentation for a senior citizens group regarding the increased suicide rates among the elderly. What is the priority content the nurse should include?
    1. Statistics about the increased incidence of suicide among the elderly.
    2. Risk factors that increase the potential for suicide among the elderly.
    3. Behaviors and/or comments from peers indicating potential suicide risk.
    4. Overview of methods used for suicide among the elderly.

14. The clinic nurse has completed teaching for a client who frequently hyperventilates in response to anxiety. What statement by the client indicates teaching was effective?
    1. "I just need to learn to get over my anxiety and forget about it."
    2. "I should try taking deep breaths when I feel my anxiety going up."
    3. "As long as I keep taking my antianxiety meds I don't need to worry."
    4. "I will just try to avoid anything that makes me anxious."

15. The nurse is implementing the plan of care for a client with a diagnosis of depression. What nursing actions are included in the plan? Select all that apply.
    1. Offer small, high caloric or high protein snacks during the day.
    2. Encourage the client to limit activities to conserve energy.
    3. Encourage the client to get dressed and stay out of bed during the day.
    4. Provide reminders regarding self-care and hygiene as needed.
    5. Encourage client to avoid intake of fluid in the evening.

16. The nurse is assessing a client with a diagnosis of bipolar disorder in the manic phase. What assessment findings could pose an immediate safety concern? Select all that apply.
    1. Distraction by environmental events.
    2. Purposeless movements.
    3. Inflated sense of self-importance.
    4. Risky, impulsive behavior.
    5. Non-compliance with medications.

17. The nurse caring for a client with a diagnosis of schizophrenia is reviewing the care plan. What nursing actions would the nurse anticipate implementing? Select all that apply.
    1. Assess the client's contact with reality as needed.
    2. Implement a planned schedule and set limits as needed.
    3. Encourage the client to independently make decisions.
    4. Monitor food and fluid intake.
    5. Focus on reality-based here and now activities.

18. The clinic nurse is assessing a client with chronic obstructive pulmonary disease (COPD) and moderate anxiety. In what order should the nurse collect assessment data? Rank order the responses.
    1. Conduct a respiratory assessment to compare with history.
    2. Review the medical record for history and prescriptions.
    3. Encourage the client to report their symptoms.
    4. Ask meaningful questions to elicit information.
    5. Assess vital signs and compliance with prescriptions.

19. The school nurse is planning a meeting with parents to talk about the risk of depression among teenagers. What risk factors will the nurse include? Select all that apply.
    1. Hormonal changes.
    2. Being on the honor roll.
    3. Cyberbullying.
    4. Loss of a significant other.
    5. Peer relationships.

20. The nurse is reviewing the medication administration record in the electronic health record for a client with Bipolar Disorder and reviews the prescription for lithium carbonate. The client preferred the elixir and is ordered 450 mg/four times/day and it is available 300 mg/5 mL. How many mL. would the client receive in one 24-hour period?

21. The nurse is discussing advanced directives with a client and his family. The family questions what it means for the client to be competent and make personal decisions. What would be the nurse's best response?
    1. "When he is able to understand risks and benefits of the decisions being made."
    2. "When he's able to legibly sign the forms."
    3. "When he is oriented to person, place and time."
    4. "When he is able to physically take care of himself."

22. A client reports difficulty sleeping and a "pounding heart." There are no abnormal findings on the physical examination. Further assessment reveals that the client is worried about being successful on a new job that he just started. What is an appropriate nursing response to this finding?
    1. "Counseling could be of much benefit to you right now."
    2. "It seems that your concern right now is about whether you can do your job."
    3. "Have you spoken with any of your family members about what concerns you?"
    4. "Anxiety is very normal whenever someone starts a job for the first time."

23. The nurse is assessing a client at the clinic. The client reports that the loss of her husband two months ago has made her anxious about life. The client reports "I really can't go on living this way." Which would be the most therapeutic response by the nurse?
    1. "That is a very common feeling and it will pass in time."
    2. "Tell me about your anxiety and how you are feeling."
    3. "Did your husband leave you in debt? Is that why you are anxious?"
    4. "You should speak to your doctor about your feelings."

24. The nurse is caring for a client at the inpatient psychiatric unit. The client tells the nurse that someone is poisoning the food and drink here and they will not eat or drink anything. What therapeutic response from the nurse would help the client?
    1. "I eat the same food and I am not poisoned."
    2. "The food is approved by the health department so it is fine."
    3. "Tell me why you feel someone is poisoning you."
    4. "All the clients eat the same food here."

25. The nurse interviews a family member after the loss of a loved one from a myocardial infarction. The family member states their loved one never took care of themselves. The nurse identifies the family member to be in what stage of the grief process?
    1. Depression.
    2. Denial.
    3. Bargaining.
    4. Anger.

26. A nurse is approached by a family member about their loved one's roommate. The family member wants to know the roommate's diagnosis and if they may be potentially violent. Which is the best response by the nurse?
    1. "Don't worry, we don't have violent people on this unit."
    2. "I cannot discuss another client with you."
    3. "I will watch out for your family member."
    4. "Perhaps you should voice your concerns with administration."

27. The nurse is caring for a client who expressed thoughts of suicide. Which is the priority nursing action?
    1. Report this to the family so the client can go home.
    2. Place the client in a locked room by himself.
    3. Place the client on the locked unit with other clients.
    4. Ensure that the client is on one-on-one surveillance.

28. The nurse is providing education information to the client regarding the risperidone the healthcare prescribed. What statement by the client demonstrates a good understanding of teaching?
    1. "I can stop taking the medication when I feel better."
    2. "I may have a dry mouth while on this medication."
    3. "I will no longer have symptoms while on this medication."
    4. "I need to eat a lot of salt and drink lots of water when on this medication."

29. The healthcare provider prescribed fluphenazine for a client diagnosed with psychosis. The prescribed dose is 10 mg/daily. The nurse has fluphenazine 2.5 mg on the unit. How many pills should the nurse administer?
    1. 2 pills.
    2. 3 pills.
    3. 4 pills.
    4. 5 pills.

30. The nurse is counseling a client at the clinic. The client states they experience panic attacks at work and they don't know what to do. What is the nurse's best response?
    1. "Medications are the most effective treatment for panic attacks."
    2. "Try to ignore the panic attacks and they may become less often."
    3. "It is best for you to go home and rest during your panic attacks."
    4. "Let's talk about suggestions to help you cope better with the panic attacks."

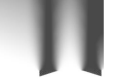

1. The nurse is assessing a client recently admitted to hospice care. When trying to determine the needs of the client, which assessment is a priority?
   1. 📍 Exploring the relationships and communication patterns within the family.
   2. Identifying the client's religious preferences and name of their spiritual counselor. *This information is available from the medical record.*
   3. Reviewing the prescribed medications with the client to see if they understand them. *Medications knowledge is no longer a priority and many medications are discontinued when a client is placed in hospice care.*
   4. Determining whether the client's insurance will pay for hospice care. *This information should be in the medical record.*

   Rationale: The nurse needs to understand the support systems available to the client by exploring family relationships and the communication patterns within the family. Gathering data such as insurance coverage and religion can be collected by reviewing the client's medical record. Many times, previously prescribed medications are discontinued when the client is placed on hospice status.

   THIN Thinking: Top Three – *Assessment of the client and family dynamics is an important part of the assessment when determining stages of the grieving process. This interaction assessment is an important part of planning care.* **NCLEX®:** Management of Care **QSEN:** Patient-centered Care

2. The spouse of a client nearing death states "she has been my whole life, I don't think I can go on without her." What is the appropriate response by the nurse?
   1. "You are a strong person and you will be able to carry on." *This statement does not allow spouse to verbalize feelings.*
   2. 📍 "Tell me more about your concern that you cannot go on without her."
   3. "Losing someone is always difficult, but it will get easier with time." *This statement does not allow spouse to verbalize feelings.*
   4. "Tell me more about those many years you have shared with her." *While giving the spouse the chance to talk about his wife, it does not give information about spouse's current feelings and possible safety issues.*

   Rationale: Feeling hopeless and powerless when a loved one is near death are common feelings. Exploring what those feelings mean to family members can assess the safety of the spouse left behind or if they may be potentially suicidal.

   THIN Thinking: Nursing Process – *Therapeutic communication needs to be empathetic, open-ended, and caring. Asking clients to restate and clarify their feelings are parts of this process.* **NCLEX®:** Psychosocial Integrity **QSEN:** Patient-centered Care

3. The interprofessional team is planning end-of-life care for a client with terminal cancer. The client's young children recently climbed into bed to snuggle their mom which is an infection control concern. What suggestion by the nurse would be appropriate?
   1. "We may need to limit the time the client's young children visit." *This would not meet families need to spend time together.*
   2. "The kids need to touch their mother, maybe we could encourage holding hands." *Small children won't understand this restriction and need to be in close contact with loved one.*
   3. 📍 "If the kids wash their hands before snuggling, short periods should be fine."
   4. "We could encourage the client's spouse to snuggle with the kids at home." *This is not meeting the need for physical contact for the children or the dying parent.*

   Rationale: One of the primary goals for end-of-life care is to meet the physical and emotional needs of the client and their family. Therefore, allowing opportunities for closeness, touch and physical contact can help alleviate the fear of abandonment and dying alone.

   THIN Thinking: Top Three – *Given the setting and situation, adjustments to the infection control policy is acceptable. Meeting the psychosocial needs of the client and family are more important than the risk of infection.* **NCLEX®:** Safety and Infection Control **QSEN:** Patient-centered Care

4. The nurse is delegating the care of a client with bipolar disorder to an unlicensed assistive personnel (UAP). What instruction is critical to a successful plan of care?
   1. "Allow the client to maintain as much control as possible." *Clients with bipolar disorder require guidelines.*
   2. "Do not argue with the client if they don't want to eat lunch." *While arguing with the client may not be the best option, strongly encouraging the client to eat would be important.*
   3. 📍 "Be sure to consistently implement the limits set for the client."
   4. "Encourage the client to play card games to keep them busy." *Group activities may be too much stimuli for this client.*

   Rationale: Consistency among staff is imperative if the limit setting is to be effectively implemented. Using a calm, firm manner is effective with bipolar clients rather than encouraging independent decision making. Group activities can result in too much stimuli for a bipolar client.

   THIN Thinking: Top Three – *The top priority for clients with bipolar disorder is to implement limits. Distracting them and arguing will not create a therapeutic environment.* **NCLEX®:** Psychosocial Integrity **QSEN:** Evidence-based Practice

5. The hospice nurse is visiting a client who is terminally ill. What assessment is the priority when caring for a client on hospice care?

    1. Level of consciousness. *LOC is expected to decrease when experiencing the dying process.*
    2. ◉ Pain management.
    3. Intake and output. *Intake and output is expected to decrease as the organs begin to fail.*
    4. Respiratory rate. *Respirations are expected to decrease as the condition deteriorates.*

    Rationale: The goal of hospice care is to provide palliative care with a primary focus on keeping the client comfortable. Therefore, assessing pain management is the priority assessment.

    THIN Thinking: Top Three – *In a palliative/hospice situation, pain management is the priority assessment. Assessment of the LOC, I/O and Respirations will help determine when the end is near, but pain management is the priority.* **NCLEX®:** Basic Care and Comfort **QSEN:** Patient-centered Care

6. The client with a diagnosis of major depression states "I have been on these antidepressant medications for a week now and I don't feel any better." What statement by the nurse would appropriate?

    1. "It took you a long time to get this depressed, don't expect an immediate turnaround." *This statement doesn't give the client any real information as to how long the drug will take to be effective.*
    2. "Oh, I see improvements in your mood every day since you started the prescription." *This is a false reassurance.*
    3. ◉ "Sometimes the antidepressant medications take up to 3 weeks before you see a change."
    4. "I will check with your healthcare provider, maybe we need to change medications." *This is unnecessary as it will just take a couple more weeks for a change to be seen.*

    Rationale: One of the drawbacks of antidepressant medications is that it can take up to three weeks before an effective blood level is reached. Telling the client that they seem better when the client doesn't feel it can interfere with the therapeutic relationship.

    THIN Thinking: Top Three – *Because it can take longer for a client to feel the effects of antidepressants they need to be cautioned that the depression will continue until the medication takes effect.* **NCLEX®:** Pharmacology and Parenteral Therapies **QSEN:** Evidence-based Practice

7. While the nurse is caring for a client with a diagnosis of schizophrenia, the client states "I keep hearing those voices telling me to run away." What response by the nurse is appropriate?

    1. "Those voices are just in your head and the medication will help in a few days." *Does not redirect client to focus on reality.*
    2. "Can you tell me who the voice sounds like and what you think you need to do?" *Does not redirect client to focus on reality.*
    3. "Sometimes those voices tell you things that don't make any sense just ignore them." *Doesn't encourage client to focus on reality.*
    4. ◉ "Try to listen to me and the others around you that you can see."

    Rationale: Hallucinations are very real to the schizophrenic client, do not negate them. Encourage the client to focus on the reality of here and now.

    THIN Thinking: Help Quick – *For the client experiencing hallucinations, it is important to have them focus on reality* **NCLEX®:** Psychosocial Integrity **QSEN:** Patient-centered Care

8. While walking through the dining room the nurse overhears a client with a diagnosis of paranoid schizophrenia whisper to another client "they are all out to get us and probably poisoned the food too." What would be the priority nursing action?

    1. "Don't worry you are safe here. Watch I will take a bite of the food to prove it." *This statement can derail trust as the nurse was eavesdropping on a private conversation.*
    2. "This is a safe place and no one is going to poison your food here." *This statement may feed into the client's paranoia.*
    3. ◉ "Can I sit down and join you while you eat? What are you having for lunch?"
    4. "Don't be silly all of the food here is safe. The staff have the same meals." *This is shutting down the client's concerns.*

    Rationale: The nurse needs to be careful not to feed into the client's sense of paranoia such as eavesdropping on their conversations. By offering to sit with the clients provides an opportunity for the nurse to further assess the conversation before intervening. When clients are expressing delusions, the nurse needs to continue to work on building trust.

    THIN Thinking: Help Quick – *The immediate intervention would be to assess further, being present in the discussion will allow for this.* **NCLEX®:** Psychosocial Integrity **QSEN:** Patient-centered Care

9. The nurse is planning care for client with a history of anxiety disorder who is admitted for pneumonia. What would be the priority goal for the care plan?
   1. ⊙ Client will participate in care planning.
   2. Anxiety levels will be managed. *This is not a client-centered goal.*
   3. Client will be compliant with treatment plan. *To help relieve the client's anxiety, the client needs to be involved in the plan of care.*
   4. Anti-anxiety medications will be administered as needed. *This is an intervention, not a goal.*

   Rationale: Whenever possible, encourage the client to participate actively in planning care. Participating in decision making can help to control anxiety and increases the potential for positive outcomes.

   THIN Thinking: Nursing Process – *Establishing client-centered goals that are obtainable needs to include the client in the process.* **NCLEX®:** Management of Care **QSEN:** Patient-centered Care

10. The nurse has completed the admission assessment of a client with a diagnosis of acute bipolar disorder. Based on the assessment, what is the priority focus for the nursing plan of care?
    1. Control the client's hyperactivity. *The nurse does not focus on controlling the hyperactivity, but rather maintaining safety.*
    2. Monitor relevant lab values. *This is important but not as important as maintaining hydration and nutrition.*
    3. ⊙ Hydration and nutrition.
    4. Client teaching. *Teaching may not be appropriate during an acute episode.*

    Rationale: During the acute phase of a bipolar episode the priority outcomes should focus on both the physiologic and psychologic aspects of care. Priority issues to reduce risk of physiologic complications is maintaining adequate hydration and nutrition. The priority psychologic focus is on keeping the client safe from harm.

    THIN Thinking: Top Three – *Hydration and nutrition are concerns during an acute bipolar phase. Both hyperactivity and depression will impact hydration and nutrition.* **NCLEX®:** Basic Care and Comfort **QSEN:** Patient-centered Care

11. The nurse is meeting with the interdisciplinary team to discuss the care plan for a client with a diagnosis of depression. What statement by the nurse indicates that the care needs to be re-evaluated?
    1. "We have been letting the client make decisions about activities of daily living." *This is a positive statement and encouraged.*
    2. ⊙ "The client has lost another 2 pounds and reports being constipated."
    3. "The family says that the client is more talkative when they come to visit." *This is a positive statement and encouraging.*
    4. "Antidepressant medications were started 10 days ago but no apparent effect." *It will take longer for antidepressant medications to take effect.*

    Rationale: When implementing care for a client with depression it is important to be aware of vegetative signs of depression such as lack of appetite. Changes in bowel habits are common and constipation is often a result of psychomotor retardation with depression. Antidepressant medications can take 2 – 3 weeks to reach an effective blood level.

    THIN Thinking: Nursing Process – *Evaluation of client statements and family interactions will help the nurse to recognize if the current treatment plan needs revision.* **NCLEX®:** Basic Care and Comfort **QSEN:** Teamwork and Collaboration

12. The nurse is instructing an unlicensed assistive personnel (UAP) who will be caring for a client with a diagnosis of schizophrenia. The UAP has asked how to deal with the client who reports hearing voices. What is the appropriate response by the nurse?
    1. "Just ignore the client's report of hearing voices." *Doing this can put client in danger.*
    2. "Tell the client that the voices are just in his head." *This prevents client from sharing information.*
    3. "Distract the client by changing the subject." *This prevents client from sharing information.*
    4. ⊙ "Ask the client what the voices are saying."

    Rationale: It is important to assess the content of the client's hallucinations to determine if there is the potential for the client to harm him/herself or if they feel in danger. Do not discount the hallucination but acknowledge that they are very real to the client while conveying empathy and telling the client you do not hear the voices.

    THIN Thinking: Nursing Process – *The nurse needs to identify the most important interventions that will assist in the care of clients with mental health issues.* **NCLEX®:** Psychosocial Integrity **QSEN:** Teamwork and Collaboration

13. **The nurse is preparing a presentation for a senior citizens group regarding the increased suicide rates among the elderly. What is the priority content the nurse should include?**
    1. Statistics about the increased incidence of suicide among the elderly. *This may be helpful but isn't as important as sharing means of identifying suicide risk.*
    2. Risk factors that increase the potential for suicide among the elderly. *This is helpful, but not as important as information on identifying suicide risk behaviors.*
    3. 💡 Behaviors and/or comments from peers indicating potential suicide risk.
    4. Overview of methods used for suicide among the elderly. *This can be important but not the priority information.*

    Rationale: Identification and suicide risk is the key to suicide prevention. Informing senior citizens regarding behaviors to be alert for can be the first step in getting help for an elderly person who is depressed and considering suicide.

    THIN Thinking: Help Quick – *The highest priority to prevent suicide would be early identification of behaviors by peers. Knowing the statistics will not prevent it from occurring.* **NCLEX®:** Safety and Infection Control **QSEN:** Safety

14. **The clinic nurse has completed teaching for a client who frequently hyperventilates in response to anxiety. What statement by the client indicates teaching was effective?**
    1. "I just need to learn to get over my anxiety and forget about it." *Does not indicate an effective coping mechanism.*
    2. 💡 "I should try taking deep breaths when I feel my anxiety going up."
    3. "As long as I keep taking my antianxiety meds I don't need to worry." *Does not indicate an understanding of how to deal with hyperventilation.*
    4. "I will just try to avoid anything that makes me anxious." *May be impossible to avoid all causes of anxiety.*

    Rationale: Teaching the client relaxation techniques such as deep breathing can be a first defense against rising anxiety. Also teaching the client alternate coping skills when their anxiety level continues to escalate can be an effective strategy to improve the client's quality of life.

    THIN Thinking: Help Quick – *Relaxation techniques and deep, slow breaths can help to calm the client during an anxiety attack.* **NCLEX®:** Psychosocial Integrity **QSEN:** Patient-centered Care

15. **The nurse is implementing the plan of care for a client with a diagnosis of depression. What nursing actions are included in the plan? Select all that apply.**
    1. 💡 Offer small, high caloric or high protein snacks during the day.
    2. Encourage the client to limit activities to conserve energy. *Activity is shown to benefit the client with depression.*
    3. 💡 Encourage the client to get dressed and stay out of bed during the day.
    4. 💡 Provide reminders regarding self-care and hygiene as needed.
    5. Encourage client to avoid intake of fluid in the evening. *This would have no effect on the client's depression.*

    Rationale: Anorexia and lack of interest in food is a common symptom of depression. Therefore, encouraging small (not overwhelming) high calorie or high protein snacks is a strategy to boost the client's nutritional intake. Encouraging the client to get dressed and stay out of bed during the day minimizes sleeping during the day to increase the likelihood of sleeping at night.

    THIN Thinking: Nursing Process – *Identification of beneficial interventions is important to the development of the plan of care.* **NCLEX®:** Psychosocial Integrity **QSEN:** Patient-centered Care

16. **The nurse is assessing a client with a diagnosis of bipolar disorder in the manic phase. What assessment findings could pose an immediate safety concern? Select all that apply.**
    1. 💡 Distraction by environmental events.
    2. 💡 Purposeless movements.
    3. Inflated sense of self-importance. *Typically does not cause an immediate safety risk.*
    4. 💡 Risky, impulsive behavior.
    5. Non-compliance with medications. *This is a concern but doesn't cause an immediate safety risk during a manic phase.*

    Rationale: Clients experiencing the manic phase of bipolar disorder often perform meaningless movements and are easily distracted which could pose safety concerns on the unit. Also, they are prone to risky, impulsive behaviors not considering any potential safety risks linked to those behaviors. An inflated sense of importance and non-compliance with medications are also nursing concerns but they typically do not pose a safety risk.

THIN Thinking: Identify Risk to Safety – *The client experiencing the manic phase of bipolar disorder is at risk for injuring self and others. The nurse needs to identify immediate safety concerns and keep the client safe.* **NCLEX®:** Safety and Infection Control **QSEN:** Safety

17. **The nurse caring for a client with a diagnosis of schizophrenia is reviewing the care plan. What nursing actions would the nurse anticipate implementing? Select all that apply.**
    1. 🔵 Assess the client's contact with reality as needed.
    2. 🔵 Implement a planned schedule and set limits as needed.
    3. Encourage the client to independently make decisions. *This client is incapable of making decisions independently.*
    4. 🔵 Monitor food and fluid intake.
    5. 🔵 Focus on reality-based here and now activities.

    Rationale: The nurse needs to assess the client's contact with reality to determine whether they are experiencing hallucinations and/or delusions. Encouraging a planned schedule and setting limits can help the client feel safe and secure. If the client is psychotic, food and fluid intake may not be of concern to them or may be incorporated in their delusions such as thinking the food is poisoned. Therefore, the nurse needs to monitor food and fluid intake to make sure the client has adequate nutrition. Focusing on reality-based, here and now activities can distract the client from hallucinations and/or delusions.

    THIN Thinking: Nursing Process – *The nurse needs to understand appropriate interventions for the client with schizophrenia.* **NCLEX®:** Psychosocial Integrity **QSEN:** Patient-centered Care

18. **The clinic nurse is assessing a client with chronic obstructive pulmonary disease (COPD) and moderate anxiety. In what order should the nurse collect assessment data? Rank order the responses.**
    1. Review the medical record for history and prescriptions.
    2. Encourage the client to report their symptoms.
    3. Ask meaningful questions to elicit information.
    4. Assess vital signs and compliance with prescriptions.
    5. Conduct a respiratory assessment to compare with history.

    Rationale: Review the medical record in advance to understand the client's history and prescriptions. The client is the expert on their experience and allowing them to tell their story will help to build trust. The assessment should be meaningful and client-centered, therefore, asking meaningful questions will decrease anxiety. Client with anxiety often experiences increased anxiety with physical contact. Therefore, assessing vital signs is less invasive than a respiratory assessment.

THIN Thinking: Top Three – *With the history of anxiety, the assessment will be performed to meet the needs of the client and to minimize anxiety. There is no indication that the client is in distress so physiological needs are not the priority.* **NCLEX®:** Physiological Adaptation **QSEN:** Patient-centered Care

19. **The school nurse is planning a meeting with parents to talk about the risk of depression among teenagers. What risk factors will the nurse include? Select all that apply.**
    1. 🔵 Hormonal changes.
    2. Being on the honor roll. *This is not a risk factor for depression.*
    3. 🔵 Cyberbullying.
    4. 🔵 Loss of a significant other.
    5. 🔵 Peer relationships.

    Rationale: Depression can occur at any point across the lifespan. Teenagers are experiencing hormonal changes as well as stress in their environment, such as peer relationships and bullying, that can result in depression. Loss of a significant other whether it is a parent, grandparent or a peer can lead to depression.

    THIN Thinking: Nursing Process – *When planning a teaching session, it is important to understand the risk factors associated with a condition and share that as a part of the teaching session.* **NCLEX®:** Reduction of Risk **QSEN:** Patient-centered Care

20. **The nurse is reviewing the medication administration record in the electronic health record for a client with Bipolar Disorder and reviews the prescription for lithium carbonate. The client preferred the elixir and is ordered 450 mg/four times/day and it is available 300 mg/5 mL. How many mL. would the client receive in one 24-hour period?**

    Answer: 30 mL.

    Rationale: Each dose = 450 mg which = 7.5 mL. 7.5 mL is to be administered four times/day for a total of 30 mL.

    THIN Thinking: Identify Risk to Safety – *In order to safely administer medications, the nurse must perform accurate calculations.* **NCLEX®:** Pharmacological and Parenteral Therapies **QSEN:** Safety

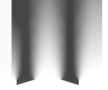

21. **The nurse is discussing advanced directives with a client and his family. The family questions what it means for the client to be competent and make personal decisions. What would be the nurse's best response?**
    1. 🔘 "When he is able to understand risks and benefits of the decisions being made."
    2. "When he's able to legibly sign the forms." *Does not reflect cognitive ability.*
    3. "When he is oriented to person, place and time." *Person can be oriented to person place and time and still be unable to make sound decisions.*
    4. "When he is able to physically take care of himself." *Being able to perform ADLs does not mean the client can cognitively make sound decisions.*

    Rationale: The client must be able to understand the benefits, risk, and implications of decisions in order to be considered competent. In order for the advanced directive to be used, the client must be declared mentally incompetent, or lacking capacity to make decisions.

    THIN Thinking: Nursing Process – *The nurse needs a clear understanding of the circumstances when explaining advanced directives to the client and family.* **NCLEX**®: Management of Care - **QSEN:** Patient-centered Care

22. **A client reports difficulty sleeping and a "pounding heart." There are no abnormal findings on the physical examination. Further assessment reveals that the client is worried about being successful on a new job that he just started. What is an appropriate nursing response to this finding?**
    1. "Counseling could be of much benefit to you right now." *This does not indicate that the nurse is trying to help the client.*
    2. 🔘 "It seems that your concern right now is about whether you can do your job."
    3. "Have you spoken with any of your family members about what concerns you?" *Does not demonstrate that the nurse is being an attentive listener.*
    4. "Anxiety is very normal whenever someone starts a job for the first time." *This statement shuts down communication.*

    Rationale: The answer conveys listening and being attentive to the client's concerns. Using reflection ensures that the client knows their thoughts are received and accepted and builds a foundation for ongoing conversation.

    THIN Thinking: Top Three – *Therapeutic communication needs to be empathetic, caring, and with open-ended questions that encourage further communication.* **NCLEX**®: Psychosocial Integrity **QSEN:** Patient-centered of Care

23. **The nurse is assessing a client at the clinic. The client reports that the loss of her husband two months ago has made her anxious about life. The client reports "I really can't go on living this way." Which would be the most therapeutic response by the nurse?**
    1. "That is a very common feeling and it will pass in time." *This statement shuts down communication.*
    2. 🔘 "Tell me about your anxiety and how you are feeling."
    3. "Did your husband leave you in debt? Is that why you are anxious?" *This is jumping to conclusions.*
    4. "You should speak to your doctor about your feelings." *This statement shuts down communication.*

    Rationale: The answer conveys listening and being attentive to the client's concerns while validating that the nurse wants to assist. The word "tell" opens up the client, allowing the client to take initiative in the conversation and emphasizes the importance of client perceptions.

    THIN Thinking: Nursing Process – *The nurse needs to identify and use a therapeutic, empathetic, and caring response to clients.* **NCLEX**®: Psychosocial Integrity **QSEN:** Patient-centered Care

24. **The nurse is caring for a client at the inpatient psychiatric unit. The client tells the nurse that someone is poisoning the food and drink here and they will not eat or drink anything. What therapeutic response from the nurse would help the client?**
    1. "I eat the same food and I am not poisoned." *This response is based on logic, and client is not thinking logically.*
    2. "The food is approved by the health department so it is fine." *Does not address client's concern.*
    3. 🔘 "Tell me why you feel someone is poisoning you."
    4. "All the clients eat the same food here." *Does not address client's concern.*

    Rationale: This answer invites the client to open up to the nurse and express their feelings about why they feel the food and drink is poisoning them. It conveys acceptance of the client perceptions and encourages them to share components of the hallucination, but does not reinforce the reality of the sensory experience.

    THIN Thinking: Nursing Process – *The nurse should not argue or disagree with the client's statements but allow them to verbalize more of what they are feeling.* **NCLEX**®: Psychosocial Integrity **QSEN:** Patient-centered Care

25. The nurse interviews a family member after the loss of a loved one from a myocardial infarction. The family member states their loved one never took care of themselves. The nurse identifies the family member to be in what stage of the grief process?
   1. Depression. *Client's in this stage are sad and feel hopeless.*
   2. Denial. *Client's in this stage do not believe the loss occurred.*
   3. Bargaining. *Client's in this phase try to find a way to change the loss.*
   4. 🔘 Anger.

   Rationale: This is the correct answer as the family member is eluding to the fact that maybe if the loved one took better care of themselves they would still be alive. The family member is expressing anger regarding the loved one's behavior. The anger phase is characterized by self-blame and blame of others.

   THIN Thinking: Nursing Process – *Assessment of the stages of grief can allow the nurse to create a more effective plan of care.* **NCLEX**®: Psychosocial Integrity **QSEN:** Patient-centered Care

26. A nurse is approached by a family member about their loved one's roommate. The family member wants to know the roommate's diagnosis and if they may be potentially violent. Which is the best response by the nurse?
   1. "Don't worry, we don't have violent people on this unit." *No information should be shared.*
   2. 🔘 "I cannot discuss another client with you."
   3. "I will watch out for your family member." *Implies the roommate is violent and doesn't instruct family on importance of HIPAA.*
   4. "Perhaps you should voice your concerns with administration." *Does not instruct family on importance of HIPAA.*

   Rationale: HIPAA indicates that no information can be shared with other clients, other client's family members, or other members of the health care team who are not involved in the client's care.

   THIN Thinking: Top Three – *Confidentiality of health information is the top priority when dealing with clients in the health care setting.* **NCLEX**®: Management of Care **QSEN:** Patient-centered Care

27. The nurse is caring for a client who expressed thoughts of suicide. Which is the best response by the nurse?
   1. Report this to the family so the client can go home. *Client needs one-on-one observation in health care setting.*
   2. Place the client in a locked room by himself. *This alone would not address safety needs.*
   3. Place the client on the locked unit with other clients. *This alone would not address safety issues.*
   4. 🔘 Ensure that the client is on one-on-one surveillance.

   Rationale: Suicidal ideations warrant that suicide precautions be implemented, including taking away potentially dangerous items (belts, utensils, writing implements), placing on heightened surveillance, including one-on-one observations, and encouraging visitors to monitor what is brought into the room. A prevention of suicide contract may be indicated.

   THIN Thinking: Identify Risk for Safety – *When a client voices thoughts of suicide ideation, the top concern is to not leave the client alone. They should be under constant observation by a health care employee.* **NCLEX**®: Management of Care **QSEN:** Patient-centered Care

28. The nurse is providing education information to the client regarding the risperidone the healthcare prescribed. What statement by the client demonstrates a good understanding of teaching?
   1. "I can stop taking the medication when I feel better." *Client needs to take medication as prescribed.*
   2. 🔘 "I may have a dry mouth while on this medication."
   3. "I will no longer have symptoms while on this medication." *Client may still have some symptoms while on this medication.*
   4. "I need to eat a lot of salt and drink lots of water when on this medication." *This is not required for this medication.*

   Rationale: Risperidone is an antipsychotic that elicits anti-cholinergic side effects, including dry mouth, urinary retention, and constipation. It may not relieve all symptoms and may need to be continued to control psychotic symptoms. Salt and water are indicated for lithium.

   THIN Thinking: Nursing Process – *Teaching clients about medications, including side effects, is an important nursing intervention.* **NCLEX**®: Pharmacological and Parenteral Therapies **QSEN:** Patient-centered Care

29. The healthcare provider prescribed fluphenazine for a client diagnosed with psychosis. The prescribed dose is 10 mg/daily. The nurse has fluphenazine 2.5 mg on the unit. How many pills should the nurse administer?
   1. 2 pills.
   2. 3 pills.
   3. ⦿ 4 pills.
   4. 5 pills.

   Rationale: Fluphenazine is an antipsychotic. 2.5 X 4 = 10 mg.

   THIN Thinking: Identify Risk for Safety – *The nurse must safely calculate medication dosing in order not to commit medication errors.* **NCLEX®**: Pharmacological and Parenteral Therapies **QSEN:** Safety

30. The nurse is counseling a client at the clinic. The client states they experience panic attacks at work and they don't know what to do. What is the nurse's best response?
   1. "Medications are the most effective treatment for panic attacks." *Behavioral techniques are often more effective in managing panic attacks.*
   2. "Try to ignore the panic attacks and they may become less often." *Ignoring will not make a panic attack go away.*
   3. "It is best for you to go home and rest during your panic attacks." *This may not be a safe or feasible option.*
   4. ⦿ "Let's talk about suggestions to help you cope better with the panic attacks."

   Rationale: Panic attacks are temporary disruptions in coping. The nurse should calmly discuss coping options with the client, such as deep breathing, meditation, exercise, or prayer. In severe panic attacks, medications may be indicated but coping strategies are explored first.

   THIN Thinking: Nursing Process – *Creating a plan and discussing coping mechanisms is beneficial to achieving a positive outcome.* **NCLEX®**: Psychosocial Integrity **QSEN:** Patient-centered Care

Cognition

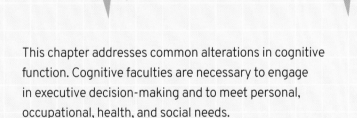

This chapter addresses common alterations in cognitive function. Cognitive faculties are necessary to engage in executive decision-making and to meet personal, occupational, health, and social needs.

Nurses provide care to clients that suffer cognitive issues which are reversible or irreversible, progressive or temporary, represent a wide range of cognitive abilities and disabilities, and may occur in clients across the lifespan.

Re-orientation therapy for clients with advanced dementia/Alzheimer's disease is controversial because of short-term memory deficits in the presence of intact long-term crystallized memories. Recent events as part of fluid memories are fragile and difficult to retrieve for clients with dementia.

Research demonstrates that attempting to reorient the client to the present may add to the client's frustration and poor self-esteem. Validation therapy allows client to "live in" the time they are remembering and validates the client's currently perceived emotions and feelings. Nurses should not argue or try to reorient the client but allow the client to be comfortable in their memories. What a great example of client-centered, evidence-based practice!

Priority Exemplars:

> Delirium
> Dementia/Alzheimer's disease
> Autism
> Attention-deficit/hyperactivity disorder

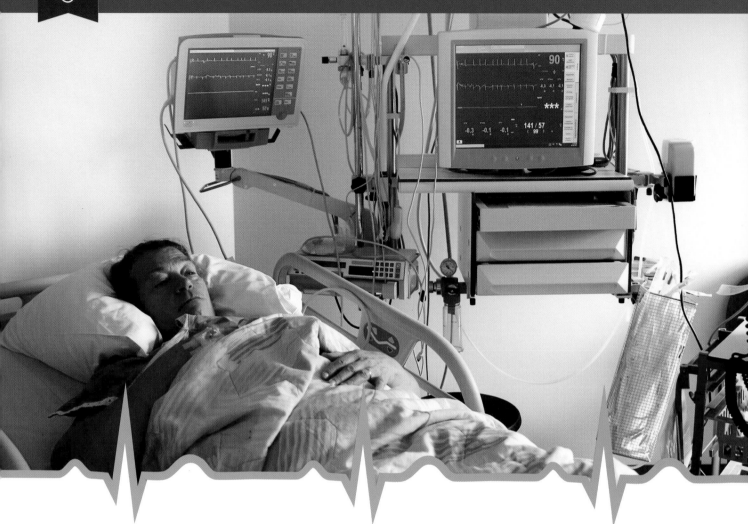

Go To Clinical Case 1

G.R. is a 53-year-old client in the surgical intensive care unit. G.R. sustained a traumatic brain injury in a motor vehicle accident. G.R. is operated on to evacuate a large intracranial hematoma. Following return from the operating room, G.R. is extubated and slowly regains consciousness. On post-op day 3 G.R. remains disoriented, agitated, and restless. He became combative and is hallucinating about people coming into his room and touching him and his medical equipment.

The client has sustained high blood pressure well above his baseline since the accident. His wife and children are at his bedside. Although the family received reassurance that the client's deficits were thought to be temporary and the client is anticipated to sustain a full recovery, they are confused and angered by his slow recovery and behavior. G.R. is slowly able to communicate some of his needs but often becomes agitated when trying to communicate. Each day G.R. makes slow progress and once his blood pressure is under control, discharge to a rehabilitation facility is anticipated.

NurseThink® Time

Using the NurseThink® system, complete the priorities. Check your answers designated by 💡 in the Delirium Priority Exemplar.

NurseThink® Time

✏️ Priority Assessments or Cues

1.

2.

3.

🧪 Priority Laboratory Tests/Diagnostics

1.

2.

3.

⚠️ Priority Interventions or Actions

1.

2.

3.

🚩 Priority Potential & Actual Complications

1.

2.

3.

🩺 Priority Nursing Implications

1.

2.

3.

💧 Priority Medications

1.

2.

3.

👤 Priority Education/Discharge Issues

1.

2.

3.

Delirium

Pathophysiology/Description

> Changes in cognitive function, awareness, and ability to attend to stimuli. Occurs rapidly over a short period

> Cognitive impairment is manifested by changes in attention span, speech patterns, orientation, and decision-making

> Most often in older adults or those with serious illnesses

> May have hallucinations (false, sensory experiences) and illusions (misperceptions of environment)

> Symptoms may present immediately after the precursor (head injury, seizure) or more slowly (if related to electrolyte imbalance or medical condition)

> Causes and related factors include infections, seizures, electrolyte imbalances, hypercarbia, hypoxia, pain, hypoglycemia, and experiences of social isolation. Clients with a history of stroke, burns, migraine headaches, nutritional deficiencies (thiamine), hepatic or renal failure, a brain tumor, heat stroke, head trauma, or having surgery may also be at risk

> Other etiologies include:
  - Substance intoxication delirium
  - Substance withdrawal delirium
  - Medication-induced delirium
  - Delirium due to another medical condition

Priority Assessments or Cues

> Observe vital signs for elevated heart rate and hypotension

> Assess for distractibility, lack of ability to attend to conversations, restlessness

> Assess speech patterns. Verbalizations may be rambling, pressured, incoherent, or irrelevant. Client may change topics frequently

> Assess level of orientation. Clients may be disoriented to time and place and lacking in short-term memory

> Assess sleep patterns, client may have distorted sleep, wakefulness, insomnia, day sleeping, hypersomnia, ask about dreams and nightmares

> Assess for changes in state of awareness. Client may rapidly progress from hypervigilance to stupor to coma

> Observe physical behavior for restlessness, hyperactivity, hitting, tremoring, agitation, appearing to pick/pinch at air with fingers or punch objects that are not real; may also become stuporous

> Assess emotional stability. Client may be fearful, anxious, depressed, irritable, angry, euphoric, and lacking in response. Observe for crying, laughter, calling for help, muttering, moaning, violent acts against self or others, cursing, and trying to flee agency

> Observe physical signs including diaphoresis, facial flushing, dilated pupils

> Assess safety risks and potential for injury for self and others

Priority Laboratory Tests/Diagnostics

> Monitor serum electrolyte levels for abnormalities that may cause delirium

> Monitor blood glucose level

> Arterial blood gases for oxygenation and ventilation

> Assess for sexually transmitted infections and HIV as indicated

> Assess for thyroid dysfunction, nutritional/Vitamin B12 deficiencies, and liver and renal function studies

> Implement drug/alcohol screens for new admissions

> Lumbar puncture to assess for infection

Priority Interventions or Actions

> Determine and manage the underlying cause

> Ensure that electrolytes, oxygenation, serum sodium levels, and blood glucose levels are within normal limits

> Maintain an environment of low stimulation

> Employ interventions to manage behaviors including distractibility

> Remain calm and assume an undemanding attitude.

> Engage client in anxiety-reducing behaviors, such as dance or movement therapy

> Assume physical care and feeding for client
  - Allow client to be as independent as possible, allowing time as needed
  - Provide a structured schedule recognizing the individual's routine
  - Frequently assess client's self-care abilities. Ensure that clients have eyeglasses and hearing aids, as indicated

> For clients who are disoriented
  - Introduce yourself by name and use the client's name with each interaction
  - Use touch when appropriate
  - Approach client from the front and use simple words or single questions
  - Use clocks and calendars
  - Provide signs on doors for separate rooms
  - Encourage use of personal items, a favorite chair, and pictures
  - Encourage visits from loved ones and friends, when appropriate
  - Encourage television, radio, and other diversions
  - Provide reminiscence therapy with movies, pictures, and photo albums
  - Keep staffing consistent

> Ensure client is safe
  - Keep the bed in the lowest position and follow agency policy about side rails and bed alarm for safety
  - Consider putting the client in a bed closest to the nurses' station for safety and close observation
  - Consider one-on-one observation as needed
  - Pad head and foot boards as needed

Priority Potential & Actual Complications

- Potential for injury or safety threats to others
- Hazards of immobility associated with lack of movement/being bedridden
- Potential for malnutrition/dehydration/electrolyte imbalance

Priority Nursing Implications

- Monitor for side effects of new and previously taken medications
- Deal with complications of immobility including contractures, skin breakdown, constipation, depression, and pneumonia
- Instruct family on causes and management of delirium, may be very concerning due to rapid onset and troubling symptoms

Priority Medications

- haloperidol
  - Antipsychotic
  - To manage psychotic symptoms
  - Monitor cardiac status-may prolong QT intervals
- lorazepam
  - Anti-anxiety agent
  - For substance withdrawal and anxiety
  - Client may become physically dependent and tolerant

- melatonin
  - Homeopathic mood stabilizer
  - Available over-the-counter
  - May be combined with ramelteon (for insomnia)
  - Used to prevent and treat delirium
  - Additonal studies are needed to confirm this as an evidence-based practice

Priority Education/Discharge Issues

- Ensure that family understands progress of illness, safety interventions, and other treatments
- Ensure that family has support and means to share feelings and frustrations with the disease process
- Refer to community organizations for adult day care, respite services, and hospice services (when appropriate)
- > Evaluate family's ability to cope with delirium. This condition may be very frustrating due to the unpredictable nature and unknown outcome of delirium

Go To Clinical Answers

Text designated by 💡 are the top answers for the Go To Clinical related to Delirium.

Briefly review a couple of different resources on the differences and similarities between delirium, dementia, and depression. Complete this table to help you Save Time Studying.			
	DELIRIUM	**DEMENTIA**	**DEPRESSION**
Onset			
Duration			
Reversible			
Awareness			
Attention			
Hallucinations			
Memory			
Sleep			
Thoughts			

Table 17-1: Compare and Contrast

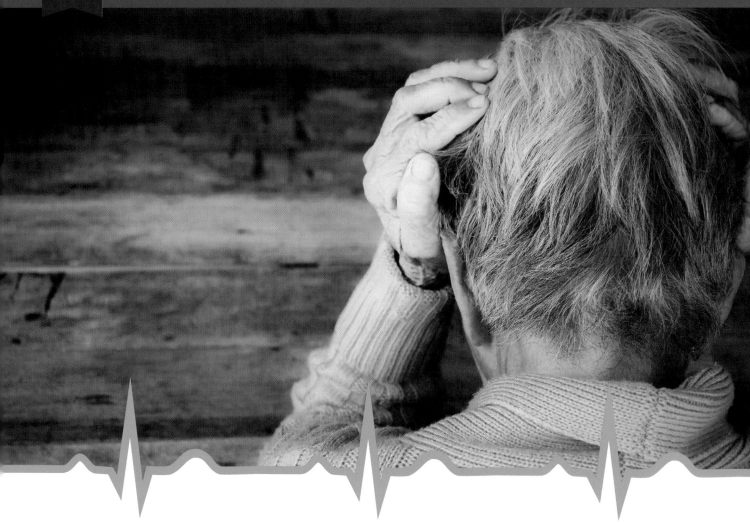

Go To Clinical Case 2

You are a nurse in a memory care unit of a continuing care facility. You are the case manager for H.F., an 81-year-old woman with Stage 5 Alzheimer's disease. The nursing staff are expressing several new care needs as part of H.F.'s care. She wanders frequently, usually during the nighttime hours and has begun to fall. She is restless when in her chair and the no-restraint policy of the agency precludes her from being restrained. H.F. refuses to sit still at the table and walks around during mealtimes. She has experienced weight loss and is dehydrated. She is incontinent of urine and stool and often pulls off the protective briefs. She has been fainting related to low blood glucose and orthostatic hypotension.

As you are working during a night shift, you find H.F. leaning on the wall in the hallway outside her room.

You escort her to the nearest chair and obtain a set of vital signs. They are 98.5°F—124-26-96/62.

NurseThink® Time

Using the NurseThink® system, complete the priorities. Check your answers designated by 💡 in the Dementia/ Alzheimer's disease Priority Exemplar.

Next Gen Clinical Judgment

The increasing incidence of Alzheimer's Disease has been widely studied. What do you think contributes to the increased incidence of this difficult disease? What influence does the growing life expectancy have on this increased prevalence?

✏ Priority Assessments or Cues

1.

2.

3.

⚗ Priority Laboratory Tests/Diagnostics

1.

2.

3.

⚠ Priority Interventions or Actions

1.

2.

3.

⚑ Priority Potential & Actual Complications

1.

2.

3.

☿ Priority Nursing Implications

1.

2.

3.

◗ Priority Medications

1.

2.

3.

👤 Priority Education/Discharge Issues

1.

2.

3.

Dementia/Alzheimer's disease

Pathophysiology/Description

> Dementia is the insidious and progressive decline in cognitive capacity and function while the client is conscious, these changes cause social and occupational dysfunction

> Categorized as neurocognitive disorders and classified based on severity of symptoms

- Major Neurocognitive Disorder
  - Previously described as dementia
  - Significant decline in cognitive function
  - Conflict with ADLs and IADLs
- Minor Neurocognitive Disorder
  - Mild cognitive impairment from previous level of functioning
  - May be responsive to early intervention
  - Still able to complete ADLs and IADLs but may employ compensatory mechanisms (writing lists, accommodations, or increased effort)
- If disease is progressive, minor may precede major

> Causes/Associated pathologies including Alzheimer's disease (AD), Huntington's disease, Parkinson's disease, HIV, substance/medication use, traumatic brain injury, vascular disease, Lewy body disease, frontotemporal lobar degeneration, or Prion disease

> May also be primary (such as AD) or secondary (to another disease or cause)

> Alzheimer's increase in incidence associated with increased life expectancy

> Stages of Alzheimer's Disease

- Stage 1—no apparent symptoms-changes in brain function
- Stage 2—forgetfulness-lose things or forget names
- Stage 3—mild cognitive decline-interference with work, getting lost
- Stage 4—mild to moderate cognitive decline-forgetfulness, depression, withdrawal, confabulation (making up stories to cover up memory loss)
- Stage 5—moderate cognitive decline-lose ability to perform ADLs, disoriented
- Stage 6—moderate to severe decline-disoriented, unable to do ADLs, sleeping problems, sundowners (agitation at nighttime), unable to communicate, institutionalization
- Stage 7—severe cognitive decline-bedfast, aphasia, deteriorated cognitive function

Priority Assessments or Cues

- Administer standardized cognitive assessment tests
> Assess for changes in personal hygiene habits/ability to accomplish ADLs
> Assess for changes in judgment, abstract thinking, and impulse control

> Assess speech and language-difficulty labeling objects, aphasia (inability to talk)

> Inquire of family members about personality changes, reports of wandering, changes in cognitive function, orientation, language difficulties, social issues

- Assess nutritional and hydration status
  - Ability to swallow
  - Ability to coordinate eating functions
  - Toleration of feedings
  - Measures of hydration including skin turgor, intake and output, mucous membranes, weight

> Determine history of drug or alcohol use

> Assess for signs of potential abuse or neglect

> Assess ability to move, risk for wandering, or for apraxia (inability to initiate motor function). Assess pain level

> Assess for incontinence/skin integrity

> Assess potential for injury, self-harm, and falls

Priority Laboratory Tests/Diagnostics

- Monitor serum electrolyte levels for abnormalities
- Serum albumin to assess nutritional status
- Urine specific gravity for hydration status
> Monitor blood glucose level
> Assess for sexually transmitted infections and HIV as indicated
> Assess for thyroid dysfunction, nutritional/Vitamin B12 deficiencies, and liver and renal function studies
> Implement drug/alcohol screens for new admissions
> Lumbar puncture to assess for infection
> CT scanning and MRI to assess for atrophy
> Positron emission tomography (PET)-assess metabolic activity of brain

Priority Interventions or Actions

> Determine and manage the underlying cause and assess reversibility of potential causes

> Ensure that electrolytes, oxygenation, and blood glucose levels are within normal limits

- Provide nutritional interventions
  - Encourage favorite foods
  - Provide finger foods and easy-to-eat foods when agitated
  - Thicken liquids as tolerated
    - Ascertain client's wishes about tube feedings/potential for nasogastric or percutaneous endoscopic gastrostomy (PEG) tube feedings/hydration

> Gradually assume more physical care and feeding for client as condition deteriorates
  - Allow client to remain as independent as possible, allowing time as needed

- Provide a structured schedule recognizing the individual's routine
- Frequently assess client's self-care abilities

- Prevent injury
  - Ensure the client's environment is arranged for convenience and safety
  - Keep highly used items close to the client, including call light
  - Keep the bed in the lowest position or place a mattress on the floor and follow agency policy about side rails for safety. Pad head and foot boards as needed.
  - Ensure client is supervised with ambulation, apply a bed alarm if appropriate
  - Move client to a room easily observed by nursing staff
  - Ensure nightlights are used
  - Consider use of soft restraints if indicated

- Re-orient client
  - Introduce yourself by name and use the client's name with each interaction
  - Use touch when appropriate
  - Approach client from the front and use simple words or single questions
  - Use clocks and calendars
  - Provide signs on rooms as indicated
  - Encourage use of personal items, a favorite chair, and pictures
  - Encourage visits from loved ones and friends, when appropriate
  - Encourage television, radio, and other diversions
  - Provide reminiscence therapy with movies, pictures, and photo albums
  - Keep staffing consistent

- Keep client safe when wandering
  - Maintain a structured time schedule for sleeping, meals, toileting, and hygiene
  - Provide a safe location to allow for pacing and wandering
  - When wanderer is a distance from the unit, walk with the client for a while and then redirect back to the unit
  - Ensure locking and alarm systems are in place

- If client has delusions and/or hallucinations
  - Do not reinforce or discuss false beliefs or experiences
  - Reinforce client safety
  - Change the subject or distract to another activity
  - Lavender oil may reduce anxiety and promote sleep

Priority Potential & Actual Complications

- Potential for hazards of immobility
- Malnutrition
- Dehydration
- May be fatal when confronted with potential co-morbidities

Priority Nursing Implications

- Falls are prime risk as motor function deteriorates
- Ensure hearing aids and eyeglasses are at optimal functioning
- Some research indicates that use of ginkgo (an herbal supplement) may delay loss of memory
- Ensure that medications are reviewed for polypharmacy noting potential drug interactions and side effects

Priority Medications

- rivastigmine
  - Off-label use of antipsychotics to manage behavioral symptoms
  - Decrease memory loss
  - Slows disease progress, does not cure or stop the disease
- memantine
  - Improve cognitive function
  - Increases ability to conduct ADLs
- risperidone
  - To treat psychotic symptoms
  - Black box warning-associated with cardiac deaths in elder adults
- paroxetine
  - SSRI
  - First line treatment for depression
  - Older adults should be assessed for hyponatremia
- lorazepam
  - Anti-anxiety agent
  - Anxiety associated with loss of cognitive functioning
  - Shorter half-life anti-anxiety agents preferable with the elderly
- zolpidem
  - Hypnotic
  - To enhance sleep
  - Watch for daytime sleeping, increased risk for falls, cognitive impairment, and paradoxical effects

Priority Education/Discharge Issues

- Ensure that family understands progress of illness, safety interventions, and other treatments
- Ensure that family has support and means to share feelings and frustrations with the disease process
- Refer to community organizations for adult day care, respite services, disease-specific information, and hospice services (when appropriate)

Go To Clinical Answers

Text designated by 💡 are the top answers for the Go To Clinical related to Dementia/Alzheimer's disease.

Autism spectrum disorders (ASD)

📋 Pathophysiology/Description

> A varied set of neurodevelopmental syndromes characterized by a wide range of communication impairments, social withdrawal, lack of social interaction, and repetitive/unusual physical behaviors. May cause significant social impairment

> The spectrum includes autistic disorder, Rett syndrome, childhood disintegrative disorder, pervasive developmental disorder, and Asperger's disorder

> May be associated with other conditions including epilepsy, genetic disorders, and intellectual disabilities

> Incidence in the US is increasing. It is five times more common in males, ½ have average or above average intelligence

> Diagnosed early in childhood with chronic symptoms persisting into adulthood

> Etiology unknown, may have genetic and perinatal causal influences

✏️ Priority Assessments or Cues

> Assessment depends upon where client is on the spectrum and level of functionality

> Assess eye contact, social interactions, interest in others, capacity to imitate others, demonstration and receipt of affection, attachment, and intro/extroversion

> Assess ability to empathize and process feelings of others, ability to hold a reciprocal conversation, verbal/non-verbal skills or echolalia, for idiosyncratic utterances or monotone speech, presence of facial expressions/gestures, lack of response to or overreaction to noise/sounds/stimuli

> Assess imaginative activity and ability/capacity to play alone and with others and for friendships, assess for internal imaginative play

> Assess intelligence and age-appropriate development (accelerated, delayed, or on par)

> Assess restricted/stereotyped physical activities/interests including response to stimuli, irritability, compulsivity, fascination with objects, repetitive body movements (clapping, banging, rocking), self-injurious behaviors, restricted food choices/acceptance of foods, repetitive verbalizations, and need for strict routine and sameness of surroundings

🧪 Priority Laboratory Tests/Diagnostics

> Diagnosed based on symptoms and reports of child, family, and others

> Early diagnosis increases effectiveness of interventions

> Diagnostic tests for potential co-morbidities (epilepsy)

⚠️ Priority Interventions or Actions

> Ensure safety related to high levels of physical activity without cognitive controls

> Create a safe, consistent environment for learning and play. Use safety devices to protect from self-injury. Provide familiar foods, objects, and routines

> Support client's interactions with others

> Set realistic goals for success and provide clear, concrete instructions

> Form trusting relationships and ensure consistent caregivers/limit number of caregivers, convey acceptance, positive regard, and provide positive feedback/reinforce positive behaviors, eye contact, socially acceptable behavior, appropriate use of touch, and communication using the client's own methods of communicating

> Expose to group learning and play as tolerated

> Only touch client when they appear receptive, follow client cues for hugging, etc.

> Encourage self-care and capitalize on individual, personal strengths to meet future goals

🚩 Priority Potential & Actual Complications

> Potential exists for misdiagnosis and incorrect treatment

> Assumption of lower cognitive function related to communication impairment

⚕️ Priority Nursing Implications

> Provide support with symptoms of self-injury, aggression, hyperactivity, impulsivity, and temper tantrums

> Be aware of savants who may excel in music, art, puzzles/patterning, design, or memory

> Children with autism may seek healthcare related to other physical needs/diagnoses. Nurses need to be sensitive to and capable of working with clients with autism across the lifespan

💧 Priority Medications

> risperidone
  - Use for irritability controversial
  - Ages 5-15 years
  - Assess for neuroleptic malignant syndrome, tardive dyskinesia, and hyperglycemia/diabetes

> aripiprazole
  - Use for irritability controversial
  - Ages 6-17 years
  - May cause sedation, fatigue, weight gain, drooling, and tremoring

👤 Priority Education/Discharge Issues

> Complex care requires ongoing healthcare and behavioral surveillance and collaboration with the school, family, caregivers, and healthcare providers

> Support family and client as the child grows and needs change

> Reinforce principles of safety

> Refer client/family to community resources, schools, and respite services. Consider legal rights afforded to clients with disabilities during planning of care

Attention-deficit/hyperactivity disorder (ADHD)

📋 Pathophysiology/Description

> Characterized by behaviors of inattention and/or hyperactivity with impulsivity (may be mild to severe)

> Hyperactivity is defined as increased psychomotor activity, may or may not be purposeful, may include rapid physical movements and verbal activity. May be inattentive or highly distractible

> Impulsivity is defined as acting without reflection or thought to consequences, unable to resist acting

> Difficult to diagnose in children less than 4 years of age, most often recognized when child enters school

> More common in boys, prevalence about 10% (among children in the US)

> May persist into adolescence and adulthood

> May have genetic, biochemical, anatomical, psychosocial, environmental, and perinatal origins of causality

> May occur with co-morbidities such as disruptive mood dysregulation, sleep disorders, oppositional defiance disorder, bipolar disorder, conduct disorder, learning disorders, and anxiety

✏️ Priority Assessments or Cues

> Assessment includes observation of child and accessing history with family, teachers, and caregivers

> Often assessed using standardized psychiatric testing methods

> Assess ability to perform age-appropriate tasks, complete activities, and stay with activities until completed

> Assess ability to attend, length of attention span, ability to cooperate, ability to tolerate frustration, and level of distractibility

> Assess ability to form relationships with peers, siblings, and classmates

> Assess level of activity, including fidgeting with hands/ fingers, squirming in seat, or engagement in risky or dangerous behaviors

> Assess ability to hear and listen to others, assess for excessive talking or frequently using interruption to dominate conversation

⚗️ Priority Laboratory Tests/Diagnostics

> Diagnosed based on symptoms and reports of child, family, teachers, and others

> Early diagnosis increases effectiveness of interventions

> Diagnostic tests for potential co-morbidities (sleep disorders)

⚠️ Priority Interventions or Actions

> Ensure safety related to high levels of physical activity without cognitive controls

> Create a safe, consistent environment for learning and play. Consider distractibility and impulsivity

> Set realistic goals for success and provide clear, concrete instructions

> Encourage a highly nutritious diet, eat early in day to avoid impact of anorexia, and, although the role of sugar and caffeine in diet is unknown, these are limited in diet

> Reinforce the need for family/individual therapy along with medication management

> Form trusting relationships and ensure consistent caregivers, convey acceptance, positive regard, and provide positive feedback

> Develop a behavior plan with logical consequences for engagement in high-risk behaviors

> Expose to group learning and play as tolerated

🚩 Priority Potential & Actual Complications

> Potential exists for misdiagnosis and incorrect treatment

> Exacerbation of behavioral issues due to mismanagement

⚕️ Priority Nursing Implications

> Ensure that families understand the need for therapy along with medications such that children are managed as they grow and their needs change

> Children with ADHD may seek healthcare related to other physical needs/diagnoses. Nurses need to be sensitive to and capable of working with clients with ADHD

💧 Priority Medications

> dextroamphetamine/amphetamine
  - Stimulant that calms hyperactivity and increases attentiveness
  - High-risk for dependence
  - Appetite depressant-give early in day and monitor for weight loss
  - May cause hypertension-monitor blood pressure and avoid over-the-counter medications

> methylphenidate
  - Stimulant that calms hyperactivity and increases attentiveness
  - May disturb sleep so given in morning or at least 6 hours before bedtime (14 hours for extended-release)
  - Appetite depressant-give early in day and monitor for weight loss
  - May cause growth retardation such that clients are encouraged to take a "drug holiday" to allow for growth during summer or breaks from school

> bupropion
  - To manage depression and mood swings
  - May cause headache, sedation, and dizziness

👤 Priority Education/Discharge Issues

> Requires ongoing healthcare and behavioral surveillance and collaboration with the school, family, caregivers, and healthcare providers

1. A nurse is caring for a client who is at end-of-life. What assessment finding is consistent with delirium associated at the end-of-life?
   1. The client is oriented x 1 and sees bugs on the wall.
   2. The client's spouse states, "He seems so weak and tired now. He sleeps a lot."
   3. Cheyne-stokes respirations.
   4. Withdrawing from the physical environment but can still hear.

2. The nurse is assessing a client with a new prescription for antipsychotic medications focusing on the potential extrapyramidal side effects. What symptoms would the nurse expect to see if the client was experiencing extrapyramidal side effects?
   1. Restlessness, hypotension and headache.
   2. Stiffening of muscles and impaired gait.
   3. Lethargy, anorexia, and aphasia.
   4. Confusion, nausea and constipation.

3. The nurse is reviewing the medical record before starting to assess a client experiencing confusion. The medical record indicates that the client is experiencing apraxia. What behaviors will the nurse expect to find during the assessment?
   1. Inability to find the correct word when answering an assessment question.
   2. Irritability and inability to focus on the conversation during the assessment.
   3. Inability to perform routine, familiar tasks while the nurse is doing the assessment.
   4. Loss of orientation to person, place and time while able to converse.

4. The nurse is delegating care of a client with a diagnosis of dementia to an unlicensed assistive personnel (UAP). What instruction will facilitate the implementation of the plan of care?
   1. "Encourage the client to make decisions regarding when to complete activities of daily living."
   2. "Keep the client's routine as structured as possible to decrease the potential that the client will act out."
   3. "Discourage the family from bringing in more personal items as the client just gets more confused."
   4. "Introduce yourself and call the client by name even if you were only out of the room for a short time."

5. The home care nurse is doing a weekly visit to a client with Alzheimer's disease. What statement by the client would be of greatest concern?
   1. "When I go to the grocery store to get a few things, it takes me a really long time to get home."
   2. "My daughter organizes my medications and I have an alarm that goes off to let me know when to take them."
   3. "Sometimes when the phone rings I am not sure how to answer it so I just let it ring until it stops."
   4. "I thought you were going to come to see me last week but you didn't come until I called you today."

6. The nurse is teaching family members strategies for communicating with their loved one with dementia. What strategy should the nurse include?
   1. Speak slowly and loudly, repeating everything.
   2. Focus on one piece of information at a time.
   3. Talk to the person about the news to keep them oriented.
   4. Remove pictures that remind the client of the past.

7. The home care nurse is doing an initial assessment for a client with a diagnosis of Alzheimer's disease and congestive heart failure. What assessment findings indicate a potential risk to the client's safety? Select all that apply.
   1. Lives with daughter who works outside the home all day.
   2. Struggles with telling time on the large wall clock.
   3. Able to ambulate without assistive devices.
   4. Often disoriented to place and time.
   5. Has meals delivered when daughter is at work.

8. The nurse is instructing an unlicensed assistive personnel (UAP) regarding effective communication strategies when caring for a confused client. What strategies will the nurse encourage the UAP to implement? Select all that apply.
   1. Offer the client choices to maintain independent decision making.
   2. Identify yourself and call the client by name every time you enter the room.
   3. Refer to personal objects in the client's room such as pictures to start conversations.
   4. Encourage the client to tell you about happy times from their past.
   5. If the person becomes verbally agitated, leave the room and get the nurse.

9. The nurse is preparing to administer the prescribed 2 mg of haloperidol IM to an acutely psychotic adult client in the emergency department. The vial directions indicate 5 mg/mL. How much will the nurse draw up to administer the prescribed dose?

_____

10. The nurse for the evening shift has just arrived on the memory care unit. Based on the change of shift report about the clients assigned, how would the nurse prioritize the clients' safety needs? Rank Order the Responses.
    1. Elderly client who is quiet and stays in his room most of the day watching TV.
    2. Newly admitted client who wanders into other client's rooms.
    3. Client with early onset Alzheimer's disease who was admitted for assessment.
    4. Agitated client who has paranoid delusions and thinks she is being held prisoner.
    5. Confused client who keeps trying to leave the unit whenever the door is opened.

11. **The home care nurse is visiting a client with a history of confusion. The health care provider recently prescribed lorazepam to control the client's anxiety level at home. What statement by the client's family member indicates the prescription is effective?**
    1. "My dad is much calmer in the evening when he takes the lorazepam and he is able to get to sleep when he goes to bed."
    2. "My dad naps in the afternoons now rather than pacing but when I get home he seems to be confused about where I have been."
    3. "I am really afraid that my dad will become dependent on the lorazepam and not use his coping skills anymore."
    4. "I worry that my dad may get confused and not take the medications as prescribed and possibly overdose."

12. **When debriefing the nursing staff after a confused client has fallen, the nurse stresses the need for client safety. The nurse knows the staff understands safety when they make which statement?**
    1. The client should eat a balanced diet.
    2. The client should not receive pain medicine.
    3. The client should have all four side rails up at all times.
    4. The client should wear non-skid footwear when ambulating.

13. **The home health nurse is talking with a family of an elderly client. The client is experiencing episodes of confusion. What client behavior should the nurse educate the family to be observant for?**
    1. Repeating questions or statements.
    2. Getting up at night to urinate.
    3. Requesting the same foods for meals.
    4. Excessive irritability and violent behavior.

14. **The nurse is doing a home visit for a client diagnosed with moderate cognitive deficits secondary to dementia. The nurse stresses basic care and comfort of the client. What would be a priority action for the family when caring for the client?**
    1. Put the light on at night.
    2. Remove clutter from the rooms.
    3. Do not allow the client in the kitchen.
    4. Do not leave the client home alone.

15. **Which action by a client indicates to the nurse the client has moderate cognitive deficits?**
    1. Doing activities twice when completing activities of daily living.
    2. Snoring when sleeping and waking up frequently in the night.
    3. Writing lists and important dates in a planner.
    4. Not eating when directed to do so.

16. **The daughter brings her mother into the clinic for an evaluation. The mother is a widow of three years and still talks to her late husband. What is the nurse's best response?**
    1. "We need to do tests to see if your mother is having auditory hallucinations."
    2. "This is all part of the normal grieving process and you should leave her alone."
    3. "Let me talk with your mother and find out if she is having excessive stress."
    4. "Everyone grieves differently and it is important to give your mother her space."

17. **The nurse is attempting to educate the family of a client experiencing memory loss, on care of the client. Which statement by the family demonstrates understanding of appropriate care?**
    1. "He can't dress himself."
    2. "He can't manage his medications."
    3. "He can't feed himself."
    4. "He can't take a bath or brush his teeth."

18. **The school nurse is reassessing a child with attention-deficit/hyperactivity disorder (ADHD) who has recently been placed on a stimulant medicine (methylphenidate). What behaviors might demonstrate a lack of therapeutic dosage?**
    1. Child now eats meals in the cafeteria without throwing food.
    2. Parents report that the child angers easily and hits younger siblings with toys.
    3. Parents report that the child sleeps 6 hours at night in one stretch.
    4. Teachers say the child now works alone quietly in a corner.

19. **A child with autism spectrum disorder is admitted for placement of tympanostomy tubes. Which nursing interventions should the nurse include when planning the care of the child? Select all that apply.**
    1. Rotate nurses so that the child doesn't become dependent on one provider.
    2. Quickly transition to new activities to engage the child's imagination.
    3. Determine and utilize the best ways to communicate with the child.
    4. Inquire and incorporate the child's routines, habits and preferences.
    5. Use picture boards to enhance communication with the child.

20. An 8-year-old client with attention-deficit/hyperactivity disorder (ADHD) is attending a new school. The school nurse and teacher work together to develop a plan of care for the client. Which would be included in this plan? Select all that apply.
    1. Administration of central nervous system stimulants.
    2. Counseling sessions with the client and family.
    3. Benzodiazepines to sedate the child as prescribed.
    4. Limiting caffeine and excess sugar in diet.
    5. Using a rewards system for positive behaviors and outcomes.
    6. Providing weekly updates and progress reports to parents.

21. A parent questions the nurse about the link between autism and immunizations. Which response should the nurse include in teaching the parent this material?
    1. "There is some evidence that immunizations are linked with autism, but the benefits of protecting against these diseases outweigh the risks."
    2. "There is a small risk to having the immunizations but the risks associated with these diseases is far greater."
    3. "You need to decide whether the risks of these immunizations, along with your family history, outweighs the risk of the diseases."
    4. "There is no current evidence that links autism with immunizations. The causes of autism are very complex and represent many factors."

1. **A nurse is caring for a client who is at end-of-life. What assessment finding is consistent with delirium associated at the end-of-life?**
    1. 🔵 The client is oriented x 1 and sees bugs on the wall.
    2. The client's spouse states, "He seems so weak and tired now. He sleeps a lot." *This is not a symptom of delirium.*
    3. Cheyne-stokes respirations. *This is not a symptom of delirium.*
    4. Withdrawing from the physical environment but can still hear. *This is not a symptom of delirium.*

    Rationale: All assessment findings listed are common at the end-of-life. Delirium is characterized by confusion, restlessness and hallucinations. It is important to assess for possible causes of delirium which include pain, constipation, and urinary retention.

    THIN Thinking: Nursing Process – *The nurse should understand the physical and psychological changes that occur at end-of-life. Recognition of the assessment changes will assist with the plan of care.* **NCLEX**®: Basic Care and Comfort **QSEN:** Patient-centered Care

2. **The nurse is assessing a client with a new prescription for antipsychotic medications focusing on the potential extrapyramidal side effects. What symptoms would the nurse expect to see if the client was experiencing extrapyramidal side effects?**
    1. Restlessness, hypotension and headache. *Headache is not a common side effect of antipsychotic medications. Hypertension is a common side effect not hypotension.*
    2. 🔵 Stiffening of muscles and impaired gait.
    3. Lethargy, anorexia, and aphasia. *Aphasia is not a side effect of antipsychotic medications. Weight gain is a common side effect not anorexia.*
    4. Confusion, nausea and constipation. *Nausea and confusion are not side effects of antipsychotic medications.*

    Rationale: Extrapyramidal side effects include acute dystonia (sustained muscle contractions), akathisia (psychomotor restlessness) and pseudoparkinsonism (tremors, impaired gait and stiffening of muscles).

    THIN Thinking: Identify Risk to Safety – *The nurse must be able to recognize side effects that impact safety, like mobility issues.* **NCLEX**®: Pharmacological and Parental Therapies **QSEN:** Safety

3. **The nurse is reviewing the medical record before starting to assess a client experiencing confusion. The medical record indicates that the client is experiencing apraxia. What behaviors will the nurse expect to find during the assessment?**
    1. Inability to find the correct word when answering an assessment question. *This is a cognitive skill not related to apraxia.*
    2. Irritability and inability to focus on the conversation during the assessment. *Concentration is a cognitive skill unrelated to apraxia.*
    3. 🔵 Inability to perform routine, familiar tasks while the nurse is doing the assessment.
    4. Loss of orientation to person, place and time while able to converse. *Another unrelated change in the client's orientation.*

    Rationale: Apraxia is the loss of purposeful movements in the absence of motor or sensory impairments. The client is unable to perform routine tasks independently such as dressing.

    THIN Thinking: Top Three – *Recognizing anticipated assessments will allow the nurse to prioritize care.* **NCLEX**®: Reduction of Risk Potential **QSEN:** Patient-centered Care

4. **The nurse is delegating care of a client with a diagnosis of dementia to an unlicensed assistive personnel (UAP). What instruction will facilitate the implementation of the plan of care?**
    1. "Encourage the client to make decisions regarding when to complete activities of daily living." *Client's with dementia struggle with making choices, therefore, encouraging decision making would be frustrating for the client.*
    2. "Keep the client's routine as structured as possible to decrease the potential that the client will act out." *Clients with dementia typically do not demonstrate acting out behaviors and too much structure can cause anxiety.*
    3. "Discourage the family from bringing in more personal items as the client just gets more confused." *Encouraging the family to bring in personal items may help the client with orientation.*
    4. 🔵 "Introduce yourself and call the client by name even if you were only out of the room for a short time."

    Rationale: Always introduce yourself and call the client by name each time you meet. Bringing in personal items can provide comfort and help to reorient the client. Keeping the environment overly structured can cause added anxiety for a client with dementia.

    THIN Thinking: Top Three – *Dementia often causes memory loss. Frequent reminders are a priority in the plan of care.* **NCLEX**®: Management of Care **QSEN:** Patient-centered Care

5. The home care nurse is doing a weekly visit to a client with Alzheimer's disease. What statement by the client would be of greatest concern?

1. "When I go to the grocery store to get a few things, it takes me a really long time to get home."

2. "My daughter organizes my medications and I have an alarm that goes off to let me know when to take them." *This is a sound strategy to ensure that the client takes the medications as prescribed.*

3. "Sometimes when the phone rings I am not sure how to answer it so I just let it ring until it stops." *This is not a significant concern.*

4. "I thought you were going to come to see me last week but you didn't come until I called you today." *Forgetting schedules is a common factor with Alzheimer's disease and this would not be a significant concern.*

Rationale: As Alzheimer's disease progresses the client may forget his/her own address and how to get from one place to another. The fact that it is taking a long time to get home could suggest that the client is getting lost which is a safety issue that needs to be addressed first.

THIN Thinking: Identify Risk to Safety – *This statement supports the fact that the client could be getting lost and jeopardizing their safety.* **NCLEX®:** Safety and Infection Control **QSEN:** Safety

6. The nurse is teaching family members strategies for communicating with their loved one with dementia. What strategy should the nurse include?

1. Speak slowly and loudly, repeating everything. *Just because a client has dementia that does not mean they are hard of hearing.*

2. Focus on one piece of information at a time.

3. Talk to the person about the news to keep them oriented. *Bringing in too much information can increase confusion and anxiety.*

4. Remove pictures that remind the client of the past. *Pictures and memorabilia from the past can help the client reminisce about their life.*

Rationale: When communicating with a client with dementia it is important to keep the communication short, simple and focus on one piece of information at a time. Do not confuse dementia with being hard of hearing. Use familiar objects that will help the client stay oriented.

THIN Thinking: Top Three – *Sensory overload and memory loss is a priority concern.* **NCLEX®:** Health Promotion and Maintenance **QSEN:** Evidence-based Practice

7. The home care nurse is doing an initial assessment for a client with a diagnosis of Alzheimer's disease and congestive heart failure. What assessment findings indicate a potential risk to the client's safety? Select all that apply.

1. Lives with daughter who works outside the home all day.

2. Struggles with telling time on the large wall clock.

3. Able to ambulate without assistive devices. *If the client is able to ambulate safely this is not a safety concern.*

4. Often disoriented to place and time.

5. Has meals delivered when daughter is at work. *Having meal delivered routinely ensures that client has nutritious food available.*

Rationale: If the client is disoriented to time and place, being home alone during the day is a potential safety risk. They may wander outside the home and get lost. Also, if they are disoriented to time and struggle with reading the clock there is the potential that they will not be able to follow prescribed medication schedules for congestive heart failure or any other medications.

THIN Thinking: Identify Risk to Safety – *The nurse must identify risks to safety both inside and outside of the home.* **NCLEX®:** Reduction of Risk Potential **QSEN:** Safety

8. The nurse is instructing an unlicensed assistive personnel (UAP) regarding effective communication strategies when caring for a confused client. What strategies will the nurse encourage the UAP to implement? Select all that apply.

1. Offer the client choices to maintain independent decision making. *Choices may cause anxiety and frustration.*

2. Identify yourself and call the client by name every time you enter the room.

3. Refer to personal objects in the client's room such as pictures to start conversations.

4. Encourage the client to tell you about happy times from their past.

5. If the person becomes verbally agitated, leave the room and get the nurse. *If the client becomes verbally agitated the UAP should stay with the client and try to help calm him/her.*

Rationale: Identify yourself and call the client by name is a strategy to promote reality orientation. Referring to personal items in the room provides an opportunity for the client to reminisce about people or events that were important to them. Long-term memory often stays intact when the client is confused about day to day things and talking about the past promotes self-esteem.

THIN Thinking: Top Three – *Recognize things that will allow the client to feel at home and recall fond memories.* **NCLEX®:** Basic Care and Comfort **QSEN:** Patient-centered Care

9. The nurse is preparing to administer the prescribed 2 mg of haloperidol IM to an acutely psychotic adult client in the emergency department. The vial directions indicate 5 mg/mL. How much will the nurse draw up to administer the prescribed dose?

Answer: 0.4 mL

Rationale: The recommended dose for adults is 2 – 5 mg. every 1 – 8 hours not to exceed 100 mg per day. 2/5 X 1= 0.4

THIN Thinking: Identify Risk to Safety – *The nurse must correctly perform medication calculations to provide safe care.* **NCLEX®:** Pharmacological and Parental Therapies **QSEN:** Safety

10. **The nurse for the evening shift has just arrived on the memory care unit. Based on the change of shift report about the clients assigned, how would the nurse prioritize the clients' safety needs? Rank Order the Responses.**
    1. Agitated client who has paranoid delusions and thinks she is being held prisoner.
    2. Confused client who keeps trying to leave the unit whenever the door is opened.
    3. Newly admitted client who wanders into other client's rooms.
    4. Client with early onset Alzheimer's disease who was admitted for assessment.
    5. Elderly client who is quiet and stays in his room most of the day watching TV.

    Rationale: The agitated client with paranoid delusions is the greatest safety risk both to herself and to others. Because the confused client tries to leave the unit, the nurse needs to know the client's whereabouts and make sure someone is assigned to monitor the client when the unit door is opened for any reason. The client who wanders into other's room is a mild safety risk because of how others may respond to the intrusion. The client can then be assessed (early onset would suggest little safety risk) and the client who stays in his room watching TV is of little safety risk at this time.

    THIN Thinking: Identify Risk to Safety – *The highest concern is the client with a risk for safety of self or others.* **NCLEX®:** Safety and Infection Control **QSEN:** Safety

11. **The home care nurse is visiting a client with a history of confusion. The health care provider recently prescribed lorazepam to control the client's anxiety level at home. What statement by the client's family member indicates the prescription is effective?**
    1. 🏵 "My dad is much calmer in the evening when he takes the lorazepam and he is able to get to sleep when he goes to bed."
    2. "My dad naps in the afternoons now rather than pacing but when I get home he seems to be confused about where I have been." *Confusion is a cause for concern with lorazepam and does not indicate effectiveness.*
    3. "I am really afraid that my dad will become dependent on the lorazepam and not use his coping skills anymore." *Dependency occurs with long-term use and at the moment the priority is to treat the client's anxiety at home.*
    4. "I worry that my dad may get confused and not take the medications as prescribed and possibly overdose." *This*

would be a concern that should be discussed with the health care provider but is not related to the effectiveness of the prescription.

Rationale: Prescribing an antianxiety medication for a client with a history of confusion is to decrease the anxiety level and promote sleep at night. Antianxiety medications can potentially increase confusion which needs to be monitored.

THIN Thinking: Identify Risk to Safety – *The nurse must be able to identify when a medication causes a positive affect or poses a risk for safety.* **NCLEX®:** Pharmacological and Parental Therapies **QSEN:** Safety

12. **When debriefing the nursing staff after a confused client has fallen, the nurse stresses the need for client safety. The nurse knows the staff understands safety when they make which statement?**
    1. The client should eat a balanced diet. *Balanced diets are not directly related to client safety.*
    2. The client should not receive pain medicine. *If pain medication is needed and prescribed appropriately there should not be any safety risk.*
    3. The client should have all four side rails up at all times. *Side rails can be perceived as restraints and may be a bigger safety risk if the client tries to climb over them.*
    4. 🏵 The client should wear non-skid footwear when ambulating.

    Rationale: The client has less of a chance of falling where using safe footwear. Pain medication is needed. Having side rails up at all times is considered restraint and may actually cause the client to fall while trying to get out of bed.

    THIN Thinking: Identify Risk to Safety – *Non-skid footwear is a way to prevent client falls.* **NCLEX®:** Reduction of Risk Potential **QSEN:** Safety

13. **The home health nurse is talking with a family of an elderly client. The client is experiencing episodes of confusion. What client behavior should the nurse educate the family to be observant for?**
    1. 🏵 Repeating questions or statements.
    2. Getting up at night to urinate. *The client may be disoriented when he/she gets up in the middle of the night.*
    3. Requesting the same foods for meals. *The client may have preferences and this is not a significant concern.*
    4. Excessive irritability and violent behavior. *Irritability and acting out behaviors are not common with bouts of confusion.*

    Rationale: this action usually is a sign of impaired short-term memory and if observed this should be reported to the nurse and physician.

    THIN Thinking: Identify Risk to Safety – *Early recognition of confusion could prevent a client injury.* **NCLEX®:** Reduction of Risk Potential **QSEN:** Safety

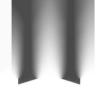

14. **The nurse is doing a home visit for a client diagnosed with moderate cognitive deficits secondary to dementia. The nurse stresses basic care and comfort of the client. What would be a priority action for the family when caring for the client?**
    1. Put the light on at night. *The light may further confuse the client about the time of day.*
    2. Remove clutter from the rooms. *The client's ability to ambulate is not impaired.*
    3. Do not allow the client in the kitchen. *Allowing the client to participate in activities of daily living helps to maintain independence.*
    4. 💡 Do not leave the client home alone.

    Rationale: Leaving a client alone would increase the risk for injury. The client with moderate cognitive decline (Stage 4-5) is unable to care for self, make safe decisions, and control impulses.

    THIN Thinking: Identify Risk to Safety – *The nurse needs to recognize that a client with dementia, if left alone, is a safety risk.* **NCLEX®:** Basic Care and Comfort **QSEN:** Patient-centered Care

15. **Which action by a client indicates to the nurse the client has moderate cognitive deficits?**
    1. 💡 Doing activities twice when completing activities of daily living.
    2. Snoring when sleeping and waking up frequently in the night. *Sleep is not impacted by cognitive deficits.*
    3. Writing lists and important dates in a planner. *This is a healthy coping skill.*
    4. Not eating when directed to do so. *The client may not be hungry at the time and appetite is not directly related to cognitive deficits.*

    Rationale: A client with moderate cognitive deficits may repeat activities because they do not remember doing them the first time. This may impact ADLs and other routine activities.

    THIN Thinking: Identify Risk to Safety – *A lack of cognitive function can place the client at a risk for safety issues.* **NCLEX®:** Basic Care and Comfort **QSEN:** Patient-centered Care

16. **The daughter brings her mother into the clinic for an evaluation. The mother is a widow of three years and still talks to her late husband. What is the nurse's best response?**
    1. "We need to do tests to see if your mother is having auditory hallucinations." *Dealing with grief is not related to hallucinations.*
    2. "This is all part of the normal grieving process and you should leave her alone." *Gathering further assessment data is important, so leaving her alone is not the best response.*
    3. 💡 "Let me talk with your mother and find out if she is having excessive stress."

    4. "Everyone grieves differently and it is important to give your mother her space." *Everyone grieves at a different pace and in different manners. This is may be her coping strategy yet 3 years is a long time and gathering additional data is important.*

    Rationale: The nurse needs to assess the client to determine the symptoms and the client's perspectives on these conversations. They may be associated to stressors which has caused her to regress in her grief, or are their changes in cognition that led to hallucinations. The nurse needs to assess the client to determine the symptoms and signs prior to determining the cause and treatment.

    THIN Thinking: Top Three – *The nurse needs to recognize examples of normal and excessive grieving.* **NCLEX®:** Psychosocial Integrity **QSEN:** Patient-centered Care

17. **The nurse is attempting to educate the family of a client experiencing memory loss, on care of the client. Which statement by the family demonstrates understanding of appropriate care?**
    1. "He can't dress himself." *Despite a memory loss, the client should be able to dress himself.*
    2. 💡 "He can't manage his medications."
    3. "He can't feed himself." *Psychomotor skills related to feeding self is not related to memory loss.*
    4. "He can't take a bath or brush his teeth." *The client may forget to take care of his personal hygiene but despite a memory loss he should be able to conduct his ADLs.*

    Rationale: Since memory loss is present the client should not manage his medications. This could lead to over medication or under medication, including omitting or repeating dosages.

    THIN Thinking: Nursing Process – *Evaluation of understanding is an important part of the nurse role when determining care.* **NCLEX®:** Psychosocial Integrity **QSEN:** Patient-centered Care

18. **The school nurse is reassessing a child with attention-deficit/hyperactivity disorder (ADHD) who has recently been placed on a stimulant medicine (methylphenidate). What behaviors might demonstrate a lack of therapeutic dosage?**
    1. Child now eats meals in the cafeteria without throwing food. *Eating appropriately in a group setting would indicate the prescription is effective.*
    2. 💡 Parents report that the child angers easily and hits younger siblings with toys.
    3. Parents report that the child sleeps 6 hours at night in one stretch. *Client's with ADHD usually struggle to sleep for any blocks of time so this would indicate effectiveness of the prescription.*

4. Teachers say the child now works alone quietly in a corner. *This is a good indicator that the medication is effective in controlling the child's behaviors.*

Rationale: The goal of therapeutic management is to reduce frequency and intensity of unsocialized behaviors. This requires a balance between the child's temperament and environmental demands, expectations, and supports. Treatment interventions are targeted at enhancing the child's capabilities and self-esteem. Goals and expectations are set in realistic and measurable terms. The nurse documents (before medication and again after) the parent's or teacher's description of the child's typical behavior, while playing alone or with others, during mealtimes, while the parent is occupied otherwise, and ability to perform dressing and other ADLs.

THIN Thinking: Nursing Process – *Assessment of therapeutic and non-therapeutic effects of medication is important to the nurse's plan of care.* **NCLEX®:** Pharmacological and Parenteral Therapies **QSEN:** Teamwork and Collaboration

19. **A child with autism spectrum disorder is admitted for placement of tympanostomy tubes. Which nursing interventions should the nurse include when planning the care of the child? Select all that apply.**
    1. Rotate nurses so that the child doesn't become dependent on one provider. *Providing continuity will help to build the child's trust.*
    2. Quickly transition to new activities to engage the child's imagination. *Sudden changes may trigger anxiety and/or frustration especially for a child with autism spectrum disorder.*
    3. ⊕ Determine and utilize the best ways to communicate with the child.
    4. ⊕ Inquire and incorporate the child's routines, habits and preferences.
    5. ⊕ Use picture boards to enhance communication with the child.

Rationale: Nurses must determine an autistic child's usual routines, habits and preferences to decrease the child's anxiety and increase the level of cooperation. Include families when developing a plan of care to include the best ways for communicating with the child. Using the same nurses and transitioning from an activity slowly decreases anxiety.

THIN Thinking: Nursing Process – *Understanding appropriate interventions based on the child's needs is important to planning care.* **NCLEX®:** Physiological Adaption **QSEN:** Evidence-based Practice

20. **An 8-year-old client with attention-deficit/hyperactivity disorder (ADHD) is attending a new school. The school nurse and teacher work together to develop a plan of care for the client. Which would be included in this plan? Select all that apply.**
    1. ⊕ Administration of central nervous system stimulants.
    2. ⊕ Counseling sessions with the client and family.
    3. Benzodiazepines to sedate the child as prescribed. *Benzodiazepines are not appropriate for an 8-year-old child with ADHD.*
    4. ⊕ Limiting caffeine and excess sugar in diet.
    5. ⊕ Using a rewards system for positive behaviors and outcomes.
    6. ⊕ Providing weekly updates and progress reports to parents.

Rationale: CNS stimulants sustain paradoxical effects on children and a calming effect. Therapy is recommended for clients and families, rewards systems and periodic updates are suggested. Although not proven, restrictions of caffeine and sugar are part of the plan of care. Benzodiazepines are not recommended.

THIN Thinking: Nursing Process – *Planning care needs to be focused around the specific needs of a client based on age and diagnosis.* **NCLEX®:** Psychosocial Integrity **QSEN:** Evidence-based Practice

21. **A parent questions the nurse about the link between autism and immunizations. Which response should the nurse include in teaching the parent this material?**
    1. "There is some evidence that immunizations are linked with autism, but the benefits of protecting against these diseases outweigh the risks." *The evidence linking immunizations to autism is not supported by research.*
    2. "There is a small risk to having the immunizations but the risks associated with these diseases is far greater." *This response may frighten the parents.*
    3. "You need to decide whether the risks of these immunizations, along with your family history, outweighs the risk of the diseases." *This is not providing the parents with evidence for decision making.*
    4. ⊕ "There is no current evidence that links autism with immunizations. The causes of autism are very complex and represent many factors."

Rationale: There is no current evidence linking autism with immunizations. Current evidence points to complex perinatal, genetic, and neurological factors. There are familial and medical condition links, but no connections have been established with specific medications or immunizations.

THIN Thinking: Nursing Process – *It is important for the nurse to identify components of care based on evidence-based practice.* **NCLEX®:** Pharmacological and Parenteral Therapies **QSEN:** Evidence-based Practice

SECTION 3

Closing

Health Promotion

Across the Lifespan

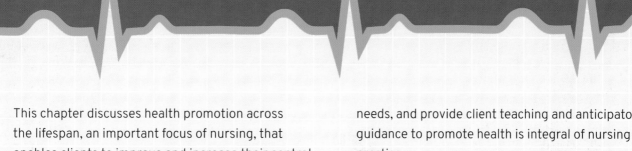

This chapter discusses health promotion across the lifespan, an important focus of nursing, that enables clients to improve and increase their control over health. Health is defined many ways, but most definitions describe a holistic state of physical, spiritual, social, emotional, relational, and sexual well-being. Wellness is the positive state of health of individuals, families, or communities.

This chapter also addresses development or the sequence of change over a person's lifetime in several domains (we address physical, motor, cognitive, psychoemotional, language, and play). Individuals across the lifespan may experience developmental delays in any of these domains, requiring nursing assessment and planning of client-centered care. The ability to address clients on their developmental, not just chronological level, meet their health promotion needs, and provide client teaching and anticipatory guidance to promote health is integral of nursing practice.

As you read through this chapter, consider how principles of growth and development and health promotion may influence your answers to NCLEX® questions.

Priority Exemplars:

> Infants

> Toddlers

> Preschoolers

> School-age children

> Adolescents

> Adults

> Older adults

Infants

📋 Pathophysiology/Description

> Includes ages from birth to 12 months (some sources indicate 18 months)

> Is a critical period for development in multiple domains, and infancy is the most rapid period of growth and development in the lifespan

✏️ Priority Assessments or Cues

> Assess vital signs including newborn ranges (heart rate 120-160 bpm, respirations 30-60 bpm, blood pressures 80-90/40-50 mmHg) and infant ranges (heart rate 90-130 bpm, respirations 20-40 bpm, blood pressure 90/56 mmHg), temp. approximately 97-99°F axillary. For infants, cardiac output is heart rate dependent so bradycardia may markedly decrease perfusion

> Assess developmental milestones in a variety of domains

- Physical
  - Infants double birth weight by six months, triple birth weight by 12 months
  - Infant length increases by 50% at 1 year of age
  - Infants' heads are proportionally larger than the rest of the body
  - Assess infant reflexes (see Newborn Care Priority Exemplar)
  - Assess appearance to include muscle tone, behavior, level of consciousness, and mood. Assess for developmentally appropriate smile

- Motor
  - Fine motor skills demonstrated in infants as they learn reflexive movements, move from reflexive to simple repetitive movements, are able to bring toys to mouth, are able to use a pincer grasp, perform hand to hand transfer, and hold a pencil
  - Gross motor skills demonstrated in infants as they gain head control, learn to roll (front to back/back to front), sit, crawl, stand, and walk

- Cognitive
  - Piaget's stage of sensorimotor phase in which learning begins by trial and error and learning through reflexive to purposeful movements
  - Infants learn object permanence as they develop a memory and understand disappearing/reappearing (peek-a-boo)

- Psychoemotional
  - Erikson's phase of trust versus mistrust, as they form attachments, learn to trust caregivers, and negative feelings in response when needs are not met; infants learn to develop hope and faith. Lack of trust may contribute to attachment disorders and emotional strain
  - Learn boundaries of self with social games, responsive smiling, and understanding of self as separate from others
  - Assess eye contact, social smiling, and responsive hugging
  - Parents/caregivers are center of social circle
  - Separation anxiety is manifested and progresses from protest to despair to detachment to adjustment

- Language
  - Progresses from crying to cooing to laughing to imitating sounds
  - Progresses to comprehending simple commands and repeating words

- Play
  - Largely about manipulation of toys
  - Exploratory and solitary play

> Assess for child maltreatment including abuse and neglect

🧪 Priority Laboratory Tests/Diagnostics

> Newborn screening (see Newborn Care Priority Exemplar)

> Screening during infancy for congenital hip dysplasia

> Health screening and monitoring

> Length, weight, and head circumference and plot on a growth chart

⚠️ Priority Interventions or Actions

> Provide health education

- Teach infant care including bathing and bath safety, dressing, safe handling, and infant developmental milestones

- Sleeping is a significant concern for many parents
  - Infants often establishing sleep patterns and many parents/caregivers may deal with sleep refusal, frequent waking, and mix up days and nights
  - Usually sleep about 9-11 hours a night with 1-2 naps/day
  - Teach safe sleep practices, including back-to-sleep, pacifiers, dressing lightly, no bumpers/pillows/blankets in bed, no co-bedding

- Teach about nutrition and feeding practices including bottle/breastfeeding, introducing solid foods at about 6 months
  - No whole cow's milk, egg whites, or honey until 12 months
  - Begin with well-cooked table foods, offer new foods one at a time
  - Encourage water between meals
  - Limit juice, use a cup to avoid bottle mouth caries
  - Use care with microwave, do not microwave bottles

- Teach about dental care, teeth begin to appear 6-10 months
  - Assist parents/caregivers to deal with irritability related to teething
  - Use of cold teething rings, over-the-counter topical pain relievers, and oral analgesics

- Teach parents about infant's body self-exploration and infant's tendency to touch their genitals

Priority Potential & Actual Complications

> Poor attachment with lack of a secure caregiver
> Development delay
> Unintentional or intentional injury or illness

Priority Nursing Implications

> For hospitalized infants, nurses should:
  • Cuddle and hold infants
  • Encourage parent/caregivers to participate in care
  • Stimulate with toys
  • Allow for security objects
  • Encourage parent/caregiver involvement in care and rooming in
> Provide for non-nutritive sucking and oral stimulation if NPO or agitated
> Teach toy safety with hand to mouth infant behaviors, inquisitiveness, and lack of cognitive understanding of consequences
> Provide infant stimulation and teach parents/caregivers means to stimulate learning
> Nurses need to consider the cultural and spiritual aspects that may affect developmental care

Priority Medications

> Discuss the need for multivitamins with healthcare provider
> Assess the need for iron supplementation (after 6 months, may get iron from solids/cereals)
> Assess the need for Vitamin D
> Supplemental fluoride or access to fluoridated water
> Assess immunization needs which are very high in the infant period (see www.aap.org)

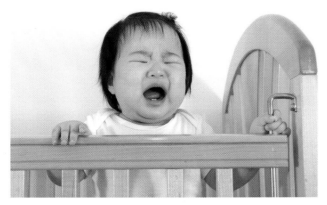

Image 18-1: The nurse is often the front-line when it comes to addressing an abuse situation.

Priority Education/Discharge Issues

> Anticipatory guidance for infant care with caregivers
  • Car seats and safe transporting of infants. Children less than two should be in a rear-facing car seat in the back seat. Provide access to information about state laws concerning passenger safety
  • Safety as infants become more mobile
  • Assist parents to choose and work with childcare arrangements
  • Assess for achievement of developmentally appropriate milestones
> For infants with health issues and developmental delay, ensure early intervention into services and use of the multidisciplinary team to optimize development
> Encourage parents to post Poison Control Center Number

Next Gen Clinical Judgment

You are a nurse in a pediatric clinic. A parent brings in a 9-month-old infant. The parent states that the baby has been irritable, crying all the time, and has some unexplained new bruises on her leg. The infant was cared for today by a new caregiver.

1. What are priority nursing assessments?

2. Based on these potential issues, what assessments should the nurse implement?

3. How does this scenario demonstrate the critical need for accurate and comprehensive assessments and analysis in clinical judgment?

_____

_____

_____

_____

_____

_____

_____

Toddlers

🗀 Pathophysiology/Description

> Includes ages 12 to 36 months

> Stage is characterized by growing mobility, independence, and learning

✎ Priority Assessments or Cues

> Assess vital signs including toddler ranges (heart rate 80-120 bpm, respirations 20-30 bpm, blood pressures 92/55 mmHg) temp. approximately 97.5-98.6°F axillary

> Assess developmental milestones in a variety of domains

- Physical
  - Toddlers gain 4-6 kg/year
  - Body begins to thin-out as child becomes mobile
- Motor
  - Gross motor development progresses such that toddlers learn to manage stairs, tricycles, running, and jumping
  - Fine motor skills typically progress to drawing circles and crosses, using blocks, using crayons, turning book pages, and turning door knobs
- Cognitive
  - Toddlers progress from sensorimotor period to pre-operational phase (Piaget)
  - Beginning reasoning skills based on own experiences
  - Begin to use symbols, imitate behaviors, and pretend
  - Enjoy completion of age-related tasks, beginning to learn chores and simple jobs
  - Beginning to master self-care, including feeding, dressing, and toileting
  - Begin to understand the past and the future
  - Are highly curious and "into everything." Need to provide safe supervision
- Psychoemotional
  - Erikson's phase of autonomy versus shame and doubt. Lack of mastery of self-control/care may elicit feelings of shame and self-doubt
  - Learn self-control, willpower, and a sense of adequacy
  - Learn to increase independence in self-care including potty training
  - Often have negative behaviors (favorite word is "no") and may have temper tantrums
  - Can separate self from others, but can't empathize
  - Begin to assert self
  - Parents/caregivers are center of social circle
- Language
  - Begin to use language to communicate
  - Usually have 10 words at 18 months to about 300 words at 24 months
  - Begin to use 2 words sentences
  - Understands language before able to use words to express needs
- Play
  - Play moves from solitary to parallel where children play beside but not with others
  - Begin to have an imagination and participate in pretend play
  - Short attention span results in changing toys and activities often
- Assess for child maltreatment including abuse and neglect

⚗ Priority Laboratory Tests/Diagnostics

> Lead screening is indicated for all children, especially those in old homes with lead-based paint or where the water supply may include unhealthy levels of lead

> The Denver II Developmental Screening test assesses children ages 1-6 for gross motor, fine motor, adaptive/self-care, and social/language skills

> Health screening and monitoring

> Length/height, weight, and head circumference all plotted on a growth chart

⚠ Priority Interventions or Actions

> Provide health education

- Toddlers are at risk for injury due to their increased mobility and lack of judgment
- Provide parents/caregivers with education about graded independence, dealing with negativism and temper tantrums, and addressing discipline
- Guide parents through toilet training to include readiness for toilet training, the child recognizing they need to void or defecate, mobility skills, language skills to express personal needs, and consistency in process
- Provide safety education about ingestions and poisoning, including household child-proofing, safe storage of harmful products, and child supervision. Discuss electrical, medication, stairway, toilet, pool, household cleaners, and other hazards
- Address safe toys and age-appropriate play, including safe supervision
- Nutrition
  - Toddlers may be "fussy" and go on "food jags"
  - Assist caregivers in providing a nutritious diet of grains, fruits, vegetables, dairy, and protein
  - Ensure table food is cut into small pieces to avoid choking and allow for self-feeding
  - Toddlers often go through physiological anorexia, if toddler refuses to eat, provide finger foods and nutritious snacks
  - Limit milk to 2-3 cups/day to prevent decreasing appetite and inadequate iron and other nutrient consumption
  - Low-fat or skim milk not to be used until after 2 years of age
  - Dilute juices to prevent diarrhea and excessive intake of sugar

- Teach parents about toddler's body self-exploration and toddler's tendency to touch their genitals, begin to teach body parts using appropriate names and about body privacy

🚩 Priority Potential & Actual Complications

> Unintentional or intentional injury or illness

> Toddlers may be prone to poisoning, ingestions, lead poisoning, water accidents, and motor vehicle accidents (risk for unrestrained toddlers who may react violently to confinement)

℧ Priority Nursing Implications

> For hospitalized toddlers, provide choices and convey a positive attitude to child

- Allow child to express protest and accept regressive behaviors

- Provide favorite objects and activities that allow for mobility

- Choose words carefully because toddlers take words very literally

- Assess for pain carefully, toddlers may react to pain, restraint, and frustration with aggressive responses

- Toddlers are at risk for falls and require injury prevention care while hospitalized

- Hospitalized toddlers fear loss of control, injury, and pain

- Encourage parent/caregiver involvement in care and rooming in

> Encourage parents to see positive sides of toddler learning, including curiosity and exploration while providing safe supervision

> Nurses need to consider the cultural and spiritual aspects that may affect developmental care

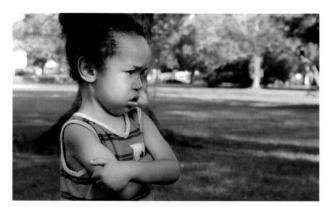

Image 18-2: Toddlers come in all different shapes, sizes, and temperaments. Parents often look to nurses for guidance in parenting. On NCLEX®, this question will ask "The parent of a toddler is asking the nurse for advice on handling temper tantrums. What is the nurse's best response?"

💧 Priority Medications

> Assess for need for multivitamins and iron

> Assess immunization needs in the toddler period (see www.aap.org)

👤 Priority Education/Discharge Issues

> Anticipatory guidance for toddler care with caregivers

- Car seats and safe transporting of toddlers. Children less than two should be in a rear-facing car seat in the back seat. Children over two should be in a front facing car seat in the back seat. Provide access to state laws and encourage caregivers to consult car seat manufacturer recommendations regarding placement of children in car seats

- Assist parents to deal with the issues associated with toddlerhood, including negativism, temper tantrums and use of "no" and "me do it"

- Safety as toddlers become more mobile. This may include risks for poisoning/ingestions, falls, drowning (bath/pool), choking, and car safety

- Assist parents to choose and work with childcare arrangements

- Assess for achievement of developmentally appropriate milestones

- Encourage strategies that foster language skills

- Reinforce the importance of reading to children on a daily basis

- Ensure that family has ready access to Poison Control center number

Next Gen Clinical Judgment

You are providing anticipatory guidance to a parent of a 2-year-old. The parent expresses frustration with the child's stubbornness and negativism. List 3-4 ideas that may be helpful to this parent:

1. _____

2. _____

3. _____

4. _____

Preschoolers

📋 Pathophysiology/Description

> Ages 3-5 years

✏️ Priority Assessments or Cues

> Assess vital signs preschool ranges (heart rate 70-110 bpm, respirations 16-22 bpm, blood pressures 95/57 mmHg), temp. approximately 97.5-98.6°F axillary

> Assess developmental milestones in a variety of domains

- Physical
  - Few physical changes in the preschool years
  - Preschoolers gain about 5 pounds/year and double birth length at four years
- Motor
  - Develop mastery of body
  - Gross motor skills include jumping rope, skating, swimming, going up and down steps, skipping, and running; children able to build coordination skills
  - Increase in fine motor skills; skills include copying squares and crosses, scribbling, drawing letters or numbers, and ability to work with fine/small toys
- Cognitive
  - Preoperational stage of development including prelogical thinking and understanding of the past/present/future. Thinking is concrete and egocentric
  - Preschool children learn to plan, categorize, and classify
  - Children beginning to learn to empathize and to socialize with peers
  - Increase in understanding of cause and effect and reasoning. Preschool children are curious and frequently ask "Why?"
  - Increase in magical thinking and belief of personal role in illness, negative effects, and impacts on siblings/peers
  - Increase in fears of things they do not understand
  - High levels of energy may be manifested as episodes of anger or tantrums
- Psychoemotional
  - Period of initiative versus guilt wherein children develop a sense of purpose and initiate activities. Children may over-anticipate their ability, do new activities, but may fail, leading to guilt
  - Develop new skills in making and keeping friends; child's world moves from the family to the neighborhood/community
  - Less negative in demeanor
  - Preschoolers often want to please adults and authority figures
  - Stressors may begin related to school, siblings, illness, moving, or other life changes. Mutilation anxiety (fear of pain and injury) begins
  - Regression is normal

- Language
  - Shares thoughts, interacts, and communicates
  - Take words at their literal meaning, may misinterpret messages
  - Vocabulary contains 8000-14000 words
  - Children ask lots of questions
- Play
  - Social/associative play
  - Begin to demonstrate cooperative play behaviors
  - Develop imaginative play, pretending, and imaginary playmates
  - Pretend play very critical for dealing with stress and learning new skills
  - Like to build and create things

> Assess for child maltreatment including abuse and neglect

🧪 Priority Laboratory Tests/Diagnostics

> The Denver II Developmental Screening test assesses children ages 1-6 for gross motor, fine motor, adaptive/self-care, and social/language skills

> Health screening and monitoring

> Height and weight assessment plotted on a growth chart

⚠️ Priority Interventions or Actions

> Provide health education

- Potty training is completed, teach parents to ensure child is clean and how to reinforce hygienic toileting in preschool children

- Dental health and hygiene habits begin, teach children to brush and floss. Ensure routine dental examinations and care

- Reinforce safe car seat use and need for continued car seat use. Children should be in the back seat. State laws differ about the use of booster seats. Provide access to information about state laws concerning passenger safety

- As their world expands, encourage child to try diversified foods. Preschoolers are known for food jags and frequent changing favorite and detested foods. Often focus on social aspects of eating and mealtime

- Encourage water consumption

- Teach parents about child's body self-exploration and children's tendency to touch their genitals, begin to teach body parts using appropriate names and encourage preschooler to use those names, teach about body privacy, introduce concepts of other gender, and safe and appropriate touching by others. Introduce concepts of safe touch and stranger safety

- Preschool children may experience sleep problems, encourage the use of pre-sleep routines, nightlights, and security blankets or objects

Priority Potential & Actual Complications

> Unintentional or intentional injury or illness

> Preschoolers may be prone to water accidents, pedestrian/bicycle, and motor vehicle accidents if not properly restrained

Priority Nursing Implications

> For hospitalized preschoolers

- Magical thinking and fears make illness and injury particularly stressful during this time frame

- Regression is a normal manifestation. May be unable to separate from parents

- Fear bodily harm and pain

- Fear invasive procedures and loss of control

- Try to continue normal routines as much as possible and allow for self-care activities

- Provide simple medical play using dolls, puppets, pictures, and harmless medical equipment. Teach to the child's level of understanding using simple words and concepts

- Allow for play and diversional activities

- Avoid invasive procedures as much as possible

- Allow child to wear underwear and own clothes if possible, allow favorites toys and books to be part of child's life during hospitalization

- Encourage parent/caregiver involvement in care and rooming in

> Teach children about strangers and personal body safety. Teach about the need to seek out assistance from a trusted adult

> Encourage swimming lessons and water safety

> Nurses need to consider the cultural and spiritual aspects that may affect developmental care

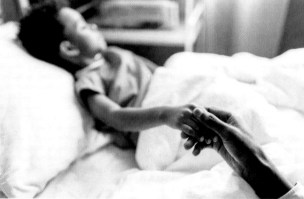

Image 18-3: Consider searching the internet for a couple of videos on how to start an IV on a child. Look for parts of their technique that address developmental needs of the child.

Priority Medications

> Consult healthcare provider about use of multivitamins

> Assess immunization needs in the preschool period (see www.aap.org)

Priority Education/Discharge Issues

> Recommend judicious use of television, computers, and video games

> Teach parents/caregivers how to prepare child for the rigors and schedule of school

> Encourage creative arts, drawing, reading, and quiet play, in addition to time outdoors building skills in gross motor activities

> Teach parents/caregivers how to foster independent self-care in their preschool child

> Teach child their full name, parents'/caregivers' names, phone number, address, and how to dial 911

Next Gen Clinical Judgment

A 4-year-old client on your unit is being treated for sickle cell anemia. He is in sequestration crisis and his iron levels are increased. His intravenous line has infiltrated and he requires a new intravenous line for chelation therapy and hydration. Consider these issues:

1. How can we best gain cooperation from this child to insert the new intravenous line?

2. How can we best teach this client at his developmental level?

3. How can we assist the client and family to prevent future complications and hospitalizations?

_____

_____

_____

_____

_____

_____

School-age children

📋 Pathophysiology/Description

> Ages 6-12 years

> This is a period of rapid changes in skills, thoughts, and behaviors with expanded physical, psychoemotional, social, and cognitive skills

✏️ Priority Assessments or Cues

> Assess vital signs including school-age children ranges (heart rate 60-100 bpm, respirations 18-20 bpm, blood pressures 107/64 mmHg) temp. approximately 97.5-98.6°F axillary

> Assess developmental milestones in a variety of domains

- Physical
  - Period of slowed physical growth until the pre-puberty growth spurt
  - Gains about 4-7 pounds/year and grows about 2 inches/year. Girls tend to be taller and heavier than boys until puberty
- Motor
  - Gross motor skills become increasingly graceful with running, jumping, balancing, throwing, and catching. Enjoy games and activities
  - Fine motor skills develop as children have more control over their wrists and fingers. Able to draw, paint, write, and manipulate computer games
  - Develop increased strength and endurance
- Cognitive
  - In Piaget's stage of concrete operational thought. Children use logical thought and problem solving
  - May progress to formal operational thought with abstract reasoning at the end of the school-age period
  - Beginning to make decisions and accept responsibility
  - Learn to function within the rules and expectations of school and other settings. Able to attend to content, adjust to school routine, control activity, and control impulsivity. Increased concentration
  - Learn conservation of size, shape, and volume
  - Can categorize and put objects in series. Begin to collect and sort objects. Collections are valued possessions of school-age children
  - Assess for learning disabilities and differences and the potential for accommodations to aid in learning
- Psychoemotional
  - The child's world becomes broadened to include friends and the community, church, school, and neighborhood
  - Erikson's task of industry versus inferiority includes achieving competency, learning to learn and work, taking on tasks and mastering activities, ongoing development of self-esteem and sense of worth

  - Increasingly empathic, less egocentric, and able to see the perspectives of others
  - Desire to please adults and authority figures
  - Developing personal preferences to meet needs and independence in activities and routine. Still need guidance in making good choices
  - Peers become more important. Emphasis is on same-gender peers. Develop "best friends" and small groups. Increase in group identity as they near adolescence
- Language
  - Rapid language acquisition
  - Learning to use the rules of grammar
  - Learning to understand jokes and meaning of content when out of context
- Play
  - Play in small or large groups
  - Play is cooperative with rules. Breaking rules is reacted to with anger and frustration
  - Interest in competition and sports

> Assess for child maltreatment including abuse and neglect

⚗️ Priority Laboratory Tests/Diagnostics

> Scoliosis screening in children 11-12 years (preteen screening)

> Health screening and monitoring

> Vision and hearing screening usually completed at school

> Height and weight assessment and calculation of body mass index (BMI)

⚠️ Priority Interventions or Actions

> Provide health education

- Teach about safe car restraints including children 8-16 in a properly fitted seatbelt. Children less than 12 years of age should be in the back seat. Provide access to information about state laws concerning passenger safety

- Teach about bike, car, fire, and water safety

- Provide sexuality education at an age appropriate level to include forms of sexual identity, sexual self-esteem, and about impending puberty with physical, psychoemotional, and social impacts. Teach parents about school-age children's sexual curiosity, using appropriate names, about body privacy, concepts of other gender, and safe and appropriate touching by others. Reinforce concepts of safe touch and stranger safety

- Ensure teaching about dental care and routine dental examinations

- Begin focusing health education at the child as they assume greater levels of self-care

- Reinforce nutritious diet habits and drinking adequate water. Ensure that eating and exercise habits lay the foundation to avoid obesity later in life. Encourage new and different food

- Begin to discuss peer pressure with child and parents/caregivers and explore family values and means to deal with pressure from friends, the media, and other sources

- Teach about judicious use of television, computer, and video games; encourage active exercise, time outdoors, and sports

🚩 Priority Potential & Actual Complications

> Unintentional or intentional injury or illness

> School-age children are capable of self-care but still require the monitoring and supervision of a caring adult

> Beginning of risk behaviors that may result in accidents (pedestrian, car, bicycle, fires)

> Increased exposure to infections as world broadens

♻ Priority Nursing Implications

> For hospitalized school-age children

- May fear separation from parents/caregivers, stress may cause regressed behavior

- Miss school, peers, and routine

- Fear bodily injury, illness, and disability

- Fear immobilization and restrictions

- Provide choices whenever possible, provide limits on behaviors

- Teaching using medical play, body diagrams, pictures, and movies

- Provide privacy when warranted

- Encourage visitation of peers, siblings, and pets

- Encourage parent/caregiver involvement in care and rooming in

> School-age children are stressed about peers, parental expectations, school expectations, and self-care after school if they spend time alone (latch-key issues). Teach children stress management techniques such as exercise, hobbies, music, care of pets, and other diversional activities

> Bullying and dealing with bullies are two areas prompting an increased focus by nurses and others working with school-age children

> Nurses need to consider the cultural and spiritual aspects that may affect developmental care

💧 Priority Medications

> Consult healthcare provider about use of multivitamins

> Human papilloma vaccine recommended in girls ages 11-12, boys ages 9-26 (may be earlier in cases of sexual abuse)

> Assess immunization needs in the school-age period (see www.aap.org)

👤 Priority Education/Discharge Issues

> School-age children are highly responsive to environmental stimuli and enrichment. Teach parents/caregivers to provide diversified experiences during this period

> Teach children how to call 911

Next Gen Clinical Judgment

As a school nurse you are teaching a group of 6th grade, 11-13-year-old children about sexual health.

1. What topics might be included for this age group?

2. What issues might the nurse confront related to parent/caregiver consent?

3. A female student comes to you after the class and asks how she would know if she was pregnant. How should the nurse proceed? How does the child's age of 12 influence your nursing care? What assessments are indicated? What other professionals should the nurse consult?

_____

_____

_____

_____

_____

_____

Adolescents

📋 Pathophysiology/Description

> Ages 13-20 years

> Begins around puberty, when reproduction is possible

> Often a healthy period, with teens needing encouragement and teaching to obtain physical examinations and routine care

✏️ Priority Assessments or Cues

> Assess vital signs including adolescent ranges (heart rate 55-90 bpm, respirations 12-20 bpm, blood pressure 121/70 mmHg) temp. approximately 97.5-98.6°F axillary

> Assess developmental milestones in a variety of domains

- Physical
  - During pre-pubertal growth spurt, teens may grow 4-12 inches and gain 15-65 pounds
  - Period of increased growth, gender specific changes, secondary sexual organ development and changes, and changes in the distribution of fat and muscle.
  - Adolescents begin to complain of acne and body odor apparent
  - Onset of secondary sexual characteristics and menstruation begins
- Motor
  - Continue to develop fine and gross motor skills
  - Puberty may be a period of awkwardness
  - Determine personal talents in motor areas
  - Increasing strength and endurance
- Cognitive
  - Able to engage in future-oriented, deductive reasoning
  - Can base new knowledge on past experiences
  - Engages in abstract, formal operations according to Piaget characterized by logical thinking and maturing problem solving. Able to determine and rank options.
  - The developing prefrontal cortex provides cognitive controls when faced with risk, temptation, impulsiveness, and new sensations or stimuli
  - Standardized assessment tools provide assessments of intelligence and cognitive functioning
  - Need opportunities for independent decision-making to build skills
  - Assess for learning disabilities and differences and the potential for accommodations to aid in learning
- Psychoemotional
  - Erikson identified as identity versus role confusion where teens develop a sense of personal identity. Inability to master this task may lead to decreased self-esteem/decreased self-awareness, and frustration or depression related to role confusion
  - Become independent from parents/family and depend more on peers

- Preoccupied with body and body image, imagine everyone is looking at them with a critical eye
- Developing a sexual and gender identity, and family, health, and group identity
- Usually skilled in empathy though may regress when stressed
- May no longer be focused on pleasing adults or adhering to the rules of authority
- Language
  - Vocabulary continues to develop and expand
  - Language is often regionalized or based on local word choice or syntax, peer, and media influences
  - Beginning to articulate thoughts and feelings to family, teachers, peers, and others
  - Building personal communication skills and style
- Play
  - Building talents and interests into hobbies
  - Games and athletics are common forms of play, friends are key in age-appropriate play and activities
  - May begin to work outside the home for money
  - Importance of chores, value of money, and budgeting explored with adolescents
  - May need assistance to schedule time for diversional activities along with routine or scheduled ones

> Assess for child maltreatment including abuse and neglect, intimate partner violence, and other threats to home safety

⚗️ Priority Laboratory Tests/Diagnostics

> Standardized nutrition screening, including body mass index

> Testing for sexually transmitted diseases in sexually active teens

> Screen for depression, anxiety, or other mental health issues, including risk for suicide (see Priority Exemplars)

> Screen for eating disorders (see Priority Exemplar)

> Teach self-breast and self-testicular exams

⚠️ Priority Interventions or Actions

> Provide health education

- Teach parents and teens about the changes and characteristics inherent of adolescence

- Address mental health during the teen years and importance of early detection and intervention. Assess for suicide and make immediate referrals. Be attuned to such signs of suicide as absenteeism, social withdrawal, verbalization of suicidal ideations, and changes in sleep or eating patterns. Directly ask about ideas, methods, or intent of self-harm

- Provide and support education related to car safety/ seatbelts, avoiding risk behaviors, and the hazards of tobacco, alcohol, and illicit drugs

- Provide sexual education including the pleasures and responsibilities associated with sexual activity, understanding consent, prevention of sexually transmitted diseases, and contraception

- Provide risk reduction and harm reduction education related to substances, smoking, driving, activities, swimming, firearms, biking, and other threats to safety

- Discuss with teens and parents about privacy and confidentiality

- Teach about stress of adolescents (peers, school, etc.) and coping mechanisms. Identify less constructive coping methods (cutting, substances) and refer or address as needed while exploring healthy coping mechanisms

- Teach teens to sleep about eight hours per night. Most teens lack adequate rest

- Instruct teens on the importance of an adequate diet. Most teens lack calcium, zinc, iron, folic acid, and protein in their usual diet. Teach about the avoidance of empty calories and the need for high protein/moderate carbohydrate food choices

> Assess teen's receptivity to teaching and learning

⚑ Priority Potential & Actual Complications

> Adolescents who are not provided with opportunities to make and learn from mistakes may remain dependent on adults in their world

> High-risk behaviors, related to dopamine surges and desire for risk, may lead to accidents or injury

> Unintentional or intentional illness or injuries

> Injuries related to substance use, motor vehicles, and other high-risk behaviors

> Homicide and suicide are two common causes of mortality in teens

℧ Priority Nursing Implications

> The hospitalized adolescent

- May vacillate between dependence on and independence from parents

- May miss peers and be concerned about missing school

- Fear being different from peers

- May not admit to being fearful of procedures or healthcare

- May respond with anger, withdrawal, or uncooperativeness

- May seek help and then reject it

- Nurses should provide complete explanations and support positive coping

- Allow clients to wear their own clothes, make some choices in care, provide an appropriate warning prior to treatments, and allow favorite foods

- Ensure privacy and confidentiality are respected. This may cause difficulty with parents or caregivers. Ensure conditional confidentiality, wherein one must divulge any information that reflects harm of self or others. Explore state laws related to minors, emancipated minors, and mature minors and their implications for consent, confidentiality, and care

- Provide books, apps, websites, and videos as appropriate to provide health teaching

- Encourage parent/caregiver involvement in care and assess teens' need for parent/caregiver rooming in

> Nurses may encounter teens who are pregnant or parenting. Teens who have prenatal care, receive adequate nutrition, and avoid risk behaviors have the capacity to have healthy pregnancies. Teen parents may require health supervision, psychosocial support, and assistance with the logistics of parenting, such as childcare and managing school and children

> Bullying and dealing with bullies are two areas prompting an increased focus by nurses and others working with teens

> Peers are often a positive force in teens' lives. Consider using peer or group focused interventions when working with teens

> There is growing concern that teens may be homeless, living in poverty, lack access to healthcare, or are subjected to intimate partner violence or human trafficking. Nurses need to be vigilant in assessing and managing the needs of these teens. For example, School Based Health Centers provide access to teen-friendly, convenient, low/no cost, and comprehensive healthcare

> Nurses need to consider the cultural and spiritual aspects that may affect developmental care

◉ Priority Medications

> Human papilloma vaccine if not previously vaccinated; may be given to girls 13-26 and boys 9-26 (see school age Priority Exemplar)

> Consult healthcare provider about use of multivitamins

> Assess immunization needs in the adolescent period (see www.aap.org)

👤 Priority Education/Discharge Issues

> Adolescents may begin to self-advocate and manage their health care needs, with the support of parents, caregivers, and healthcare providers

> Previously considered only a period of stress and conflict, adolescence is a time to gain knowledge and skills, learn about self, and learn to manage in the world.

Adults

📋 Pathophysiology/Description

> 18-25-year-old individuals comprise a new category of emerging adults. This is a newly defined category, wherein individuals are increasingly independent of parental control but may be dependent on them for support and financial assistance

> Young adult defined as 18-35 years

> Middle adult defined as 36-64 years

> This cohort of individuals is more racially/ethnically diverse than ever before

> This is a growing cohort as the life expectancy increases

✎ Priority Assessments or Cues

> Assess vital signs including adult ranges (heart rate 55-90 bpm, respirations 12-18 bpm, blood pressures 128/80 mmHg) temp. approximately 97.5-98.6°F axillary. Need to know client baseline vital signs

> Assess developmental milestones in a variety of domains

- Physical
  - Assess height, weight, and body mass index
  - Completes physical growth around 20 years of age (except for childbearing and breastfeeding women)
  - Changes in weight associated with nutrition and lifestyle issues
  - Physical strength peaks in the young adult years
  - Body function may begin to decline in the middle adult years
  - Tend to be active during the adult years with few illnesses, chronic and other illnesses increase in incidence as adults age
  - Changes in appearance to include wrinkling of skin, graying of hair, decreased hearing and visual acuity, and body composition
  - Posture may change

- Motor
  - Fine and gross motor skills are mature and may change with decreased muscle mass, decreased bone strength, and increase in fat deposits
  - Adulthood is a time to cultivate hobbies and talents and use fine and grow motor skills (sports, golf, hobbies, gardening, crafts, and walking, among others)

- Cognitive
  - Ability to reason using formal operations, decision-making is stable, although adults may still make poor choices
  - Critical thinking improves throughout the adult years with experience and increased contextual thinking
  - Flexibility with life changes, responses to aging, and cognitive function associated with temperament and personality characteristics
  - Education, life experiences, and occupation impact thinking skills

- Psychoemotional
  - Young adults in Erikson's stage of intimacy versus isolation, individuals develop the ability to love and commit one's self; establish intimate bonds of love and friendship. Lack of achievement may lead to anger, bitterness, and isolation
  - Middle adults are in Erikson's stage of generativity versus stagnation wherein efforts are devoted to life goals for family, career, and community; giving care to others is a priority. Focus is on passing on qualities and assets to the next generation and providing support to the previous generation. Failure to meet the goals of this stage may lead to lack of personal growth and egocentricity
  - Roles have changed as male and female roles in intimate relationships, parenting, and gender responsibilities/expectations, have changed
  - Adult years are ones of personal and career achievement, as adults deal with biological changes of the body
  - Described as the "sandwich generation" in the caring of and balancing of the needs of aging parents and children and/or grandchildren
  - Changes in social norms related to marriage, parenting, and aging may impact adult development; influenced also by social media, technology, and current social issues
  - In these years adults address and resolve social and personal tasks, from ages 23-28, adults may focus on self-perception and intimacy, ages 29-34 years may focus on achievement and mastery, and ages 35-43 may assess life goals and relationships
  - Mid-life crises may occur in career, marriage, parenting, and lifestyles
  - Adults deal with changes in career, mobility, sexual performance, family and marital transitions, and depression and anxiety

- Language
  - Adults are generally articulate
  - May require support with local/regional language
  - May speak better than able to read and illiteracy continues to persist in modern society

- Play
  - Usually a financially stable period, but current economic conditions may jeopardize this stability
  - Time for building hobbies and diversional activities

> Assess family history of disease as it may impact personal disease trajectory

> Assess functional assessment as one grows older and assess ability to care for self and others

> Assess for exposure to occupational and environmental hazards

> Assess life satisfaction, hobbies, interests, habits (sleep, diet, exercise, sexual activity, alcohol, cigarettes, caffeine, substances, home, and pets)

> Assess for personal safety, violence in the home, and intimate partner violence

Priority Laboratory Tests/Diagnostics

> Screen using self-breast and self-testicular exams
> Screen for hypertension, hypercholesterolemia, blood glucose levels, and conduct genetic screening
> Screen for drug use
> Screen for sexually transmitted infections
> Screen for exposure to occupational or environmental factors
> Screen for eating disorders
> Conduct mammograms (annually after age 40 years), colonoscopies (every 10 years after age 50), and other assessments as recommended

Priority Interventions or Actions

> Provide health education
  - Consider lifestyle enhancements including diet, exercise, healthy sleep, balancing stress, smoking, risky and under-the-influence driving, binge drinking, use of seatbelts, sun safety, age related changes, and healthy stress management
  - Provide sexual health education to promote healthy sexual behaviors, contraception, protection, consent, sexual pleasure and responsibilities, and the psychodynamic aspects of sexual activity. Also address pregnancy, birth, and childbearing
  - Provide support during the perimenopausal period in women (decreased menses, sleep disturbances, weight changes, hot flashes, and mood changes) and the climacteric period in men (less rigid erections, fatigue, mood changes, longer refractory periods between erections)
  - Identify modifiable risk factors and provide teaching to assist with lifestyle change
> Provide assistance with minor or chronic health issues (see appropriate Priority Exemplars)
> Assist clients to deal with unplanned pregnancy or infertility
> Encourage adequate sleep and encourage use of sleep hygiene interventions
> Ensure that adults are able to deal with life stresses, including family and job stressors

Priority Potential & Actual Complications

> Unintentional or intentional injury or illness
> Accidental injury including motor vehicle accidents, suicide, and homicide
> Potential for intimate partner violence, including physical, verbal and emotional aspects

Priority Nursing Implications

> Many young adults are healthy and active, they tend to postpone health seeking and ignore symptoms. As adults age, they may be more inclined to seek care
> Nurses may be involved in encouraging preconception health (those behaviors that enhance the positive outcomes of pregnancies)
> Nurses need to consider the cultural and spiritual aspects that may affect developmental care

Priority Medications

> Folic acid during the preconception years to prevent neural tube defects
> Travel immunizations to selected areas
> Multivitamins to enhance nutrition
> Calcium and Vitamin D supplements to prevent osteoporosis

Priority Education/Discharge Issues

> Encourage adults to establish internal and external support systems to assist them into the older adult years
> Assess client's ability to learn and grow and desire to adhere to recommendations of a healthy lifestyle
> Assess for health literacy and ability to understand health instruction and recommendations

Next Gen Clinical Judgment

A 52-year-old client enters the crisis intervention clinic with her spouse. The female client is caring for her 78-year-old mother who is bedridden following a cerebrovascular accident. The client's spouse works two jobs to meet the financial needs of the family. The couple's single daughter and her two children just moved in and the house is crowded. The client is crying, shaking, and states "I am exhausted... I can't do this anymore... I can't take it anymore."

List three recommendations the nurse can provide to assist this family:

1. _____

   _____

2. _____

   _____

3. _____

   _____

Older adults

Pathophysiology/Description

> Young-old adult ages 65-75 years

> Middle-old adult 76-85 years

> Old-old adult over 85 years

> High degree of variability in how each individual ages

> Increasing percentages of the population are older adults, increasing diversity of this cohort

> Most older adults live in non-institutional settings, or at home, despite common misperceptions

Priority Assessments or Cues

> Recognize that a comprehensive assessment of an older adult may take a long time and require more detail as a person ages

> Assess vital signs including older adult ranges (heart rate 55-90 bpm, respirations 12-18 bpm, blood pressures 130/80 mmHg) temp. approximately 97.5-98.6°F axillary. Need to know client baseline vital signs

> Assess developmental milestones in a variety of domains

- Physical
  - Assess weight and height, with the knowledge that height will decrease, and body mass index will decrease
  - Changes include loss of pigment and wrinkling of skin, slowed reflexes, decreased balance, decreased short-term memory, decreased muscle mass, brittle bones, changes in gait, decreased cardiac output, decreased exercise tolerance, decreased pulmonary function, suppressed cough, decreased immune function, decreased need for calories, decreased thirst, constipation, dehydration, decreased glucose tolerance, decreased metabolic rate, decreased continence and bladder capacity, and decreased visual/hearing acuity, among other changes
  - Assess for impact of changes in hearing and vision. Changes in taste cause older adults to want salt and sweets. Changes in smell and taste hamper appetite

- Motor
  - May deteriorate with changes in muscle tone, strength, bone structure, and balance
  - Tremors, arthritis, stiffness, or pain may change fine motor abilities
  - Changes in visual acuity may alter fine motor abilities

- Cognitive
  - Assess level of consciousness and orientation
  - Confusion is often related to physical illness, including urinary tract infections
  - Assess for depression, delirium, and dementia (See Priority Exemplars)
  - Assess for sudden changes in neurological status or functional/cognitive status

- Psychoemotional
  - Erikson's period of integrity versus despair, when one looks back over one's life, accepts meaning out of life, and finds integrity and fulfillment or becomes sad and full of despair
  - Psychological adjustment to deterioration and threats to independent living
  - Dealing with loss of income and loss of skills
  - Changes in role function
  - Coping with loss (spouse, friends, job, body image, functioning), depression, grief, potential for suicide, and isolation/loneliness
  - Changes in memory
    - Fluid knowledge is acquired recently and may be forgotten
    - Crystallized knowledge is learned long ago and often remembered by older adults

- Language
  - Remain articulate
  - Language may be hampered by hearing impairment

- Play/work/functional assessment
  - ADLs (Activities of daily living) including hygiene, self-feeding, moving, and meeting personal needs
  - IADLs (Instrumental activities of daily living) including procuring and preparing food, shopping, paying bills, and talking via the phone

> Assess health history, genetic history, and for co-morbidities

> Assess for pain and impact of pain on functional abilities

> Assess lifestyle and habits, including alcohol, cigarettes, diet, exercise, drugs, sleep, and stress management

Priority Laboratory Tests/Diagnostics

> Assess renal, hepatic, and cardiac function

> Assess serum calcium levels

> Assess serum albumin levels to determine nutritional status

> Screen for hypertension, depression, changes in vision or hearing acuity, skin changes, and other health alterations

> Conduct mammograms (annually after age 40 years), colonoscopies (every 10 years after age 50), and other assessments as recommended

Priority Interventions or Actions

> Goals are to stabilize chronic conditions, promote health, and promote independence

> Provide health education as individuals adjust to changes of aging

- Teach about dental health and means to maintain teeth or substitutes

- Counsel about proper weight, exercise, low-fat diet, moderate alcohol use, smoking cessation, stress management, and handwashing

- Provide nutrition counseling to include small, frequent feedings. Older adults often eat most for breakfast and appetite decreases throughout the day

- Provide sleep hygiene interventions because older adults tend to experience sleep disturbances; older adults frequently sleep during day, making nighttime sleep difficult; older adults require moderate levels of sleep and rest

- For clients with incontinence, provide instruction on hygiene, protection, and Kegel exercises

- Assist clients to deal with constipation including fluids, fiber, exercise, and laxatives. Some clients experience diarrhea, encourage fluids and analyze diet

- Assist client to deal with changes in housing, social situation, sexuality, grieving, and life transitions

> With decreased thirst, encourage adequate fluid intake except at night when trips to the bathroom may precipitate falls

> Provide opportunities for reality orientation, validation, and reminiscence

> Educate as clients are able to manage and comprehend information

Priority Potential & Actual Complications

> Unintentional or intentional injury or illness

> Elder abuse (assess and refer/manage related to domestic, institutional or self) emotional financial, physical, verbal, financial, or sexual abuse or neglect or abandonment

> Older adults are highly prone to infections related to suppressed immune systems

> At risk for dehydration and clients may become malnourished, but dehydration is a greater concern

> Social isolation, despair, unresolved pain, and other sorrows may drive older adults to suicide

> Multiple co-morbidities may tax the client's ability to live a quality life

Priority Nursing Implications

> Hospitalized older adults

- Protect from hospital-acquired infections and falls, assess continence, skin for breakdown, mobility issues, and for poor nutrition/hydration

- Provide favorite foods and fluids and use restraints sparingly

- Round hourly for assessments, toileting, and meeting client needs

- Encourage sterile technique and handwashing, use invasive procedures only when needed

> Increased incidence of falls related to physical and other factors

> Nurses need to consider the cultural and spiritual aspects that may affect developmental care

> Consider ageism and person bias toward older adults as it impacts care

Priority Medications

> Assess older adult medications and for polypharmacy, medication errors, interactions, side effects, non-compliance, use of over-the-counter medications, and use of complementary or alternative medications

> Assess effects and use lower dosages, understanding the potential for accumulation and toxicity

> Assess for changes in neurological status as it may relate to medications

> Immunizations to include influenza, shingles, tetanus, diphtheria, pertussis (if around young children), and pneumococcal disease. Older adults may need boosters of selected immunizations if titers are not adequate

> Assess use of probiotics to regulate bowel function

Priority Education/Discharge Issues

> Ensure safety aspects for clients with decreased cognitive function

> Ensure home safety including lighting, limiting of physical obstacles, moving of throw rugs, limit use of heat therapies such as heating pads, easy access to phone, home set up for current living needs and desires, and ability to adapt home to physical limitations

> Encourage case management to ensure safe and adequate home environment, access to resources, and healthcare surveillance

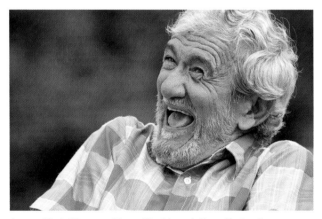

Image 18-4: When working with older adults suffering from dementia, asking about their past, their skills, interests may help improve their sense of well-being.

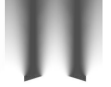

1. A nurse is planning to educate a 40-year-old female client to administer her own insulin injections. Which method would be most effective in teaching the client this skill?
   1. Provide the client with a brochure.
   2. Utilize the educational library at the hospital.
   3. Demonstrate the technique and have the client practice.
   4. Provide the client with a video to watch.

2. A nurse is completing a safety assessment on an 80-year-old client. The nurse is assessing the client's home. Which is the most significant risk that may be present?
   1. Electrical hazards.
   2. Inadequate smoke detectors.
   3. Broken windows.
   4. Loose rugs or uneven floors.

3. A toddler is clinging to his parent to resist entering the procedure room to have an intravenous line inserted. Which statement by the nurse would be most appropriate at this time?
   1. "We need to get into the procedure room to ensure your child's intravenous line is inserted immediately."
   2. "We expect toddlers to act like this, your child is going through separation anxiety."
   3. "Your child doesn't want to leave your side. Are you comfortable watching your child have an intravenous line inserted?"
   4. "Your child will not cooperate without you. Please join us in the procedure room."

4. After an educational session, a new mother is repeating the key concepts related to infant bed safety to the nurse. Which statements indicate a need for more teaching?
   1. "I will place my son on his belly to sleep."
   2. "My son can sleep with his pacifier."
   3. "I will not use bumper pads or place stuffed toys in my son's crib."
   4. "I will not sleep in the same bed as my infant son."

5. A client is receiving pre-conception education. Which statement, if made by the client, indicates priority information to ensure healthy pregnancies?
   1. "I need to make sure I get enough B complex vitamins to ensure that I can deal with stress."
   2. "I need to take fluoride to make sure that my teeth are healthy before pregnancy."
   3. "I will drink orange juice to make sure I have enough vitamin C to fight infection."
   4. "I will take a multivitamin with adequate levels of folic acid in the years prior to planning a pregnancy."

6. A nurse is providing distraction to a 4-year-old as part of pain management during intravenous device insertion. Which intervention would the nurse implement with this client?
   1. Allowing the child to listen to soothing music.
   2. Encouraging the child to watch cartoons on television.
   3. Providing a kaleidoscope for the child to peer into.
   4. Reading books to the child on a favorite topic.

7. A nurse is assessing a non-verbal, 1-year-old child's level of pain. Which would require immediate intervention with pharmacological and non-pharmacological pain management?
   1. A client whose medication is due to provide round-the-clock analgesia.
   2. The client is tachycardic and writhing and restless in bed.
   3. The client is calm and smiling, splinting his incision with his hand if moved.
   4. The client who is occasionally moaning.

8. A five-year client is hospitalized and will undergo surgery. The nurse is planning the best way to discuss the surgery experience with the client. According to the child's developmental stage, which method should the nurse choose?
   1. Show a 20-minute video about the surgery experience to the client.
   2. Allow the child to visit the operating room.
   3. Have the child read a book about the surgery experience.
   4. Use a doll to demonstrate the surgery experience and allow to play with it.

9. A client asks a nurse when her child can start riding in the front seat of the car. Which is the best nursing response?
   1. "Your child can begin riding in the front seat of the car after the age of 6."
   2. "Your child cannot ride in the front seat of the car until they weigh 30 pounds or more."
   3. "Your child can ride in the front seat of the car if they use a booster seat."
   4. "Your child can ride in the front seat after the age of 12."

10. An adolescent calls the nurse helpline at a primary care provider's office and tells the nurse that his friend mentioned a suicide plan. Which is the priority action?
    1. Determine the specifics of the plan.
    2. Tell the friend's parents about the plan.
    3. Remove any weapons from the friend.
    4. Get immediate help for the friend.

11. When providing a client with written material, which criteria should the nurse ensure are met?
    1. The material contains the appropriate medical terms.
    2. The material is written in English.
    3. The material is written at a 5th grade level.
    4. The material is written at a 12th grade level.

12. A nurse caring for a 19-year-old transgender client, recognizes that this client is at increased risk for which health outcomes? Select all that apply.
    1. Attempted suicide.
    2. Health care provider bias.
    3. Social isolation.
    4. Positive body image.
    5. Pneumonia.

13. A 6-year-old client is diagnosed with a life-threatening illness. The parents express concern over their child's prognosis. Which statement by the nurse would be most helpful initially?
    1. "Would you like another parent with the same problems to talk to?"
    2. "Would you like to meet with a chaplain to discuss your concerns?"
    3. "Do you and your spouse support each other during times of stress?"
    4. "Tell me what your current concerns are about your child."

14. A 14-year-old female enters the emergency department escorted by police following an alleged sexual assault. The nurse conducts an admission assessment and is told by the client that the partner she was dating was a 20-year-old man and she did not consent to sexual activity. In addition to comfort care and providing support to the client, what is a priority for the nurse in this situation?
    1. Determine how the client's parents want to proceed in the client's care.
    2. Ensure that the client is showered and cleaned as soon as possible.
    3. Determine local statutory rape laws and involve social services.
    4. Encourage the client to resolve issues related to her dating partner.

15. A child states, "Everyone has a mommy and a daddy except me. I have two mommies." What response does the nurse make?
    1. "That is too bad you do not have a daddy."
    2. "Two parents are best even if it is two mommies."
    3. "You must feel very special to have two mommies."
    4. "What do you do with your mommies to have fun?"

16. A nurse notes that a female client has multiple bruises on her body during a wellness exam. What nursing action would be appropriate?
    1. Assess the color of the bruises.
    2. Take photographs of the bruises.
    3. Screen the client for intimate partner violence.
    4. Conduct a comprehensive physical assessment.

17. A 16-year-old discovers she is pregnant and seeks out the assistance of the school nurse. The client has heard that teen women often do not have healthy babies. The nurse provides instruction to the young woman based on which information?
    1. Teens can have healthy babies if they have prenatal care and healthy behaviors.
    2. Teens do not have healthy babies due to their young age and lack of maturity.
    3. Teens bodies are usually not able to have healthy babies due to their pelvic size.
    4. Teens are often poorly nourished and unable to carry their pregnancies to term.

18. A 2-year-old client and her parents seek out primary care in a clinic. The nurse is providing anticipatory safety guidance for the family. Which instructions are critical based on this client's age?
    1. Providing lessons in swimming and water safety.
    2. Ensuring safe sleep practices and back to sleep positioning.
    3. Discussing ingestions and safe storage of potential poisons.
    4. Providing information on bicycle safety and use of helmets.

19. A nurse is providing education to a young adult who is sexually active and reports using no "protection." The nurse would plan to include which content in teaching about safer sexual behavior? Select all that apply.
    1. Using condoms with vaginal or anal sexual activity.
    2. Using dental dam membranes or condoms with oral sexual activity.
    3. Ensuring sexual activity is consented by all parties prior to each sexual encounter.
    4. Using double condoms with vaginal intercourse to prevent pregnancy.
    5. Vaginal douching with vinegar immediately after sexual intercourse.
    6. Using petroleum-based lubricants to avoid injury with vaginal or anal intercourse.

20. The nurse is teaching parents about the four stages of separation anxiety that children experience. Place these behaviors in the correct order from initial, to last stage.
    1. Plays quietly and does not interact with others.
    2. Cries uncontrollably when parents leave
    3. Resists when the nurse tries to comfort the child.
    4. Interacts with the nurses but ignores the parents.
    5. Plays appropriately with parents and others.

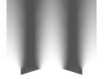

21. The nurse is caring for a hospitalized school age child. The nurse asks when the father is coming back to visit. The child states, "He is not my father, he is my mother's husband." What initial response does the nurse make?
 1. "So what you mean is that he is your stepfather."
 2. "You are so lucky to have such a nice stepfather."
 3. "What activities do you enjoy with your mother's husband?"
 4. "I bet you wish your father was here instead of your stepfather."

22. The nurse is making a home visit and observes peeling paint from the window sills on the floor of the enclosed porch where the infant's toys are stored. What follow-up action is required by the nurse?
 1. Refer to the department of social services.
 2. Discuss strategies for sudden infant death syndrome prevention.
 3. Complete a lead risk assessment.
 4. Review the immunization schedule.

23. During a well child visit, parents of a child ask the nurse about using complementary therapies that are used in their native country. What response does the nurse make?
 1. "You need to get approval from your healthcare provider before you start complementary therapies."
 2. "Let's see if the therapy can be used safely with your child's current treatments."
 3. "It sounds very expensive; do you really think it will be worth the expense?"
 4. "Did you research all the benefits and side effects in scientific literature?"

24. A Muslim female adult client is requesting a female provider to perform her physical assessment. Which response by the nurse is most appropriate?
 1. "There are only male health care providers, but I will stay with you during the exam."
 2. "You do not need to remove your clothes if I cannot find a female health care provider."
 3. "I will request a Muslim health care provider to perform your physical assessment."
 4. "I will get a female health care provider to perform your physical exam."

25. The healthcare provider orders 1 unit of packed red blood cells for a child. The nurse recalls the mother mentioning that the child is a Jehovah's Witness. What is the most appropriate next action?
 1. Tell the healthcare provider that treatment was refused by the parents due to religious beliefs.
 2. Explain the benefits and advantages of allowing the blood transfusion to the parents.
 3. Arrange an emergency meeting with healthcare provider and the ethics committee.
 4. Discuss any appropriate alternative treatments with the health care team and parents.

26. What is the most appropriate teaching that the nurse can provide to a parent who is concerned about his toddler's interactions when playing with other toddlers?
 1. Usually do not pay attention to most toys, playing only with a few of them.
 2. There is minimal conflict when toddlers play together.
 3. Toddlers like to play in the presence of other toddlers but not with them.
 4. Toddlers are good at sharing their toys with others during play.

27. A 13-month-old infant does not babble or make sounds. The nurse is screening the infant for a hearing impairment. Which assessment finding causes the nurse the greatest level of concern?
 1. The infant appears surprised when someone approaches them.
 2. The infant had a history of otitis media two months ago.
 3. The pinna of the ear is red and swollen.
 4. The baby makes eye contact and attends to faces.

28. The nurse visits an older adult home care client who is bedridden and being cared for by her family. The nurse is discussing with the client and family about the importance of changing position in bed. The nurse's teaching is direct toward preventing complications in which area when a client is immobile?
 1. Nausea.
 2. Jaundice.
 3. Atelectasis.
 4. Mental confusion.

29. A 45-year-old female adult client is being seen as part of the annual health examination. Which screening tests are recommended for this client? Select all that apply.
 1. A colonoscopy.
 2. An annual mammogram.
 3. An annual skin exam.
 4. Blood pressure screening annually.
 5. Cholesterol profile annually.
 6. Vision examination every two years.

30. A spouse of a client with a head trauma speaks with the nurse. The spouse says, "I am so tired, I don't know how much longer I can do this." Which is the best response for the nurse?
 1. "You should think about a long-term care facility for your spouse."
 2. "Your spouse can be trained to care for herself."
 3. "There are several local resources to help you, let me put you in touch with some of them."
 4. "Perhaps you need to have an examination to see why you are fatigued."

1. **A nurse is planning to educate a 40-year-old female client to administer her own insulin injections. Which method would be most effective in teaching the client this skill?**
    1. Provide the client with a brochure. *The client may not be able to read or may not learn best via reading or printed material.*
    2. Utilize the educational library at the hospital. *The client may not be motivated to use the library or know where to access resources.*
    3. ⚉ Demonstrate the technique and have the client practice.
    4. Provide the client with a video to watch. *The client may not learn via video and this is not most effective for a psychomotor skill.*

    Rationale: Demonstration and practice are the most effective methodology to teach a skill, especially a psychomotor skill.

    THIN Thinking: Nursing Process – *Part of teaching is assessing the most effective method to teach and evaluating effectiveness of the teaching session* **NCLEX®:** Health Promotion and Maintenance **QSEN:** Patient-centered Care

2. **A nurse is completing a safety assessment on an 80-year-old client. The nurse is assessing the client's home. Which is the most significant risk that may be present?**
    1. Electrical hazards. *These are not a priority concern among older adults.*
    2. Inadequate smoke detectors. *These are not a priority concern, nor specific to, older adults.*
    3. Broken windows. *These are not a priority concern, nor specific to, older adults.*
    4. ⚉ Loose rugs or uneven floors.

    Rationale: Falls are the leading cause of injury in the elderly population. Special attention should be given to any loose rugs or uneven floors that may cause a fall.

    THIN Thinking: Identify Safety Needs – *Nurses need to be able to anticipate and identify safety threats based on client characteristics* **NCLEX®:** Safety and Infection Control **QSEN:** Safety

3. **A toddler is clinging to his parent to resist entering the procedure room to have an intravenous line inserted. Which statement by the nurse would be most appropriate at this time?**
    1. "We need to get into the procedure room to ensure your child's intravenous line is inserted immediately." *This answer is not helpful and may distress the parent even more, further upsetting the child.*
    2. "We expect toddlers to act like this, your child is going through separation anxiety." *Naming the behavior is not helpful to the parent and may raise stress levels.*
    3. ⚉ "Your child doesn't want to leave your side. Are you comfortable watching your child have an intravenous line inserted?"
    4. "Your child will not cooperate without you. Please join us in the procedure room." *Not all parents can watch painful procedures performed on their children. Nurses need to ask them and put them in control of the situation.*

    Rationale: This client is experiencing separation anxiety. This is a common developmental attribute of the toddler. This child is also experiencing fear and may benefit from his parent's presence.

    THIN Thinking: Nursing Process – *Knowledge of child growth and development assists the nurse to plan/propose age-appropriate interventions.* **NCLEX®:** Basic Care and Comfort **QSEN:** Patient Care and Comfort

4. **After an educational session, a new mother is repeating the key concepts related to infant bed safety to the nurse. Which statements indicate a need for more teaching?**
    1. ⚉ "I will place my son on his belly to sleep."
    2. "My son can sleep with his pacifier." *Studies demonstrate that pacifiers are protective for sudden infant death syndrome.*
    3. "I will not use bumper pads or place stuffed toys in my son's crib." *This is a correct behavior to prevent sudden infant death syndrome.*
    4. "I will not sleep in the same bed as my infant son." *This is a positive behavior as sleeping with infants has been associated with sudden infant death syndrome.*

    Rationale: An infant should be placed on his/her back to sleep to decrease the risk of sudden infant death syndrome. A pacifier and less bedding will also reduce the risk of SIDS. Co-bedding increases the risk of suffocation.

    THIN Thinking: Identify Safety Risks – *An important part of anticipatory guidance for new parents is to teach safe sleep precautions to prevent SIDS.* **NCLEX-RN®** Safety and Infection Control **QSEN:** Safety

5. A client is receiving pre-conception education. Which statement, if made by the client, indicates priority information to ensure healthy pregnancies?
    1. "I need to make sure I get enough B complex vitamins to ensure that I can deal with stress." *This is not a priority during the preconception period.*
    2. "I need to take fluoride to make sure that my teeth are healthy before pregnancy." *Although healthy oral hygiene is important for healthy pregnancies, it is not as important as folic acid.*
    3. "I will drink orange juice to make sure I have enough vitamin C to fight infection." *There is no conclusive evidence that Vitamin C prevents infection and is not as important as folic acid.*
    4. ⊙ "I will take a multivitamin with adequate levels of folic acid in the years prior to planning a pregnancy."

    Rationale: Folic acid has been shown to decrease the incidence of neural tube defects and should ideally be included in the mother's diet or supplemented before conception.

    THIN Thinking: Top Three – *Folic acid is a critical element of preconception education to ensure healthy pregnancies and prevent neural tube defects* **NCLEX®:** Health Promotion and Maintenance **QSEN:** Evidence-based Practice

6. A nurse is providing distraction to a 4-year-old as part of pain management during intravenous device insertion. Which intervention would the nurse implement with this client?
    1. Allowing the child to listen to soothing music. *4-year-old children may not be distracted by soothing music.*
    2. Encouraging the child to watch cartoons on television. *Although television may be distracting, it is not a novel stimulus and may not last for the whole procedure.*
    3. ⊙ Providing a kaleidoscope for the child to peer into.
    4. Reading books to the child on a favorite topic. *Reading is not as distracting as the moving parts and interest stimulated by the kaleidoscope.*

    Rationale: Young children have been found to be distracted in response to kaleidoscope treatments. Although music television, music, and reading may be effective, research demonstrates age-related measures are superior.

    THIN Thinking: Nursing Process – *The nurse uses developmental principles to plan nursing interventions.* **NCLEX®:** Basic Care and Comfort **QSEN:** Patient-centered Care

7. A nurse is assessing a non-verbal, 1-year-old child's level of pain. Which would require immediate intervention with pharmacological and non-pharmacological pain management?
    1. A client whose medication is due to provide round-the-clock analgesia. *Although this medication is due, the round-the-clock nature indicates that some pain medication is on board to allow some time before administration.*
    2. ⊙ The client is tachycardic and writhing and restless in bed.
    3. The client is calm and smiling, splinting his incision with his hand if moved. *Although splinting indicates pain, the demeanor of calmness and smiling indicates the need is not immediate.*
    4. The client who is occasionally moaning. *Although moaning may be a sign of pain, it may be a form of communication not specific to distress.*

    RATIONALE: Elevated vital signs and restlessness are suggestive of pain in non-verbal clients. Non-verbal clients can't ask for pain medication. Although round the clock medication is usually an optimal means to address pain, the client's behaviors indicate immediate intervention. Splinting is a sign of pain, but not as significant as the other signs.

    THIN Thinking: Help Quick – *The nurse may quickly assess client appearance and behaviors to determine the pain level in non-verbal clients* **NCLEX®:** Basic Care and Comfort **QSEN:** Patient-centered Care

8. A 5-year-old client is hospitalized and will undergo surgery. The nurse is planning the best way to discuss the surgery experience with the client. According to the child's developmental stage, which method should the nurse choose?
    1. Show a 20-minute video about the surgery experience to the client. *A video will not be as informative for a 5-year-old, and does not allow for active play.*
    2. Allow the child to visit the operating room. *Although this will allow a sensory experience for the child, it is not as effective as play.*
    3. Have the child read a book about the surgery experience. *Although reading may be useful, it is not as effective as active play.*
    4. ⊙ Use a doll to demonstrate the surgery experience and allow to play with it.

    Rationale: The pre-school child utilizes abstract thinking. Preparation for the surgical procedure can be done with dolls and play.

    THIN Thinking: Nursing Process – *Nurses will use knowledge of growth and development to plan their care and teaching* **NCLEX®:** Basic Care and Comfort **QSEN:** Patient-centered Care

9. **A client asks a nurse when her child can start riding in the front seat of the car. Which is the best nursing response?**
   1. "Your child can begin riding in the front seat of the car after the age of 6." *Due to airbags and child size, this is not recommended.*
   2. "Your child cannot ride in the front seat of the car until they weigh 30 pounds or more." *Many children are 30 pounds prior to being the appropriate age to sit in the front seat.*
   3. "Your child can ride in the front seat of the car if they use a booster seat." *This is not true and the booster seat will not prevent airbag or other injuries.*
   4. 💡 "Your child can ride in the front seat after the age of 12."

   Rationale: It is recommended that a child does not ride in the front seat of a car until after the age of 12.

   THIN Thinking: Nursing Process – *The nurse uses evidence-based practices to provide client teaching and safety education* **NCLEX®:** Health Promotion and Maintenance **QSEN:** Safety

10. **An adolescent calls the nurse helpline at a primary care provider's office and tells the nurse that his friend mentioned a suicide plan. Which is the priority action?**
    1. Determine the specifics of the plan. *Although this may be helpful, it is more important to immediately attempt to prevent the suicide.*
    2. Tell the friend's parents about the plan. *Although parents need to know, it is more important to get immediate intervention to prevent the suicide.*
    3. Remove any weapons from the friend. *Weapon removal is important, but immediate help is critical to prevent the suicide.*
    4. 💡 Get immediate help for the friend.

    Rationale: Threats of suicide need to be taken seriously and immediate help is the priority. An appointment may be too late but is beneficial for continued follow-up. Telling his parents, learning about the plan and asking about weapons are helpful but not the priority.

    THIN Thinking: Identify Safety Needs – *The nurse should quickly identify threats to safety, including suicidal ideations and intervene quickly.* **NCLEX®:** Psychosocial Integrity **QSEN:** Safety

11. **When providing a client with written material, which criteria should the nurse ensure are met?**
    1. The material contains the appropriate medical terms. *Medical terms may be confusing or not understood by clients.*
    2. The material is written in English. *The question does not indicate that the client is English speaking or able to read English.*
    3. 💡 The material is written at a 5th grade level.
    4. The material is written at a 12th grade level. *Many clients may not be able to read at this level.*

    Rationale: According to the National Action Plan to improve health literacy, written material should be written at a 5th grade level and in the client's primary language.

    THIN Thinking: Help Quick – *Ensuring that teaching materials are at this level ensures that the nurse can quickly access materials for many clients. The nurse would need to assess if the client can read and if they can read at this level* **NCLEX®:** Health Promotion and Maintenance **QSEN:** Patient-centered Care

12. **A nurse caring for a 19-year-old transgender client, recognizes that this client is at increased risk for which health outcomes? Select all that apply.**
    1. 💡 Attempted suicide.
    2. 💡 Health care provider bias.
    3. 💡 Social isolation.
    4. Positive body image. *Transgender youth are at risk for negative body image.*
    5. Pneumonia. *There is no reason for transgender youth to be at risk for pneumonia.*

    Rationale: The transgender population may be more at risk for attempted suicide, health care provider bias, and social isolation. They are not more prone to pneumonia and may be at risk for negative body image issues.

    THIN Thinking: Nursing Process – *The nurse assesses the client's risk and plans care accordingly* **NCLEX®:** Health Promotion and Maintenance **QSEN:** Patient-centered Care

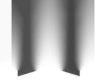

13. A 6-year-old client is diagnosed with a life-threatening illness. The parents express concern over their child's prognosis. Which statement by the nurse would be most helpful initially?
    1. "Would you like another parent with the same problems to talk to?" *Although this intervention may be helpful, it is important to first explore the parents' concerns.*
    2. "Would you like to meet with a chaplain to discuss your concerns?" *Although this is a helpful intervention, it is important to first open the conversation.*
    3. "Do you and your spouse support each other during times of stress?" *It will be important to explore support systems after the parents voice their concerns.*
    4. ⦿ "Tell me what your current concerns are about your child."

    Rationale: The initial response should address opening conversation and determining the parents' needs. After these are assessed, the nurse may suggest and explore interventions. One can't assume which interventions will be the most effective until consulting the individuals.

    THIN Thinking: Help Quick – *The initial response in a communication situation should open up conversation and allow the clients to express their concerns* **NCLEX®:** Psychosocial Integrity **QSEN:** *Patient-centered Care*

14. A 14-year-old female enters the emergency department escorted by police following an alleged sexual assault. The nurse conducts an admission assessment and is told by the client that the partner she was dating was a 20-year-old man and she did not consent to sexual activity. In addition to comfort care and providing support to the client, what is a priority for the nurse in this situation?
    1. Determine how the client's parents want to proceed in the client's care. *The local laws will determine parental notification laws.*
    2. Ensure that the client is showered and cleaned as soon as possible. *This should not be done in case evidence needs to be collected.*
    3. ⦿ Determine local statutory rape laws and involve social services.
    4. Encourage the client to resolve issues related to her dating partner. *This is not appropriate with non-consensual sexual activity.*

    Rationale: Local laws need to be explored related to age of majority and years of age difference associated with sexual assault. The social services department may assist with this process. It will also impact the parental consent laws related to age of majority, mature minors, and emancipated minors. Encouraging resolution in episodes of violence is not the nurse's prerogative. Cleaning may eradicate evidence if that is to be collected.

THIN Thinking: Top Three – *Finding out local laws and regulations is a priority in cases of potential crimes, in addition to client comfort and support* **NCLEX®:** Management of Care **QSEN:** Teamwork and Collaboration

15. A child states, "Everyone has a mommy and a daddy except me. I have two mommies." What response does the nurse make?
    1. "That is too bad you do not have a daddy." *This is judgmental and is not appropriate for the nurse.*
    2. "Two parents are best even if it is two mommies." *This comment is judgmental and is not helpful to the child.*
    3. "You must feel very special to have two mommies." *Although a positive comment, it is more important to open conversation with the client.*
    4. ⦿ "What do you do with your mommies to have fun?"

    Rationale: Use of open-ended questions help explore the child's feelings about her family structure. Making the child feel different is not appropriate. Talking with the child will allow the child to share his or her experiences and explore his developmental response to his or her family.

    THIN Thinking: Help Quick – *Open questions will open up communication and assess the client's needs* **NCLEX®:** Psychosocial Integrity **QSEN:** Patient-centered Care

16. A nurse notes that a female client has multiple bruises on her body during a wellness exam. What nursing action would be appropriate?
    1. Assess the color of the bruises. *Although this assessment is important, the client's safety is paramount.*
    2. Take photographs of the bruises. *This may be part of the protocol, but ensuring that the client is safe is most important at this time.*
    3. ⦿ Screen the client for intimate partner violence.
    4. Conduct a comprehensive physical assessment. *Although important, it is critical to conduct a screening for intimate partner violence and refer accordingly.*

    Rationale: Intimate partner violence screening is recommended to be completed on all women, especially those with bruises or signs of abuse.

    THIN Thinking: Help Quick – *The first priority is to screen this client for intimate partner violence and refer to services* **NCLEX®:** Safety and Infection Control **QSEN:** Safety

17. **A 16-year-old discovers she is pregnant and seeks out the assistance of the school nurse. The client has heard that teen women often do not have healthy babies. The nurse provides instruction to the young woman based on which information?**
    1. ⊕ Teens can have healthy babies if they have prenatal care and healthy behaviors.
    2. Teens do not have healthy babies due to their young age and lack of maturity. *This is not true and teens may have healthy babies.*
    3. Teens bodies are usually not able to have healthy babies due to their pelvic size. *This is not true, pelvic size is not only related to body size.*
    4. Teens are often poorly nourished and unable to carry their pregnancies to term. *This is not true, teens may have healthy pregnancies.*

    Rationale: Adequate prenatal care, nutrition, and avoiding high-risk behaviors are associated with positive birth outcomes among all women, especially teens. Teens are physically able to have a healthy pregnancy and birth if they receive the care they need. There is no evidence to suggest that teens are too young physically to have a child, but social norms often impact thoughts about healthy pregnancies during the teen years.

    THIN Thinking: Nursing Process – *The nurse uses science-based information to provide client teaching* **NCLEX®:** Health Promotion and Maintenance **QSEN:** Evidence-based Practice

18. **A 2-year-old client and her parents seek out primary care in a clinic. The nurse is providing anticipatory safety guidance for the family. Which instructions are critical based on this client's age?**
    1. Providing lessons in swimming and water safety. *Water safety is important, but more appropriate for parents of pre-school aged children.*
    2. Ensuring safe sleep practices and back to sleep positioning. *Safe sleeping practices are important but more appropriate for parents of infants.*
    3. ⊕ Discussing ingestions and safe storage of potential poisons.
    4. Providing information on bicycle safety and use of helmets. *This is a priority for school-aged children.*

    Rationale: Children are at risk for certain behaviors and subsequent consequences according to their developmental level and abilities. Toddlers are mobile and inquisitive, allowing them to access and want to touch, taste, and handle dangerous substances. This increases their risk for ingestions and injury.

    THIN Thinking: Identify Safety Risks – *Due to developmental characteristics, toddlers are at risk for ingestions and poisoning* **NCLEX®:** Health Promotion and Maintenance **QSEN:** Safety

19. **A nurse is providing education to a young adult who is sexually active and reports using no "protection." The nurse would plan to include which content in teaching about safer sexual behavior? Select all that apply.**
    1. ⊕ Using condoms with vaginal or anal sexual activity.
    2. ⊕ Using dental dam membranes or condoms with oral sexual activity.
    3. ⊕ Ensuring sexual activity is consented by all parties prior to each sexual encounter.
    4. Using double condoms with vaginal intercourse to prevent pregnancy. *Doubling condoms increases the risk for friction of the latex and ripping.*
    5. Vaginal douching with vinegar immediately after sexual intercourse. *There is no reason to douche after sexual activity.*
    6. Using petroleum-based lubricants to avoid injury with vaginal or anal intercourse. *Petroleum lubricants may deteriorate latex condoms.*

    Rationale: Condoms and dental dams provide safe barriers for sexual activity. Consent is critical for healthy sexual activity. Doubling up on condoms is not suggested and may lead to breakage, petroleum based lubricants may degrade condoms, and douching is not effective in preventing pregnancy and may cause yeast infections. Water-soluble lubricants are suggested as needed.

    THIN Thinking: Nursing Process – *The nurse should use evidence-based practices when implementing teaching with clients* **NCLEX®:** Health Promotion and Maintenance **QSEN:** Evidence-based Practice

20. **The nurse is teaching parents about the four stages of separation anxiety that children experience. Place these behaviors in the correct order from initial, to last stage.**
    1. Cries uncontrollably when parents leave.
    2. Resists when the nurse tries to comfort the child.
    3. Plays quietly and does not interact with others.
    4. Interacts with the nurses but ignores the parents.
    5. Plays appropriately with parents and others.

    Rationale: The stages of separation anxiety are protest, despair, detachment and a resolution with the return to a healthy parent- child attachment. The protest stage is characterized by crying and a resistance to caregivers. A child in despair is hopeless and becomes quiet and withdrawn. In the detachment stage the child may ignore the parents but interact with others. Finally, playing with parent and others indicates adjustment.

    THIN Thinking: Nursing Process – *Knowledge of growth and development allows the nurse to assess and intervene in the care of children* **NCLEX®:** Psychosocial Integrity **QSEN:** Patience Centered Care

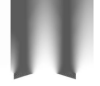

21. **The nurse is caring for a hospitalized school age child. The nurse asks when the father is coming back to visit. The child states, "He is not my father, he is my mother's husband." What initial response does the nurse make?**
    1. "So what you mean is that he is your stepfather." *This statement does not open communication with the child.*
    2. "You are so lucky to have such a nice stepfather." *This is a judgment and does not open discussion.*
    3. 📍 "What activities do you enjoy with your mother's husband?"
    4. "I bet you wish your father was here instead of your stepfather." *This is inappropriate and judgmental.*

    Rationale: Using open-ended questions will encourage conversation about the child's thoughts and feelings. These questions open discussions and allow the nurse to assess the child's family relationships. The other statements are not appropriate and will not encourage further discussion.

    THIN Thinking: Help Quick – *Using open-ended questions in initial communications stimulates sharing and allows for nursing assessment* **NCLEX®:** Psychosocial integrity **QSEN:** Patient-centered Care

22. **The nurse is making a home visit and observes peeling paint from the window sills on the floor of the enclosed porch where the infant's toys are stored. What follow-up action is required by the nurse?**
    1. Refer to the department of social services. *There is no indication for social service involvement in this case.*
    2. Discuss strategies for sudden infant death syndrome prevention. *There is no association between peeling paint and sudden infant death syndrome.*
    3. 📍 Complete a lead risk assessment.
    4. Review the immunization schedule. *This is not appropriate, there are no immunizations associated with peeling paint.*

    Rationale: Lead risk assessment begins when infants become mobile at around 6 months. Once mobile, infants can move around areas where dust and paint chips are found getting on the infant's hands where it can be easily ingested by putting their hands in their mouths. If the house was built before 1974, there may be lead in the paint.

    THIN Thinking: Identify Safety Risks – *The nurse should be aware of the health risks associated with lead-based paints* **NCLEX®:** Safety and Infection Control **QSEN:** Safety

23. **During a well child visit, parents of a child ask the nurse about using complementary therapies that are used in their native country. What response does the nurse make?**
    1. "You need to get approval from your healthcare provider before you start complementary therapies." *The parents have the right to provide care to their children and do not need the healthcare provider's approval.*
    2. 📍 "Let's see if the therapy can be used safely with your child's current treatments."
    3. "It sounds very expensive; do you really think it will be worth the expense?" *This is not helpful and does not attend to the safety of the child.*
    4. "Did you research all the benefits and side effects in scientific literature?" *This may make the parents defensive and does not assist them in ensuring the health of their child.*

    Rationale: Direct and supportive discussions about the use of complementary and alternative medical therapies (CAM) build a rapport with families. Validate the families desire to cure their child and discuss the family's goal for using CAM. Ensure families feel comfortable about discussing CAM with the health care provider.

    THIN Thinking: Top Three – *When counseling clients about alternative therapies, a top consideration is to explore potential interactions and contraindications with current therapies* **NCLEX®:** Psychosocial Integrity **QSEN:** Safety

24. **A Muslim female adult client is requesting a female provider to perform her physical assessment. Which response by the nurse is most appropriate?**
    1. "There are only male health care providers, but I will stay with you during the exam." *This is not responsive to this client's needs.*
    2. "You do not need to remove your clothes if I cannot find a female health care provider." *This does not meet the client's privacy needs.*
    3. "I will request a Muslim health care provider to perform your physical assessment." *This does not meet the client's privacy needs.*
    4. 📍 "I will get a female health care provider to perform your physical exam."

    Rationale: Muslim women prefer female health care providers and honoring this request provides culturally sensitive care. The Muslim laws of modesty are a very important part of Muslim culture and should be respected.

    THIN Thinking: Nursing Process – *The nurse will assess the cultural preferences of the client and ensure those needs are met* **NCLEX®:** Health Promotion and Maintenance **QSEN:** Patient-centered Care

25. The healthcare provider orders 1 unit of packed red blood cells for a child. The nurse recalls the mother mentioning that the child is a Jehovah's Witness. What is the most appropriate next action?
    1. Tell the healthcare provider that treatment was refused by the parents due to religious beliefs. *Although this action is correct, it does not provide a resolution to the issue.*
    2. Explain the benefits and advantages of allowing the blood transfusion to the parents. *The nurse should not impose their beliefs or those of the healthcare community on the client.*
    3. Arrange an emergency meeting with healthcare provider and the ethics committee. *This situation does not warrant an emergency meeting with the ethics committee and escalates the issue.*
    4. 🔘 Discuss any appropriate alternative treatments with the health care team and parents.

    Rationale: Although blood transfusions are prohibited for clients who are Jehovah's Witnesses, alternatives such as non-blood plasma expanders may be acceptable. Discussions with the health care team to explore what treatments are acceptable based on religious beliefs are imperative when providing culturally sensitive care. There is no need for an emergency meeting prior to exploring alternative options.

    THIN Thinking: Top Three – *A critical component of culturally competent care with children and families is to ensure that their wishes are respected and the healthcare team works together to meet their needs* **NCLEX®:** Manager of Care **QSEN:** Teamwork and Collaboration

26. What is the most appropriate teaching that the nurse can provide to a parent who is concerned about his toddler's interactions when playing with other toddlers?
    1. Usually do not pay attention to most toys, playing only with a few of them. *This behavior is typical of infants.*
    2. There is minimal conflict when toddlers play together. *Toddlers often have issues with sharing and are possessive of objects, creating conflict.*
    3. 🔘 Toddlers like to play in the presence of other toddlers but not with them.
    4. Toddlers are good at sharing their toys with others during play. *Sharing usually does not occur until the preschool years.*

    Rationale: Toddlers demonstrate parallel play which is when children play alongside each other, but do not interact with each other. Toddlers often play with many different toys and may take toys away from other children with little regard for the child's feelings. Sharing toys is learned in the preschool years.

    THIN Thinking: Nursing Process – *The nurse uses knowledge of development to implement teaching with clients and families* **NCLEX®:** Health Promotion and Maintenance **QSEN:** Patient-centered Care

27. A 13-month-old infant does not babble or make sounds. The nurse is screening the infant for a hearing impairment. Which assessment finding causes the nurse the greatest level of concern?
    1. 🔘 The infant appears surprised when someone approaches them.
    2. The infant had a history of otitis media two months ago. *Although chronic ear infections may impair hearing, this does not create the highest level of concern.*
    3. The pinna of the ear is red and swollen. *This may indicate otitis externa which does not usually impair hearing.*
    4. The baby makes eye contact and attends to faces. *These are normal infant behaviors.*

    Rationale: The inability of the infant to hear individuals approaching and being surprised by the appearance of others may be indicative of hearing impairment. This behavior should be assessed further for hearing impairment.

    THIN Thinking: Nursing Process – *The nurse assessing a child and noting these behaviors will plan care of the client to include further assessment* **NCLEX®:** Health Promotion and Maintenance **QSEN:** Patient-centered Care

28. The nurse visits an older adult home care client who is bedridden and being cared for by her family. The nurse is discussing with the client and family about the importance of changing position in bed. The nurse's teaching is direct toward preventing complications in which area when a client is immobile?
    1. Nausea. *Nausea is not associated with immobility.*
    2. Jaundice. *Liver impairment and jaundice are not associated with immobility.*
    3. 🔘 Atelectasis.
    4. Mental confusion. *Although the client may be confused while immobile, airway and breathing are higher priorities.*

    Rationale: The client and family would benefit from teaching reinforcing the need for turning and movement in bed to prevent skin breakdown, constipation, and atelectasis, among other complications. Nursing care and teaching is directed toward preventing complications.

    THIN Thinking: Identify Safety Risks – *The nurse may prevent complications by identifying and teaching the family about safety risks* **NCLEX®:** Basic Care and Comfort **QSEN:** Safety

29. A 45-year-old female adult client is being seen as part of the annual health examination. Which screening tests are recommended for this client? Select all that apply.
    1. A colonoscopy. *This is not routinely recommended until 50 years of age, except if risk factors exist.*
    2. ◉ An annual mammogram.
    3. ◉ An annual skin exam.
    4. ◉ Blood pressure screening annually.
    5. ◉ Cholesterol profile annually.
    6. ◉ Vision examination every two years.

    Rationale: Screening women in their forties includes blood pressure screening and cholesterol studies since both of these may increase in the forties. The vision screening assesses for age-related eye diseases such as cataracts and glaucoma (recommended every two years at this age) and the mammogram screens for breast cancer (recommended annually at this age). The colonoscopy is not recommended until age 50 unless there are risk factors.

    THIN Thinking: Nursing Process – *The nurse needs to be aware of the appropriate assessments and provide appropriate client teaching* **NCLEX®:** Health Promotion and Maintenance **QSEN:** Evidence-based Practice

30. A spouse of a client with a head trauma speaks with the nurse. The spouse says, "I am so tired, I don't know how much longer I can do this." Which is the best response for the nurse?
    1. "You should think about a long-term care facility for your spouse." *This is not helpful and makes a recommendation to the client rather than exploring concerns.*
    2. "Your spouse can be trained to care for herself." *It is unlikely that this is helpful since the spouse is already providing the care. This does not open conversation.*
    3. ◉ "There are several local resources to help you, let me put you in touch with some of them."
    4. "Perhaps you need to have an examination to see why you are fatigued." *Although this may be important, a more immediate need is to access resources.*

    Rationale: This spouse is experiencing caregiver role strain. Accessing local resources may provide assistance and relieve the stress and fatigue experienced by the client and spouse.

    THIN Thinking: Help Quick – *Accessing resources quickly will address the needs of the client and the spouse* **NCLEX®:** Management of Care **QSEN:** Teamwork and Collaboration

Role of the Nurse in Quality and Safety

Judgment Connections

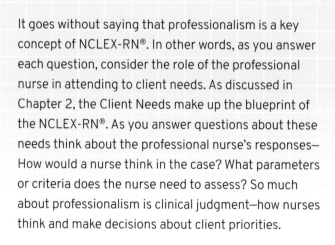

It goes without saying that professionalism is a key concept of NCLEX-RN®. In other words, as you answer each question, consider the role of the professional nurse in attending to client needs. As discussed in Chapter 2, the Client Needs make up the blueprint of the NCLEX-RN®. As you answer questions about these needs think about the professional nurse's responses— How would a nurse think in the case? What parameters or criteria does the nurse need to assess? So much about professionalism is clinical judgment—how nurses think and make decisions about client priorities.

Next Gen Clinical Judgment

A key to being the best nurse you can be is understanding the role of the nurse in safe delivery of quality care.

So what elements are critical components of professionalism? What do we need to think about when addressing professionalism on the exam? First, remember NCLEX-RN® is an examination of safety. Keeping clients safe is always a priority—both in real life and on the exam.

The QSEN competencies (Quality and Safety Education for Nurses—www.qsen.org) are designed to guide students and nurses in the safe delivery of quality care. We will discuss each competency and types of NCLEX-RN® questions that may be related to each concept. As we unpack professionalism and the NCLEX-RN®, think about how this information will enhance your success!

Patient-centered care

As you answer questions, think about the most client-centered or family-centered options. Clients and families are actively involved in decisions that impact them and are partners in care. When answering questions, consider the option that demonstrates the highest level of respect for the client and ensures that the client's and family's needs are a priority over nursing, institutional, and agency priorities. For example, review the following question and see how patient-centered care is the priority:

Q: **A nurse is assessing a client in the preoperative care unit. The client states "I am not sure I am ready to have this surgery." How would the nurse respond?**

    1. "Why don't you want to have surgery today?"
    2. "You signed the consent and the operating room is ready."
    3. "You are just nervous, the medicine will calm you down."
    4. 💡 "Would you like to speak to the surgeon about your surgery?"

The answer is 4 and is the most client-centered response. Ensuring that care is focused on the client and the client's concerns is an important role of the professional nurse as advocate. Advocacy is a fundamental role for nursing. Advocacy is speaking up for and providing support for another person or group who may not be able to speak or act for themselves. The nursing profession offers a voice for clients, ensuring that clients have their questions answered, concerns expressed, and priorities attended to while receiving care. Client-centered care also emphasizes cultural assessment and culturally aware nursing care. The client may represent the individual, family, group, or community and offers a sharp focus for nursing care!

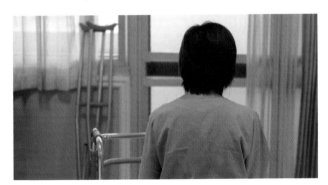

Image 19-1: A key role of the nurse is to ensure that all patients have all the information they need.

Teamwork and collaboration

Nursing does not practice alone, nor does a nurse practice nursing in solitude. Even in home care or independent practice, nurses are members of the healthcare team and nurses collaborate to attain better client outcomes. To be successful on NCLEX-RN®, you need to know the roles of members of the healthcare team, ensure that team members are informed of changes in client's needs and status, advocate for clients within the team, and coordinate the team's cohesive, well-communicated, and client-centered plan of care! Consider teamwork and collaboration as you answer this question:

Q: **A nurse is caring for a client who suffered a cerebrovascular accident two days ago with significant right-sided hemiparesis. Which referral is of highest priority at this time?**

    1. Social work for home care assistance and follow-up.
    2. Physical therapy for transfers in and out of the car.
    3. Occupational therapy for adaptive devices for meals.
    4. 💡 Speech therapy for a swallow evaluation.

The correct answer is 4. It is imperative that the client is evaluated for the ability to swallow and the strength of the oral muscles and gag reflexes are assessed to ensure safety during eating and drinking. The client would be at risk for aspiration if these capacities were not evaluated and ensured prior to eating.

Inherent with teamwork and collaborations are the concepts of leadership and delegation. As a leader, nurses guide the healthcare team, coordinate the team to enhance communication, ensure quality care, and delegate to other nurses and unlicensed assistive personnel to get the job done! As discussed in Chapter 4, NCLEX-RN® questions may pertain to delegating to UAPs, LPV/LPNs, or other registered nurses. Always consider the rights of delegation: the right task, to the right person, with the right instructions, with the right supervision, and with the right communication.

Consider the skill level required of the task and the skill level of the potential completer of the task. For example, if a test question mentions years of experience, years of working with a specific client population, special training/certification, and education level, it is asking you to consider these elements as you delegate! Think about client factors---what is the question asking you to think about prior to answering the question? Does it specify a client's age, diagnosis, or treatment that requires appropriate knowledge and skills? See how this is operationalized in this question:

Q: **A charge nurse is making assignments for a medical unit. A registered nurse from the ambulatory care center is reassigned to the unit. Which client would be the most appropriate to assign to the reassigned registered nurse?**

1. A 48-year-old who had a tracheostomy placed yesterday and is on humidified room air.
2. A 72-year-old following a transurethral prostatectomy with a triple lumen catheter.
3. 💡 A postoperative client who just arrived to the unit and requires frequent vital signs and close observation.
4. A client to be discharged on portable oxygen, an albuterol inhaler, and requires instruction.

The correct answer is option 3. The nurse in an ambulatory setting is able to take and interpret vital signs and assessments. The nurse may be less skilled with a tracheostomy, the triple lumen catheter, and portable oxygenation systems. Although teaching is the role of the registered nurse, that content needed to provide discharge teaching may not be readily available to or known by the reassigned nurse.

One exercise you may want to do is to visit the board of nursing's website in the state where you would like to be licensed. Look for the statements about delegation. They usually focus on the nursing process, nursing judgment, and the need for nurses to assess, teach, and evaluate nursing care. Although the nurse practice acts of each state are unique, they all include some statements about the role of the professional nurse and delegation. Delegation questions may ask you to consider multiple variables while making sound decisions about priority setting and client care!

Another part of teamwork and collaboration is communication! Consider the chaos of the healthcare environment if people were not communicating effectively. A current evidence-based practice being launched is bedside reporting. The practice of nurses providing shift-change, handoff reports at the client's bedside is one that is sweeping the nation. This change in practice is thought to increase client satisfaction and involvement in care, the efficacy of report, and comprehensive environmental rounds during report. You may hear some downsides, too! Confidentiality, the need to have a positive working relationship with the clients, and other issues may impede the effectiveness of bedside reporting. In an evidence-based project, researchers analyzed bedside reporting practices in their institution and validated its usefulness in enhancing client safety and promoting professionalism among the nurses. Let's do this test question about bedside reporting:

Q: **A nurse is receiving report from the previous shift's nurse at the client's bedside. Which report information requires immediate follow-up by the nurse?**

1. The client's reported oxygen saturations have been 88-90% and the monitor reads 89%.
2. The client's intravenous fluids are infusing at 100 mL/hr and the client states the site is "a little sore."
3. 💡 The client has a nasogastric tube hooked to low suction that did not drain last night, the client's abdomen is distended.
4. The client has a history of asthma with a respiratory rate of 18 breaths/minute and the head of bed is elevated.

The correct answer is 3—the tubing may be occluded and the gastric distension may indicate that the tube needs to be irrigated. The other findings validate the report. Just from this example, one can see the power of bedside reporting in allowing the nurse to be there and discuss findings with fellow colleagues and the client! A great evidence-based practice to enhance client outcomes and may serve as potential subjects of questions on your exam!

Evidence-based practices

Remember NCLEX-RN® World in Chapter 4? In NLCEX-RN® World, the nurse has nearly endless resources in terms of time, supplies, money, and friends (or help/assistance to carry out a task). When answering a question, the nurse is charged with conducting nursing practice without "cutting corners" or breaching policy standards and best practices. As such, the nurse is responsible to sustain a "spirit of inquiry" for using best practices to provide client care, to ensure that current research informs care, and continue to seek out evidence to support nursing practice. Let's review this question to see EBP concepts in action:

Q: **A 6-month-old client has a nasogastric tube. The nurse is checking placement of the tube to initiate a feeding. Which procedure is indicated?**

1. Aspirating gastric fluid with a syringe and noting fluid characteristics.
2. Auscultating abdomen and listening for air injected into the tube via syringe.
3. 💡 Assessing the pH and pepsin of aspirated gastric fluids
4. Obtaining a chest X-ray to visualize tube prior to each feeding or medication.

Research indicates that 3 is the correct answer. Although a chest X-ray may be the most definitive method, it is not feasible, nor practical, to have one done before every feeding or medication. A study found that checking both the pH (acidity) and the pepsin levels are the most definitive approaches to verifying nasogastric placement. A comprehensive review of the literature affirms this answer and demonstrates the power of and need for evidence-based practices!

These EBP are interpreted in terms of changing practices and models exist to examine and assimilate research findings into policies and procedures. On a bigger scale, changes in practice may influence health policy and make positive health status changes for people around the world! (And, specifically will be reflected in NCLEX-RN® items!)

Quality Improvement

In line with EBP, nurses are concerned with advancing the quality of care through ongoing quality improvement practices. Nurses at the bedside are able to identify client care issues, generate care practice questions, and participate in projects to determine best practices. Not every nurse can be a nurse researcher but all should be involved in quality improvement projects regardless of setting. One of the best ways to ensure safety is to carefully monitor concerns, near misses, and errors that may arise in the nurses' practice setting.

After data and trends are analyzed, an initiative is developed to address concerns. Here is an important example of quality improvement in action since SBAR is becoming more important on the NCLEX-RN®.

Many of us learned about SBAR in our nursing education. Those initials denote:

> S-situation
> B-background
> A-assessment
> R-recommendations

The SBAR model provides a framework for nurses to call healthcare providers with changes in status. The nurse is charged to provide information on each of the SBAR criteria to ensure comprehensive communication among the healthcare team and to inform healthcare providers of in-time information upon which to make decisions. You may be asked questions about SBAR, as in the following question:

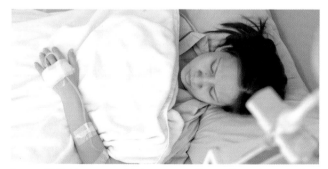

Image 19-2: Nurses need to be very cautious with post-surgical patients for any clues of a complication or worsening condition. Some clues are subtle, others are overt.

Q: A nurse is caring for a woman during the postpartum period on day 3 after a cesarean delivery. At 0400, the nurse notes that the client's temperature is 103.7°F. The client's incision is draining serosanguinous, yellow drainage and the client is restless and complaining of incisional pain, denying the nurse's attempts to bring the baby into the room. Which of these statements would provide the healthcare provider with valuable SBAR recommendation data?

1. "The client is febrile and I think she has an infection."
2. "The mother has a history of HIV and she is at risk for infection."
3. 💡 "I think we need to culture her wound and provide acetaminophen."
4. "I am concerned that she doesn't want to see or feed her baby."

The correct answer is 3 because it is a nursing recommendation. The other answers are correct for the other letters of the acronym.

One example of a quality improvement project at work is the use of SBAR within computer communication systems. Their organization placed the SBAR report within a computer platform and was found to positively impact communication practices and client safety—a nurse-led initiative effecting positive change in nursing practice. This is an example of a quality improvement project designed to increase client safety and positive client outcomes!

Safety

Nurses use their thinking skills, or clinical judgment/ clinical decision-making in order to enhance client safety! Medication errors, falls, and other safety issues are threats to our healthcare system and to clients. We've said several times that NCLEX-RN® is an examination of safety.

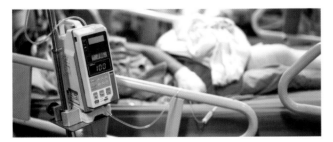

Image 19-3: Technology can bring benefit and harm. The nurse has to be mindful of the functionality of technology and always comparing the desired outcomes to reality. For instance, if the pump is set for 100 mL per hour and after 3 hours the IV bag is completely empty, the nurse needs to quickly respond.

When employed as a registered nurse you will hear more about safety in client care and organizations' goals to promote a culture of safety. For many questions, keeping the client safe is of highest priority. Let's view this question to validate the importance of safety.

Q: A client undergoes a flexible bronchoscopy under conscious sedation. The client is transferred to the medical surgical unit. The nurse is providing teaching to the client. Which instruction is of highest priority?

1. Use the call bell when needing to use the restroom.
2. 💡 Do not eat or drink for four hours after the procedure.
3. Ensure the client understands the bed alarm system.
4. Use strict handwashing and protective isolation practices.

The correct answer is option 2. The bronchoscopy procedure includes conscious sedation to ensure decreased level of consciousness and a topical anesthetic is used to allow the bronchoscope to pass through the vocal cords into the lungs. While anesthetized, the gag reflex, which protects the airway during eating or drinking, is not functioning. If a client drinks or eats before the gag reflex is functional, they could aspirate or choke. Since they are conscious, clients are especially at risk because they can access food and drink. This is an example of a question in which you need to focus on safety and think about what makes the client more at risk than other clients. Remember the client need Reduction of Risk Potential? Again, using good decision-making and clinical judgment skills while setting sound priorities will ensure that you select the correct response on questions in this domain, and others!

Informatics

Informatics is a QSEN competency that uses information and technology to enhance safe, quality care. So what is informatics? It is the use of the internet, internal intranet platforms, computers/ digital methods and new mechanisms to improve client care, safety, and outcomes. How does informatics increase communication and safety? We know that many states and agencies have adopted electronic health records (EHR) or electronic medical records (EMR). These mechanisms allow for health records to be communicated between healthcare professionals and facilities to ensure comprehensive care. Functionality such as medication reconciliation, home medication review, and holistic case management promotes safety in medication management and administration. Telehealth, or using telephones, computers, and technologies to provide healthcare at a distance or between separate settings, brings healthcare and expertise to remote locations, homes or across miles. This is another informatics role for nursing!

Nurses are involved with the use of informatics at many levels. Let's use a test question to demonstrate nursing informatics:

Q: A nurse is caring for a client following a bedside chest tube insertion. The nurse is documenting the client toleration of the procedure in the electronic health record. Which assessments would be documented? Select all that apply.

1. The depth the chest tube is inserted into the chest.
2. The vital signs following the procedure.
3. The size of the chest tube inserted.
4. The number of sutures used to anchor the chest tube.
5. The client's oxygen saturation following the procedure.
6. The client's pain level on a numeric scale.

The answers to this question are 2, 5, and 6. It would be the responsibility of the healthcare provider that inserted the tube, based on agency protocol, to document the size and depth of the tube and the number of sutures placed. This documentation question demonstrates how informatics can appear in NCLEX-RN® items. Finally, using technology to seek out information and search the literature reflects a significant use of informatics in nursing practice. Consider the breadth of information available on the world wide web to use to enhance client care and outcomes.

In this chapter we reinforced concepts of professionalism, client safety, and the role of the nurse using the QSEN framework. These topics may infuse any client need of the NCLEX-RN®, especially Management of Care, Safety and Infection Control, and Reduction of Risk Potential. Now, take the NurseThink® Quiz on these concepts.

Next Gen Clinical Judgment

Consider the principles of QSEN and leadership as you consider each of these cases!

1. Catastrophic disasters often require nurses to make hard ethical decisions. After a significant earthquake, a nurse is responding at a disaster relief shelter. The shelter is over capacity with more injured civilians crowding outside. The nurses are under-equipped and low on critical supplies. How should the nurses prioritize patients as they arrive? How does unpreparedness for this type of disaster affect the nurse's ability to provide appropriate care to victims?

2. Nurses must be able to adapt when disasters do not unfold exactly as a preparedness plan describes. A hospital emergency plan calls for the use of mobile telephones for internal communication during a disaster. However, when the disaster strikes cellular reception is interrupted. How should the nurses communicate? What emergency preparedness measures could the hospital have taken to prevent this issue?

3. As a catastrophic hurricane approaches, nurses are given orders to evacuate the hospital. What type of training would a nurse need to successfully perform an evacuation? Which patients should the staff evacuate first? How does unpreparedness for this type of disaster affect the nurse's ability to provide appropriate care to victims?

4. Nurses must be able to recognize deviations from the norm that might indicate an emergency. A school nurse notes a large amount of similar complaints that are uncommon from children in the community. Do the complaints warrant concern of an infectious disease outbreak? What emergency preparedness action should the nurse take?

1. The nurse is orienting a new graduate nurse to the unit. Reviewing the policies and procedures is included in the orientation. What statement by the nurse reinforces the importance of complying with the organization's policies and procedures?
   1. "Always refer to the policies and procedures as a reminder for how to do whatever task you are assigned."
   2. "If there is a legal question about a practice issue the policies and procedures serve as the standard of care."
   3. "The policies and procedures are a recipe for success to make sure we all do things the same way."
   4. "Administration develops the policies and procedures for us so that we are providing cost effective care."

2. The new graduate nurse is being orientated by a nurse preceptor. The new graduate asks "why do you belong to a professional nursing organization?" What is the most appropriate response by the nurse preceptor?
   1. "I was in the student nurse organization then felt like I should become a member of a professional organization when I graduated."
   2. "I get additional points at my annual performance evaluation because I can prove I am a member of one of the nursing organizations."
   3. "It is a good way to stay involved with the big picture of nursing by advocating for the profession and establishing guidelines for practice."
   4. "I really enjoy the socialization with other nurses across the county and the dues have been tax deductible as a professional expense."

3. The nurse is Facebook friends with other members of the nursing team. The nurse notes that one of the unlicensed assistive personnel (UAP) posts a comment on Facebook about a client "it was great to see my neighbor was discharged from the hospital today." Why should this be a concern that needs to be addressed?
   1. Potential legal issues.
   2. Potential HIPAA issue.
   3. Potential ethical issues.
   4. Potential malpractice issue.

4. What is the purpose of the Nurse Practice Act for any given state? Select all that apply.
   1. Define nursing for that state.
   2. Regulate nursing practice within the state.
   3. Set standards of care for the state.
   4. Differentiate practice by education.
   5. Set standards for nurse education programs.

5. The nurse witnesses another nurse bully a colleague. What is the best action for the witness to take?
   1. Confront the nurse who is bullying the colleague.
   2. Come to the rescue of the victim of the bullying.
   3. Report the observation to the charge nurse.
   4. Ignore it but watch to see if it happens again.

6. The nurse reports to work for the scheduled shift. The nurse manager tells the nurse to report to the emergency department today as a float nurse due to staffing shortages. The nurse has never worked in the emergency department. What is the best action by the nurse?
   1. Refuse to float to the emergency department.
   2. Call the supervisor to report the reassignment.
   3. Clarify the reassignment with the nurse manager.
   4. Check the policies and procedures regarding float assignments.

7. The nurse is the team leader responsible for 5 clients on the acute care unit. What client care can the nurse delegate to a Licensed Practical/Vocational Nurse? Select all that apply.
   1. Wound care for a client with a stage 2 pressure ulcer.
   2. Assessment of a postoperative client returning to the unit.
   3. Administering routine medications to assigned clients.
   4. Conducting discharge teaching for a client.
   5. Contacting the health care provider regarding lab values.

8. After receiving change of shift report, in what order would the nurse assess the assigned clients? Prioritize in rank order.
   1. Elderly client with pneumonia being discharged to long-term care later today.
   2. Client with a white count of 14,000 cells/mm^3 and a temperature of 102.8°F.
   3. Adolescent client admitted for evaluation following a motor vehicle accident.
   4. Confused elderly client with a urinary tract infection receiving IV antibiotics.
   5. Stable postoperative client who received pain medications about 30 minutes ago.

9. The nurse in long-term care is making assignments to a team that includes one LPN/LVN and 2 unlicensed assistive personnel (UAPs). What task is most appropriate for the LPN/LVN only?
   1. Monitoring vital signs.
   2. Dressing changes.
   3. Ambulating clients.
   4. Routine ADLs.

10. The charge nurse is planning the assignments for the day on an acute care unit. What factors should be considered when making the assignments? Select all that apply.
    1. Client acuity levels.
    2. Room configuration on the unit.
    3. Staff requests.
    4. Client needs.
    5. Staff preparation.

11. The nurse is delegating care for a team of clients. Which client would be most appropriately delegated to an unlicensed assistive personnel (UAP)?
    1. Client with difficulty swallowing.
    2. Client with continuous tube feedings.
    3. Client requiring a clean catch urine specimen.
    4. Client just transferred from ICU.

12. The nurse on the quality improvement committee has asked the staff nurses on the unit to participate in evaluating the new protocol. What statement by the nurse describes the role of the staff nurses?
    1. "We will be conducting a research project so each nurse will need to read the proposal."
    2. "Staff nurses on the unit will be implementing the new protocol and documenting your findings."
    3. "Each staff nurse will be responsible for identifying problems that would be barriers to implementation."
    4. "Once you have implemented the new protocol you will need to report to the committee."

13. The nurse is meeting with the interprofessional team doing discharge planning. Which statement by the nurse uses SBAR to organize the communication?
    1. "The client will be living alone and has a history of falling. The client is not confident with cane walking so I would recommend adding a walker."
    2. "Mrs. Jones has been the ideal client. She has complied with all treatment and I am sure she will follow the treatment plan."
    3. "The client continues to be confused and I have some real concerns about the discharge plans. Maybe we should add home health care."
    4. "The health care provider has provided all of the discharge prescriptions and I have completed the discharge teaching. The client seems to understand."

14. When delegating client care to an unlicensed assistive personnel (UAP) what does the nurse need to communicate? Select all that apply.
    1. The nurse action that is to be performed.
    2. What the nurse expects to have reported.
    3. Significant information regarding the client.
    4. Information about other clients in adjoining rooms.
    5. The names of the medications prescribed for the client.

15. Implementation of the electronic medical record has changed the way documentation is done. What is the primary goal for implementing the electronic medical record?
    1. Eliminate spelling and grammatical errors.
    2. Enhance the nurse ability to read prescriptions.
    3. Streamline documentation eliminating narratives.
    4. Share information across disciplines and settings.

16. The nurse manager is orienting a new nurse to the charge nurse role. What needs to be included in the orientation regarding delegation?
    1. When delegating to an LPN/LVN the nurse is also delegating accountability.
    2. The delegating nurse retains accountability for care delegated to non-RN staff.
    3. The LPN/LVN can re-delegate an assignment to an unlicensed assistive personnel (UAP).
    4. The unlicensed assistive personnel (UAP) has the authority to refuse a delegation.

17. The nurse is planning an in-service for unlicensed assistive personnel regarding being effective team members. What content should the nurse include? Select all that apply.
    1. Respect for colleagues.
    2. Identifying who agrees with you.
    3. Being open to others ideas.
    4. Communicating clearly.
    5. Avoid disagreeing with colleagues.

18. The charge nurse is reviewing another nurse's documentation for a postoperative client who just returned to the unit following abdominal surgery with a general anesthetic. The nurse caring for the client documented that active bowel sounds were heard in all 4 quadrants. What is the most appropriate action by the charge nurse?
    1. Compliment the nurse on documenting a complete post-operative assessment.
    2. Question the nurse about hearing bowel sounds when assessing this client.
    3. Go into the client's room and assess the client with a focus on an abdominal assessment.
    4. Do nothing and wait to see what the nurse documents the next time the client is assessed.

19. The unlicensed assistive personnel (UAP) reports to the nurse that the client fell when trying to get back into bed. What nursing actions will the nurse complete to follow-up? Select all that apply.
    1. Complete an assessment of the client.
    2. Reprimand the UAP for allowing the client to fall.
    3. Collaborate with the UAP to complete an incident report.
    4. Discuss the incident with the UAP as a teaching opportunity.
    5. Report the incident to the nurse manager.

20. The nurse case manager for a hospice client reviews the goals of the interprofessional team at the meeting with the family. What is the priority goal?
    1. Treatment of disease symptoms.
    2. Keeping the client at home.
    3. Providing comfort care.
    4. Providing cost effective care.

21. At change of shift the nurse is reporting off to the oncoming nurse. Which statement is an example of an effective handoff?
    1. "Mrs. Smith is ready for discharge. All of her discharge paperwork is completed and her daughter is coming soon."
    2. "Mr. Jones just returned from OR at 1500 following a total hip replacement. He is being assessed by the staff nurse now."
    3. "The client in 202 slept most of the shift so I don't have much to report. He was up all night so sleep was a good thing."
    4. "A client is being admitted from the emergency room following a motor vehicle accident. All I know so far is that he is stable."

22. The nurse is recommending a change in practice based on evidence-based practice. Which statement by the nurse reflects an understanding of evidence-based practice?
    1. "I think we should change the practice because the way I learned to do in school was different. Both my teachers and the book said to do it this way."
    2. "For the last couple years, I have done it this way and the outcomes have been good. So I would like to change the practice."
    3. "I was at a conference recently and hear about this new technique and I have two recent research publications that support it."
    4. "We keep doing the same thing and getting the same outcomes that no one is happy with so let's try something different and see what happens."

23. The charge nurse is following up with a staff nurse following a medication error. Which of the statements by the staff nurse could be the root cause for the error?
    1. "I checked the client's wristband and asked him to tell me his birthday before I administered the medications."
    2. "When I entered the room the client was on his way to the bathroom so I gave him his medications right away."
    3. "I doubled checked the medication dosage and route before I took the medication out of the package."
    4. "The client was NPO for a lab test so I held the medication until the test was completed."

24. A neighbor calls the emergency room nurse who is off-duty and at home to report "My son just fell out of a tree and his eyes are rolled back in his head. Please help me." What is the most appropriate action by the nurse?
    1. Immediately go to the neighbor's house to assess the boy.
    2. Call 911 before going over to assess the boy.
    3. Tell the mother that you are off duty and can't do anything.
    4. Tell the mother to call her primary health care provider.

25. The home care nurse is training a new unlicensed home health worker. The exhibit below includes the prescriptions for the client. What prescription(s) could be delegated to the unlicensed home health worker? Select all that apply.

> **Mary Jones (age 86)** Discharge home following hospitalization for congestive heart failure
>
> **Prescriptions:**
> 1. Monitor edema in lower extremities
> 2. Continue with previous medications
> 3. Assist with bathing once per week
> 4. Cardiac and respiratory assessments weekly
> 5. Monitor food and fluid intake

26. The nurse case manager is planning care for a client who had a total knee replacement 10 days ago and is being discharged from a rehabilitation center. What other disciplines should the nurse case manager seek input from to develop the plan of care? Select all that apply.
    1. Chaplain.
    2. Physical therapist.
    3. Home health nurse.
    4. Respiratory therapist.
    5. Pharmacist.

27. The charge nurse is notified that a new postoperative client will be coming to the unit shortly. The exhibit below identifies the beds available. What bed will the nurse hold for the new client?

Medical Surgical Unit with only beds available in double rooms	
201A Client with a white count of 17,000 and elevated temperature	1. 201B
202A Elderly client being discharged to a rehab facility later today	2. 202B
3. 203A	203B Confused Client with urinary tract infection
204A Adolescent admitted last night after motor vehicle accident	4. 204B

28. The nurse is calling the health care provider to question a medication order for a client. What statement by the nurse is using SBAR?
    1. "Ms. Jones, a 93-year-old client with a fractured femur is very lethargic and difficult to arouse at times. Her blood pressure has been 98/60 – 102/72. Do you want to continue using the narcotics for pain or would you like to order something else?"
    2. "Mary Smith was admitted this morning with pneumonia. She came here from long-term care. Do you want to continue all of the medications that she was on there?"
    3. "Mr. Green is going home today. We have completed all of his discharge teaching and have his prescriptions ready to send with him. Do you want to think about adding something for pain?"
    4. "John Potter's lab values came back a few minutes ago. His blood glucose after lunch was 220. Do you want to implement a sliding scale insulin?"

29. The charge nurse is explaining to the new nurse the role of the licensed vocation/practical nurse (LVN/LPN) on the acute care unit. What is included in the LVN/LPN's scope of practice? Select all that apply.
    1. Developing a plan of care for assigned clients.
    2. Administering routine medications to stable clients.
    3. Conducting client teaching.
    4. Collecting subjective and objective data.
    5. Analyzing assessment data for decision making.

30. The nurse is preparing a presentation for a new group of unlicensed assistive personnel (UAP) to discuss documentation. What should the nurse include in the presentation? Select all that apply.
    1. Legal aspects of documentation.
    2. Importance of documenting opinions.
    3. Need for documentation to be legible.
    4. Role of the UAP with the electronic medical record.
    5. Samples of inappropriate documentation.

1. **The nurse is orienting a new graduate nurse to the unit. Reviewing the policies and procedures is included in the orientation. What statement by the nurse reinforces the importance of complying with the organization's policies and procedures?**
   1. "Always refer to the policies and procedures as a reminder for how to do whatever task you are assigned." *Including "always review" suggests that the new nurse will not learn the process.*
   2. 🔘 "If there is a legal question about a practice issue the policies and procedures serve as the standard of care."
   3. "The policies and procedures are a recipe for success to make sure we all do things the same way." *Portraying the policies and procedures as a "recipe for success" assumes the procedure will be effective every time.*
   4. "Administration develops the policies and procedures for us so that we are providing cost effective care." *Policies and procedures focus on quality and safety and not costs.*

   Rationale: The first question that will be asked if there is a legal issue was whether the practice was consistent with the prevailing standard of care. The organization's policies and procedures are based on best practices and serve as the standard of care for practice.

   THIN Thinking: Help Quick – *The nurse needs to always be aware of legal issues that may arise from practice. Once the nurse considers the legal implications then other issues raise in priority.* **NCLEX®:** Management of Patient Care **QSEN:** Evidence-based Practice

2. **The new graduate nurse is being orientated by a nurse preceptor. The new graduate asks "why do you belong to a professional nursing organization?" What is the most appropriate response by the nurse preceptor?**
   1. "I was in the student nurse organization then felt like I should become a member of a professional organization when I graduated." *While this is a good reason, the reason for joining is not clear. She/he may have enjoyed the social aspects as a student.*
   2. "I get additional points at my annual performance evaluation because I can prove I am a member of one of the nursing organizations." *This may be a reason but it does not focus on the benefits of joining a professional organization.*
   3. 🔘 "It is a good way to stay involved with the big picture of nursing by advocating for the profession and establishing guidelines for practice."
   4. "I really enjoy the socialization with other nurses across the county and the dues have been tax deductible as a professional expense." *Socialization is not consistent with the mission of the professional organization.*

   Rationale: Nursing professional organizations advocate for the discipline on local and national levels. Organizations also are instrumental in setting standards of practice, codes of ethics and taking stands on practice issues..

   THIN Thinking: Nursing Process - *Using the nursing process the nurse will be able to look at the bigger picture of any situation to make decisions. Understanding the purpose of professional organizations should be the motivator for participation.* **NCLEX®:** Management of Patient Care **QSEN:** Teamwork and Collaboration

3. **The nurse is Facebook friends with other members of the nursing team. The nurse notes that one of the unlicensed assistive personnel (UAP) posts a comment on Facebook about a client "it was great to see my neighbor was discharged from the hospital today." Why should this be a concern that needs to be addressed?**
   1. Potential legal issues. *Nothing illegal was done.*
   2. 🔘 Potential HIPAA issue.
   3. Potential ethical issues. *This is not an ethical dilemma.*
   4. Potential malpractice issue. *This is not a practice issue so there is no malpractice.*

   Rationale: Although the UAP did not identify the client by name, others could determine who the client was the UAP was referring to in the post. Referring to a client via social media can be an infringement of privacy and potential HIPAA concern.

   THIN Thinking: Top Three- *Safe practice means that the nurse protects the confidentiality of the client to meet the HIPAA standards. Compromising HIPAA can impact the nurse's job and professional standards.* **NCLEX®:** Management of Patient Care **QSEN:** Teamwork and Collaboration

4. **What is the purpose of the Nurse Practice Act for any given state? Select all that apply.**
   1. 🔘 Define nursing for that state.
   2. 🔘 Regulate nursing practice within the state.
   3. Set standards of care for the state. *Nurse Practice Acts set qualities of practice by the nurse not quality of care.*
   4. 🔘 Differentiate practice by education.
   5. Set standards for nurse education programs. *The Nurse Practice Act may include criteria regarding developing nursing programs but it does not address standards for educational programs.*

   Rationale: The Nurse Practice Act defines nursing within that state, identifies the differentiated roles of practice such as LVN/LPN, RN and Advanced Practice, and regulates criteria for licensure in that state.

   THIN Thinking: Help Quick – *Knowledge of the Nurse Practice Act provides a framework and reference for safe nursing care.* **NCLEX®:** Management of Patient Care **QSEN:** Safety

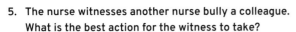

5. The nurse witnesses another nurse bully a colleague. What is the best action for the witness to take?
   1. Confront the nurse who is bullying the colleague. *Confronting the bully may make you the next victim.*
   2. Come to the rescue of the victim of the bullying. *Interfering by rescuing may exacerbate the situation.*
   3. Report the observation to the charge nurse.
   4. Ignore it but watch to see if it happens again. *Ignoring bullying will not address the problem.*

Rationale: Reporting the behavior observed to the charge nurse or nurse manager is the most appropriate behavior. Intervening or rescuing the other nurse could exacerbate the situation. Everyone is responsible for workplace safety so ignoring the situation is not an option.

THIN Thinking: Top Three - *Prioritizing strategies when observing bullying is critical for breaking the cycle of lateral violence. Recognizing that the priority is to report the observation is an opportunity for the nurse to report data so that appropriate decisions can be made.* **NCLEX®:** Safety and Infection Control **QSEN:** Safety

6. The nurse reports to work for the scheduled shift. The nurse manager tells the nurse to report to the emergency department today as a float nurse due to staffing shortages. The nurse has never worked in the emergency department. What is the best action by the nurse?
   1. Refuse to float to the emergency department. *This could be considered insubordination.*
   2. Call the supervisor to report the reassignment. *The supervisor will probably refer the nurse back to the nurse manager.*
   3. Clarify the reassignment with the nurse manager.
   4. Check the policies and procedures regarding float assignments. *Staff assignments is a management right.*

Rationale: The nurse is an employee of the organization and therefore, can be floated to another unit if needed. Refusing to go to the emergency department can be seen as insubordination. Clarifying the reassignment with the nurse manager can be an opportunity to discuss whether the nurse meets the 5 rights of delegation.

THIN Thinking: Help Quick - *The nurse is responsible for the duties delegated by the nurse manager. Therefore, the priority action would be to clarify with the nurse manager before moving to any other steps.* **NCLEX®:** Safety and Infection Control **QSEN:** Safety

7. The nurse is the team leader responsible for 5 clients on the acute care unit. What client care can the nurse delegate to a Licensed Practical/Vocational Nurse? Select all that apply.
   1. Wound care for a client with a stage 2 pressure ulcer.
   2. Assessment of a postoperative client returning to the unit. *Assessment is the responsibility of an RN.*
   3. Administering routine medications to assigned clients.
   4. Conducting discharge teaching for a client. *The RN is responsible for client teaching, the LPN can reinforce teaching as needed.*
   5. Contacting the health care provider regarding lab values.

Rationale: Assessment and client teaching are roles for the registered nurse and cannot be delegated. The LPN/LVN can collect assessment data but the analysis of the data is the responsibility of the RN. The LPN/LVN can reinforce teaching but the RN is responsible for client teaching.

THIN Thinking: Top Three - *When delegating care, the nurse needs to follow the 5 rights which includes understanding the scope of practice of each of the team members. The nurse remains accountable for the care provided, therefore, appropriate delegation is critical to safe practice.* **NCLEX®:** Management of Patient Care **QSEN:** Teamwork and Collaboration

8. After receiving change of shift report, in what order would the nurse assess the assigned clients? Prioritize in rank order.
   1. Client with a white count of 14,000 cells/mm³ and a temperature of 102.8°F.
   2. Adolescent client admitted for evaluation following a motor vehicle accident.
   3. Confused elderly client with a urinary tract infection receiving IV antibiotics.
   4. Stable postoperative client who received pain medications about 30 minutes ago.
   5. Elderly client with pneumonia being discharged to long-term care later today.

Rationale: The client with the elevated white count and temperature is the most unstable at the moment and needs to be a priority. Assessment of the client from the MVA is not complete and so more data is needed to determine that client's status. The elderly client is confused and needs to be assessed to ensure safety. It may take longer than 30 minutes for the pain medication to reach peak action. The client being discharged to long term care is the most stable at this time.

THIN Thinking: Help Quick - *The nurse needs to be able to prioritize effectively to ensure safe, quality care. When deciding which client to assess first, the nurse needs to consider the client's assessment data, stability and needs.* **NCLEX®:** Management of Patient Care **QSEN:** Patient-centered Care

9. The nurse in long-term care is making assignments to a team that includes one LPN/LVN and 2 unlicensed assistive personnel (UAPs). What task is most appropriate for the LPN/LVN only?
   1. Monitoring vital signs. *Vital signs is a task that can be done by UAPs.*
   2. 💡 Dressing changes.
   3. Ambulating clients. *UAP can ambulate clients within their scope of practice.*
   4. Routine ADLs. *The scope of practice for UAP includes routine ADLs.*

   Rationale: The LVN/LPN has the skills to perform routine nursing actions such as dressing changes. The UAP does not have the knowledge level to be able to collect data regarding wound healing while changing a dressing.

   THIN Thinking: Top Three - *When delegating care, the nurse needs to follow the 5 rights which includes understanding the scope of practice of each of the team members. The nurse remains accountable for the care provided therefore, appropriate delegation is critical to safe practice.* **NCLEX®:** Basic Care and Comfort **QSEN:** Teamwork and Collaboration

10. The charge nurse is planning the assignments for the day on an acute care unit. What factors should be considered when making the assignments? Select all that apply.
    1. 💡 Client acuity levels.
    2. Room configuration on the unit. *Client needs and safety are the key factors that need to be considered, not geography of the unit.*
    3. Staff requests. *While staff requests may be considered, following the 5 rights of delegation is the priority.*
    4. 💡 Client needs.
    5. 💡 Staff preparation.

    Rationale: The level of acuity, or degree of illness, is a factor in making assignments, as are the extensiveness of client needs and the level of expertise of the staff members. The staff member's personal requests and the physical layout of the unit are not priorities.

    THIN Thinking: Top Three - *When delegating care, the nurse needs to follow the 5 rights which includes understanding the scope of practice of each of the team members. The nurse remains accountable for the care provided therefore, appropriate delegation is critical to safe practice.* **NCLEX®:** Management of Patient Care **QSEN:** Teamwork and Collaboration

11. The nurse is delegating care for a team of clients. Which client would be most appropriately delegated to an unlicensed assistive personnel (UAP)?
    1. Client with difficulty swallowing. *Stable clients can be delegated to a UAP and a client with difficulty swallowing is at risk.*
    2. Client with continuous tube feedings. *This client requires skilled care beyond the scope of the UAP.*
    3. 💡 Client requiring a clean catch urine specimen.
    4. Client just transferred from ICU. *The client was just transferred from ICU typically are not stable.*

    Rationale: The UAP is prepared to provide care for stable clients and can assist with routine nursing actions such as specimen collection.

    THIN Thinking: Top Three - *When delegating care, the nurse needs to follow the 5 rights which includes understanding the scope of practice of each of the team members. The nurse remains accountable for the care provided therefore, appropriate delegation is critical to safe practice.* **NCLEX®:** Management of Patient Care **QSEN:** Teamwork and Collaboration

12. The nurse on the quality improvement committee has asked the staff nurses on the unit to participate in evaluating the new protocol. What statement by the nurse describes the role of the staff nurses?
    1. "We will be conducting a research project so each nurse will need to read the proposal." *The staff nurse is not required to read the research proposal.*
    2. 💡 "Staff nurses on the unit will be implementing the new protocol and documenting your findings."
    3. "Each staff nurse will be responsible for identifying problems that would be barriers to implementation." *The staff nurse will be participating in collecting data for the research project not identifying barriers.*
    4. "Once you have implemented the new protocol you will need to report to the committee." *The staff nurse will document findings and responses.*

    Rationale: The quality improvement process focuses on continual evaluation of new products, processes and procedures. The role of staff nurses is typically to implement the new product, process or procedure and document their findings.

    THIN Thinking: Nursing Process - *The nurse needs to understand the quality improvement process and the staff's role in implementation of these projects. Being on the quality improvement committee is an opportunity for the nurse to advocate for the profession and evidence-based practice.* **NCLEX®:** Management of Patient Care **QSEN:** Quality Improvement

13. The nurse is meeting with the interprofessional team doing discharge planning. Which statement by the nurse uses SBAR to organize the communication?
    1. 🔾 "The client will be living alone and has a history of falling. The client is not confident with cane walking so I would recommend adding a walker."
    2. "Mrs. Jones has been the ideal client. She has complied with all treatment and I am sure she will follow the treatment plan." *This statement does not provide any specific information using the SBAR model.*
    3. "The client continues to be confused and I have some real concerns about the discharge plans. Maybe we should add home health care." *No assessment data is included in this statement.*
    4. "The health care provider has provided all of the discharge prescriptions and I have completed the discharge teaching. The client seems to understand." *There are no recommendations included in this statement.*

    Rationale: SBAR includes describing the situation, background, assessment and recommendation.

    THIN Thinking: Help Quick - *When making decisions about communicating client needs, the nurse needs to prioritize. Communicating safety needs is almost always a priority.* **NCLEX®:** Management of Patient Care **QSEN:** Teamwork and Collaboration

14. When delegating client care to an unlicensed assistive personnel (UAP) what does the nurse need to communicate? Select all that apply.
    1. 🔾 The nurse action that is to be performed.
    2. 🔾 What the nurse expects to have reported.
    3. 🔾 Significant information regarding the client.
    4. Information about other clients in adjoining rooms. *The UAP does not need information regarding clients they are not assigned to care for that day.*
    5. The names of the medications prescribed for the client. *The UAP does not administer medications.*

    Rationale: When delegating care the nurse needs to communicate significant information about the specific client needs, what actions are to be performed and what the nurse expects to have reported back.

    THIN Thinking: Top Three - *When delegating care, the nurse needs to follow the 5 rights which includes understanding the scope of practice of each of the team members. The nurse remains accountable for the care provided therefore, appropriate delegation is critical to safe practice* **NCLEX®:** Management of Patient Care **QSEN:** Teamwork and Collaboration

15. Implementation of the electronic medical record has changed the way documentation is done. What is the primary goal for implementing the electronic medical record?
    1. Eliminate spelling and grammatical errors. *Spelling and grammatical errors are not always corrected using an EMR.*
    2. Enhance the nurse ability to read prescriptions. *While the EMR may help with poor penmanship, that is not the primary goal for implementation.*
    3. Streamline documentation eliminating narratives. *The EMR still requires some narrative documentation.*
    4. 🔾 Share information across disciplines and settings.

    Rationale: The primary goal for implementing the electronic medical record is to facilitate communication and information sharing across disciplines and settings. By sharing information the quality and continuity of care is enhanced.

    THIN Thinking: Top Three - *Understanding the priority reasons for implementing technology is important to facilitate buy-in to the process. Communicating across disciplines and settings may prevent errors.* **NCLEX®:** Management of Patient Care **QSEN:** Informatics

16. The nurse manager is orienting a new nurse to the charge nurse role. What needs to be included in the orientation regarding delegation?
    1. When delegating to an LPN/LVN the nurse is also delegating accountability. *Accountability cannot be delegated.*
    2. 🔾 The delegating nurse retains accountability for care delegated to non-RN staff.
    3. The LPN/LVN can re-delegate an assignment to an unlicensed assistive personnel (UAP). *It is not appropriate for the LPN/LVN to re-delegate an assignment.*
    4. The unlicensed assistive personnel (UAP) has the authority to refuse a delegation. *Refusing a delegation can be considered insubordination.*

    Rationale: The nurse delegating to an LPN/LVN or unlicensed personnel remains accountable for the care provided. The individual doing the delegating is personally responsible for making prudent decisions based on the 5 rights of delegation.

    THIN Thinking: Help Quick - *When delegating care, the nurse needs to follow the 5 rights which includes understanding the scope of practice of each of the team members. The nurse remains accountable for the care provided therefore, appropriate delegation is critical to safe practice.* **NCLEX®:** Management of Patient Care **QSEN:** Teamwork and Collaboration

17. The nurse is planning an in-service for unlicensed assistive personnel regarding being effective team members. What content should the nurse include? Select all that apply.
    1. 💡 Respect for colleagues
    2. Identifying who agrees with you. *Effective teams agree to disagree.*
    3. 💡 Being open to others ideas.
    4. 💡 Communicating clearly.
    5. Avoid disagreeing with colleagues. *Effective team members are open to the opinions of others even if they disagree.*

    Rationale: Effective teams require that all members respect each other's opinions and feel free to disagree in a non-judgmental manner. Team members also need to be open to ideas, listen effectively, and communicate clearly.

    THIN Thinking: Top Three - *Identifying priorities to plan an in-service is an important strategy for a successful presentation. The goal for the in-service is to develop effective teams to provide quality, safe care.* **NCLEX®:** Management of Patient Care **QSEN:** Teamwork and Collaboration

18. The charge nurse is reviewing another nurse's documentation for a postoperative client who just returned to the unit following abdominal surgery with a general anesthetic. The nurse caring for the client documented that active bowel sounds were heard in all 4 quadrants. What is the most appropriate action by the charge nurse?
    1. Compliment the nurse on documenting a complete post-operative assessment. *Rationale Providing feedback is important but it is not the priority in this situation.*
    2. 💡 Question the nurse about hearing bowel sounds when assessing this client.
    3. Go into the client's room and assess the client with a focus on an abdominal assessment. *After questioning the nurse, it may be appropriate to follow-up with another assessment but it is not the first action.*
    4. Do nothing and wait to see what the nurse documents the next time the client is assessed. *The charge nurse has the overall responsibility of the unit and needs to follow-up as needed.*

    Rationale: A client who had abdominal surgery under a general anesthesia will not have active bowel sounds immediately postoperatively. Therefore, the charge nurse is responsible for questioning the nurse in a non-threatening manner.

    THIN Thinking: Nursing Process - *The nurse needs to understand what assessment data is "normal" at various stages of recovery following a general anesthetic. The assessment may be accurate but the charge nurse should question it because it does not fit the "normal" expectation.* **NCLEX®:** Management of Patient Care **QSEN:** Evidence-based Practice

19. The unlicensed assistive personnel (UAP) reports to the nurse that the client fell when trying to get back into bed. What nursing actions will the nurse complete to follow-up? Select all that apply.
    1. 💡 Complete an assessment of the client.
    2. Reprimand the UAP for allowing the client to fall. *Reprimanding the UAP will discourage any further reporting of client incidents such as falls.*
    3. 💡 Collaborate with the UAP to complete an incident report.
    4. 💡 Discuss the incident with the UAP as a teaching opportunity.
    5. 💡 Report the incident to the nurse manager.

    Rationale: The UAP is obligated to report falls to the nurse. To follow-up the nurse must assess the client, gather additional data from the UAP about the incident, complete an incident report and most incidents need to be reported to the nurse manager.

    THIN Thinking: Nursing Process - *When the UAP reports an observation such as a fall, the nurse needs to follow-up with an assessment of the client. It is also an opportunity to implement teaching.* **NCLEX®:** Management of Patient Care **QSEN:** Patient-centered Care

20. The nurse case manager for a hospice client reviews the goals of the interprofessional team at the meeting with the family. What is the priority goal?
    1. Treatment of disease symptoms. *The primary goal for hospice care is palliative not disease focused.*
    2. Keeping the client at home. *There are multiple settings where hospice care can occur depending on the client's needs.*
    3. 💡 Providing comfort care.
    4. Providing cost effective care. *While cost effective care is always important, it is not the priority for hospice care.*

    Rationale: The nurse case manager plays a pivotal role in coordinating hospice care. At the meeting it is important to reinforce that the priority goal for a hospice client is to provide palliative care.

    THIN Thinking: Top Three - *The nurse needs to recognize the priority goals for hospice care so that planning can be done appropriately.* **NCLEX®:** Management of Patient Care **QSEN:** Teamwork and Collaboration

Next Gen Clinical Judgment

How can a nurse implement QSEN principles in daily nursing care?

How can teamwork and collaboration increase client safety in outpatient settings and home care?

21. At change of shift the nurse is reporting off to the oncoming nurse. Which statement is an example of an effective handoff?
    1. "Mrs. Smith is ready for discharge. All of her discharge paperwork is completed and her daughter is coming soon." *The information is vague.*
    2. "Mr. Jones just returned from OR at 1500 following a total hip replacement. He is being assessed by the staff nurse now." *Information is not complete.*
    3. ⊚ "The client in 202 slept most of the shift so I don't have much to report. He was up all night so sleep was a good thing."
    4. "A client is being admitted from the emergency room following a motor vehicle accident. All I know so far is that he is stable." *The information is vague.*

    Rationale: Effective change of shift report is important for continuity and quality of care. Saying the client slept most of the day is not sufficient information for the oncoming nurse to determine priorities for the upcoming shift.

    THIN Thinking: Top Three - *Identifying priorities related to safety and quality of care should direct the information communicated to the oncoming shift. Effective communication is important for continuity and quality of care.* **NCLEX®:** Management of Patient Care **QSEN:** Teamwork and Collaboration

22. The nurse is recommending a change in practice based on evidence-based practice. Which statement by the nurse reflects an understanding of evidence-based practice?
    1. "I think we should change the practice because the way I learned to do in school was different. Both my teachers and the book said to do it this way." *This is not an evidence-based decision but rather depends on authority of faculty.*
    2. "For the last couple years, I have done it this way and the outcomes have been good. So I would like to change the practice." *This is not an evidence-based decision but rather depends on "the way we have always done it."*
    3. ⊚ "I was at a conference recently and hear about this new technique and I have two recent research publications that support it."
    4. "We keep doing the same thing and getting the same outcomes that no one is happy with so let's try something different and see what happens." *This is not an evidence-based decision but rather a random guess what might work.*

    Rationale: Evidence-based Practice is based on data that is accumulated through practice protocols or research. Depending on authority to determine practice or traditional ways of providing care may not be the best practices to facilitate quality outcomes.

    THIN Thinking: Top Three - *Exploring the sources of rationale for decision making helps to determine whether or not it is evidence based. Priorities for quality outcomes are based on evidence-based practice.* **NCLEX®:** Management of Patient Care **QSEN:** Evidence-based Practice

23. The charge nurse is following up with a staff nurse following a medication error. Which of the statements by the staff nurse could be the root cause for the error?
    1. "I checked the client's wristband and asked him to tell me his birthday before I administered the medications." *This is an appropriate strategy to identifying the client before administering medications.*
    2. ⊚ "When I entered the room the client was on his way to the bathroom so I gave him his medications right away."
    3. "I doubled checked the medication dosage and route before I took the medication out of the package." *This is an appropriate strategy to identify the correct dose.*
    4. "The client was NPO for a lab test so I held the medication until the test was completed." *This is an appropriate strategy to determine if the mediation should be administered.*

    Rationale: Following up after a medication error or a near miss is an opportunity to discover the root cause so that the error can be avoided in the future. When administering medications, the nurse needs to use two methods of identifying the client. Response number 2 suggests the nurse just gave the client the medications because he was in a hurry to get to the bathroom.

    THIN Thinking: Help Quick - *Safe medication administration is a priority for quality nursing care. The nurse needs to follow the 5 rights for medication administration every time.* **NCLEX®:** Management of Patient Care **QSEN:** Safety

24. A neighbor calls the emergency room nurse who is off-duty and at home to report "My son just fell out of a tree and his eyes are rolled back in his head. Please help me." What is the most appropriate action by the nurse?
    1. Immediately go to the neighbor's house to assess the boy. *Calling for help first is a priority.*
    2. ⊚ Call 911 before going over to assess the boy.
    3. Tell the mother that you are off duty and can't do anything. *The nurse should respond as a good Samaritan.*
    4. Tell the mother to call her primary health care provider. *Contacting 911 is a priority over calling the health care provider.*

    Rationale: The first thing the nurse should do is call 911 for emergency help. Once the nurse arrives on the scene, he/she is obligated to stay until first responders arrive per the Good Samaritan Law.

THIN Thinking: Top Three - *The nurse needs to identify the top priority when the neighbor calls. The first step is to get emergency help for the child.* **NCLEX®:** Safety and Infection Control **QSEN:** Safety

25. The home care nurse is training a new unlicensed home health worker. The exhibit below includes the prescriptions for the client. What prescription(s) could be delegated to the unlicensed home health worker? Select all that apply.

Mary Jones (age 86) Discharge home following hospitalization for congestive heart failure

Prescriptions:
1. Monitor edema in lower extremities
2. Continue with previous medications *UAP does not administer medications.*
3. Assist with bathing once per week
4. Cardiac and respiratory assessments weekly *UAP does not do assessments.*
5. Monitor food and fluid intake

Rationale: The unlicensed home health worker can monitor symptoms such as edema of the lower extremities or food and fluid intake and report observations to the nurse who will make the assessment and/or clinical decision. The home health worker can also assist with bathing.

THIN Thinking: Top Three - *When delegating care, the nurse needs to follow the 5 rights which includes understanding the scope of practice of each of the team members. The nurse remains accountable for the care provided therefore, appropriate delegation is critical to safe practice.* **NCLEX®:** Basic Care and Comfort **QSEN:** Teamwork and Collaboration

26. The nurse case manager is planning care for a client who had a total knee replacement 10 days ago and is being discharged from a rehabilitation center. What other disciplines should the nurse case manager seek input from to develop the plan of care? Select all that apply.
   1. Chaplain. *The chaplain is not needed unless there are other concerns beyond the total knee replacement.*
   2. ⦿ Physical therapist.
   3. ⦿ Home health nurse.
   4. Respiratory therapist. *Typically there are not respiratory issues when a client is discharged from rehab following a knee replacement.*
   5. Pharmacist. *The medications prescribed when discharge from rehab typically are not new, therefore, the pharmacist is not needed at the planning meeting.*

Rationale: The case manager will seek input for the interprofessional team collaborating to provide care to a client in rehabilitation. The rehabilitation team usually consists of the case manager and physical therapist

following a knee replacement. A referral to home health is common after a stay in rehabilitation so the home health nurse would also be part of the discharge planning team.

THIN Thinking: Top Three - *The nurse needs to be able to prioritize who needs to participate in discharge planning meetings. Getting the right people at the meeting can facilitate an effective discharge plan.* **NCLEX®:** Management of Patient Care **QSEN:** Patient-centered Care

27. The charge nurse is notified that a new postoperative client will be coming to the unit shortly. The exhibit below identifies the beds available. What bed will the nurse hold for the new client?

Medical Surgical Unit with only beds available in double rooms	
201A Client with a white count of 17,000 and elevated temperature	1. 201B *This client has a potential infection due to assessment data.*
202A Elderly client being discharged to a rehab facility later today	2. ⦿ 202B
3. 203A *Admitting a new client to this room may increase the other client's confusion.*	203B Confused client with urinary tract infection
204A Adolescent admitted last night after motor vehicle accident	4. 204B *Keeping the adolescent in room alone recognizes developmental levels.*

Rationale: Decision making requires the nurse to evaluate all of the factors. Admitting a new postoperative client to a room where the other client has an active infection is not recommended. A postoperative client will require frequent assessments over the first few hours and that may enhance the confusion of the client in 203B. The client in 204A may also require frequent assessments, etc. due to the MVA so the postoperative client might not get much rest.

THIN Thinking: Top Three - *The nurse needs to look at all of the data when making decisions about room assignments. Establishing priorities is important for all clinical decisions.* **NCLEX®:** Management of Patient Care **QSEN:** Patient-centered Care

28. The nurse is calling the health care provider to question a medication order for a client. What statement by the nurse is using SBAR?
    1. ⊙ "Ms. Jones, a 93-year-old client with a fractured femur is very lethargic and difficult to arouse at times. Her blood pressure has been 98/60 – 102/72. Do you want to continue using the narcotics for pain or would you like to order something else?"
    2. "Mary Smith was admitted this morning with pneumonia. She came here from long-term care. Do you want to continue all of the medications that she was on there?" *The assessment is missing from this statement.*
    3. "Mr. Green is going home today. We have completed all of his discharge teaching and have his prescriptions ready to send with him. Do you want to think about adding something for pain?" *The statement includes the background and recommendation but not the assessment data to support the recommendation.*
    4. "John Potter's lab values came back a few minutes ago. His blood glucose after lunch was 220. Do you want to implement a sliding scale insulin?" *This statement includes the assessment and recommendation but the background and situation is not evident.*

    Rationale: SBAR communication includes **S**ituation **B**ackground **A**ssessment and **R**ecommendation. The statement in response #1 is the only option that includes all of the components of SBAR.

    THIN Thinking: Nursing Process - When communicating with the health care provider the nurse needs to include the data collected using the nursing process. Presenting the complete picture is important for effective communication. **NCLEX®:** Management of Patient Care **QSEN:** Teamwork and Collaboration

29. The charge nurse is explaining to the new nurse the role of the licensed vocation/practical nurse (LVN/LPN) on the acute care unit. What is included in the LVN/LPN's scope of practice? Select all that apply.
    1. Developing a plan of care for assigned clients. *LVN/LPN can implement the plan of care but the RN is responsible for planning care.*
    2. ⊙ Administering routine medications to stable clients.
    3. Conducting client teaching. *LVN/LPN can reinforce client teaching only.*
    4. ⊙ Collecting subjective and objective data.
    5. Analyzing assessment data for decision making. *The RN is responsible for analyzing assessment data.*

Rationale: The LPN/LVN works under the direct supervision of the RN in an acute care setting. The key to delegating to the LPN/LVN is the stability of the client because unstable clients tend to change more quickly requiring assessment and decision making. The RN develops the plan of care and the LPN/LVN implements the plan with activities included in their scope of practice such as collecting data and administering medications. Assessment and teaching are not in the scope of practice of the LPN/LVN.

THIN Thinking: Nursing Process - *When delegating care, the nurse needs to follow the 5 rights which includes understanding the scope of practice of each of the team members. The nurse remains accountable for the care provided therefore, appropriate delegation is critical to safe practice.* **NCLEX-RN®** Management of Patient Care **QSEN:** Teamwork and Collaboration

30. The nurse is preparing a presentation for a new group of unlicensed assistive personnel (UAP) to discuss documentation. What should the nurse include in the presentation? Select all that apply.
    1. ⊙ Legal aspects of documentation.
    2. Importance of documenting opinions. *Opinions do not have a place in the medical record which is a legal document.*
    3. ⊙ Need for documentation to be legible.
    4. ⊙ Role of the UAP with the electronic medical record.
    5. ⊙ Samples of inappropriate documentation.

    Rationale: The UAP may or may not be documenting with the electronic health record. That differs by organization so it is important that the nurse cover this organization's expectations. Documentation needs to be legible and objective, opinions are not appropriate as the chart is a legal document.

    THIN Thinking: Top three - *Prioritizing data that is included in documentation can help the UAP prepare complete, relevant information. The medical record serves as a legal document.* **NCLEX®:** Management of Patient Care **QSEN:** Informatics

Next Gen Clinical Judgment

A nurse is caring for a client on the 7pm-7am shift. The shift is short staffed and the nurse is caring for more than the usual number of patients. At 4am the nurse realized that a medication was given to the wrong patient.

1. What actions need to be taken?

2. What is included in the completion of the incident/variance report?

3. How can this type of error be prevented in the future?

Where do I go from here?

Next steps: Set your study goals—
Plan your study time and stick with it

You have been successful thus far. You've completed years of nursing school…you're dedicated to a career in nursing. Let's just get you through the next hurdle…NCLEX-RN®! We know you have a career goal…let's set up some study goals!

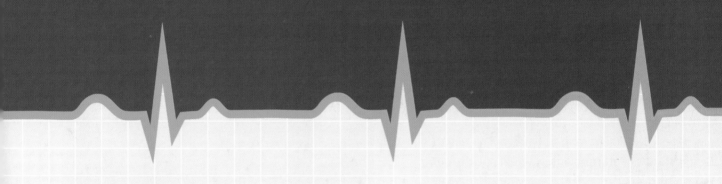

In case you are one of those people who skip to the last chapter or routinely just start at the end, let's talk about using this book. Using a calendar or your phone calendar to establish a study schedule is a good way to get started. Split this text up in sections and assign sections to days or weeks. End the week or time period with a test, from here, online, another text, or from test banks. Make sure the tests you take represent areas of study (as at the end of chapters in this text) or are based upon the NCLEX-RN® blueprint (like the quizzes available with this text).

Then, when you've read through the **Priority Exemplars**, completed the **Go To Clinical** Cases, and **NurseThink® Quizzes** you may set some additional goals for your study or prep time. First, look at your time – if you've scheduled the exam, look at the days you have until the exam. If you haven't scheduled yet—remember what we discussed in

Chapter 3. Schedule the exam with enough time to study-but soon enough to avoid memory lag! What commitments do you have in between now and then? Work? Family? Personal? Then, plot out your time. Make a commitment to study EVERY day! Some find it helpful to use a calendar, planner, or computer calendar to make a visual representation of their study plan. Remember the 50/100 study rule. Every day complete a 50-item quiz—as you check your answers, write down or take note of the topics you get wrong. Read the rationales carefully. If you still have questions, use this book or other resources to dig deeper into the topic. Remember to study the topics you don't know or you don't feel as comfortable answering questions about—don't study the material you have mastered! Look up information about the questions you don't understand—remember to study to learn, not memorize.

Once a week, complete a 100-item or more test. Longer tests allow you to maintain your "test-taking stamina" that will be needed for NCLEX-RN®. Again, focus on the questions and topics you get wrong! Also, these larger tests are also a good time to assess why you are getting items wrong. Is it a lack of knowledge? Are you missing keywords when you are reading? Did you look at the question and you believed that you knew the material—but missed the intent of the question? As discussed previously, so much of success on the NCLEX-RN® is quiet, calm reading! Taking your time is critical as you progress toward NCLEX-RN®.

Other strategies have demonstrated effectiveness in enhancing the quality of your studying. Many set apart a designated room or area for studying. Make sure it is a comfortable spot, but not too comfortable! You don't want to sleep through your study time! Surround yourself with water, plenty of pencils/pens, a computer and textbooks to look up information, and some "creature comforts." These may include your favorite slippers, soft music, heartwarming pictures of friends and family, or inspirational posters or messages. Remember, your brain responds well to the messages of affirmations, wherein positive self-talk bolsters your confidence and your test-taking abilities! Then, when you are taking a test or quiz—make sure you simulate the testing environment. Consider the testing session as a real testing event—no interruptions, no snacks, no phones, no talking, no music, no fun—just testing.

Some find that *group* studying helps reinforce concepts and information. The benefits of group studying includes the ability to garner many perspectives while studying. For example, other people may identify topics, approaches, or potential issues that you haven't thought about yet! These groups also offer the opportunity for discussion about testing and processes. Other opinions on questions, answers, and interpretations of the test plan may broaden your knowledge and the ability to prepare for NCLEX-RN®.

Your healthy NCLEX® lifestyle

We want to reiterate the importance of healthy lifestyle choices during this stressful time. Researchers tell us that the average adult needs 7-8 hours of sleep per night. Our society rewards those who don't appear to need as much sleep, posing accolades for those who sleep 3-4 hours per day. In fact, many people in our society live in chronic sleep deprivation and most people would benefit from more sleep. If you have trouble falling asleep or are wakeful during the night, investigate sleep hygiene practices. Habits such as limiting screen time a few hours before bed, a warm bath or shower, reading before bed, placing a notepad and pen near the bed to make lists of things (rather than worrying about them), listening to soft music, not studying in bed but reserving the bed for sleep, and practicing calming meditation or imagery while preparing for sleep may all assist in getting that good night's rest. Exercise is great...but make sure you complete your work-out a few hours prior to bedtime to ensure a "winding down" time before bed.

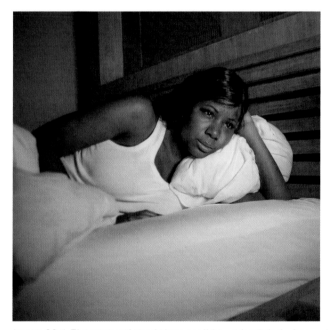

Image 20-1: The power of good sleep can't be understated when preparing for any exam, especially NCLEX®.

Neuroscience studies demonstrate that adequate sleep enhances learning by increasing our ability to attend in learning situations, in processing information to memories, and in organizing memories for later retrieval. In fact, it is during sleep that our brain transfers short-term memories into long-term storage such that we can make connections to previously learned information when exposed to new ideas and retrieve information. The implications for a sound night's rest are evident here—so sleep well!

Just as critical as sleep is the need to fuel your body for optimum functioning. Research into high protein/low carbohydrate diets and others that espouse balanced nutrition all point to the need for your body to be at its best physically when studying for and taking the exam. Many sources support the use of B-complex vitamin supplementation to enable the body to best deal with stress. Others support adequate fiber in your diet to ensure gastrointestinal regularity. Most sources affirm the universal "goodness" of adequate water intake. Think for a moment of your last busy day—during classes or on the job—if you were on day shift, somewhere around 3:00pm you may have become drowsy. You went in search of a "pick-me-up." That may have led you to a caffeinated soda or coffee, a sweet snack, or something salty. Instead many authorities contend that your "slump" was more related to dehydration than hypoglycemia (unless you have a medical diagnosis). So, try drinking 12-16 ounces of water the next time you feel lethargic and see if it really is more about hydration. Remember that caffeine and alcohol are dehydrating so imbibe within reason—this study period is not the time for excesses. That being said, also strictly avoid stimulants. Not only do they make you jittery but they may hamper your ability to make connections and think critically—essential skills in NCLEX-RN® preparation.

Other aspects of the healthy lifestyle—to put you at your best—include balancing your life. Make sure you exercise—find something you enjoy doing—running, walking, dancing, yoga, sports, swimming—and try to find time five days per week to work your muscles and enhance your oxygenation. A lot of time writing, reading, or on a computer may lead to neck and back pain—muscle stretches, twists, progressive relaxation, or even a massage, may enhance your endurance and ability to really attend as you adhere to your study goals.

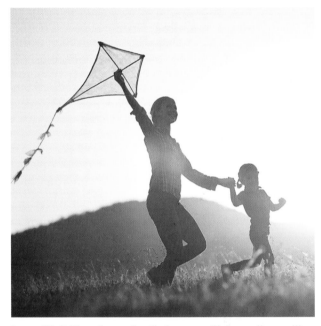

Image 20-2: The rejuvenation that comes with happy times with family can be very beneficial to you.

Now is also the time to make sure you play! Spend an afternoon with friends and family! Engage in retail therapy (within reason)! Enjoy the sunshine when you can (buildup your Vitamin D stores) and hunker down to study on rainy days. Consider your hobbies—what do you love to do? What activities help you get away from it all? Let's think about that calendar you made to study—many individuals find it helpful to identify times in the calendar for play and time with family and friends. Sometimes, it is easier to engage in hard-core studying when you know something fun is on the horizon! Still not sure of how to fill up your time? See the article on NCLEX-RN® Boot Camp listed on the reference list in the back of this book to develop your own boot camp of work, play and lifestyle activities around your studying and preparation.

That also brings up your support systems. Consider the people in your world that are also invested in your success. Think about those who have supported you throughout nursing school and, perhaps, other life crossroads. Ask them to stick with you just a few more months. Seek their assistance in managing home, family, and other obligations. Sometimes support systems need a reminder that, although you are done with school, your study time hasn't ended. Remind them that this exam is IMPORTANT and implore that they stand by you for just a little longer.

This also may be a time that your "BFFs" from nursing school (or other arenas) provide a significant amount of support. Not only do they know what you are going through, but they may be in the same situation! We all know that "misery loves company" and, although we don't want you to think of this as total misery— those in the same situation may best empathize with your current concerns. If you are working in a clinical area, engage in conversations with the staff. Talk to the registered nurses about their role, daily lives, and memories of NCLEX-RN®. This may offer some encouraging support.

Focus on your goals and the nearness of these goals! That may energize and inspire you for continued success!

Be Successful!

So now it is up to you! We have shared information on testing, studying, and nursing content. We have made suggestions on how to best prepare yourself for NCLEX-RN®. Now the hard work is up to you! We can say, unequivocally, that your time and effort, your sweat and tears, are worth it! Nursing is a privilege! No other profession can boast the assets of our life work! We reach people in so many ways, we make a difference, and we enjoy so many personal moments of success and humility every day! We wish you well and offer sincere wishes of success on the NCLEX-RN® exam! In a short period of time, we hope to welcome you to the rewarding and vital profession of nursing! Good luck on this next step of your professional life!

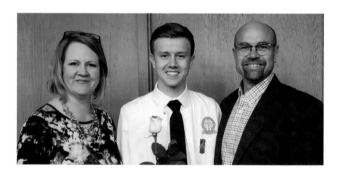

Dr. Tim Bristol with wife Christina and son Kristofer during his pinning as he graduated nursing school. The three of us wish you all the best as you pursue your dreams.

References

Altmiller, G. (2017). Content validation of quality and safety education for nurses-based clinical evaluation instrument. Nurse Educator, 42(1), 23-27.

American Automobile Association. (2018). Car seat safety laws. Retrieved from https://drivinglaws.aaa.com/tag/child-passenger-safety/

American Cancer Society. (Revised 2016). Cancer A-Z. Retrieved from https://www.cancer.org/cancer.html

American Cancer Society. (2018). Guidelines for the early detection of cancer. Retrieved from https://connection.cancer.org/Consumer/PDF/Product/P2070.00.pdf

American Cancer Society. (2018). How are Wilms tumors diagnosed? Retrieved from https://www.cancer.org/cancer/wilms-tumor/detection-diagnosis-staging/how-diagnosed.html

American Stroke Association. (2015). Complications after stroke. Retrieved from www.strokeassociation.org/letstalkaboutstroke

Bello, J., Quinn, P., & Horrell, L. (2011). Maintaining patient safety through innovation: An electronic SBAR communication tool. CIN: Computers, Informatics, Nursing, 29 (9), 481-483.

Black, B. P. (2017). Professional nursing: Concepts and challenges (8th ed.). St. Louis, MO: Elsevier.

Cancer Treatment Centers of America. (2018). About your cancer. Retrieved from https://www.cancercenter.com/cancer/

Centers for Disease Control and Prevention. (2018). Lung cancer. Retrieved from https://www.cdc.gov/cancer/lung/

Children's Hospital of Wisconsin. (2018). Hydrocephalus. Retrieved from https://www.chw.org/medical-care/fetal-concerns-center/conditions/infant-complication/hydrocephalus

Comprehensive Cancer Center, University of Michigan Health System. (2013). A Patient and family guide to blood and marrow transplant. Retrieved from http://www.med.umich.edu/cancer/files/bmt-patient-family-handbook.pdf

Cronenwett, L. & Sherwood, G. (2011). Lecture: Innovations for integrating quality and safety in education and practice: The QSEN project [Power Point slides]. Retrieved from http://www.qsen.org/docs/qsen_cronenwett_sherwood_STTI_2011_special_session.pdf

Cronenwett, L., Sherwood, G., Barnsteiner, J., Disch, J., Johnson, J., Mitchell, P., Sullivan, D., & Warren, J. (2007). Quality and safety education for nurses. Nursing Outlook, 55 (3), 122-131.

Cuellar, E.T. (2017). HESI comprehensive review for the NCLEX-RN® examination. St. Louis, MO: Elsevier.

Dickinson, P., Luo, X., Kim, D., Wood, A., Muntean, W., & Bergstrom, B. (2016). Assessing higher-order cognitive constructs by using an information-processing framework. Journal of Applied Testing Technology, 17 (1), 1-19.

Giddens, J. F. (2017). Concepts of nursing practice (2nd ed.). St. Louis, MO: Elsevier.

Giordano, S.H. (2018). Breast cancer in men. New England Journal of Medicine, 378, 2311-2320.

Halter, M.J. (2018). Varcarolis' foundations of psychiatric-mental health nursing (8th ed.). St. Louis, MO: Elsevier.

Hinkle, J.L. & Cheever, K.H. (2018). Brunner & Suddarth's textbook of medical-surgical nursing (14th ed.). Philadelphia, PA: Wolters Kluwer.

Herrman, J.W. & Johnson, A. (2009). From beta-blockers to boot camp: A nursing course approach to NCLEX® success. Nursing Education Perspectives, 30 (6), 384-388.

Hockenberry, M.J., & Wilson, D. (2015). Wong's nursing care of infants and children. St. Louis, MO: Elsevier.

Hogan, M. (2018). Comprehensive review for NCLEX-RN® (3rd ed.). New York, NY: Pearson.

Institute of Medicine. (2003). Health professions education: A bridge to quality. A. C. Greiner, & E. Knebel (Eds.). Washington, DC: Author.

Institute of Medicine of the National Academies. (2010). The future of nursing: Leading health, advancing change. Retrieved from http://nationalacademies.org/hmd/reports/2010/the-future-of-nursing-leading-change-advancing-health.aspx

Irving, S.Y., Lynam, B., Northington, L., Bartlett, J.A., & Kemper, C. (2014). Nasogastric tube placement and verification in children: A review of the current literature. Critical Care Nurse, 34 (3), 67-76.

Isaacs, D. (2017). Antibiotic prophylaxis for infective endocarditis: A systematic review and meta-analysis. Journal of Paediatrics and Child Health, 53 (9), 921-922.

Johns Hopkins Medicine, Sydney Kimmel Cancer Center, Blood and Bone Marrow Cancers Program. (n.d.). Blood and bone marrow cancer basics. Retrieved from https://www.hopkinsmedicine.org/kimmel_cancer_center/centers/blood_bone_marrow_cancers

Kaufman, J.S. (2017). Acute exacerbation of COPD: Diagnosis and management. The Nurse Practitioner, 42 (6), 1-7.

Koning, C., Young, L., & Bruce, A. (2016). Mind the gap: Women and acute myocardial infarctions: An integrated review of literature. Canadian Journal of Cardiovascular Nursing, 26 (3), 8-14.

Lewis, S.L., Dirksen, S.R., Heitkemper, M.M., & Bucher, L. (2017). Medical-surgical nursing: Assessment and management of clinical problems (10th ed.). St. Louis, MO: Elsevier.

Lilley, L.L., Collins, S.R., & Snyder, J.S. (2017). Pharmacology and the nursing process (8th ed.). St. Louis, MO: Mosby.

Lim, C.L., Byrne, C., & Lee, J.K. (2008). Human thermoregulation and measurement of body temperature in exercise and clinical settings. Annals Academy of Medicine Singapore, 37(4), 347-353.

Lowdermilk, D.L., Perry, S.E., Cashion, M.C., & Alden, K.R. (2015). Maternity and women's healthcare. St. Louis, MO: Elsevier.

Mangin, D. et al. (2012). Chlamydia trachomatis testing sensitivity in midstream compared with first void specimens. Annals of Family Medicine, 10 (1), 50-53.

Mayo Clinic. (2018). Amyotrophic lateral sclerosis. Retrieved from https://www.mayoclinic.org/diseases-conditions/amyotropic-lateral-sclerosis/diagnosis-treatment/drc-20354027

Mayo Clinic. (2018). Cleft lip and cleft palate. Retrieved from https://www.mayoclinic.org/diseases-conditions/cleft-palate/symptoms-causes/syc-20370985

Mayo Clinic. (2018). Diseases and conditions. Retrieved from https://www.mayoclinic.org/diseases-conditions

Mayo Clinic. (2018). Guillain-Barré syndrome. Retrieved from https://www.mayoclinic.org/diseases-conditions/guillain-barre-syndrome/symptoms-causes/syc-20362793

Mayo Clinic. (2018). Pyloric stenosis. Retrieved from https://www.mayoclinic.org/diseases-conditions/pyloric-stenosis/symptoms-causes/syc-20351416

Mayo Clinic. (2018). Spina bifida. Retrieved from https://www.mayoclinic.org/diseases-conditions/spina-bifida/symptoms-causes/syc-20377860

McAllister, T.W. (2011). Neurobiological consequences of traumatic brain injury. Dialogues in Clinical Neuroscience, 13(3), 287-300.

McCuistion, L., Vuljoin-DiMaggio, K., Winton, M.B., & Yeager, J.J. (2018). Pharmacology: A patient-centered nursing process approach (9th ed.). St. Louis, MO: Elsevier.

McKinney, E., James, S., & Murray, S. (2018). Maternal-child nursing (5th ed.). Philadelphia, PA: W.B. Saunders.

Metheny, N.A., Pawluszka, A., Lulic, M., Hinyard, L.J., & Meert, K.L. (2017). Testing placement of gastric feeding tubes in infants. American Journal of Critical Care, 26(6), 466-473.

Nagel, D.A. & Penner, J.L. (2016). Conceptualizing telehealth in nursing practice. Journal of Holistic Nursing, 34 (1), 91-104.

National Council of State Boards of Nursing. (2017). Next generation NCLEX® news. Retrieved from www.ncsbn.org/NCLEX_Next_Fall17_Eng.pdf

National Council of State Boards of Nursing. (2017). Exam to licensure: Your career gateway. Retrieved from www.ncsbn.org

National Council of State Boards of Nursing. (2018). Next generation NCLEX® news. Retrieved from https://www.ncsbn.org/11435.htm

National Institute of Neurological Disorders and Stroke. (2018). All disorders. Retrieved from https://www.ninds.nih.gov/Disorders/All-Disorders?title=&page=6

National Institute of Diabetes and Digestive and Kidney Diseases. (2018). Cushing's syndrome. Retrieved from https://www.niddk.nih.gov/health-information/endocrine-diseases/cushings-syndrome

National Institute of Health and Care Excellence, NICE guideline [NG14]. (2015). Melanoma: Assessment and management. Retrieved from https://www.nice.org.uk/guidance/ng14

O'Grady, N.P., Alexander, M., & Burns, L.A. (2011). Guidelines for the prevention of intravascular catheter-related infections. Atlanta, GA: Centers for Disease Control and Prevention. Retrieved from www.cdc.gov/hicpac/pdf/guidelines/bsi-guidelines-2011.pdf

Pearson Education. (2019). Nursing: A concept-based approach to learning (Vol. 1-3). Minneapolis, MN: Author.

Perry, S.E., Lowdermilk, D.L., Cashion, K., Alden, K.R., Olshansky, E.F., Hockenberry, M.J., Wilson, D., & Rodgers, C.C. (2018). Maternal child nursing care (6th ed.). St. Louis, MO: Elsevier.

Pop, V., & Badaut, J. (2011). A neurovascular perspective for long-term changes after brain trauma. Translational Stroke Research, 2(4), 533-545.

Potter, P.P., Perry, A.G., Stockert, P.A., Hall, A.M., & Ostendorf, W. (2017). Fundamentals of nursing. St. Louis, MO: Elsevier.

QSEN Institute. (2018). Quality and safety education for nurses. Retrieved from www.qsen.org

Ricci, S. (2017). Essentials of maternity, newborn, and women's health nursing (4th ed.). Philadelphia, PA: Wolters Kluwer.

Schirm, V., Banz, G., Swartz, C., & Richmond, M. (2018). Evaluation of bedside shift report: A research and evidence-based practice. Applied Nursing Research, 40, 20-25.

Sherwood, G. & Zomorodi, M. (2014). Anew mindset for quality and safety: The QSEN competencies redefine nurses' roles in practice. Nephrology Nursing Journal, 41, 15-23.

Silvestri, L.A. & Silvestri, A. (2017). Saunders comprehensive review for the NCLEX-RN® examination (7th ed.). St. Louis, MO: Elsevier.

Stalter, A. & Mota, A. (2018). Using systems thinking to envision quality and safety in healthcare (QSEN). Nursing Management, 49(2), 32-39.

Stanhope, M. & Lancaster, J. (2016). Public health nursing: Population-centered health care in the community (9th ed.). St. Louis, MO: Elsevier.

St Jude's Children's Research Hospital. (2018). Wilms tumor. Retrieved from https://www.stjude.org/disease/wilms-tumor.html

Taylor, C., Lillis, C., Lynn, P., & LeMone, P. (2015). Fundamentals of nursing (8th ed.). Philadelphia, PA: Wolters Kluwer.

Townsend, M. (2015). Psychiatric mental health nursing: Concepts of care in evidence-based practice. Philadelphia, PA: FA Davis.

University of California San Francisco (2018). Acute lymphoblastic leukemia treatment. Retrieved from https://www.ucsfhealth.org/conditions/acute_lymphoblastic_leukemia/treatment.html

U.S. Department of Health and Human Services, Centers for Disease Control and Prevention. (2018). Bacterial meningitis. Retrieved from https://www.cdc.gov/meningitis/bacterial.html

U.S. Department of Health and Human Services, Centers for Disease Control and Prevention. (2018). Information on avian influenza. Retrieved from https://www.cdc.gov/flu/avianflu/index.htm

U.S. Department of Health and Human Services, Centers for Disease Control and Prevention. (2018). Information on swine influenza/variant influenza virus. Retrieved from https://www.cdc.gov/flu/swineflu/index.htm

U.S. Department of Health and Human Services, Centers for Disease Control and Prevention. (2018). Pink eye: Usually mild and easy to treat. Retrieved from https://www.cdc.gov/Features/Conjunctivitis/

U.S. Department of Health and Human Services, Centers for Disease Control and Prevention. (2018). Prevention strategies for seasonal influenza in healthcare settings. Retrieved from https://www.cdc.gov/flu/professionals/infectioncontrol/healthcaresettings.htm

U.S. Department of Health and Human Services, Centers for Disease Prevention and Control. (2016). The ABCs of hepatitis. Retrieved from https://www.cdc.gov/hepatitis/resources/professionals/pdfs/abctable.pdf

U.S. Department of Health and Human Services, National Institute of Diabetes and Digestive and Kidney Disease. (2018). Adrenal insufficiency and Addison's disease. Retrieved from https://www.niddk.nih.gov/health-information/endocrine-diseases/adrenal- insufficiency- addisons- disease

U.S. Department of Health and Human Services, National Institute of Diabetes and Digestive and Kidney Disease. (2018). Cushing's syndrome. Retrieved from https://www.niddk.nih.gov/health-information/endocrine-diseases/cushings-syndrome

U.S. Department of Health and Human Services, National Institutes of Health, National Cancer Institute. (2018). Cancer types. Retrieved from https://www.cancer.gov/types

U.S. Department of Health and Human Services, National Institutes of Health, National Heart, Lung, and Blood Institute. (2018). Polycythemia Vera. Retrieved from https://www.nhlbi.nih.gov/health-topics/polycythemia-vera

U.S. Department of Health and Human Services National Institutes of Health, National Institute of Neurological Disorders and Stroke. (2018). Myasthenia gravis fact sheet. Retrieved from https://www.ninds.nih.gov/disorders/patient-caregiver-education/fact-sheets/myasthenia-gravis-fact-sheet

U.S. Department of Health and Human Services National Institutes of Health, National Institute of Neurological Disorders and Stroke. (2018). Peripheral neuropathy fact sheet. Retrieved from https://www.ninds.nih.gov/Disorders/Patient-Caregiver-Education/Fact-Sheets/Peripheral-Neuropathy-Fact-Sheet#3208_1

Vallerand, A.H., Sanoski, C.A., & Deglin, J.H. (2017). Davis's drug guide for nurses (15th ed.). Philadelphia, PA: FA Davis.

Varcarolis, E.M. (2017). Essentials of psychiatric mental health nursing (3rd ed.). St. Louis, MO: Elsevier.

Venes, D. (Ed). (2017). Taber's cyclopedic medical dictionary (23rd ed.). Philadelphia, PA: FA Davis.

Whelton, P.K, & Carey, R.M. (2017). The 2017 guideline for high blood pressure. JAMA: Journal of the American Medical Association, 318(21). 2073-2074.

Wilmot Cancer Institute. (2018). Blood and marrow transplantation. Retrieved from https://www.urmc.rochester.edu/cancer-institute/services/bmt/patient-discharge.aspx

World Health Organization. (2017). Fact sheets: Hepatitis E. Retrieved from http://www.who.int/en/news-room/fact-sheets/detail/hepatitis-e

Yan, S., Wang, X., Lv, C., Wang, Y., Wang, J., Yang, Y., & Wu, N. (2017). Intermittent chest tube clamping may shorten chest tube duration and postoperative hospital stay. Journal of Thoracic Oncology, 12 (1), S1402-S1403.

Yoder-Wise, P. (2014). Leading and managing in nursing (5th ed.). St. Louis, MO: Elsevier.

Index

A

Abortion, 37-39, 50
Abuse
    in adolescents, 504
    in children, 496-498, 500, 502, 504
    focused assessment, 433
    in older adults, 509
    substance, 220, 428, 434-435, 458
Acetaminophen, 98, 145, 182
Acetazolamide, 202-203
Acute coronary syndrome, 72
Acute kidney injury, 151, 275
Acute lymphocytic leukemia, 204, 206
Acute pain, 400-403
Acute respiratory distress syndrome
    (ARDS), 103, 167, 178
Acute traumatic brain injury, 214
Addison's disease, 318-319
Adolescents, 456, 504-505
Adults, 506-508
Aflibercept, 263, 369
Alendronate, 309, 348
Alfuzosin, 274
Allopurinol, 109
Alzheimer's disease, 480, 482-483
Aminoglutethimide, 317
Amitriptyline, 353, 355, 429, 457
Amoxicillin, 48, 107, 182, 251, 375
Ampicillin, 98, 123, 125
Amputation, 211, 357
Amyotrophic lateral sclerosis, 358
Anagrelide, 217
Analgesics
    in benign prostatic hypertrophy
      surgery, 273
    in carpal tunnel surgery, 356
    in cataract surgery, 366
    in glaucoma surgery, 367
    manage pain in pediatric surgery,
      245, 269
    in otitis media, 374
Anemia
    aplastic, 108-109
    in chronic kidney disease, 278
    iron deficiency, 185
    pernicious, 248
    screening of, in newborn, 32
    screening of, in pregnancy, 36
    sickle cell, 108, 151, 174, 186
    in Wilms tumor, 324-325

Anorexia
    in cancer, 206, 212, 262
    in cirrhosis, 264
    in chronic kidney disease, 275
    in hepatitis, 266
    in tuberculosis TB, 179
Anorexia nervosa, 424-425
Antacids, 146, 151, 247
Antibiotics
    in ear infection, 374
    for meningitis, 97
    in MRSA, 124
    for peritonitis, 104
    in respiratory infections, 180, 182-
      183
    for septic abortion, 39
    for urinary infections, 120-123
    in valvular heart disease, 70
    for wound infection, 107
Anticholinesterase, 362-363
Anticoagulant, 78-83, 111, 213,
350
Anticonvulsant, 346-347, 406, 408,
    429, 461
Antidepressant, 271, 436, 451, 457
Antihistamine, 109, 117, 365, 372-373,
    398
Antihypertensives, 35
Antipsychotic, 455, 460, 479
Antipyretic, 145, 182, 401
Antiseizure, 98
Anxiety disorders, 424, 436, 450
Appendicitis, 104-105
Asthma, 116-117, 170, 177, 404
Atenolol, 75, 78, 313
Atorvastatin, 278
Atropine, 65, 145, 255, 363
Attention-deficit/hyperactivity disorder
    (ADHD), 460, 485
Autism spectrum disorders (ASD), 484
Azathioprine, 111, 240-241

B

Belimumab, 111
Benign prostatic hypertrophy, 272, 274
Benzodiazepines, 372
Bereavement, 429, 456, 463
Betamethasone, 29, 39, 44
Bevacizumab, 213, 263
Bipolar disorders, 460

Bisphosphonate, 348
Bone cancer, 211-213, 311
Bradycardia
    in electrolyte imbalances, 146-147,
      149
    in heart failure, 68
    with infants, 496
    in MI/Acute coronary syndrome, 72
    in neurological conditions, 358-359,
      378-379
    in postpartum hemorrhage, 46
    in shock, 64-65
Brain cancer, 211-213
Breast cancer, 211-213
Breastfeeding, 42, 47, 114
Bronchiolitis, 181
Bronchodilators, 171, 174
Buerger's disease and raynaud's
    phenomenon, 74
Bupropion, 271, 457
Burns, 398-399, 430
Buspirone, 451
Busulfan, 217

C

Calcitonin, 146, 213, 309
Calcium carbonate, 151, 155, 311
Cancer
    blood-borne, 206-207
    bone, 211-213
    breast, 211-213
    brain, 211-213
    cervical, 49
    colorectal, 262-263
    lung, 211-213
    lymph, 210
    prostate, 272-274
    skin, 208-209
Carbachol, 367
Carbamazepine, 322, 347, 355, 429
Cardiomyopathy, 70, 78
Carisoprodol, 351
Carpal tunnel, 356
Ceftazidime, 98, 105
Ceftriaxone, 98, 105
Celiac disease, 253
Cellulitis, 106-107, 394
Cephalexin, 107
Cephalosporins, 97-98, 105
Cerebral palsy, 340, 342-343

Cervical cancer, 49
Chemotherapy
    in blood-borne cancers, 206-207
    for breast cancer, 213
    in colorectal cancer, 263
    in polycythemia, 216
    in prostate cancer, 274
    for skin cancer, 209
    for Wilms tumor, 325
Chest trauma, 176
Chlamydia, 33, 36, 48, 368
Chlorpropamide, 322
Chronic kidney disease, 122, 185, 275, 278, 281
Chronic obstructive pulmonary disease, 170, 405
Chronic pain, 186, 401-403
Cilostazol, 73-74
Ciprofloxacin, 121, 123, 375
Cirrhosis, 264-265, 435
Clarithromycin, 251
Cleft lip, 242, 244-245
Cleft palate, 244
Clomipramine, 436
Clonazepam, 347, 355, 406
Clonidine, 403
Clopidogrel, 71, 73, 77
Clotting, 61, 64, 80, 110-111, 146
Clozapine, 452, 455
Codeine, 182, 401
Colchicine, 109
Colorectal cancer, 258, 262-263
Conjunctivitis, 48, 368
Constipation, 256
    in colorectal cancer, 262
    in diverticular disease, 260-261
    in hypoparathyroidism, 315
    with iron intake, 185
    in older adults, 508-509
    with opioid use, 401, 403
    in pregnancy, 37, 42
Contact dermatitis, 116, 404
Contraception, 34, 42, 505, 507
Contraceptives, 34, 76, 79-80, 110, 254
Coronary artery disease (CAD), 68, 71, 75, 275
Corticosteroids
    in hypersensitivity reactions, 116
    in cancers, 207, 210, 213
    in inflammatory bowel disease, 241
    in celiac disease, 253
    in Cushing's disease, 319
    in systemic lupus erythematosus, 111
    in rheumatoid arthritis, 113

Crisis intervention, 187, 429, 432-434, 457
Crohn's disease, 238-241, 258
Croup syndromes, 183
Cushing's syndrome, 316-317
Cyclobenzaprine, 351, 406
Cystic fibrosis, 172, 174-175

D

Dapsone, 111
Death and dying, 462
Dehydration, 144-145
    in diabetic insipidus, 322
    in diabetic ketoacidosis, 296
    in diverticular disease, 260
    in hyperthermia, 219
    in hyperosmolar hyperglycemic syndrome, 306
    in intestinal obstruction, 258
    in inflammatory bowel disease, 238
Delirium, 178, 399, 408, 435, 478-479
Dementia, 482-483, 508-509
Depression, 456
    in acquired immune-deficiency syndrome (AIDS), 115
    in Addison's disease, 318-319
    in chronic pain, 402-403
    in Cushing's syndrome, 316-317
    in human immunodeficiency virus, 115
    in hypothyroidism, 314
    postpartum, 458
Desmopressin acetate, 322-323
Dexamethasone, 98, 109, 183, 213, 218, 375
Diabetes insipidus, 150, 321-322
Diabetes mellitus, 300-303, 326, 352
Diabetic ketoacidosis, 147-148, 152, 296-297, 302
Dialysis
    in acute kidney injury, 281
    hemodialysis, 275-278
    peritoneal, 275-279
Diphenhydramine, 365, 373, 455
Disseminated intravascular coagulation (DIC), 29, 44, 46, 81-82
Disulfiram, 435
Diuretics
    in acute traumatic brain injury, 215
    in cirrhosis, 70
    in diabetes insipidus, 323
    in fluid overload, 141
    in hypertension, 75
    in sudden inappropriate antidiuretic hormone, 320-321

Diverticular disease, 258, 260-261
Docusate sodium, 72
Dopamine, 65, 178, 364-365, 408, 505
Doxycycline, 48
Dronabinol, 403
Dual-energy x-ray absorptiometry (DXA), 348
Dutasteride, 273-274
Dystocia, 43, 46

E

Eating disorders, 422, 424-425, 504, 507
Edrophonium, 362-363
Encephalitis, 96-98, 155, 267
End-stage renal disease, 119, 122, 275-278
Enoxaparin, 79-81, 379, 399
Epiglottitis, 183
Epinephrine, 65, 117, 183, 186
Epoetin, 207, 213
Erectile dysfunction, 35, 272, 274
Erythromycin, 33, 48, 180
Escitalopram, 458
Ethambutol, 179
Etoposide, 210, 213, 325
Ezetimibe, 71

F

Fatigue, 406
    in acute hepatitis, 266
    with autoimmune conditions, 110-113
    in cancers, 206-210, 213
    with heart disease, 68, 70, 73
    with neuromuscular conditions, 358, 360, 362
    in pregnancy, 36-37, 39
    with respiratory conditions, 118, 177, 179
Febuxostat, 109
Fentanyl, 42, 403, 462
Ferrous gluconate, 185
Ferrous sulfate, 45, 185, 406
Fibromyalgia, 402, 405-406
Filgrastim, 207, 210, 213
Finasteride, 273
Fluid deficit, 144-145
Fluid overload, 140-141, 277-278, 280-281, 296
Flumazenil, 435
Fluoxetine, 425, 436, 457-458
Fosfomycin, 121

Fractures, 350
  in bone cancer, 211-213
  in hypocalcemia, 146
  in newborns, 32
  in osteoporosis, 348
Furosemide, 69, 141, 178, 202-203, 215, 320-321

G

Gabapentin, 353, 355
Gallbladder conditions, 254
Gastritis, 185, 248-249, 434-435
Gastroesophageal reflux, 174, 246
Gemfibrozil, 278
Gestational diabetes, 37, 304-305
Gestational hypertension, 28, 37
Glaucoma, 367
Glucagon, 301
Glucocorticoids, 146, 318-319
Gout, 108-109, 179, 349
Guillain-barré syndrome, 359

H

Haloperidol, 479
Hearing impairment, 370, 508
Heart failure, 68-69
  in acute kidney disease, 280
  in cardiomyopathy, 70
  in chronic kidney disease, 275
  related to fluid overload, 140-141
  in pulmonary hypertension, 184
HELLP syndrome, 81
Heparin, 79-81, 218, 278, 378-379
Hepatitis, 33, 36, 264, 266-268
HIV/AIDS, 114-115
  assessment for, in delirium, 478
  assessment of, in pregnancy, 36, 41
  co-infection with hepatitis, 267
  comorbidity with tuberculosis (TB), 179
  existing with other sexually transmitted infections (STI), 48, 50
Hodgkin's, 210, 253
Hydrocephalus, 202-203, 212, 377
Hydrochlorothiazide, 66, 75, 150, 373
Hydrocodone, 401, 403
Hydrocortisone, 109, 241, 317-319
Hydroxychloroquine, 111, 113
Hydroxyurea, 187, 217
Hypercalcemia, 146, 211-212, 308-309, 311
Hyperglycemic hyperosmolar syndrome, 297, 300, 306
Hyperkalemia, 147, 275, 277-278, 398

Hypermagnesemia, 29, 45, 149
Hypernatremia, 144, 150
Hyperparathyroidism, 278, 308-309, 311
Hyperphosphatemia, 151, 155
Hypersensitivity reactions, 116, 404
Hypertension
  in coronary artery disease, 71
  with chronic kidney disease, 275
  with heart failure, 68-69
  portal, 265
  in pregnancy, 28-29, 36-37
  pulmonary, 184
  in stroke, 76
Hypertensive disorders of pregnancy, 26, 28-29
Hyperthermia, 33, 219, 313
Hyperthyroidism, 312-314, 348
Hypocalcemia, 146, 149, 151, 308, 310
Hypokalemia, 147-148, 153, 296, 398
Hyponatremia, 150, 174, 264-265, 296, 320
Hypoparathyroidism, 151, 310-311
Hypophosphatemia, 151, 296, 308
Hypotension
  with heart failure, 68-69
  orthostatic, 71, 74-75, 144, 147, 264, 323
  in shock, 64-65
  supine, in pregnancy and labor, 37, 40, 42
Hypothermia, 64, 180, 220-221, 424
Hypothyroidism, 220-221, 256, 313-315, 352
Hypovolemia, 144-145, 152, 278, 280
Hypovolemic shock, 46, 104, 251, 399

I

Ibandronate, 348
Immunomodulators, 111, 404
Immunosuppressants, 111, 206, 404
Impetigo, 404
Infant, 496-497
  assessment and care of, 32-33, 40-41
  breastfeeding of, 47
  bronchiolitis in, 181
  care of, in postpartum depression, 458
  dehydration of, 144
  developmental stages, 496-497
  hydrocephalus in, 202-203
  spina bifida in, 377
Infections
  hospital-acquired, 3, 509

  in meningitis, 96
  MRSA/VRE, 124-125
  opportunistic, human immunodeficiency virus (HIV), 114-115
  in pregnancy, 36-37
  respiratory, 174-175, 180-183
  sexually transmitted, 34, 50
  urinary tract, 119-120, 122
  wound, 106-107
Inflammatory bowel disease, 236, 238-241, 262
Influenza, 118, 171, 206, 509
Insulin, 151-152, 296-297, 300-307, 326
Intestinal obstruction, 175, 258, 324
Iron-deficiency anemia, 185
Isoniazid, 179

K

Ketorolac, 366, 401

L

Labetalol, 77
Labyrinthitis, 372-373
Laxatives, 147, 256-257, 261, 424, 509
Leflunomide, 113
Leukotriene, 117, 177
Levodopa, 365, 408
Levofloxacin, 121, 123, 180
Levothyroxine, 315
Linezolid, 125
Liraglutide, 271, 301
Lisinopril, 69-70, 75
Lithium carbonate, 461
Loperamide, 145
Lorazepam, 347, 373, 435, 451, 479, 483
Lower airway infections, 181
Lung cancer, 211-213

M

Macular degeneration, 369
Mannitol, 141, 174, 213, 215
Meclizine, 373
Memantine, 483
Meniere's disease, 372-373
Meningitis, 96-99, 180, 368, 373, 376-377
Mesalamine, 241
Metabolic acidosis, 152, 154, 275, 280, 297
Metabolic alkalosis, 153-155
Metabolic syndrome, 71, 267, 326
Metformin, 298, 300-301

Methadone, 435

Methicillin-resistant staphylococcus aureus, 124

Methotrexate, 111, 113, 207, 240-241

Methylergonovine, 46

Methylphenidate, 485

Methylprednisolone, 109, 111, 183

Metoprolol, 70, 313

Mifepristone, 317

Milrinone, 69

Mineralocorticoids, 318-319

Modafinil, 408

Morphine, 69, 72, 102-103, 182, 399

Moxifloxacin, 368

Multiple sclerosis, 360-361

Mupirocin, 404

Myasthenia gravis, 362-363

Myocardial infarction, 68, 70, 72, 185

N

Nalbuphine, 42

Naloxone, 42, 401, 435

Narcotics, 42

Neostigmine, 363

Newborn care, 32-33, 40, 48, 496

Niacin, 71

Nifedipine, 29, 39, 70, 74-75

Nitrazine, 36

Nitrofurantoin, 121

Nitroglycerin, 35

Nutrition
    assessment of, in cancer, 211
    assessment of, with cleft lip and palate, 244-245
    in eating disorders, 424-425
    in children, 496, 498, 504
    in irritable bowel disease, 239, 241
    assessment, in older adults, 509
    parenteral and enteral, 102, 178
    planning, in diabetes, 300, 302, 304
    in pregnancy, 36-37, 42
    to promote wound healing, 107, 394-395

O

Obesity, 270-272, 298, 300, 304, 316, 326, 424-425

Obsessive-compulsive disorder (OCD), 436

Older adults, 144-145, 430, 508-509

Olsalazine, 241

Oseltamivir, 118

Osteoarthritis, 349

Osteoporosis, 112, 253, 316-317, 348, 351

Otitis externa, 374-375

Otitis media, 374-375

Overhydration, 41, 138, 140-141

Oxybutynin, 274, 379

Oxygenation, 176, 178, 220, 312, 346

Oxytocin, 38, 41-42, 46

P

Palivizumab, 181

Pamidronate, 146

Pancrelipase, 103

Pancreatitis, 102-103, 146, 250, 301

Parkinson's disease, 364-365, 482

Paroxetine, 429, 436, 458, 483

Pegloticase, 109

Penicillin, 50, 97-98, 107, 404

Pentoxifylline, 74

Peptic ulcer, 248, 250-252

Peripheral artery disease, 73

Peripheral neuropathy, 110, 275, 352-353, 435

Peritonitis, 104-105, 238, 240, 260-263, 277-279

Phenazopyridine, 121

Phenobarbital, 347

Phentermine, 271

Phenytoin, 97-98, 213, 215, 317, 346

Placental abruption, 29, 44, 46

Placenta previa, 44-46

Pneumonia, 180
    acquired immune deficiency syndrome (AIDS) in, 114
    in acute respiratory distress syndrome ARDS, 178
    with bronchiolitis, 181
    as a complication of burns, 399
    human immunodeficiency virus (HIV) in, 114
    as a complication of influenza, 118
    neonatal, 48

Pneumothorax, 174, 176, 180

Polycystic kidney, 119

Polycythemia, 170, 184, 216

Postpartum depression (PPD), 458

Postpartum hemorrhage, 39, 41

Post-traumatic stress disorder (PTSD), 428

Potassium chloride, 69, 147-148

Prazosin, 274, 429

Prednisone
    in benign prostatic hypertrophy BPH, 274

    in cancer, 207, 210, 212-213
    in chronic obstructive pulmonary disease (COPD), 171
    in gout, 109
    in labyrinthitis/Meniere's disease, 373
    in multiple sclerosis, 361
    in thrombocytopenia, 218

Preeclampsia, 8, 28-29

Pregabalin, 353, 406

Pregnancy, 36-37
    acquired immune deficiency syndrome (AIDS) in, 114-115
    disseminated intravascular coagulopathy (DIC) in, 81
    gestational diabetes in, 304-305
    human immunodeficiency virus HIV in, 114-115
    hypertension in, 28-29
    physiological changes in, 36
    prevention of, 34, 507
    risk conditions related to, 28-29, 38-39, 44-45
    sexually transmitted infections (STI) in, 48-49

Preschoolers, 500-501

Pressure ulcers, 350, 360, 364, 378, 392, 394-395

Preterm labor, 36, 39, 174

Probenecid, 109

Prochlorperazine, 105, 373

Professionalism, 521, 523, 526

Promethazine hcl, 145

Prostate cancer, 272-274

Proton pump inhibitors, 103, 247-248, 251

Psyllium, 71, 257, 261

Pulmonary embolism, 79-80, 154-155, 213, 218

Pulmonary hypertension, 78, 170, 178, 184

Pyelonephritis, 120, 122-123

Pyloric stenosis, 269

Pyrazinamide, 179

R

Ranibizumab, 369

Ranitidine, 399

Rape, 428, 430-431

Respiratory acidosis, 152-154, 170, 177, 183

Respiratory alkalosis, 146, 151, 153, 155, 178

Rheumatoid arthritis, 112, 116, 348, 356, 407

Ribavirin, 181
Rifampin, 179
Risperidone, 452, 455, 483-484
Rivaroxaban, 80
Rivastigmine, 483
Ropinirole, 365

S

SBAR, 524-525
Schizophrenia, 452, 454-455
School-age children, 502-503
Scoliosis, 371, 376, 502
Seizures, 346-347
    priority concern in cerebral palsy,
      342-343
    with brain conditions, 96-98, 202,
      211, 214-215
    assessment for, in diabetes insipidus
      DI, 322
    with electrolyte imbalances, 146,
      149, 151, 153, 160
    in pregnancy, 28-29
    assessment for, in sudden
      inappropriate antidiuretic
      hormone, 320
    monitoring for, in systemic lupus
      erythematosus, 110
Selegiline, 365
Septicemia, 81, 106-107, 122, 124-125
Sertraline, 436, 458
Sexual assault, 429-431
Sexually transmitted infections (STI)
    Chlamydia, 48
    Human papillomavirus (HPV), 49
    Syphilis, 50
Shock, 64-65
    anaphylactic, 117
    cardiogenic, 68, 72
    in disseminated intravascular
      coagulopathy (DIC), 81
    hypovolemic, 104, 145, 251, 296,
      399
    neurogenic, 379
    in postpartum hemorrhage, 46
    septic, 106, 258
    spinal, 378-379
Sickle cell anemia (SSA), 186
Sildenafil, 35, 184
Simvastatin, 66, 71, 77
Sinus, 96, 118, 374
Skin cancers, 208
Sleep disorders, 403, 407-408
Sofosbuvir, 268
Spina bifida, 36, 376-377

Spinal cord injury, 64, 378-379, 394
Spironolactone, 66, 265
Stages of labor, 40, 42
Stroke, 75-78, 141, 216, 346, 379
Substance abuse, 220, 431, 434-435,
    450
Sulfasalazine, 113, 240-241
Syndrome of inappropriate antidiuretic
    hormone, 140, 150, 320-321
Syphilis, 36, 50, 342
Systemic lupus erythematosus, 110-111,
    116

T

Tachycardia
    in anxiety disorder, 450
    in fluid imbalances, 140, 144
    with hyperthyroidism, 312-313
    in labor and delivery, 42-43, 46
    with pulmonary embolism, 80-81
    in shock, 64-65
    fetal tachycardia, 41, 43
Tacrolimus, 111
Tadalafil, 35, 274
Tapentadol, 403
Temozolomide, 208-209
Tetracycline, 251-252
Thrombocytopenia, 79, 110, 218, 435
Tobramycin, 123, 172, 175
Toddlers, 495, 498-499
Tolvaptan, 265, 321
Topiramate, 271
Trigeminal neuralgia, 354-355
Trimethoprim, 121, 123
Tropicamide, 366
Tuberculosis, 36-37, 179
Tympanoplasty tubes, 375

U

Ulcerative colitis, 235-236, 238-241
Upper airway infections, 182
Urinary tract infection, 77, 119-123, 306
Ursodeoxycholic acid, 255

V

Valproic acid, 461
Valvular heart disease, 78
Vancomycin, 97-98, 123-125
Vancomycin resistant enterococcus, 124
Vasopressin, 321
Venous thromboembolism, 77, 79, 378-
    379, 399
Vinblastine, 210
Vincristine, 207, 210, 213, 325

W

Warfarin, 78-80, 111, 317, 408
Wilms tumor, 324-325
Wound infection, 105-107, 271

Z

Zanamivir, 118
Zoledronic acid, 348
Zolpidem, 406, 408, 483

NurseThink® Quick Laboratory and Diagnostics

LAB TEST	NORMAL RANGE	CRITICAL CONCERNS	INCREASED	
HEMATOLOGY				
CBC				
*Red Blood Cells / Erythrocytes (RBC)	4.2 - 5.9 cells/L		(Polycythemia), Hemoconcentration	
Reticulocytes	0.5 - 1.5%		Acute Hemorrhage	
*Hemoglobin (Hgb)	12 - 17 g/dL	< 5.0 g/dL or > 20 g/dL		
*Hematocrit (Hct)	36 - 51%	< 15% or > 60%		
*White Blood Cells / Leukocytes (WBC)	4,000-10,000 µL or mm^3	< 2,500 or > 30,000 µL or mm^3	Infections, Inflammation, Stress	
*Neutrophils (polys/segs)	> 75%		Bacterial Infections	
Bands	< 10%	> 10%	Acute Bacterial Infection	
*Absolute Neutrophil Count (ANC)	> 1000 µL or mm^3	< 1000 µL or mm^3		
*Platelets	150,000-350,000 µL or mm^3	< 50,000 or > 1 million µL or mm^3	Malignancies	
COAGULATION				
Bleeding time	Less than 10 minutes	> 10 minutes	Low Platelets, DIC, ASA	
Prothrombin Time (PT)	11 - 12.5 seconds	> 20 seconds	Liver dysfunction, Coumadin, Vit K Deficiency	
*International Normalized Ratio (INR)	0.8 - 1.1	> 5.5	Liver dysfunction, Coumadin, Vit K Deficiency	
Activated Partial Thromboplastin Time (aPTT)	25 - 35 seconds	> 70 seconds	Coagulation Deficiencies, Heparin	
Partial Thromboplastin Time (PTT)	60 - 70 seconds	> 100 seconds	Coagulation Deficiencies, Heparin	
D-dimer	< 0.5 mcg/mL		Thrombus	
IMMUNE & INFLAMMATORY				
C-Reactive Protein (CRP)	< 1.0 mg/dL		Bacterial Infection, Inflammation	
Erythrocyte Sedimentation Rate (ESR)	0 - 20 mm/h		Inflammation, Renal Failure, Malignancy	
FLUID, ELECTROLYES & RENAL				
URINE				
*Urine Specific Gravity	1.005 - 1.030		Dehydration, SIADH	
METABOLIC PANEL				
*Blood Urea Nitrogen (BUN)	8 - 20 mg/dL	> 100 mg/dL	Renal Failure, Dehydration, ↑Protein Intake	
*Creatinine	0.7 - 1.3 mg/dL	> 4 mg/dL	Renal Disease	
Electrolytes				
*Potassium (K)	3.5 - 5.0 mEq/L	< 2.5 mEq/L or > 6.5 mEq/L	Acidosis, Renal Failure	
*Sodium (Na)	136 - 145 mEq/L	< 120 mEq/L or > 160 mEq/L	Diabetes Insipidus, Cushing's, HHNK	
*Calcium (Ca)	9 - 10.5 mg/dL	< 6 mg/dL or > 13 mg/dL	Hyperparathyroidism, Renal Failure	
Chloride (Cl)	98 - 106 mEq/L	< 80 mEq/L or > 115 mEq/L	Dehydration, Metabolic Acidosis	
*Magnesium (Mg)	1.5 - 2.4 mEq/L	< 0.5 mEq/L or > 3 mEq/L	Renal Failure	
Phosphorus (Ph)	3.0 - 4.5 mg/dL	< 1 mg/dL	Hypoparathyroidism, Renal Failure	
*Glucose	70 - 100 mg/dL	< 50 mg/dL or > 400 mg/dL	Diabetic Ketoacidosis, HHNK	
*Protein - Total	6 - 7.8 g/dL		Hemoconcentration	
*Protein - Albumin	3.5 - 5.0 g/dL		Dehydration	
FLUID STATUS				
* Serum Osmolality	275 - 295 mOsm/kg	< 265 or > 320 mOsm/kg	Diabetes Insipidus, HHNK, Hyperglycemia	
CARDIOPULMONARY				
ABG's				
*pH	7.35 - 7.45	< 7.25 or > 7.55	Alkalosis (resp/metabolic)	
*pO$_2$	80 - 100 mmHg	< 40 mmHg	Hyperoxygenation	
*pCO$_2$	35 - 45 mmHg	< 20 mmHg or > 60 mmHg	Hypoventilation	
*HCO$_3$	22- 26 mEq/L	< 15 mEq/L or > 40 mEq/L	Metabolic alkalosis	
*O$_2$ saturation	> 94%	< 75%		
Brain natriuretic peptide (BNP)	< 100 pg/mL		Heart failure	
METABOLISM & WASTE				
Ammonia	40 - 80 mcg/dL		Liver dysfunction	
Bilirubin - Total	0.3 - 1.2 mg/dL	Adult: > 12 mg/dL	Liver failure, RBC hemolysis, GB obstruction	
Thyroid Stimulating Hormone (TSH)	0.5 - 5 mU/L		Thyroid dysfunction	
ENZYMES				
Alkaline Phosphatase (ALP.)	36 - 92 U/L	Enzymes will be released and rise with cell damage. Once the damage stops, the enzymes will return to normal.	Liver, Biliary Tract, Bone	
Aminotransferase, Alanine (ALT)	0 - 35 U/L		Liver, (Less in Kidneys, Heart, Muscles)	
Aminotransferase, Aspartate (AST)	0 - 35 U/L		Liver	
Amylase	0 - 130 U/L		Pancreas	
Creatine Kinase (CPK)	30 - 170 U/L		Heart, Brain, Muscle	
Lactic Dehydrogenase (LDH)	60 - 100 U/L		Heart, Liver, Kidneys, Muscles, Brain, Lungs	
Lipase	< 95 U/L		Pancreas	
Troponin I & T	< 0.5ng/mL & < 0.10 ng/mL		Cardiac	
THERAPUETIC DRUG LEVELS				
Peak and Trough				
Digoxin	0.8-2.0 ng/mL	> 2.4 ng/mL = toxic level		
Lithium	0.6- 1.2 mEq/L	> 1.5 mEq/L = toxic level	Renal Failure, ↓consciousness, ECG changes	

* Know APPROXIMATE Normal for NCLEX® Exam   References: American College of Physicians & Mosby's Diagnostic and Laboratory Test Reference, 10th ed.

Do not memorize specific lab numbers - they vary greatly.
It is more important to know **approximate** normal and recognize **critical concerns** - this is when a nursing action is required.

DECREASED	SPECIAL NOTES	PRIORITY LABS
		Infection, Inflammation & Immunity
		WBCs, Segs, Bands, ANC, CRP, ESR
(Anemia), Blood Loss, Hemodilution	↑ with Epoetin; Too High = Clot formation; Too Low = O₂ Transport	**Liver Disorders**
Bone Marrow Failure	Immature RBCs	Liver Enzymes; PT/PTT/INR; Albumin; Ammonia, Bilirubin Na, K, Glucose
	Oxygen Carrying Capacity; PRBC < 7 g/dL	**Renal Disorders**
	Hydration Dependent	BUN; Creatinine; Osmolality, K, Na, Ca, Ph, RBCs, Urine SG
Chemo, Bone Marrow Failure	↑ with Filgrastim	**Cardiac Disorders**
Chemo, Bone Marrow Failure	Poly/Segs are Mature WBCs	Cardiac Enzymes, BNP, ABGs, Digoxin Level
Bone Marrow Failure	Increase = Left Shift	**Pancreas Disorders**
(Neutropenia)	ANC = WBC x (% Neutrophils + % Bands); < 1000 = Isolation	Amylase, Lipase, Ca, Glucose
ITP, Leukemia, Chemo	< 20,000: = Spontaneous Bleed; ↑ with Oprelvekin	**Hemorrhage - DIC**
		RBCs, Reticulocytes, Hgb, Hct, Platelets, Coagulation Studies
		Fluid Imbalance
	Therapeutic is > 1.5 - 2 times control with warfarin therapy	Protein, Albumin, Na, Urine SG, Osmolality, RBCs, Hgb, Hct, BUN
	Therapeutic is 1.5 to 4 with warfarin therapy	
	Therapeutic is 1.5-2.5 times the control with heparin therapy	
	Cardiac marker but not specific to myocardium	
Sickle Cell Anemia, Polycythemia Vera		
Excessive Diuresis, Diabetes Insipidus	Fluctuates Fluid Status	
Hepatic Failure, Overhydration	End By-Product of Protein Breakdown	
Decreased Muscle Mass	Doubling of level indicates 50% reduction in the GFR	
Diuretics, Gastrointestinal Loss	Abnormal level leads to arrhythmias, muscle cramps	
SIADH, Addison's	↓ = Lethargy, Stupor, Coma, Seizures; ↑ = Agitation, Seizures	
Hypoparathyroidism, Pancreatitis, Low Protein	↓ = Tetany; ↑ = Osteomalacia, Dehydration	
Gastrointestinal Loss, Low Na Diet	↓ = Hyperexcitability; ↑ = Weakness, Lethargy	
Alcoholism; Renal Disease	Abnormal level leads to arrhythmias, muscle irritability	
Hyperparathyroidism, Vit D Deficiency	↓ = Osteomalacia; ↑ Hypocalcemia (tetany)	
↓ Glucose intake or absorption, Exercise		
Malnutrition, Burns, Blood Loss	Needed for wound healing	
Liver Dysfunction, Nephrotic Syndrome	Impacts fluid shift in and out of the vascular space	
SIADH, Overhydration	Measures concentration of dissolved particles in blood	
Acidosis(resp/metabolic)	pH is inversely proportional to H+ concentration	
Hypoxemia (pneumonia, etc.)	Indirect measure of O₂ concentration in arterial blood	
Hyperventilation	Measurement of ventilation	
Metabolic acidosis	Measures metabolic component of acid-base balance	
Hypoxemia/Anemia	Indication of the % of Hgb saturated with oxygen	
	The higher the number the weaker the left ventricular contractions	
	Product of protein breakdown; Neurotoxic; Treated with Lactulose	
	Neurotoxic to newborns	
Pituitary dysfunction, Hyperthyroidism	T3, T4, T7 often needed to rule out thyroid dysfunction	
	Biochemical Markers for Cardiac Disease	
	Monitors therapeutic drug levels of nephrotoxic medications	
Subtherapeutic	Cardiac Glycoside	
Subtherapeutic: symptoms poorly controlled	Lithium clearance from the body is increased during pregnancy	

Go To Clinical Cases — Patient Assignments

Chapter 5: Sexuality

Case 1: Hypertensive Disorders of Pregnancy

Case 2: Newborn Care

Chapter 6: Circulation

Case 1: Shock

Case 2: Heart Failure

Chapter 7: Protection

Case 1: Meningitis

Case 2: Pancreatitis

Chapter 8: Homeostasis

Case 1: Overhydration/Fluid Overload

Case 2: Dehydration/Fluid Deficit

Chapter 9: Respiration

Case 1: Chronic Obstructive Pulmonary Disease

Case 2: Cystic Fibrosis

Chapter 10: Regulation

Case 1: Hydrocephalus

Case 2: Blood-borne Cancers

Chapter 11: Nutrition

Case 1: Inflammatory Bowel Disease:
Crohn's Disease/Ulcerative Colitis

Case 2: Cleft Lip and Palate

Chapter 12: Hormonal

Case 1: Diabetic Ketoacidosis

Case 2: Diabetes Mellitus Type 2

Chapter 13: Movement

Case 1: Cerebral Palsy

Case 2: Seizures

Chapter 14: Comfort

Case 1: Pressure Ulcers

Case 2: Burns

Chapter 15: Adaptation

Case 1: Eating Disorders

Case 2: Post-traumatic Stress Disorder (PTSD)

Chapter 16: Emotions

Case 1: Anxiety Disorders

Case 2: Schizophrenia

Chapter 17: Cognition

Case 1: Delirium

Case 2: Dementia/Alzheimer's Disease